Teratogenic Effects of Drugs

TERATOGENIC EFFECTS OF DRUGS

A Resource for Clinicians

(TERIS)

J. M. FRIEDMAN, M.D., Ph.D.

Professor and Head, Department of Medical Genetics
University of British Columbia
Vancouver, British Columbia

AND

JANINE E. POLIFKA, Ph.D.

TERIS Project Coordinator, Department of Pediatrics
University of Washington
Seattle, Washington

THE JOHNS HOPKINS UNIVERSITY PRESS
Baltimore and London

©1994 The Johns Hopkins University Press
All rights reserved
Printed in the United States of America on acid-free paper

The Johns Hopkins University Press
2715 North Charles Street, Baltimore, Maryland 21218-4319
The Johns Hopkins Press Ltd., London

Library of Congress Cataloging-in-Publication Data

Friedman, J. M. (Jan Marshall), 1947-
  Teratogenic effects of drugs : a resource for clinicians : TERIS /
J.M. Friedman and Janine E. Polifka.
  p. cm.
Includes bibliographical references and index.
ISBN 0-8018-4800-8 (hc : alk. paper)
  1. Teratogenic agents--Handbooks, manuals, etc. 2. Drugs--
Toxicology--Handbooks, manuals, etc. I. Polifka, Janine E. II. Title.
[DNLM: 1. Teratogens--toxicity--handbooks. 2. Abnormalities, Drug-
Induced--handbooks. QS 639 F911t 1994]
QM691.F75 1994
615'.704--dc20
DNLM/DLC
for Library of Congress   93-33818

A catalog record for this book is available from the British library.

Acknowledgments

This book is derived from the TERIS database, an electronic resource that was originally developed under a grant from the U.S. Public Health Service Bureau of Maternal and Child Health. Additional financial support for the development of TERIS was provided by the Department of Pediatrics and the School of Medicine at the University of Washington.

We wish to thank the members of the TERIS Advisory Board, Drs. Robert Brent, Jose Cordero, James Hanson, Richard Miller, and Thomas Shepard, for their invaluable expertise in assessing the teratogenic risks associated with the agents discussed in this book. Our summaries could not have been developed without their advice and support.

Dr. Bert Little served as Project Coordinator for TERIS during the first two years of its development. He helped write the initial summaries and design the database. Barbara Brownfield performed many of the bibliographic searches for TERIS and assisted in the preparation of this book. Her contributions are greatly valued. Dr. Gerald Barnett, of the University of Washington Office of Technology Transfer, generously provided his time and advice to further development of the TERIS project. We have enjoyed collaborating with him over the past four years and particularly appreciate his vision for the future of TERIS.

Automation of the TERIS database was originally accomplished under the direction of William Singleton at the Medical Computing Resources Center of the University of Texas Southwestern Medical Center. For the past five years, the TERIS database has been maintained by Gerard Pence at the University of Washington's Locke Computer Center. We are grateful for his expertise, especially in times of crisis.

A computer program was created by Delores Boldrin, who is also at the Locke Computer Center, which enabled a subset of synonyms to be selected for the book from the 38,000 chemical and trade names currently on the system. Her program has greatly simplified this selection process, and we appreciate the time she spent in generating the seemingly endless lists of synonyms.

We are indebted to Dr. Glen Cooper, of Glen Cooper & Associates Ltd., in Vancouver, B.C., for designing a program that easily and efficiently converts the computerized database into printed output for the book. Dr. Cooper also developed the microcomputer version of TERIS, which has been in production since 1988.

We also wish to thank Jenny Nakahara, Marci Ameluxen, Gail Provo, Cora Gluckhertz, Elizabeth Lustig, Margaret Carlisle, and Joby Isaac for the many hours they have invested in collecting and preparing materials for the TERIS database and this book.

Finally, we wish to express special thanks to Tom Shepard for his friendship, support, and wisdom. He is the grandfather of this book.

Introduction

Every infant has at least a 5 percent risk of being born with a serious congenital anomaly. This includes not only malformations but also mental retardation and other important functional deficits that may not become apparent until later in life. The cause of most congenital anomalies is unknown. Purely genetic factors (i.e., chromosomal aberrations and abnormalities of a single gene or gene pair) account for about one-quarter of all congenital anomalies; environmental factors by themselves probably account for no more than one-tenth (Beckman & Brent, 1984). Nevertheless, congenital anomalies caused by environmental agents are especially important because they are potentially preventable.

A teratogen may be defined as an agent that can produce a permanent abnormality of structure or function in an organism exposed during embryonic or fetal life. The identification of human teratogens requires careful interpretation of data obtained from several kinds of studies (Brent, 1982; Cordero & Oakley, 1983). The first evidence that an agent is teratogenic in humans often comes from clinical case reports. Case reports are most useful if they reveal a recurrent pattern of anomalies in children who experienced similar well-defined exposures at similar points during embryonic or fetal development. Case reports cannot provide reliable quantitative estimates of the risk of anomalies in an exposed pregnancy. While case reports are important in raising causal hypotheses, most such hypotheses are incorrect. The coincidental occurrence of an environmental exposure in a pregnant woman and congenital anomalies in her child is very common, especially if the exposure or the defects or both are relatively frequent.

Epidemiologic studies provide the only means of obtaining quantitative estimates regarding the strength and statistical significance of associations between agent exposures in pregnant women and abnormalities in their children.

Epidemiologic investigations used in teratology are primarily of two types: cohort studies and case-control studies. In cohort studies, the frequencies of certain anomalies are compared in the children of women exposed and unexposed to the agent in question. In case-control studies, the frequency of prenatal agent exposure is compared among children with and without a given anomaly. If a teratogenic agent increases the risk of anomalies only slightly, very large studies may be necessary to demonstrate the increase. On the other hand, spurious associations often occur in investigations involving large numbers of comparisons between exposed and unexposed or affected and unaffected subjects. In interpreting epidemiologic studies, one must remember that the maternal disease or situation that occasioned the exposure rather than the agent itself may be responsible for an observed association. Biases of ascertainment and recall may also produce spurious associations. One can never assume that a statistically significant association in an epidemiologic study indicates causality without adducing other evidence to support such a conclusion. Moreover, the usefulness of most published epidemiological studies is limited by a failure to consider the etiologic heterogeneity of human congenital abnormalities or the subtle patterns of anomalies characteristic of many human teratogens.

Although human investigations are necessary to demonstrate that an agent is teratogenic in humans, such studies are not informative until the agent has already damaged many children. Experimental animal studies sometimes provide a means of identifying agents with teratogenic potential before humans have been harmed. Unfortunately, it is usually impossible to extrapolate findings in animals to a clinical situation involving an individual pregnant woman. Species differences in placentation, pharmacodynamics, embryonic development, and innate predisposition to various fetal anomalies are well recognized. Moreover, teratology experiments in animals often employ agent dosages that are many times greater than those likely to occur in humans, and maternal toxic effects may confound the interpretation of fetal outcome. It is even more difficult to assess the relevance of in vitro teratology assays to pregnant women.

In the summaries in this book, the analysis of each agent's teratogenicity has been made on the basis of the reproducibility, consistency, and biological plausibility of available clinical, epidemiological, and experimental data. Reproducibility is judged by whether similar findings have been obtained in independent studies. Concordance is considered to be particularly important if the studies are of different design and if the types of anomalies observed in various studies are consistent. Effects seen in animal investigations are weighed more heavily if the exposure is similar in dosage and route to that encountered clinically and if the species tested are closely related phylogenetically to humans.

Of critical importance is that observed associations make biological sense. Exposures that produce malformations in the embryo or fetus should do so only during organogenesis or histogenesis, and affected structures should be susceptible to the teratogenic action of an agent only at specific gestational times. Systemic absorption of the agent by the mother and its presence at susceptible sites in the embryo or placenta should be demonstrable. In most cases, exposure to a greater quantity of the agent should increase the likelihood of abnormalities. Such dose-response relationships are expected in experimental studies but are often not demonstrable in human data because of the limited dose range encountered clinically. Finally, a causal inference is supported if a reasonable pathogenic mechanism can be established for the observed effect.

The agent summaries in this book were developed for TERIS, an automated teratogen information resource that is used by more than 900 specialized centers throughout the world. The summaries include data on teratogenicity, transplacental carcinogenesis, embryonic or fetal death, and fetal and perinatal pharmacologic effects of drugs and selected environmental agents. Information regarding the pharmacodynamics of the agents, their excretion in breast milk, and their

maternal and neonatal pharmacology is not included but is available elsewhere (Briggs et al., 1990; Gilman et al., 1990; Windholtz et al., 1983). The mutagenicity of agents is also usually excluded. Although many agents have been shown to be mutagenic in experimental systems (Lewis & Sweet, 1982; Shepard, 1992), there is no evidence in humans that the exposure of an individual to any mutagen measurably increases the risk of congenital anomalies in his or her offspring (Crow & Denniston, 1985).

Each agent summary is based on a thorough review of published data identified through a Toxline bibliographic search. References provided in Catalog of Teratogenic Agents (Shepard, 1992), Drugs in Pregnancy and Lactation: A Reference Guide to Fetal and Neonatal Risks (Briggs et al., 1990), and Chemically Induced Birth Defects (Schardein, 1993) are also used extensively. Statements regarding the absence of published studies are made on the basis of this literature review and are true to the best of our knowledge. Unpublished studies, such as those submitted by pharmaceutical or chemical companies to regulatory agencies, are not included because their unpublished state precludes conventional peer review and assessment. Mention of these unpublished studies is often included in package inserts, the Physician's Desk Reference, and similar information provided by manufacturers. Such sources should be consulted to obtain a broader perspective on the teratogenicity of an agent.

Although every effort has been made to make certain that the agent summaries contained in this book are up-to-date at the time they are written, new information is continually accumulating. The use of computer bibliographic databases such as National Library of Medicine's Toxline service is an effective way to identify more recent publications regarding particular agents. Online clinical teratology databases such as TERIS and REPROTOX and regional Teratology Information Services may also provide more recent information.

Lists of agent names and synonyms included in the index were obtained from Martin-dale: The Extra Pharmacopoeia (Reynolds et al., 1989), USP Drug Information (1993), and the Chemline and RTECS files of the National Library of Medicine Toxicology Information Program.

Near the beginning of each agent summary is an aphorism printed entirely in italics. *It should be noted that the risk rating in the aphorism refers only to the risk of teratogenic effects after maternal exposure to commonly encountered doses.* Exposures to unusually high doses, especially to doses that are toxic to the mother, may be associated with a higher risk. Other adverse effects, such as alterations of perinatal adaptation or transplacental carcinogenesis, are considered separately in the narrative and, if deemed sufficiently important, are also mentioned in the aphorism under "Comments."

The aphorism rates the risk of teratogenic effects in the children of women exposed to the agent during pregnancy as None, Minimal, Small, Moderate, High, or Undetermined. In some instances, this rating is amplified by a comment. For example, an agent may be given a risk of minimal with a comment that it is unlikely to pose a substantial teratogenic risk if available data are negative but insufficient to conclude that there is no risk. Similarly, the risk of teratogenic effects may be rated as undetermined with a comment that a small risk cannot be excluded, but there is no indication that the risk of congenital anomalies in the children of women treated with this agent during pregnancy is likely to be great. Such statements are made on the basis of general pharmacology, animal data, or analogy to a closely related agent that has been studied more thoroughly.

In general, risks that are minimal or less ought not to alter decisions regarding the continuation or termination of an exposed pregnancy. Moderate or high risks may be considered important enough to influence such decisions, at least in some cases.

The aphorism also rates the quality and quantity of the data on which the risk assessment is based as None, Poor, Fair, Good, or Excellent. Risk assessments based on evidence that is poor or fair ought to be considered tentative and may change as more information becomes available. Even with good data, only crude estimates of the magnitude of the risk are possible.

The aphorism for each agent is based on a consensus of ratings by the authors and five internationally recognized authorities in clinical teratology. These five individuals, who comprise the TERIS Advisory Board, are Drs. Robert Brent, Jose Cordero, James Hanson, Richard Miller, and Thomas Shepard.

The aphorism is followed by a brief discussion of the data upon which it is based. Emphasis has been placed primarily on information obtained from human studies. Experimental animal data are also included to amplify and clarify the analysis, but, in general, only experiments in mammals are considered. The aphorism should always be read in context of the discussion that follows it.

The references included in the agent summaries have been selected for their quality and accessibility. Each key reference is classified as a review [R], human case report [C], human epidemiological study [E], human clinical series [S], animal study [A], or other [O]. These references are intended not to provide a comprehensive bibliography but rather to help the clinician obtain a broader understanding of the agent's effects on the embryo and fetus.

This book is not a guide for prescribing medications to pregnant women. Physicians should consult approved package inserts for such guidance. Proprietary names are used only for purposes of identification, and such use does not imply any recommendation regarding the agent.

The agent summaries are designed to assist physicians and other health professionals in counseling pregnant patients who have concerns about possible effects of drugs and other agents on their developing babies. *The agent summaries comprise only part of the comprehensive pregnancy risk assessment that is necessary to provide counseling for such patients.* It is always necessary to determine as accurately as possible what the route and dose of the exposure were and whether there were concurrent exposures to other agents. Accurate assessment of when the exposure occurred is critical. The greatest risks of teratogenesis exist during the period of organogenesis (i.e., between about 18 and 60 days after conception). Before this period, malformations are less likely to be induced, but death of the embryo can be caused by certain exposures. Later in pregnancy, insults to the fetus are unlikely to produce malformations but can cause death, growth retardation, disruptions, or functional deficits.

The evaluation of each patient must also include obtaining information on her state of health, previous and current pregnancy history, and family history. Counseling provided as the result of this comprehensive risk assessment should be tailored to each patient's intellectual, educational, psychosocial, and cultural back-ground. The risk associated with an exposure should be presented with reference to the background risk of congenital anomalies which attends every pregnancy for every woman. Decisions regarding prenatal diagnosis and the continuation or termination of pregnancy should be made by the patient in consultation with her physician, family, and other appropriate individuals.

Counseling a pregnant woman about possible effects of a drug or environmental exposure on her developing embryo or fetus is an important component of her medical care. Such counseling should be provided by physicians and other health professionals with competence in clinical teratology. Difficult or complex cases should be referred to appropriate specialists.

References

Beckman DA, Brent RL: Mechanisms of teratogenesis. Ann Rev Pharmacol Toxicol 24:483-500, 1984.

Brent RL: Drugs and pregnancy: Are the insert warnings too dire? Contemp Obstet Gynecol 20:42-49, 1982.

Briggs GG, Freeman RK, Yaffe SJ: Drugs in Pregnancy and Lactation: A Reference Guide to Fetal and Neonatal Risk, 3rd ed. Baltimore: Williams and Wilkins, 1990.

Cordero JF, Oakley GP: Drug exposure during pregnancy: Some epidemiologic considerations. Clin Obstet Gynecol 26:418-428, 1983.

Crow JF, Denniston C: Mutation in human populations. Adv Hum Genetics 14:59-121, 1985.

Gilman AG, Goodman LS, Gilman A: The Pharmacological Basis of Therapeutics, 8th ed. New York: Macmillan Publishing Company, 1990.

Physician's Desk Reference, 47th ed. Montvale, N.J.: Medical Economics Data, 1993.

Reynolds JEF, Parfitt K, Parsons AV, Sweetman SC (eds): Martindale: The Extra Pharmacopoeia, 29th ed. London: Pharmaceutical Press, 1989.

Schardein JL: Chemically Induced Birth Defects, 2nd ed. New York: Marcel Dekker, 1993.

Shepard TH: Catalog of Teratogenic Agents, 7th ed. Baltimore: Johns Hopkins University Press, 1992.

USP Drug Information, 13th ed. Rockville, Md.: The United States Pharmacopeial Convention, 1993.

Windholz M, Budavari S, Blumetti RF, Otterbein ES (eds): The Merck Index, 10th ed. Rathway, N.J.: Merck and Company, 1983.

Teratogenic Effects Of Drugs

ACEBUTOLOL

Synonyms

Acecor, Alol, Diasectral, Molson, Naptall, Neptal, Prent, Rhodiasectral, Sectral, Wesfalin

Summary

Acebutolol is a beta-adrenoreceptor blocking agent used in the treatment of hypertension and cardiac arrhythmias.

Magnitude of Teratogenic Risk

None To Minimal

Quality and Quantity of Data

Poor To Fair

Comment

None

No adequate epidemiological studies of congenital anomalies among infants born to women treated with acebutolol during pregnancy have been reported. One of 56 infants born to women treated with acebutolol had congenital anomalies in one series, but only six of these pregnancies were treated in the first trimester (Dubois et al., 1982). Treatment began in the 24th week in the mother of an affected infant (Dubois et al., 1980).

The frequency of malformations was not increased among the offspring of rats treated with acebutolol in doses 1-25 times that used orally or 1-12 times that used intravenously in humans (Yokoi et al., 1978).

Bradycardia and low blood pressure have been observed among infants born to women treated with acebutolol late in pregnancy (Dumez et al., 1981; Bavoux et al., 1982; Brosset et al., 1985).

Key References

Bavoux F, Huault G, Lanfranchi C, Olive G: Risk assessment of drugs in perinatal period. Therapie 37:337-345, 1982. [C]

Brosset P, Ronayette D, Negrier S, Bouquier JJ: Low-heart-rate collapse in two newborn infants from mothers treated with beta-blockers. Presse Med 14:105-106, 1985. [C]

Dubois D, Petitcolas J, Temperville B, Klepper A: Treatment of hypertension in pregnant women with beta-blockers. 60 cases. Nouv Presse Med 9(38):2807-2810, 1980. [S]

Dubois D, Petitcolas J, Temperville B, Klepper A, et al.: Treatment of hypertension in pregnancy with beta-adrenoceptor antagonists. Br J Clin Pharmacol 13:375S-378S, 1982. [S]

Dumez Y, Tchobroutsky C, Hornych H, Amiel-Tison C: Neonatal effects of maternal administration of acebutolol. Br Med J 283(6299):1077-1079, 1981. [S]

Yokoi Y, Yoshida H, Hirano K, et al.: Teratological studies of acebutolol hydrochloride in rats. Oyo Yakuri 15:885-904, 1978. [A]

ACETALDEHYDE

Synonyms

Acetaldehido, Acetaldehyd, Acetic Aldehyde, Acetylaldehyde, Ethyl Aldehyde

Summary

Acetaldehyde is used as a solvent in the tanning, rubber, and paper industries. Acetaldehyde is produced in the body during metabolism of ethanol or paraldehyde.

Magnitude of Teratogenic Risk

Undetermined

Quality and Quantity of Data

Poor

None

No epidemiological studies of congenital anomalies in children of women exposed directly to acetaldehyde during pregnancy have been reported. Acetaldehyde produced from the metabolism of ethanol has been suggested as an important teratogenic factor in fetal alcohol syndrome (Veghelyi, 1983; Randall, 1987; Fisher & Karl, 1988).

Increased frequencies of various congenital anomalies have been observed among the offspring of mice or rats treated during pregnancy with 50-100 mg/kg or more of acetaldehyde, respectively (Sreenathan et al., 1982, 1984; Webster et al., 1983). In mice, treatment during pregnancy with lower doses of acetaldehyde has produced inconsistent results, with increased frequencies of fetal death and growth retardation being observed in some studies but not others (O'Shea & Kaufman, 1979, 1981; Blakley & Scott, 1984). The relevance of these observations to the risks associated with human exposure to acetaldehyde during pregnancy is unknown.

Please see agent summaries on alcohol and paraldehyde for information on metabolically related agents that have been more thoroughly studied.

Key References

Blakley PM, Scott WJ: Determination of the proximate teratogen of the mouse fetal alcohol syndrome. 1. Teratogenicity of ethanol and acetaldehyde. Toxicol Appl Pharmacol 72:355-363, 1984. [A]

O'Shea KS, Kaufman MH: Effect of acetaldehyde on the neuroepithelium of early mouse embryos. J Anat 132:107-118, 1981. [A]

O'Shea KS, Kaufman MH: The teratogenic effect of acetaldehyde: Implications for the study of the fetal alcohol syndrome. J Anat 128:65-76, 1979. [A]

Sreenathan RN, Padmanabhan R, Singh S: Teratogenic effects of acetaldehyde in the rat. Drug Alcohol Depend 9:339-350, 1982. [A]

Webster WS, Walsh DA, McEwen SE, Lipson AH: Some teratogenic properties of ethanol and acetaldehyde in C57BL/6J Mice: Implications for the study of the fetal alcohol syndrome. Teratology 27:231-243, 1983. [A]

ACETAMINOPHEN

Synonyms

Acephen, Anacin-3, Datril, Panadol, Paracetamol, Tempra, Tylenol, Valadol

Summary

Acetaminophen is an oral analgesic and antipyretic agent.

Magnitude of Teratogenic Risk

None

Quality and Quantity of Data

Good

Comment

1) The assessment given above is based on exposure to usual therapeutic doses of acetaminophen.

2) The risk of fetal toxicity or death may be substantial when the mother takes a toxic overdose of acetaminophen during pregnancy (see below).

The frequency of congenital anomalies was no greater than expected among the children of 493 and 350 women who took acetaminophen during the first trimester of pregnancy in two cohorts of the Boston Collaborative Drug Surveillance Program (Jick et al., 1981; Aselton et al., 1985). Similarly, there was no increase in the frequency of congenital anomalies among the infants of 226 women who took acetaminophen during the first four lunar months of pregnancy or of 781 women who took this drug anytime during gestation in the Collaborative Perinatal Project (Heinonen et al., 1977). In a case-control study of 458 infants with various congenital anomalies, the frequency of maternal use of acetaminophen during the first trimester or anytime during pregnancy was no greater than expected (Nelson & Forfar, 1971). In another case-control study which included 298 children with congenital heart disease, the frequency of maternal use of acetaminophen during the first trimester of pregnancy was not increased (Zierler & Rothman, 1985). Streissguth et al. (1987) found no association between maternal use of acetaminophen during the first half of pregnancy and IQ of 421 children at 4 years of age.

Among 51 women who were treated for acetaminophen overdose in pregnancy in one series, there were nine spontaneous abortions or fetal deaths; six of the spontaneous abortions occurred among the 11 patients with first-trimester overdoses (Riggs et al., 1989). Thirty-two liveborn infants were delivered in this series; the only one with a congenital anomaly was a child with positional deformity of the feet whose mother had taken an overdose of acetaminophen at 30 weeks gestation. All five infants born to mothers who had taken acetaminophen overdoses in the first trimester of pregnancy appeared normal at birth. In another series of 41 cases of acetaminophen overdose in pregnancy, there was one infant with cleft lip and palate (overdose at 28 weeks gestation), one with spina bifida occulta and strabismus (overdose at 26 weeks), and one who developed pyloric stenosis (overdose at 36 weeks) (McElhatton et al., 1990). Among 14 cases with first-trimester acetaminophen overdose in this series, there were two spontaneous abortions and 12 normal liveborn infants.

Hepatotoxicity and nephrotoxicity occur as complications of acetaminophen overdosage in adults. Similar effects have been observed among infants born to women who took large therapeutic or toxic doses of acetaminophen late in pregnancy (Char et al., 1975; Haibach et al., 1984; Riggs et al., 1989; Kurzel, 1990). Fetal distress has been demonstrated in a pregnant woman who took a toxic overdose of acetaminophen in the third trimester (Rosevear & Hope, 1989).

In one study in mice, the frequency of malformations was not increased among the offspring of animals treated during pregnancy with a combination containing acetaminophen, ethenzamide, and caffeine in doses 1-5 times those used in humans (Ogawa et al., 1982). The frequency of fetal death and eye anomalies was increased among the offspring of mice treated with 5-7.5 times the maximal human dose of acetaminophen in another investigation (Popp et al., 1979).

Key References

Aselton PA, Jick H, Milunsky A, Hunter JR, et al.: First-trimester drug use and congenital disorders. Obstet Gynecol 65:451-455, 1985. [S]

Char VC, Chandra R, Fletcher AB, Avery GB: Polyhydramnios and neonatal renal failure--a possible association with maternal acetaminophen ingestion. J Pediatr 86:638, 1975. [C]

Haibach H, Akhter JE, Muscato MS, Cary PL, et al.: Acetaminophen overdose with fetal demise. Am J Clin Pathol 82:240-242, 1984. [C]

Heinonen OP, Slone D, Shapiro S: Birth Defects and Drugs in Pregnancy. Littleton, Mass.: John Wright-PSG, 1977, pp 286-288, 434. [E]

Jick H, Holmes LB, Hunter JR, Madsen S, et al.: First-trimester drug use and congenital disorders. JAMA 246:343-346, 1981. [S]

Kurzel RB: Can acetaminophen excess result in maternal and fetal toxicity? South Med J 83(8):953-955, 1990. [C]

McElhatton PR, Sullivan FM, Volans GN, Fitzpatrick R: Paracetamol poisoning in pregnancy: An analysis of the outcomes of cases referred to the Teratology Information Service of the National Poisons Information Service. Hum Exp Toxicol 9:147-153, 1990. [S]

Nelson MM, Forfar JO: Associations between drugs administered during pregnancy and congenital abnormalities of the fetus. Br Med J 1:523-527, 1971. [E]

Ogawa H, Arakawa E, Morobushi A, et al.: Reproductive studies of NB-6. Kiso to Rinsho 16:683-695, 1982. [A]

Popp RA, Owens S: Effect of acetaminophen in mice. Environ Mutagen 1:117, 1979. [A]

Riggs BS, Bronstein AC, Kulig K, et al.: Acute acetaminophen ovcrdose during pregnancy. Obstet Gynecol 74(2):247-253, 1989. [S]

Rosevear Sk, Hope PL: Favourable neonatal outcome following maternal paracetamol overdose and severe fetal distress. Case Report. Br J Obstet Gynecol 96:491-493, 1989. [C]

Streissguth AP, Treder RP, Barr HM, Shepard TH, et al.: Aspirin and acetaminophen use by pregnant women and subsequent child IQ and attention decrements. Teratology 35:211-219, 1987. [E]

Zierler S, Rothman KJ: Congenital heart disease in relation to maternal use of Bendectin and other drugs in early pregnancy. New Engl J Med 313:347-352, 1985. [E]

ACETAZOLAMIDE

Synonyms

Atenezol, Defiltran, Diamox, Didoc, Diuramid, Edemox, Glaucomide, Glaupax, Inidrase, Oratrol

Summary

Acetazolamide is a carbonic anhydrase inhibitor used as a diuretic and in the treatment of glaucoma and certain kinds of epilepsy.

Magnitude of Teratogenic Risk

None To Minimal

Quality and Quantity of Data

Poor To Fair

Comment

None

Congenital anomalies were no more frequent than expected among the children of 1024 women treated with acetazolamide during pregnancy in the Collaborative Perinatal Project, but only 12 of these mothers were treated during the first four lunar months of gestation (Heinonen et al., 1977). An association was claimed between maternal acetazolamide treatment in the first trimester of pregnancy and malformations in the offspring in a Japanese cohort study (Nakane et al., 1980), but this investigation included only 19 pregnancies exposed to acetazolamide, and the data presentation does not permit evaluation of the biological significance of the association.

Acetazolamide produces an unusual and specific limb malformation when administered to rats, mice, or hamsters early in pregnancy in doses many times those used clinically (Layton & Hallesy, 1965; Layton, 1971; Ellison & Maren, 1972; Vickers, 1976; Scott et al., 1981; Hirsch et al., 1983; Biddle, 1988; Holmes et al., 1988; Beck & Urbano, 1991). These doses are often toxic to the mothers. Typical dependence of the teratogenic effect on dose and gestational timing of the exposure as well as on genetic background has been demonstrated (Layton & Hallesy, 1965; Layton, 1971; Vickers, 1976; Scott et al., 1981; Biddle, 1988; Brown et al., 1989; Biddle et al., 1991; Beck & Manabat, 1992). Rabbits and rhesus monkeys appear to be relatively resistant to acetazolamide teratogenesis (DeSesso & Jordan, 1977; Scott et al., 1981), but maternal plasma and embryonic tissue levels of acetazolamide with a given dose are substantially lower in monkeys than in rats (Scott et al., 1981). Craniofacial and central nervous system malformations have also been reported, although less consistently, among the offspring of pregnant mice treated with acetazolamide in doses 25 to 50 times those used clinically (Castro-Correia et al., 1974; Scott et al., 1984). The relevance, if any, of these observations to the therapeutic use of acetazolamide in human pregnancy is unknown.

Key References

Beck SL, Manabat N: Dependence of acetazolamide teratogenesis on fetal and not maternal genotypes. Reprod Toxicol 6:63-67, 1992. [A]

Beck SL, Urbano CM: Potentiating effect of caffeine on the teratogenicity of acetazolamide in C57BL/6J mice. Teratology 44:241-250, 1991. [A]

Biddle FG: Genetic differences in the frequency of acetazolamide-induced ectrodactyly in the mouse exhibit directional dominance of relative embryonic resistance. Teratology 37:375-388, 1988. [A]

4

Biddle FG, Mulholland LR, Eales BA: Time-response and dose-response to acetazolamide in the WB/ReJ and C57BL/6J mouse strains: Genetic interaction in the ectrodactyly response. Teratology 44:107-120, 1991. [A]

Brown NA, Hoyle CI, McCarthy A, Wolpert L: The development of asymmetry: The sidedness of drug-induced limb abnormalities is reversed in situs inversus mice. Development 107:637-642, 1989. [A]

Castro-Correia J, Sousa-Nunes A, Silva-Bacelar A: Teratogenic action of acetazolamide in mice. Teratology 10:221-226, 1974. [A]

DeSesso JM, Jordan RL: Drug-induced limb dysplasias in fetal rabbits. Teratology 15:199-212, 1977. [A]

Ellison AC, Maren TH: The effect of potassium metabolism on acetazolamide-induced teratogenesis. Johns Hopkins Med J 130:105-115, 1972 [A]

Heinonen OP, Slone D, Shapiro S: Birth Defects and Drugs in Pregnancy. Littleton, Mass.: John Wright-PSG, 1977, p 495. [E]

Hirsch KS, Wilson JG, Scott WJ, O'Flaherty EJ: Acetazolamide teratology and its association with carbonic anhydrase inhibition in the mouse. Teratogenesis Carcinog Mutagen 3:133-144, 1983. [A]

Holmes LB, Kawanishi H, Munoz A: Acetazolamide: Maternal toxicity, pattern of malformations, and litter effect. Teratology 37:335-342, 1988. [A]

Layton WM: Teratogenic action of acetazolamide in golden hamsters. Teratology 4:95-102, 1971. [A]

Layton WM, Hallesy DW: Deformity of forelimb in rats: Association with high doses of acetazolamide. Science 149:306-308, 1965. [A]

Nakane Y, Okuma T, Takahashi R, Sato Y, et al.: Multi-institutional study on the teratogenicity and fetal toxicity of antiepileptic drugs: A report of a collaborative study group in Japan. Epilepsia 21:663-680, 1980. [E]

Scott WJ, Hirsch KS, DeSesso JM, Wilson JG: Comparative studies on acetazolamide teratogenesis in pregnant rats, rabbits, and rhesus monkeys. Teratology 24:37-42, 1981. [A]

Scott WJ, Lane PD, Randall JL, Schreiner CM: Malformations in nonlimb structures induced by acetazolamide and other inhibitors of carbonic anhydrase. Ann NY Acad Sci 429:447-456, 1984. [A]

Vickers TH: Concerning so-called sexual dimorphism in acetazolamide-induced dysmelia of rats. Teratology 13:305-308, 1976. [A]

ACETIC ACID

Synonyms

Acetum, Etanoico, Ethanoic Acid, Ethylic Acid, Glacial Acetic Acid, Methanecarboxylic Acid, Vinegar Acid, Vosol

Summary

Acetic acid is a simple organic acid. It is used topically as an antibacterial agent, as a caustic, and as a vaginal douche. Vinegars contain diluted solutions of acetic acid.

Magnitude of Teratogenic Risk

Undetermined

Quality and Quantity of Data

Poor

Comment

A small risk cannot be excluded, but a substantial risk of congenital anomalies in the children of women exposed to acetic acid during pregnancy is unlikely.

No epidemiological studies of congenital anomalies among infants born to women who ingested or were exposed to unusually large amounts of acetic acid during pregnancy have been reported.

No teratogenic effects were observed among the offspring of mice, rats, or rabbits that had been given very large doses of apple cider vinegar (containing acetic acid) during pregnancy (Food and Drug Research Laboratories, Inc., 1974).

5

Key References

Food and Drug Research Laboratories, Inc.: Teratologic evaluation of FDA 71-78 (apple cider vinegar [acetic acid]; table strength 5%) in mice, rats and rabbits. NTIS (National Technical Information Service) Report/PB-234 869) 1974. [A]

ACETOHEXAMIDE

Synonyms

Dimelor, Dymelor, Gamadiabet, Metaglucina, Minoral, Ordimel

Summary

Acetohexamide is a sulphonylurea compound used as an oral hypoglycemic agent.

Magnitude of Teratogenic Risk

Undetermined

Quality and Quantity of Data

None

Comment

None

No epidemiological studies of congenital anomalies among the infants of women treated with acetohexamide during pregnancy have been reported.

No animal teratology studies of acetohexamide have been published.

Neonatal hypoglycemia has been observed in the infant of a woman treated with acetohexamide throughout pregnancy (Kemball et al., 1970).

Please see agent summary on chlorpropamide for information on a related agent that has been studied.

Key References

Kemball ML, McIver C, Milner RDG, Nourse CH, et al.: Neonatal hypoglycaemia in infants of diabetic mothers given sulphonylurea drugs in pregnancy. Arch Dis Child 45:696-701, 1970. [S]

ACETOHYDROXAMIC ACID

Synonyms

Lithostat, Uronefrex

Summary

Acetohydroxamic acid is an organic acid that is given orally to prevent the formation of renal calculi.

Magnitude of Teratogenic Risk

Undetermined

Quality and Quantity of Data

Poor

Comment

Although the risk of this agent is undetermined, it may be substantial since experimental animals show adverse effects at therapeutic levels.

No epidemiological studies of congenital anomalies among infants born to women treated with acetohydroxamic acid during pregnancy have been reported.

Increased frequencies of skeletal anomalies, encephalocele, and other malformations were observed among the offspring of pregnant rats treated with 25-33 but not 17 times the maximal human therapeutic dose of acetohydroxamic acid (Chaube & Murphy, 1966). Cardiovascular, skeletal, and abdominal wall defects were observed with increased frequency among the offspring of dogs treated during pregnancy with acetohydroxamic acid in doses within the human therapeutic range (Bailie et al., 1986).

Key References

Bailie NC, Osborne CA, Leininger JR, et al.: Teratogenic effect of acetohydroxamic acid in clinically normal beagles. Am J Vet Res 47:2604-2611, 1986. [A]

Chaube S, Murphy ML: The effects of hydroxyurea and related compounds on the rat fetus. Cancer Res 26:1448-1457, 1966. [A]

ACETYL TRIBUTYL CITRATE

Synonyms

Citroflex A, Tributyl Acetylcitrate, Tributyl Citrate Acetate

Summary

Acetyl tributyl citrate is used in protective skin dressings.

Magnitude of Teratogenic Risk

Undetermined

Quality and Quantity of Data

None

Comment

A small risk cannot be excluded, but a high risk of congenital anomalies in the children of women treated with acetyl tributyl citrate during pregnancy is unlikely.

No epidemiological studies of congenital anomalies among infants born to women treated with dressings containing acetyl tributyl citrate during pregnancy have been reported.

No animal teratology studies of acetyl tributyl citrate have been published.

Key References

None available.

ACETYLCYSTEINE

Synonyms

Airbron, Brunac, Eurespiran, Fabrol, Ilube, Mucomyst, Mucosal, Mucret, Parvolex, Tixair

Summary

Acetylcysteine is a mucolytic agent. It is administered by direct instillation into the respiratory tract or by nebulization. Acetylcysteine is also used in ophthalmic preparations to treat dry eyes and systemically to treat acetaminophen poisoning.

Magnitude of Teratogenic Risk

Undetermined

Quality and Quantity of Data

None

Comment

None

No epidemiological studies of congenital anomalies among infants born to women treated with acetylcysteine during pregnancy have been reported.

No animal teratology studies of acetylcysteine have been published.

Key References

None available.

ACETYLDIGITOXIN

Synonyms

Acedoxin, Acetildigitoxin, Acylanid, Adicin

Summary

Acetyldigitoxin is a cardiac glycoside used to treat heart failure.

Magnitude of Teratogenic Risk

Undetermined

Quality and Quantity of Data

None

Comment

None

No epidemiological studies of congenital anomalies in infants whose mothers took acetyldigitoxin during pregnancy have been reported.

No animal teratology studies of acetyldigitoxin have been published.

Please see agent summary on digoxin for information on a closely related agent that has been studied.

Key References

None available.

ACTODIGIN

Synonyms

Actodigine, Actodigino, Actodiginum

Summary

Actodigin is a cardiotonic drug.

Magnitude of Teratogenic Risk

Undetermined

Quality and Quantity of Data

None

Comment

None

No epidemiological studies of congenital anomalies in infants born to women treated with actodigin during pregnancy have been reported.

No animal teratology studies of actodigin have been published.

Key References

None available.

ACYCLOVIR

Synonyms

Acyvir, Cusiviral, Maynar, Vipral, Virherpes, Virmen, Zovirax

Summary

Acyclovir is a synthetic purine nucleoside analog that is used topically and systemically to treat herpes and other viral infections (Brown & Baker, 1989; Brown & Watts, 1990). Systemic absorption of the topical preparation appears to be minimal through normal skin but may occur to a moderate degree through diseased skin.

Magnitude of Teratogenic Risk

Undetermined

Quality and Quantity of Data

Poor

Comment

None

In an international Acyclovir in Pregnancy Registry, nine of 168 infants born to women treated with acyclovir systemically during the first trimester and followed prospectively to birth were found to have congenital anomalies (Andrews et al., 1988, 1992). No recurrent pattern of anomalies was seen among these affected infants or among nine other infants with congenital anomalies born to women who took systemic acyclovir during the first trimester of pregnancy and reported to the registry after delivery. No congenital anomalies attributable to acyclovir were observed among the children of 73 women treated systemically with acyclovir in the second or third trimester of pregnancy and reported to the registry before delivery.

Maternal systemic treatment with acyclovir near term has been used to prevent recurrent genital herpes and perinatal transmission (Stray-Pedersen et al., 1990; Frenkel et al., 1991). No "short-term side-effects" of acyclovir were noted among the newborns in a controlled trial in which 92 women received such treatment (Stray- Pedersen et al., 1990).

No teratogenic effect was observed among the offspring of mice, rats, or rabbits treated systemically with acyclovir during pregnancy in doses, respectively, 2.5-22, <1-2.5, and <1-2.5 times those used in humans (Moore et al., 1983). In contrast, increased frequencies of fetal death, growth retardation, and malformations were observed among the offspring of rats treated with 5-15 times the usual human dose of acyclovir (Neubert et al., 1986; Stahlmann et al., 1988; Chahoud et al., 1988). Craniofacial and skeletal anomalies were observed most often. The relevance of these observations to the therapeutic use of acyclovir in women is unknown.

Key References

Andrews EB, Tilson HH, Hurn BAL, et al.: Acyclovir in Pregnancy Registry. An observational epidemiologic approach. Am J Med 85(Suppl 2A):123-128, 1988. [E]

Andrews EB, Yankaskas BC, Cordero JF, et al.: Acyclovir in pregnancy registry: Six years' experience. Obstet Gynecol 79:7-13, 1992. [E]

Brown ZA, Baker DA: Acyclovir therapy during pregnancy. Obstet Gynecol 73(3):526-531, 1989. [R]

Brown ZA, Watts DH: Antiviral therapy in pregnancy. Clin Obstet Gynecol 33:276-289, 1990. [R]

Chahoud I, Stahlmann R, Bochert G, et al.: Gross-structural defects in rats after acyclovir application on day 10 of gestation. Arch Toxicol 62:8-14, 1988. [A]

Frenkel LM, Brown ZA, Bryson YJ, et al.: Pharmacokinetics of acyclovir in the term human pregnancy and neonate. Am J Obstet Gynecol 164(2):569-576, 1991. [S]

Moore HL, Szczech GM, Rodwell DE, Kapp RW, et al.: Preclinical toxicology studies with acyclovir: Teratologic, reproductive and neonatal tests. Fundam Appl Toxicol 3:560-568, 1983. [A]

Neubert D, Blankenburg G, Chahoud I, Franz G, et al.: Results of in vivo and in vitro studies for assessing prenatal toxicity. Environ Health Perspect 70:89-103, 1986. [A]

Stahlmann R, Klug S, Lewandowski C, et al.: Prenatal toxicity of acyclovir in rats. Arch Toxicol 61:468-479, 1988. [A]

Stray-Pedersen B: Acyclovir in late pregnancy to prevent neonatal herpes simplex. Lancet 336:756, 1990. [E]

AFLATOXINS

Synonyms

Aflatoxin B_1

Summary

Aflatoxins are toxic metabolites produced by the growth of fungus of the genus Aspergillus.

They combine with DNA and inhibit DNA and RNA synthesis. Aflatoxin contamination may occur in many foods, such as cereals and peanuts.

Magnitude of Teratogenic Risk

Undetermined

Quality and Quantity of Data

Poor

Comment

There may be a substantial risk of fetal damage or transplacental carcinogenesis with exposure to aflatoxins during pregnancy in doses sufficient to cause overt maternal toxicity.

No epidemiological studies of congenital anomalies among the infants of women exposed to large amounts of aflatoxins during pregnancy have been reported. In one study, the mean birth weight of 24 female infants born to women in whom aflatoxins were detected in the blood at delivery was significantly lower than among female infants born to women in whom aflatoxins were not found (de Vries et al., 1989). No correlation between birth weight and the presence of aflatoxins in maternal blood was observed among male infants. Overall, 37 of 101 cord bloods in this series were found to contain aflatoxins. There were two unexplained stillbirths; both these cord bloods contained aflatoxins.

Increased frequencies of fetal death, growth retardation, and eye, central nervous system, and other anomalies have been observed among the offspring of mice and hamsters treated with 4 mg/kg/d or more of aflatoxin during pregnancy, a dose that generally produces maternal hepatic toxicity as well (Elis et al., 1967; Schmidt & Panciera et al., 1980; Arora et al., 1981; Tanimura et al., 1982; Hood & Szczech, 1983; Roll et al., 1990). Fetal growth retardation but no increase in malformations was observed among the offspring of rats treated during pregnancy with 3.5-7 mg/kg/d of aflatoxin (Sharma & Sahai, 1987).

Rats born to mothers treated with aflatoxins in doses of 0.5-4 mg/kg/d during pregnancy develop benign and malignant neoplastic lesions of the liver, nervous system, and other organs much more frequently than expected (Grice et al., 1973; Goerttler et al., 1980). Similar lesions also occur in the mother animals.

Key References

Arora RG, Frolen H, Nilsson A: Interference of mycotoxins with prenatal development of the mouse. Acta Vet Scand 22:524-534, 1981. [A]

De Vries HR, Maxwell SM, Hendrickse RG: Foetal and neonatal exposure to aflatoxins. Acta Paediatr Scand 78:373-378, 1989. [E]

Elis J, DiPaolo JA: Aflatoxin B_1. Induction of malformations. Arch Pathol 83:53-57, 1967. [A]

Goerttler K, Lohrke H, Schweizer H-J, Hesse B: Effects of aflatoxin B_1 on pregnant inbred Sprague-Dawley rats and their F1 generation. A contribution to transplacental carcinogenesis. J Natl Cancer Inst 64:1349-1354, 1980. [A]

Grice HC, Moodie CA, Smith DC: The carcinogenic potential of aflatoxin or its metabolites in rats from dams fed aflatoxin pre- and postpartum. Cancer Res 33:262-268, 1973. [A]

Hood RD, Szczech GM: Teratogenicity of fungal toxins and fungal-produced antimicrobial agents. Handb Nat Toxin 1:201-235, 1983. [R]

Roll R, Matthiaschk G, Korte A: Embryotoxicity and mutagenicity of mycotoxins. J Environ Pathol Toxicol Oncol 10(1-2):1-7, 1990. [A]

Schmidt RE, Panciera RJ: Effects of aflatoxin on pregnant hamsters and hamster foetuses. J Comp Path 90:339-347, 1980. [A]

Sharma A, Sahai R: Teratological effects of aflatoxin on rats (Rattus Norvegicus). Indian J Anim Res 21(1):35-40, 1987. [A]

Tanimura T, Kihara T, Yamamoto Y: Teratogenicity of aflatoxin B_1 in the mouse. Kankyo Kagaku Kenkyusho Kenkyu Hokoku (Kinki Daigaku) 10:247-256, 1982. [A]

ALANINE

Synonyms

Alpha-Alanine, Alpha-Aminopropionic Acid, 2-Aminopropionic Acid

Summary

Alanine is a non-essential amino acid. It is sometimes used in elemental diets and nutritional supplements.

Magnitude of Teratogenic Risk

Undetermined

Quality and Quantity of Data

None

Comment

A small risk cannot be excluded, but a high risk of congenital anomalies in the children of women treated with alanine during pregnancy is unlikely.

No epidemiological studies of congenital anomalies among infants born to women who ingested exceptionally large amounts of alanine during pregnancy have been reported.

No animal teratology studies of high-dose alanine have been published.

Key References

None available.

ALBUMIN

Synonyms

Enteroquanil, Ovalbumin

Summary

Albumin is the major plasma protein in human blood. Albumin is administered intravenously in the treatment of shock, burns, hepatic cirrhosis, and nephrosis.

Magnitude of Teratogenic Risk

Undetermined

Quality and Quantity of Data

None

Comment

A small risk cannot be excluded, but a substantial risk of congenital anomalies in the children of women treated with albumin during pregnancy is unlikely.

No epidemiological studies of congenital anomalies among infants born to women treated with intravenous albumin during pregnancy have been reported.

No animal teratology studies of albumin have been published.

Key References

None available.

ALBUTEROL

Synonyms

Aerolin, Asmaven, Asmidon, Cobutolin, Proventil, Salbulin, Salbutamol, Ventodisks, Ventolin, Volmax

Summary

Albuterol is a beta-sympathicomimetic used as a bronchodilator and to arrest premature labor.

Magnitude of Teratogenic Risk

Undetermined

Quality and Quantity of Data

Poor

Comment

None

No epidemiological studies of congenital anomalies among infants born to women treated with albuterol during pregnancy have been reported.

Pregnant rabbits given albuterol at thousands of times the usual human dose produced offspring with no increased frequency of malformations (Szabo et al., 1975). An increased frequency of malformations (mostly cleft palates) was observed among the offspring of pregnant mice given albuterol in doses many times that used in humans (Szabo et al., 1975). The relevance of this finding to the therapeutic use of albuterol in pregnant women is unknown.

Maternal albuterol treatment in late pregnancy produces fetal tachycardia, but this has not been associated with any important neonatal problems (Ryden, 1977; Hastwell et al., 1978).

Key References

Hastwell GB, Halloway CP, Taylor TLO: A study of 208 patients in premature labour treated with orally administered salbutamol. Med J Aust 1:465-469, 1978. [S]

Ryden G: The effect of salbutamol and terbutaline in the management of premature labour. Acta Obstet Gynecol Scand 56:293-296, 1977. [S]

Szabo KT, Difebbo ME, Kang YJ: Effects of several beta-receptor agonists on fetal development in various species of laboratory animals: Preliminary report. Teratology 12:336-337, 1975. [A]

ALCLOMETASONE DIPROPIONATE

Synonyms

Aclovate, Vaderm

Summary

Alclometasone dipropionate is a corticosteroid that is used topically.

Magnitude of Teratogenic Risk

Undetermined

Quality and Quantity of Data

None

Comment

A small risk cannot be excluded, but a high risk of congenital anomalies in the children of women treated with alclometasone dipropionate during pregnancy is unlikely.

No epidemiological studies of congenital anomalies among infants born to women treated with alclometasone dipropionate during pregnancy have been reported.

No animal teratology studies of alclometasone dipropionate have been published.

Please see agent summary on triamcinolone for information on a related agent that has been studied.

Key References

None available.

ALCOHOL

Synonyms

Aethanolum, Alcool, Ethanol, Ethyl Alcohol, Spiritus

Summary

Alcohol is a central nervous system depressant that is widely consumed in beverages for its intoxicating effect. Alcohol is frequently used in pharmaceuticals as a solvent and preservative; it is also employed as a surface disinfectant.

Magnitude of Teratogenic Risk

Heavy Drinking (More than six drinks, glasses of wine, or beer per day): Moderate To High

Moderate Drinking (Less than two drinks, glasses of wine or beer per day): None To Minimal

Quality and Quantity of Data

Heavy Drinking: Good To Excellent

Moderate Drinking: Fair To Good

Comment

1) Alcohol-related birth defects (arbd) represent a continuum. At any given amount of maternal alcohol intake during pregnancy, more children will have arbd that do not constitute full fetal alcohol syndrome (defined below) than will have the classical syndrome. The risk of arbd of any severity decreases with decreasing alcohol use, but no safe level during pregnancy has been determined.

2) The risk associated with drinking alcohol in amounts that fall between those classified as heavy and moderate above is presumed to be intermediate.

3) The amounts given above for heavy and moderate drinking are approximate and will vary somewhat from person to person. Genetic differences are likely to be a factor in this variability.

4) The risk associated with binge drinking is unclear, but animal studies suggest that even a single heavy binge at a critical time in pregnancy may cause fetal damage.

A pattern of congenital anomalies called the fetal alcohol syndrome occurs in infants born to women who suffer from chronic alcoholism during pregnancy (Jones et al., 1973; Clarren & Smith, 1978; Streissguth et al., 1985; Jones, 1986; Abel & Sokol, 1988; Streissguth & LaDue, 1987; Burd & Martsolf, 1989; Hill et al., 1989; Ginsburg et al., 1991; Streissguth et al., 1991). Typical fetal alcohol syndrome is usually seen among the children of women who drink more (and often much more) than 3 ounces of absolute alcohol daily throughout pregnancy. This is the equivalent of about six beers, six glasses of wine, or six mixed drinks a day. Fetal alcohol syndrome is defined by: (a) prenatal and/or postnatal growth retardation; (b) central nervous system dysfunction, including microcephaly, neurological impairment, developmental delay, and neurobehavioral deficits; and (c) facial anomalies such as short palpebral fissures, indistinct philtrum, thin upper lip vermillion, elongated and flat midface (Sokol & Clarren, 1989). Congenital heart disease and brain malformations are common, but other major malformations are less frequent.

Full fetal alcohol syndrome occurs in about 6% of children of women who drink heavily during pregnancy (Day & Richardson, 1991). The risk is probably higher for women with chronic severe alcoholism during pregnancy. Less severe manifestations of alcohol embryopathy occur in a larger proportion of these children, but the estimated frequency varies widely in different studies (Abel & Sokol, 1988; Day & Richardson, 1991). The risk of full fetal alcohol syndrome is much higher for alcoholic women who have already had an affected child (Abel, 1988). The effects appear to be less severe among the children of alcoholic women who stop drinking early in pregnancy (Rosett et al., 1983; Aronson & Olegard, 1987; Autti-Ramo & Granstrom, 1991a, b; Coles et al., 1991; Autti-Ramo et al., 1992).

Lower levels of maternal alcohol consumption during pregnancy have been associated with a variety of less severe but persistent manifestations in children (Ouellette et al., 1977; Hanson et al., 1978; Streissguth et al., 1989; Day et al., 1990; Day & Richardson, 1991; Forrest & Florey, 1991). Among the "normal" children of women who drink an average of more than 1 to 2 ounces of absolute al-

13

cohol a day during pregnancy (the equivalent of about two to four beers, glasses of wine, or mixed drinks), minor anomalies, growth deficiency, intellectual deficits, and behavioral abnormalities occur with increased frequency. The risks of maternal episodic ("binge") drinking have not been clearly defined, but may be substantial (Streissguth et al., 1989; see also animal data below). No safe level of maternal drinking during pregnancy has been established.

Maternal alcohol use during pregnancy has also been associated with an increased risk of miscarriage and stillbirth (Kline et al., 1980; Abel & Sokol, 1988; Ginsburg et al., 1991).

Several animal models of fetal alcohol syndrome have been developed (Streissguth et al., 1980; Abel, 1982; Fabro et al., 1982; Leonard, 1988; West & Goodlett, 1990). Species studied include rodents, rabbits, ferrets, swine, dogs, and primates. Various physical and behavioral abnormalities similar to those seen in human fetal alcohol syndrome have been induced with administration of alcohol in dosages equivalent to those used by human chronic alcoholics. Typical dose-response relationships are demonstrable in some cases. Exposure of rodents, ferrets, and primates to alcohol under conditions similar to "binge" drinking in humans produces increased frequencies of anomalies in the offspring (Sulik & Johnston, 1983; Padmanabhan et al., 1984; McLain & Roe, 1984; Scott & Fradkin, 1984; Inouye et al., 1985; Clarren et al., 1988).

At least a dozen children with fetal alcohol syndrome who also have malignant neoplasms of various kinds have been reported (Kiess et al., 1984). Such observations appear to be surprisingly frequent, raising the possibility that maternal alcohol abuse during pregnancy may increase the risk of malignancy in children.

Transient withdrawal symptoms such as tremors, hypertonia, and irritability have been observed among infants born to women who chronically drank alcohol late in pregnancy (Coles et al., 1984; Beattie, 1986).

Key References

Abel EL: Consumption of alcohol during pregnancy: A review of effects on growth and development of offspring. Hum Biol 54:421-453, 1982. [R]

Abel EL: Fetal alcohol syndrome in families. Neurotoxicol Teratol 10:1-2, 1988. [O]

Abel EL, Sokol RJ: Alcohol use in pregnancy. In: Niebyl JR, Drug Use in Pregnancy. Philadelphia: Lea & Febiger, 1988, pp 193-202. [R]

Aronson M, Olegard R: Children of alcoholic mothers. Pediatrician 14(1-2):57-61, 1987. [E]

Autti-Ramo I, Granstrom M-L: The effect of intrauterine alcohol exposition in various durations on early cognitive development. Neuropediatrics 22:203-210, 1991b. [E]

Autii-Ramo I, Granstrom M-L: The psychomotor development during the first year of life of infants exposed to intrauterine alcohol of various duration. Fetal alcohol exposure and development. Neuropediatrics 22:59-64, 1991a. [E]

Autti-Ramo I, Korkman M, Hilakivi-Clarke L, et al.: Mental development of 2-year-old children exposed to alcohol in utero. J Pediatr 120(5):740-746, 1992. [E]

Beattie JO: Transplacental alcohol intoxication. Alcohol Alcohol 21:163-166, 1986. [C]

Burd L, Martsolf JT: Fetal alcohol syndrome: Diagnosis and syndromal variability. Physiol Behav 46:39-43, 1989. [R]

Clarren SK, Astley SJ, Bowden DM: Physical anomalies and developmental delays in nonhuman primate infants exposed to weekly doses of ethanol during gestation. Teratology 37:561-569, 1988. [A]

Clarren SK, Smith DW: The fetal alcohol syndrome. N Eng J Med 298:1063-1067, 1978. [R]

Coles CD, Brown RT, Smith IE, et al.: Effects of prenatal alcohol exposure at school age. I. Physical and cognitive development. Neurotoxicol Teratol 13:357-367, 1991. [E]

Coles CD, Smith IE, Fernhoff PM, Falek A: Neonatal ethanol withdrawal: Characteristics in clinically normal, nondysmorphic neonates. J Pediatr 105:445-451, 1984. [E]

Day NL, Richardson GA: Prenatal alcohol exposure: A continuum of effects. Semin Perinatol 15(4):271-279, 1991. [R]

Day NL, Richardson G, Robles N, et al.: Effect of prenatal alcohol exposure on growth and morphology of offspring at 8 months of age. Pediatrics 85(5):748-752, 1990. [E]

Fabro S, Brown NA: In utero alcohol exposure: Threshold for effects? Reprod Toxicol 1:11-13, 1982. [R]

Forrest F, du V Florey C: The relation between maternal alcohol consumption and child development: The epidemiological evidence. J Public Health Med 13(4):247-255, 1991. [R]

Ginsburg KA, Blacker CM, Abel EL, Sokol RJ: Fetal alcohol exposure and adverse pregnancy outcomes. Contrib Gynecol Obstet 18:115-129, 1991. [R]

Hanson JW, Streissguth AP, Smith DW: The effects of moderate alcohol consumption during pregnancy on fetal growth and morphogenesis. J Pediatr 92:457-460, 1978. [E]

Hill RM, Hegemier S, Tennyson LM: The fetal alcohol syndrome: A multihandicapped child. Neurotoxicology 10:585-596, 1989. [R]

Inouye RN, Kokich VG, Clarren SK, Bowden DM: Fetal alcohol syndrome: An examination of craniofacial dysmorphology in Macaca nemestrina. J Med Primatol 14:35-48, 1985. [A]

Jones KL: Fetal alcohol syndrome. PIR Rev 8:122-126, 1986. [R]

Jones KL, Smith DW, Ulleland CN, Streissguth AP: Pattern of malformation in offspring of chronic alcoholic mothers. Lancet 1:1267-1271, 1973. [C]

Kiess W, Linderkamp O, Hadorn HB, Haas R: Fetal alcohol syndrome and malignant disease. Eur J Pediatr 143:160-161, 1984. [C]

Kline J, Shrout P, Stein Z, et al.: Drinking during pregnancy and spontaneous abortion. Lancet 2:176-180, 1980. [E]

Leonard BE: Alcohol as a social teratogen. Prog Brain Res 73:305-317, 1988. [R]

McLain DE, Roe DA: Fetal alcohol syndrome in the ferret (Mustela putorius). Teratology 30:203-210, 1984. [A]

Ouellette EM, Rosett HL, Rosman NP, Winer L: Adverse effects on offspring of maternal alcohol abuse during pregnancy. N Eng J Med 297:528-530, 1977. [E]

Padmanabhan R, Hameed MS, Sugathan TN: Effects of acute doses of ethanol on pre- and postnatal development in the mouse. Drug Alcohol Depend 14:197-208, 1984. [A]

Rosett JL, Weiner L, Lee A, et al.: Patterns of alcohol consumption and fetal development. Obstet Gynecol 61(5):539-546, 1983. [E]

Scott WJ, Fradkin R: The effects of prenatal ethanol in cynomolgus monkeys. Teratology 29:49-56, 1984. [A]

Sokol RJ, Clarren SK: Guidelines for use of terminology describing the impact of prenatal alcohol on the offspring. Alcohol Clin Exp Res 13(4):597-598, 1989. [O]

Streissguth AP, Aase JM, Clarren SK, et al.: Fetal alcohol syndrome in adolescents and adults. JAMA 265(15):1961-1967, 1991. [S]

Streissguth AP, Clarren SK, Jones KL: Natural history of the fetal alcohol syndrome: A 10-year follow-up of eleven patients. Lancet 2:85-91, 1985. [C]

Streissguth AP, LaDue RA: Fetal Alcohol. Teratogenic causes of developmental disabilities. Monogr Am Assoc Ment Defic 8:1-32, 1987. [R]

Streissguth AP, Landesman-Dwyer S, Martin JC, Smith DW: Teratogenic effects of alcohol in humans and laboratory animals. Science 209:353-361, 1980. [R]

Streissguth AP, Sampson PD, Marr HM: Neurobehavioral dose-response effects of prenatal alcohol exposure in humans from infancy to adulthood. Ann NY Acad Sci 562:145-158, 1989. [E]

Sulik KK, Johnston MC: Sequence of developmental alterations following acute ethanol exposure in mice: Craniofacial features of the fetal alcohol syndrome. Am J Anat 166:257-269, 1983. [A]

West JR, Goodlett CR: Teratogenic effects of alcohol on brain development. Ann Med 22:319-325, 1990. [R]

ALDICARB

Synonyms

Temik

Summary

Aldicarb is a carbamate pesticide that is used in agriculture to kill insects, mites, and nematodes. Aldicarb is readily absorbed through the gastrointestinal tract and skin and may cause acute toxic symptoms by transient inhibition of cholinesterase activity (Risher, et al., 1987). The acceptable daily intake of aldicarb established by the US Environmental Protection Agency is 0.003 mg/kg/d (EPA, 1988).

Magnitude of Teratogenic Risk

Undetermined

Quality and Quantity of Data

None To Poor

Comment

None

No epidemiological studies of congenital anomalies among infants born to women exposed to large amounts of aldicarb during pregnancy have been published. Two stillbirths and two neonatal deaths were observed in 27 pregnant women who developed an illness that was probably or possibly due to eating watermelon contaminated with aldicarb (Goldman et al., 1990). However, neither aldicarb nor its metabolites could be identified in tissues of either stillbirth, and other causes appear to account for the neonatal deaths.

No teratogenic effect was reportedly observed among the offspring of rats or rabbits treated with aldicarb during pregnancy in doses of 0.04-1.0 or 0.1-0.5 mg/kg/d, respectively (Risher et al., 1987).

Key References

EPA: Pesticide Fact Handbook. Park Ridge, NJ: Noyes Publications, 1988, pp 6-18. [O]

Goldman LR, Smith DF, Neutra RR, et al.: Pesticide food poisoning from contaminated watermelons in California, 1985. Arch Environ Health 45(4):229-236, 1990. [S]

Risher JF, Mink FL, Stara JF: The toxicologic effects of the carbamate insecticide aldicarb in mammals: A review. Environ Health Perspect 72:267-281, 1987. [R]

ALFENTANIL

Synonyms

Alfenta

Summary

Alfentanil is a short-acting narcotic analgesic that is administered parenterally.

Magnitude of Teratogenic Risk

Undetermined

Quality and Quantity of Data

None To Poor

Comment

A small risk cannot be excluded, but a high risk of congenital anomalies in the children of women treated with alfentanil during pregnancy is unlikely.

No epidemiological studies of congenital anomalies among infants born to women treated with alfentanil during pregnancy have been reported.

No teratogenic effects were observed among the offspring of rats treated continuously in pregnancy with alfentanil in doses about twice those used for brief infusions in humans (Fujinaga et al., 1988).

Alterations of neonatal behavior were observed among the offspring of rhesus monkeys given alfentanil analgesia during labor (Golub et al., 1988).

Please see agent summary on morphine for information on a related agent.

Key References

Fujinaga M, Mazze RI, Jackson EC, Baden JM: Reproductive and teratogenic effects of sufentanil and alfentanil in Sprague-Dawley rats. Anesth Analg 67:166-169, 1988. [A]

Golub MS, Eisele JH Jr, Donald JM: Obstetric analgesia and infant outcome in monkeys: Neonatal measures after intrapartum exposure to meperidine or alfentanil. Am J Obstet Gynecol 158:1219-1225, 1988. [A]

ALIFLURANE

Synonyms

Aliflurano, Alifluranum

Summary

Aliflurane is a general anesthetic administered by inhalation.

Magnitude of Teratogenic Risk

Undetermined

Quality and Quantity of Data

None

Comment

None

No epidemiological studies of congenital anomalies in children born to women exposed to aliflurane during pregnancy have been reported.

No investigations of teratologic effects of aliflurane in experimental animals have been published.

Key References

None available.

ALLANTOIN

Synonyms

Allantol, Cordianine, Glyoxyldiureide, Sebical, Uniderm A

Summary

Allantoin is a vulnerary agent that is used topically to treat psoriasis and promote wound healing.

Magnitude of Teratogenic Risk

None To Minimal

Quality and Quantity of Data

Poor To Fair

Comment

Risk assessment is for topical use only

The frequency of congenital anomalies was no greater than expected among the children of 51 women treated with allantoin during the first four lunar months of pregnancy in the Collaborative Perinatal Project (Heinonen et al., 1977).

No animal teratology studies of allantoin have been published.

Key References

Heinonen OP, Sloane D, Shapiro S: Birth Defects and Drugs in Pregnancy. Littleton, Mass.: John Wright-PSG, 1977, pp 410-411. [E]

ALLOPURINOL

Synonyms

Aloral, Aluline, Caplenal, Cosuric, Hamarin, Ketanrift, Lopurin, Novopurol, Uricemil, Zyloprim

Summary

Allopurinol is a xanthine oxidase inhibitor. It is used in the treatment of chronic gout and hyperuricemia, which may result from leukemia, radiotherapy, or systemic antineoplastic therapy.

Magnitude of Teratogenic Risk

Undetermined

Quality and Quantity of Data

None To Poor

Comment

None

No epidemiological studies of infants born to women who used allopurinol during pregnancy have been published.

The frequency of malformations was not increased among the offspring of pregnant rats treated with a single injection of allopurinol at 4-63 times the usual human dose (Bragonier et al., 1964, Chaube & Murphy, 1968).

Key References

Bragonier JR, Roesky N, Carver MJ: Teratogenesis: Effects of substituted purines and the influence of 4-hydroxyprazolo-pyrimidine in the rat. Proc Soc Exp Biol Med 116:685-688, 1964. [A]

Chaube S, Murphy ML: The teratogenic effects of the recent drugs active in cancer chemotherapy. Adv Teratol 3:181-237, 1968. [A]

ALOE

Synonyms

Aroe, Nature's Remedy

Summary

Aloe is made from the juice of Aloe (Liliaceae) plants. It is used orally as a purgative and topically in creams and lotions as a moisturizer and for the treatment of minor burns.

Magnitude of Teratogenic Risk

Undetermined

Quality and Quantity of Data

None To Poor

Comment

None

No epidemiological studies of congenital anomalies in infants whose mothers used aloe during pregnancy have been reported.

Increased frequencies of embryonic death and skeletal anomalies among the offspring were observed when rats were given 125 mg/kg/d of dried aloe orally during early pregnancy (Nath et al., 1992).

Key References

Nath D, Sethi N, Singh RK, Jain AK: Commonly used Indian abortifacient plants with special reference to their teratologic effects in rats. J Ethnopharmacol 36:147-154, 1992. [A]

ALPHA INTERFERON

Synonyms

Alferon, Roferon A

Summary

Alpha interferons are a group of proteins produced mainly by lymphocytes. They are thought to have a physiologic role in modifying cellular responses to viral infections. Alpha interferon is given parenterally in the treatment of some neoplasms.

Magnitude of Teratogenic Risk

Undetermined

Quality and Quantity of Data

None To Poor

Comment

None

No epidemiological studies of congenital anomalies among infants born to women treated with alpha interferon during pregnancy have been reported. One woman who was treated with alpha interferon throughout pregnancy who had a normal child has been reported (Baer, 1991).

No teratogenic effect was observed among the offspring of rats or rabbits treated during pregnancy with human alpha interferon in doses 17-170 times those used clinically (Matsumoto et al., 1986a, b; Shibutani et al., 1987). The biological relevance of these observations is uncertain because the activity of interferons may be species-specific.

Key References

Baer MR: Normal full-term pregnancy in a patient with chronic myelogenous leukemia treated with alpha-interferon [letter]. Am J Hematol 37(1):66, 1991. [C]

Matsumoto T, Nakamura K, Imai M, Aoki H, et al.: Reproduction studies of human interferon alfa (Interferol alpha). I. Teratological study in rabbits. Iyakuhin Kenkyu 17:397-404, 1986a. [A]

Matsumoto T, Nakamura K, Imai M, Aoki H, et al.: Reproduction studies of human interferon alfa (Interferol alpha). III. Teratological study in rats. Iyakuhin Kenkyu 17:417-438, 1986b. [A]

Shibutani Y, Hamada Y, Kurokawa M, Inoue K, et al.: Toxicity studies of human lymphoblastoid interferon alfa. Teratogenicity study in rats. Iyakuhin Kenkyu 18:60-78, 1987. [A]

ALPHA-KETOGLUTARIC ACID

Synonyms

2-Ketoglutaric Acid, 2-Oxopentanedioic Acid

Summary

Alpha-ketoglutaric acid is an organic acid that is involved in the Kreb's cycle of intermediary metabolism. Alpha-ketoglutaric acid is sometimes used as a nutritional supplement.

Magnitude of Teratogenic Risk

Undetermined

Quality and Quantity of Data

None

Comment

A small risk cannot be excluded, but a high risk of congenital anomalies in the children of women treated with alpha-ketoglutaric acid during pregnancy is unlikely.

No epidemiological studies of congenital anomalies among infants born to women who took large amounts of alpha-ketoglutaric acid during pregnancy have been reported.

No animal teratology studies of alpha-ketoglutaric acid have been published.

Key References

None available.

ALPHA-1-PROTEINASE INHIBITOR

Synonyms

Prolastin

Summary

Alpha-1-proteinase inhibitor is a preparation made from human plasma that is administered intravenously to treat alpha-1-antitrypsin deficiency.

Magnitude of Teratogenic Risk

Undetermined

Quality and Quantity of Data

None

Comment

A small risk cannot be excluded, but a high risk of congenital anomalies in the children of women treated with alpha-1-proteinase inhibitor during pregnancy is unlikely.

No epidemiological studies of congenital anomalies among infants born to women treated with alpha-1-proteinase inhibitor during pregnancy have been reported.

No animal teratology studies of alpha-1-proteinase inhibitor have been published.

Key References

None available.

ALPHAXALONE/ ALPHADOLONE

Synonyms

Alfatesin, Alfathesin

Summary

A mixture of the two drugs alphaxalone and alphadolone has been used as an intravenous general anesthetic.

Magnitude of Teratogenic Risk

Undetermined

Quality and Quantity of Data

None To Poor

Comment

None

No epidemiological studies of congenital anomalies in children born to women exposed to alphaxalone/alphadolone during pregnancy have been reported.

The frequency of malformations was no greater than expected among the offspring of Rhesus monkeys, mice, or rats repeatedly anesthetized during pregnancy with alphaxalone/alphadolone in doses substantially greater than those used in humans (Esaki et al., 1976; Tanioka et al., 1977).

Key References

Esaki K, Oshio K, Yoshikawa K: Effects of intravenous administration of alphaxolone on the fetuses of mouse and rat. Kitchuken, Zenrinsho Kenkuho 2:229-236, 1976. [A]

Tanioka Y, Koizumi H, Inaba K: Teratogenicity test by intravenous administration of CT-1341 in Rhesus monkeys. CIEA (Cent Inst Exp Anim) Preclin Rep 3(1):35-45, 1977. [A]

ALPRAZOLAM

Synonyms

Xanax

Summary

Alprazolam is a benzodiazepine used orally for treatment of anxiety.

Magnitude of Teratogenic Risk

Undetermined

Quality and Quantity of Data

None To Poor

Comment

None

No epidemiological studies of congenital anomalies among infants born to women treated with alprazolam during pregnancy have been reported.

The frequency of malformations was no greater than expected among the offspring of rats or rabbits treated with alprazolam at a dose 8 times that used in humans (Esaki et al., 1981a, b). At higher doses, increased frequencies of minor skeletal anomalies and fetal mortality were seen, but such doses also produced maternal toxicity in the rabbits (Esaki et al., 1981a, b).

Transient neonatal withdrawal symptoms similar to those seen with other benzodiazepines have been observed among infants whose mothers took aprazolam throughout pregnancy (Barry & St. Clair, 1987; Anderson & McGuire, 1989).

Please see agent summary on diazepam for information on a closely related agent that has been more thoroughly studied.

Key References

Anderson PO, McGuire GG: Neonatal alprazolam withdrawal--possible effects of breast feeding. DICP Ann Pharmacother 23:614, 1989. [C]

Barry WS, St. Clair SM: Exposure to benzodiazepines in utero. Lancet 1:1436-1437, 1987. [O]

Esaki K, Oshio K, Yanagita T: Effects of oral administration of alprazolam (TUS-1) on the rat fetus--experiment on drug administration during the organogenesis period. Jitchuken Zenrinsho Kenkyuho 7:65-77, 1981a. [A]

Esaki K, Sakai Y, Yanagita T: Effect of oral administration of alprazolam (TUS-1) on rabbit fetus. Jitchuken Zenrinsho Kenkyuho 7:79-90, 1981b. [A]

ALPRENOLOL

Synonyms

Apllobal, Aptin, Aptol, Betacard, Gubernal, Regletin, Vasoton

Summary

Alprenolol is a beta-adrenergic receptor blocking agent that is used in the treatment of hypertension and cardiac disease.

Magnitude of Teratogenic Risk

Undetermined

Quality and Quantity of Data

None To Poor

Comment

None

No epidemiological studies of congenital anomalies among infants born to women treated with alprenolol during pregnancy have been reported.

Increased frequencies of fetal death and growth retardation were observed among the offspring of rats treated during pregnancy with alprenolol in doses smaller than those used in humans; parturition was also delayed in the treated animals (Chimura, 1985).

Please see agent summary on propranolol for information on a related agent that has been more thoroughly studied.

Key References

Chimura T: [Effects of beta-adrenocepter blockade on parturition and fetal cardiovascular and metabolic system]. Nippon Sanka Fujinka Gakkai Zasshi (J Jpn Obstet Gynecol) 37:691-695, 1985. [A]

ALPROSTADIL

Synonyms

PGE_1, Prostaglandin E_1, Prostin VR Pediatric

Summary

Alprostadil, prostaglandin E_1, is a vasodilator and inhibitor of platelet aggregation. It is administered intravenously or intra-arterially to prevent closure of the ductus arteriosus in newborn infants with congenital heart disease.

Magnitude of Teratogenic Risk

Undetermined

Quality and Quantity of Data

None To Poor

Comment

None

No epidemiological studies of congenital anomalies among infants born to women treated with alprostadil during pregnancy have been reported.

The frequency of malformations was not increased among the offspring of rats treated during pregnancy with alprostadil by continuous intravenous infusion in doses 3.5-28 times those used in humans or by single subcutaneous doses 3.5-7 times those administered daily by continuous infusion in humans (Marks et al., 1987). Substantial maternal toxicity occurred with all but the lowest intravenous dose, and maternal death was frequent with intravenous doses of 14 or 28 times those used in humans. An increased frequency of congenital anomalies including edema, eye malformations, and hydrocephalus was seen among the offspring of pregnant rats treated subcutaneously with single doses of alprostadil 14 times greater than those infused daily in humans.

Key References

Marks TA, Morris DF, Weeks JR: Developmental toxicity of alprostadil in rats after subcutaneous administration or intravenous infusion. Toxicol Appl Pharmacol 91:341-357, 1987. [A]

ALTEPLASE

Synonyms

Activase

Summary

Alteplase is a tissue plasminogen activator produced by recombinant DNA technology. Alteplase is administered intravenously in the treatment of acute myocardial infarction.

Magnitude of Teratogenic Risk

Undetermined

Quality and Quantity of Data

None

Comment

None

No epidemiological studies of congenital anomalies among infants born to women treated with alteplase during pregnancy have been reported.

No animal teratology studies of alteplase have been published.

Neonatal death with extensive intracranial hemorrhage has been reported in an infant born at 35 weeks gestation to a woman with antithrombin III deficiency who had been treated the day before delivery with alteplase for pulmonary embolism (Baudo et al., 1990).

Key References

Baudo F, Caimi TM, Redaelli R, et al.: Emergency treatment with recombinant tissue plasminogen activator of pulmonary embolism in a pregnant woman with antithrombin III deficiency. Am J Obstet Gynecol 163:1274-1275, 1990. [C]

AMANTADINE

Synonyms

Amantadin, Amantan, Antadine, Contenton, Mantadan, Mantadine, Mantadix, Protexin, Solu-Contenton, Symmetrel, Virofral

Summary

Amantadine is used in the prophylaxis and treatment of influenza, multiple sclerosis, and parkinsonism.

Magnitude of Teratogenic Risk

Undetermined

Quality and Quantity of Data

Poor

Comment

None

One child born to a woman who was treated with amantadine throughout the first trimester of pregnancy had pulmonary atresia and a single cardiac ventricle (Nora et al., 1975). Another child born to a treated woman had an inguinal hernia (Golbe, 1987). Three apparently normal infants who were born to treated women have also been reported (Golbe, 1987; Levy et al., 1991). No epidemiological studies of congenital anomalies among infants born to women who took amantadine during pregnancy have been published.

Increased frequencies of fetal death and malformations were observed among the offspring of pregnant rats treated with 6-12 times the human therapeutic dose of amantadine in one study (Lamar et al., 1970). No teratogenic effect was observed among the offspring of rats treated during pregnancy with 1-5 times the human therapeutic dose or among the offspring of rabbits treated during pregnancy with 1-12 times the human therapeutic dose of amantadine (Lamar et al., 1970; Vernier et al., 1969).

Key References

Golbe LI: Parkinson's disease and pregnancy. Neurology 37:1245-1249, 1987. [S]

Lamar JK, Calhoun FJ, Darr AG: Effects of amantadine hydrochloride on cleavage and embryonic development in the rat and rabbit. Toxicol Appl Pharm 17:272, 1970. [A]

Levy M, Pastuszak A, Koren G: Fetal outcome following intrauterine amantadine exposure. Reproductive Toxicology 5:79-81, 1991. [R] & [C]

Nora JJ, Nora AH, Way GL: Cardiovascular maldevelopment associated with maternal exposure to amantadine. Lancet 2:607, 1975. [C]

Vernier VG, Harmon JB, Stump JM, Lynes TW, Marvel JP, Smith DH: The toxicologic and pharmacologic properties of amantadine hydrochloride. Toxicol Appl Pharmacol 15:642-665, 1969. [A]

AMBRUTICIN

Synonyms

Antibiotic Acid S

Summary

Ambruticin is an antifungal agent.

Magnitude of Teratogenic Risk

Undetermined

Quality and Quantity of Data

None

Comment

None

No epidemiological studies of congenital anomalies in infants born to women treated with ambruticin during pregnancy have been reported.

No animal teratology studies of ambruticin have been published.

Key References

None available.

AMCINONIDE

Synonyms

Amciderm, Amcinonido, Amcinonidum, Amicla, Cyclocort, Penticort

Summary

Amcinonide is a corticosteroid that is used topically. Substantial systemic absorption may occur after topical use, particularly when applied to large areas, under occlusive dressings, or to broken skin.

Magnitude of Teratogenic Risk

Undetermined

Quality and Quantity of Data

None

Comment

A small risk cannot be excluded, but a high risk of congenital anomalies in the children of women treated topically with amcinonide during pregnancy is unlikely.

No epidemiological studies of congenital anomalies among infants born to women treated with amcinonide during pregnancy have been reported.

No animal teratology studies of amcinonide have been published.

Please see agent summary on triamcinolone for information on a related agent that has been studied.

Key References

None available.

AMDINOCILLIN/ PIVAMDINOCILLIN

Synonyms

Amdinocillin Pivoxil, Coactabs, Coactin, Hexacillin, Mecillinam, Penicillin Hx, Pivamdinocillin, Pivmecillinam

Summary

Amdinocillin is a beta lactam antibiotic that is administered parenterally. Pivamdinocillin is a pivaloyloxymethylester of amdinocillin that is used orally. Pivamdinocillin is hydrolyzed to amdinocillin during or immediately after its absorption.

Magnitude of Teratogenic Risk

Undetermined

Quality and Quantity of Data

Poor

Comment

A small risk cannot be excluded, but a high risk of congenital anomalies in the children of women treated with amdinocillin/ pivamdinocillin during pregnancy is unlikely.

No epidemiological studies of congenital anomalies among infants born to women treated with amdinocillin or pivamdinocillin during pregnancy have been reported. In one clinical series, no drug-related abnormalities were apparent among the infants of 41 women who were treated for bacteriuria during pregnancy with pivamdinocillin (Sanderson & Meday, 1984).

No animal teratology studies of amdinocillin or pivamdinocillin have been published.

Please see agent summary on penicillin for information on a related agent that has been more thoroughly studied.

Key References

Sanderson P, Menday P: Pivmecillinam for bacteriuria in pregnancy. J Antimicrob Chemother 13:383-388, 1984. [S]

AMIKACIN

Synonyms

Amicacin, Amikacina, Amikacine, Amikacinum, Amikin, Biklin

Summary

Amikacin is a semisynthetic aminoglycoside antibiotic used parenterally in the treatment of bacterial infections.

Magnitude of Teratogenic Risk

Undetermined

Quality and Quantity of Data

None To Poor

Comment

None

No epidemiological studies of congenital anomalies among infants born to women treated with amikacin during pregnancy have been reported.

The frequency of malformations was not increased among the offspring of mice or rats treated during pregnancy with 2-27 times the usual human dose of amikacin (Matsuzaki et al., 1975b). Decreased fetal weight was observed in the mice at all doses tested. In the rats, increased fetal death was seen at all doses, and generalized fetal edema, subcutaneous hemorrhages, and skeletal anomalies were frequently observed at the highest dose, which also produced maternal toxicity. Similarly, increased rates of fetal death but not of malformations were found among the offspring of rabbits treated during pregnancy with <1-11 times the usual human dose of amikacin (Matsuzaki et al., 1975a).

Please see agent summary on streptomycin for information on a related drug that has been more thoroughly studied.

Key References

Matsuzaki M, Akutsu S, Mukogawa H, Aizawa T: Teratological studies of amikacin (BB-K8) in rabbit. Jpn J Antibiot 28:366-371, 1975a. [A]

Matsuzaki M, Akutsu S, Mukogawa H, Shimamura T: Teratological studies of amikacin (BB-K8) in mice and rats. Jpn J Antibiot 28:372-384, 1975b. [A]

AMILORIDE

Synonyms

Amipramizide, Arumil, Midamor, Modamide, Nirulid, Pandiuren

Summary

Amiloride is a potassium-sparing diuretic that is administered orally.

Magnitude of Teratogenic Risk

Undetermined

Quality and Quantity of Data

Poor

Comment

None

No epidemiological studies of malformations in the infants of women treated with amiloride during pregnancy have been published.

No malformations were observed among the offspring of rats or mice treated with 10 times the human dose of amiloride during pregnancy (Nelson et al., 1989; Scott et al., 1990). Concomitant amiloride treatment did increase the frequency of malformations caused by 2-methoxyethanol and acetazolamide under conditions in which these agents exhibit teratogenic effects in rodents.

Key References

Nelson BK, Vorhees CV, Scott WJ Jr, Hastings L: Effects of 2-methoxyethanol on fetal development, postnatal behavior, and embryonic intracellular pH of rats. Neurotoxicol Teratol 11:273-284, 1989. [A]

Scott WJ, Duggan CA, Schreiner CM, Collins MD: Reduction of embryonic intracellular pH: A potential mechanism of acetazolamide-induced limb malformations. Toxicol Appl Pharmacol 103:238-254, 1990. [A]

AMINACRINE

Synonyms

Aminoacridine, Aminopt, Izoacridina, Minocrin, Monacrin, Quench Cream

Summary

Aminacrine is an acridine derivative that is used as a topical disinfectant, usually in combination with other agents, in the treatment of vaginal infections.

Magnitude of Teratogenic Risk

None To Minimal

Quality and Quantity of Data

Poor To Fair

Comment

Risk assessment is for topical use only

Prescriptions for aminacrine during the first trimester of pregnancy were not found to have been given more frequently than expected to mothers of 6564 infants with a variety of congenital anomalies, or 2326 spontaneous abortuses in a case-control study of linked Michigan Medicaid records (Rosa et al., 1987). Similarly, the frequency of congenital anomalies was no greater than expected among the infants of 59 women treated with aminacrine during the first four lunar months of pregnancy in the Collaborative Perinatal Project (Heinonen et al., 1977).

No experimental animal teratology studies of aminacrine have been published.

Key References

Heinonen OP, Slone D, Shapiro S: Birth Defects and Drugs in Pregnancy. Littleton, Mass.: John Wright-PSG, 1977, pp 300-302. [E]

Rosa FW, Baum C, Shaw M: Pregnancy outcomes after first-trimester vaginitis drug therapy. Obstet Gynecol 69:751-755, 1987. [E]

AMINOBENZOATE (PARA-AMINOBENZOIC ACID)

Synonyms

Amben, Aminobenzoic Acid, Hill-Shade, PABA, Pabagel, Pabanol, Para-Aminobenzoic Acid, Paraminol, Sodium Benzoate

Summary

Aminobenzoate is sometimes considered a vitamin of the B complex although it does not appear to be essential for humans. Aminobenzoate is used topically as a sunscreen.

Magnitude of Teratogenic Risk

Undetermined

Quality and Quantity of Data

None To Poor

Comment

A small risk cannot be excluded, but a substantial risk of congenital anomalies in the children of women treated topically with aminobenzoate during pregnancy is unlikely.

No epidemiological studies of congenital anomalies among the infants of women who took large doses of aminobenzoate during pregnancy have been reported.

No teratogenic effect was observed among the offspring of mice treated with aminobenzoate in a dose of 50 mg/kg/d during pregnancy (Kato, 1973). The frequency of fetal resorption was increased in pregnant rats fed aminobenzoate in a dose of about 125 mg/kg/d (Telford et al., 1962) but not in pregnant rats fed diets containing 1% aminobenzoate (Ershoff, 1946).

Key References

Ershoff BH: Effects of massive doses of p-aminobenzoic acid and inositol on reproduction in the rat. Soc Exper Biol Med 63:479-480, 1946. [A]

Kato T: Effect of folate metabolism-related factors on the teratogenic action of sulfonamide in mice. Cong Anom 13:85-92, 1973. [A]

Telford IR, Woodruff CS, Linford RH: Fetal resorption in the rat as influenced by certain antioxidants. Am J Anat 110:29-36, 1962. [A]

AMINOCAPROIC ACID

Synonyms

Amicar, Capramol, Epsamon, Epsikapron, Epsilon-Aminocaproic Acid, Hemocaprol, Ipsilon, Respramin

Summary

Aminocaproic acid is used in the prevention and treatment of hemorrhage associated with excessive fibrinolysis. Aminocaproic acid is also used to prevent attacks of hereditary angioedema.

Magnitude of Teratogenic Risk

Undetermined

Quality and Quantity of Data

None To Poor

Comment

None

No epidemiological studies of congenital anomalies among infants born to women treated with aminocaproic acid during pregnancy have been reported.

No teratogenic effect was observed among the offspring of rabbits treated during pregnancy with aminocaproic acid in a dose similar to that used therapeutically in humans (Howorka et al., 1970).

Key References

Howorka E, Olasinski R, Wyrzykiewicz T: The effect of EACA administered to female rabbits during pregnancy on the fetuses. Patol Pol 21:311-314, 1970. [A]

AMINOGLUTETHIMIDE

Synonyms

Cytadren, Elipten

Summary

Aminoglutethimide blocks the synthesis of adrenal steroid hormones and the physiological conversion of androgens to estrogens. Aminoglutethimide is given orally in the treatment of Cushing syndrome and breast carcinoma.

Magnitude of Teratogenic Risk

Undetermined

Quality and Quantity of Data

Poor To Fair

Comment

The pharmacological activity of this agent makes it likely that virilization of the external genitalia would frequently occur among female fetuses of women treated with aminoglutethimide during pregnancy. The risk would be expected to be related to the dose and length of treatment.

No epidemiological studies of congenital anomalies among infants born to women treated with aminoglutethimide during pregnancy have been reported. Virilization of the external genitalia has been described in three girls whose mothers were treated with aminoglutethimide during pregnancy (Iffy et al., 1965; German et al., 1970; LaMaire et al., 1972).

Virilization of female external genitalia, feminization of male external genitalia, various other congenital anomalies, growth retardation, and fetal death have been observed among the offspring of rats treated during pregnancy with aminoglutethimide in doses 5-15 times those used in humans (Goldman, 1970a, b). Premature delivery was noted after treatment of rabbits late in pregnancy with aminoglutethimide in doses smaller than those used therapeutically in humans (Torres & First, 1976).

Key References

German J, Kowal A, Ehlers KH: Trimethadione and human teratogenesis. Teratology 3:349-362, 1970. [C] & [S]

Goldman AS: Experimental congenital lipoid adrenal hyperplasia: Prevention of anatomic defects produced by aminoglutethimide. Endocrinology 87:889-893, 1970a. [A]

Goldman AS: Production of congenital lipoid adrenal hyperplasia in rats and inhibition of cholesterol side-chain cleavage. Endocrinology 87:1245-1251, 1970b. [A]

Iffy L, Ansell JS, Bryant JS, Herrmann WL: Nonadrenal female pseudohermaphroditism: An unusual case of fetal masculinization. Obstet Gynecol 20:59-65, 1965. [R] & [C]

LeMaire WJ, Cleveland WW, Bejar RL, et al.: Aminoglutethimide: A possible cause of pseudohermaphroditism in females. Am J Dis Child 124:421-423, 1972. [C]

Torres CAA, First NL: Gestation length in rabbits - effect of aminoglutethimide phosphate, dexamethasone, pregnenolone, and progesterone. J Anim Sci 42:131-137, 1976. [A]

AMINOHIPPURATE

Synonyms

Aminohippuric Acid, PAHA, Sodium-para-Aminohippurate

Summary

Aminohippurate (PAH) is given intravenously as a diagnostic test of renal plasma flow.

Magnitude of Teratogenic Risk

Undetermined

Quality and Quantity of Data

None

Comment

None

No epidemiological studies of congenital anomalies among infants born to women who had been given aminohippurate during pregnancy have been reported.

No animal teratology studies of aminohippurate have been published.

Key References

None available.

AMINOPTERIN

Synonyms

4-Aminopteroylglutamate

Summary

Aminopterin is an antagonist of folic acid. It is used as a rodenticide and has been administered to pregnant women to induce abortion. It has also been employed in the treatment of cancer.

Magnitude of Teratogenic Risk

Moderate To High

Quality and Quantity of Data

Good

Comment

Malformations have been observed among the children of women who ingested aminopterin in doses of 1-3 mg or more per day during the first trimester of pregnancy. The effects on the fetus of exposure later in pregnancy are unknown.

A very uncommon but strikingly similar pattern of congenital anomalies has been observed in more than a dozen children born to women who took aminopterin during the first trimester of pregnancy (Reich et al., 1977; Warkany, 1978; Char, 1979; Warkany, 1981). Characteristic features of this syndrome include short stature, delayed calvarial ossification, craniosynostosis, hydrocephalus, abnormal auricles, ocular hypertelorism, micrognathia, and cleft palate (Thiersch, 1952; Warkany, 1978). Limb and digital anomalies and neural tube defects have also been reported. Death in infancy may occur. Although developmental delay is seen during childhood, the few affected adults who have been reported appear to have normal intelligence or only mild mental retardation (Howard & Rudd, 1977; Reich et al., 1977; Shaw & Rees, 1980). Similar features have been observed in babies born after first-trimester maternal treatment with methotrexate, another folic acid antagonist (Milunsky et al., 1968; Powell & Ekert, 1971). The precise risk of congenital anomalies in babies born after maternal exposure to aminopterin during early pregnancy is unknown but appears to be relatively high (Warkany, 1978).

Treatment of pregnant rats, mice, and cats with aminopterin in doses several times those used in humans causes fetal loss (Thiersch & Philips, 1950; Baranov, 1966; Khera, 1976). Malformations of the calvarium, face, eyes, abdominal wall, and limbs have been observed after such exposures in rats (Baranov, 1966), and similar malformations occur in rabbits with doses smaller than those used in humans (Goeringer & DeSesso, 1990).

Key References

Baranov VS: Characteristics of the teratogenic effect of aminopterin compared with that of other teratogenic agents. Bull Exp Biol Med (USSR) 61:77-81, 1966. [A]

Char F: Denouement and discussion: Aminopterin embryopathy syndrome. Am J Dis Child 133:1189-1190, 1979. [C]

Goeringer GC, DeSesso JM: Developmental toxicity in rabbits of the antifolate aminopterin and its amelioration by leucovorin. Teratology 41(5):560-561, 1990. [A]

Howard NJ, Rudd NL: The natural history of aminopterin-induced embryopathy. Birth Defects 13 (3C):85-93, 1977. [C]

Khera KS: Teratogenicity studies with methotrexate, aminopterin, and acetylsalicylic acid in domestic cats. Teratology 14:21-27, 1976. [A]

Milunsky A, Graef JW, Gaynor MF: Methotrexate-induced congenital malformations. J Pediatr 72:790-795, 1968. [C]

Powell HR, Ekert H: Methotrexate-induced congenital malformations. Med J Aust 2:1076-1077, 1971. [C]

29

Reich EW, Cox RP, Becker MH, Genieser NB, et al.: Recognition in adult patients of malformations induced by folic-acid antagonists. Birth Defects 14 (6B):139-160, 1977. [C]

Shaw EB, Rees EL: Fetal damage due to aminopterin ingestion: Follow-up at 17-1/2 years of age. Am J Dis Child 134:1172-1173, 1980. [C]

Thiersch JB: Therapeutic abortions with a folic acid antagonist, 4-aminopteroylglutamic acid (4-amino P.G.A.) administered by the oral route. Am J Obstet Gynecol 63:1298-1304, 1952. [S]

Thiersch JB, Philips FS: Effect of 4-aminopteroylglutamic acid (aminopterin) on early pregnancy. Proc Soc Exp Biol Med 74:204-208, 1950. [A]

Warkany J: Aminopterin and methotrexate: Folic acid deficiency. Teratology 17:353-358, 1978. [R]

Warkany J: Teratogenicity of folic acid antagonists. Cancer Bull 33(2):76-77, 1981. [R]

AMIODARONE

Synonyms

Amjodaronum, Atlansil, Cardilor, Corbionax, Cordarex, Cordarone, Coronovo, Ortacrone, Ritmocardyl, Rythmarone

Summary

Amiodarone, a benzofuran derivative, is an adrenergic receptor antagonist used to treat cardiac arrhythmias. The drug contains a large amount of iodine (37% by weight).

Magnitude of Teratogenic Risk

Neonatal Goiter: Undetermined

Congenital Anomalies: Undetermined

Quality and Quantity of Data

Neonatal Goiter: Poor

Congenital Anomalies: None

Comment

1) Although the risk of neonatal goiter following chronic maternal treatment with amiodarone is unknown, it may be substantial since amiodarone contains a large amount of iodine, and several cases of neonatal goiter have been reported (see below).

2) Risk for neonatal goiter is after about 10 weeks of pregnancy when iodine is concentrated in fetal thyroid gland, and is related to dose and length of maternal treatment.

No epidemiological studies of congenital anomalies among infants born to women treated with amiodarone during pregnancy have been reported. Neonatal goiter and abnormal thyroid function have been observed among infants of women treated chronically with amiodarone during pregnancy (Laurent et al., 1987; de Wolf et al., 1988; Tubman et al., 1988; Foster & Love, 1988).

No animal teratology studies of amiodarone have been published, but unpublished studies are said to have shown no increase in malformations among the offspring of mice, rats, or rabbits treated during pregnancy with doses <1-6 times those used clinically (Foster & Love, 1988). Maternal and fetal death are said to have been frequent at the higher doses in some of these studies.

Successful treatment of fetal tachycardia by administration of amiodarone to the mother has been reported (Rey et al., 1985; Arnoux et al., 1987).

Key References

Arnoux P, Seyral P, Llurens M, et al.: Amiodarone and digoxin for refractory fetal tachycardia. Am J Cardiol 56:166-167, 1987. [C]

de Wolf D, De Schepper J, Verhaaren H, et al.: Congenital hypothyroid goiter and amiodarone. Acta Paediatr Scand 77:616-618, 1988. [C]

Foster CJ, Love HG: Amiodarone in pregnancy. Case report and review of the literature. Int J Cardiol 20:307-316, 1988. [C] & [R]

Laurent M, Betremieux P, Biron Y, et al.: Neonatal hypothyroidism after treatment by amiodarone during pregnancy. Am J Cardiol 60:942, 1987. [C]

Rey E, Duperron L, Gauthier R, et al.: Transplacental treatment of tachycardia-induced fetal heart failure with verapamil and amiodarone: A case report. Am J Obstet Gynecol 153(3):311-312, 1985. [C]

Tubman R, Jenkins J, Lim J: Neonatal hyperthyroxinaemia associated with maternal amiodarone therapy: Case report. Ir J Med Sci 157:243, 1988. [C]

AMITRIPTYLINE

Synonyms

Amitril, Domical, Elavil, Endep, Levate, Limbatril, Meravil, Novotriptyn, SK-Amitriptyline

Summary

Amitriptyline is a tricyclic antidepressant with marked anticholinergic and sedative properties.

Magnitude of Teratogenic Risk

None To Minimal

Quality and Quantity of Data

Fair

Comment

None

Available epidemiologic data on malformations in the offspring of women treated with amitriptyline during the first trimester of pregnancy are sparse. The Collaborative Perinatal Study included 21 pregnancies exposed to amitriptyline in the first four lunar months; none of the resulting infants had malformations (Heinonen et al., 1977). One case-control study of 1370 infants with malformations found a statistically significant association between maternal use of amitriptyline in the first trimester of gestation, but this association was based on the observation of only three exposed children with malformations (Bracken & Holford, 1981). Anecdotal case reports of limb reduction defects in the offspring of women who took amitriptyline early in pregnancy are unlikely to represent a causal relationship (Morrow, 1972).

Dose-dependent increased frequencies of central nervous system and skeletal malformations have been observed among the offspring of hamsters treated during pregnancy with amitriptyline in doses 10-17 times those used therapeutically in humans (Guram et al., 1982; Beyer et al., 1984). Maternal toxicity was frequently seen with such doses. Increased frequencies of similar anomalies and of fetal death were found among the offspring of pregnant mice and rabbits treated with about 10 times the usual human dose of amitriptyline (Jurand, 1980; Khan & Azam, 1969). In contrast, the frequency of malformations was not increased among the offspring of pregnant rats treated with 1-4 times the usual human dose of amitriptyline (Jelinek et al., 1967; DiCarlo et al., 1971; Henderson & McMillen, 1990). Behavioral alterations have been observed among the offspring of pregnant rats treated with 1-2 times the human therapeutic dose of amitriptyline (Bigl et al., 1982; Henderson & McMillen, 1990). The relevance of these observations to the clinical use of amitriptyline in human pregnancy is unknown.

Transient central nervous system depression has been observed in the infant of a woman treated with amitriptyline throughout pregnancy (Vree & Zwart, 1985). Serum amitriptyline levels were found to be in the moderately toxic range in the mother and in the severely toxic range in the child.

Key References

Beyer BE, Guram MS, Geber WF: Incidence and potentiation of external and internal fetal anomalies resulting from chlordiazepoxide and amitriptyline alone and in combination. Teratology 30:39-45, 1984. [A]

Bigl V, Dalitz E, Kunert F, et al.: The effect of d-amphetamine and amitriptyline administered to pregnant rats on the locomotor activity and neuro-

31

transmitters of the offspring. Psychopharmacology 77:371-375, 1982. [A]

Bracken MB, Holford TR: Exposure to prescribed drugs in pregnancy and association with congenital malformations. Obstet Gynecol 58:336-344, 1981. [E]

Di Carlo R, Pagnini G, Pelagalii GV: Effect of amitriptyline and butriptyline on fetal development in rats. J Med 2:271-275, 1971. [A]

Guram MS, Gill TS, Geber WF: Comparative teratogenicity of chlordiazepoxide, amitriptyline, and a combination of the two compounds in the fetal hamster. Neurotoxicology 3:83-90, 1982. [A]

Heinonen OP, Slone D, Shapiro S: Birth Defects and Drugs in Pregnancy. Littleton, Mass.: John Wright-PSG, 1977, pp 336-337. [E]

Henderson MG, McMillen BA: Effects of prenatal exposure to cocaine or related drugs on rat developmental and neurological indices. Brain Res Bull 24:207-212, 1990. [A]

Jelinek V, Zikmund E, Reichlova R: The influence of some psychotropic medications on the development of the rat fetus. Therapie 22:1429-1433, 1967. [A]

Jurand A: Malformations of the central nervous system induced by neurotropic drugs in mouse embryos. Dev Growth Differ 22:61-78, 1980. [A]

Khan I, Azam A: Study of teratogenic activity of trifluoperazine, amitriptyline, ethionamide and thalidomide in pregnant rabbits and mice. Excerpta Med Int Cong Ser 181:235-242, 1969. [A]

Morrow AW: Limb deformities associated with iminodibenzyl hydrochloride. Med J Aust 1:658-659, 1972. [O]

Vree PH, Zwart P: A newborn infant with amitryptyline poisoning. Ned Tijdschr Geneeskd 129:910-912, 1985. [C]

AMMONIUM LACTATE

Synonyms

Lac-Hydrin

Summary

Ammonium lactate is used in moistening lotions for the treatment of dry scaly skin.

Magnitude of Teratogenic Risk

Undetermined

Quality and Quantity of Data

None

Comment

A small risk cannot be excluded, but a high risk of congenital anomalies in the children of women treated with ammonium lactate during pregnancy is unlikely.

No epidemiological studies of congenital anomalies among infants born to women treated with ammonium lactate during pregnancy have been reported.

No animal teratology studies of ammonium lactate have been published.

Key References

None available.

AMOXAPINE

Synonyms

Asendin, Demolox

Summary

Amoxapine is a tricyclic antidepressant.

Magnitude of Teratogenic Risk

Undetermined

Quality and Quantity of Data

None

Comment

None

No epidemiological studies of congenital anomalies in infants whose mothers took amoxapine during pregnancy have been reported.

No animal teratology studies of amoxapine have been published.

Please see agent summaries on amitriptyline and imipramine for information on related agents that have been studied.

Key References

None available.

AMOXICILLIN

Synonyms

Amoxidin, Amoxil, Larotid, Polymox, Robamox, Trimox, Utimox, Wymox

Summary

Amoxicillin, a penicillin derivative, is a widely used antibiotic.

Magnitude of Teratogenic Risk

Undetermined

Quality and Quantity of Data

None

Comment

A small risk cannot be excluded, but there is no indication that the risk of congenital anomalies in the children of women treated with amoxicillin during pregnancy is likely to be great.

No epidemiological studies of congenital anomalies in infants born to women who took amoxicillin during pregnancy have been reported.

No animal teratology studies of amoxicillin have been published.

Please see agent summaries on penicillin and ampicillin for information on related drugs that have been more thoroughly studied.

Key References

None available.

AMPHOTERICIN B

Synonyms

Amfotericina B, Ampho-Moronal, Amphozone, Fungilin, Fungizone, Mysteclin-F

Summary

Amphotericin B is an antifungal agent used intravenously to treat systemic mycotic infections and topically to treat mycotic external otitis and dermatoses. Topical preparations are poorly absorbed.

Magnitude of Teratogenic Risk

Undetermined

Quality and Quantity of Data

None To Poor

Comment

None

No epidemiological studies of congenital anomalies in children born to women who took amphotericin B during pregnancy have been reported. No malformations have been observed among some two dozen anecdotal reports of infants born to women treated with this drug during pregnancy (Ismail & Lerner, 1982; Cohen, 1987; Peterson, 1989).

No animal teratology studies of amphotericin B have been published.

Key References

Cohen I: Absence of congenital infection and teratogenesis in three children born to mothers with blastomycosis and treated with amphotericin B during pregnancy. Pediatr Infect Dis 6:76-77, 1987. [C]

Ismail MA, Lerner SA: Disseminated blastomycosis in a pregnant woman: Review of amphotericin B usage during pregnancy. Am Rev Respir Dis 126:350-353, 1982. [C] & [R]

Peterson CM, Johnson SL, Kelly JV, Kelly PC: Coccidiodal meningitis and pregnancy: A case report. Obstet Gynecol 73:835-836, 1989. [C]

AMPICILLIN

Synonyms

Amcill, Ampicin, Ampilean, Deripen, Omnipen, Pen A/N, Penbritin, Polycillin, Principen, Totacillin

Summary

Ampicillin is a widely used antibiotic that is derived from penicillin.

Magnitude of Teratogenic Risk

None

Quality and Quantity of Data

Fair To Good

Comment

None

The frequency of congenital anomalies among the infants of 309 and 409 women treated with ampicillin during the first trimester of pregnancy was no greater than expected in two separate cohorts of the Boston Collaborative Drug Surveillance Program (Jick et al., 1981; Aselton et al., 1985). Rothman et al. (1979) observed an association with maternal ampicillin treatment "about the time pregnancy began" in a case-control study of 390 infants with congenital heart disease. This finding was not confirmed in a follow-up study of similar design by the same investigators (Zierler & Rothman, 1986) or in an independent case-control study of about the same size (Bracken, 1986). In two of these studies but not in the third, a significant association of maternal ampicillin use with one particular kind of heart malformation, transposition of the great arteries, was observed.

No increase in the frequency of malformations was reported among the offspring of rats treated with ampicillin during pregnancy in doses similar to those used in humans (Bachev et al., 1974; Korzhova et al., 1981).

Key References

Aselton P, Jick H, Milunsky A, Hunter JR, et al.: First-trimester drug use and congenital disorders. Obstet Gynecol 65:451-455, 1985. [E]

Bachev S, Petrova L, Voicheva V, Shishkova N, et al.: Experimental studies on the teratogenic effect, acute and chronic toxicity of ampicillin. Savremenna Medicina 25:29-32, 1974. (In Russian.) [A]

Bracken MB: Drug use in pregnancy and congenital heart disease in offspring. N Engl J Med 314:1120, 1986. [E]

Jick H, Holmes LB, Hunter JR, Madsen S, et al.: First-trimester drug use and congenital disorders. JAMA 246:343-346, 1981. [E]

Korzhova VV, Lisitsyna NT, Mikhailova EG: Effect of ampicillin and oxacillin on fetal and neonatal development. Bull Exp Biol Med 91:169-171, 1981. [A]

Rothman KJ, Fyler DC, Goldblatt A, Kreidberg MB: Exogenous hormones and other drug exposures of children with congenital heart disease. Am J Epidemiol 109:433-439, 1979. [E]

Zierler S, Rothman KJ: Congenital heart disease in relation to maternal use of Bendectin and other drugs in early pregnancy. N Engl J Med 313:347-352, 1985. [E]

AMRINONE

Synonyms

Inocor

Summary

Amrinone is an inotropic agent administered intravenously to treat heart failure.

Magnitude of Teratogenic Risk

Undetermined

Quality and Quantity of Data

None To Poor

Comment

None

No epidemiological studies of congenital anomalies among infants born to women treated with amrinone during pregnancy have been reported.

Increased frequencies of fetal death and skeletal anomalies were observed among the offspring of rats treated during pregnancy with amrinone in doses 5-10 times those used in humans, but such doses were toxic to the mothers (Frosch & Mannel, 1986; Komai et al., 1990a). At maternal doses 1-3 times those used clinically, increased frequencies of fetal skeletal variants were noted. The frequency of fetal death but not of malformations was increased among the offspring of rabbits treated during pregnancy with amrinone in doses similar to those used clinically (Komai et al., 1990b). The relevance of these observations to the therapeutic use of amrinone in human pregnancy is unknown.

Key References

Frosch I, Mannel S: Effects of Cordemcura on the prenatal development in the rat. Pharmazie 41:214-216, 1986. [A]

Komai Y, Hattori M, Inoue S, et al.: Teratology study of amrinone administered intravenously in rabbits. Kiso To Rinsho 24(2):15-21, 1990b. [A]

Komai Y, Iriyama K, Ito I, et al.: Teratology study of amrinone in rats by subcutaneous treatment. Kiso To Rinsho 24(4):351-360, 1990a. [A]

AMSACRINE

Synonyms

Acridinylanisidide, Amekrin, Amsa, Amsidine, Amsidyl

Summary

Amsacrine is an antineoplastic agent that inhibits nucleic acid synthesis. Amsacrine is given intravenously in the treatment of leukemia.

Magnitude of Teratogenic Risk

Undetermined

Quality and Quantity of Data

Poor

Comment

Although the teratogenic risk of amsacrine in humans is undetermined, the fact that this drug is cytotoxic raises concern that the risk could be substantial.

No epidemiological studies of congenital anomalies among infants born to women treated with amsacrine during pregnancy have been reported. One pregnancy in which the mother was treated with amsacrine and other antineoplastic agents during the first trimester is reported to have produced a normal child (Blatt et al., 1980).

Increased frequencies of congenital anomalies (particularly malformations of the eye and jaw) and embryonic or fetal death were observed among the offspring of pregnant rats treated with amsacrine in a dose that was not maternally toxic and was less than that used therapeutically in humans (Anderson et al., 1986; Ng et al., 1987).

Key References

Anderson JA, Petrere JA, Sakowski R, et al.: Teratology study in rats with amsacrine, an antineoplastic agent. Fundam Appl Toxicol 7:214-220, 1986. [A]

Blatt J, Mulvihill JJ, Ziegler JL, et al.: Pregnancy outcome following cancer chemotherapy. Am J Med 69:828-832, 1980. [S]

Ng WW, Anderson JA, Sakowski R: Teratogenicity of amsacrine lactate given IP to rats during the entire organogenesis period. Teratology 35(2):76, 1987. [A]

AMYL NITRITE

Synonyms

Amilnitrit, Aspiral, Isoamyl Nitrite, Isopentyl Nitrite, 3-Methylbutanol Nitrite, Nitramyl, Vaporole

Summary

Amyl nitrite is a vasodilator that is administered by inhalation of the vapor. Amyl nitrite is used in the acute treatment of angina pectoris and in the therapy of cyanide poisoning. Amyl nitrite is also used as a "recreational" drug to induce euphoria and enhance sexual stimulation.

Magnitude of Teratogenic Risk

Undetermined

Quality and Quantity of Data

None

Comment

None

No epidemiological studies of congenital anomalies among infants born to women treated with amyl nitrite during pregnancy have been reported.

No animal teratology studies of amyl nitrite have been published.

Please see agent summary on nitroglycerin for information on a related agent that has been studied.

Key References

None available.

AMYLASE

Synonyms

Amylolytic Enzyme, Amylopol P, Amzyme TX 8, Diastase, Glycogenase, Mylase 100

Summary

Amylases are a class of enzymes that break down starches and similar complex carbohydrates. Amylases are widely distributed in nature and are normal components of human salivary and pancreatic secretions. Amylase is used industrially in brewing and fermentation and is sometimes taken as a digestive aid.

Magnitude of Teratogenic Risk

Undetermined

Quality and Quantity of Data

None To Poor

Comment

A small risk cannot be excluded, but a high risk of congenital anomalies in the children of women exposed to exogenous amylase during pregnancy is unlikely.

No epidemiological studies of congenital anomalies among infants born to women

treated with amylase during pregnancy have been reported.

No teratogenic effect was observed among the offspring of pregnant rabbits given 65-260 mg/kg/d of a pancreatic preparation containing amylase and other enzymes (Nemec et al., 1986). Fetal growth and survival were normal in pregnant rats fed diets containing very large amounts of bacterial amylase (MacKenzie et al., 1989a, b).

Key References

MacKenzie KM, Petsel SRW, Weltman RH, Zeman NW: Subchronic toxicity studies in dogs and in utero-exposed rats fed diets containing bacillus megaterium amylase derived from a recombinant dna organism. Food Chem Toxicol 27(5):301-305, 1989a. [A]

MacKenzie KM, Petsel SRW, Weltman RH, Zeman NW: Subchronic toxicity studies in dogs and in utero rats fed diets containing bacillus stearothermophilus alpha-amylase from a natural or recombinant dna host. Food Chem Toxicol 27(9):599-606, 1989b. [A]

Nemec MD, Krayer J, Merz E, Rodwell DE: A capsule teratology study in rabbits with pancrease. Teratology 33(3):71C, 1986. [A]

AMYLOCAINE

Synonyms

Amyleinii Chloridum,   Chlorhydrate d'Amyleine, Phenolaine

Summary

Amylocaine is a local anesthetic of the ester class that has been used topically in ophthalmology.

Magnitude of Teratogenic Risk

Undetermined

Quality and Quantity of Data

None

Comment

None

No epidemiological studies of congenital anomalies in children born to women exposed to amylocaine during pregnancy have been reported.

No investigations of teratologic effects of amylocaine in experimental animals have been published.

Please see agent summary on procaine for information on a related agent that has been studied.

Key References

None available.

ANISOTROPINE

Synonyms

Anisotropine Methylbromide, Valpin 50

Summary

Anisotropine is a quaternary ammonium anticholinergic agent that is given orally in the treatment of peptic ulcer disease.

Magnitude of Teratogenic Risk

Undetermined

Quality and Quantity of Data

None

Comment

None

No epidemiological studies of congenital anomalies among infants born to women treated with anisotropine during pregnancy have been reported.

No animal teratology studies of anisotropine have been published.

Please see agent summary on atropine for information on a related drug that has been more thoroughly studied.

Key References

None available.

ANTHRALIN

Synonyms

Anthra-Derm, Batridol, Chrysodermol, Cignolin, Cigthranol, Dithranol, Ditranol, Lasan, Psoradrate

Summary

Anthralin is used in the topical treatment of psoriasis. Absorption of anthralin through the skin does occur, but only to a small extent.

Magnitude of Teratogenic Risk

Undetermined

Quality and Quantity of Data

None

Comment

A small risk cannot be excluded, but a high risk of congenital anomalies in the children of women treated with anthralin during pregnancy is unlikely.

No epidemiological studies of congenital anomalies among infants born to women treated with anthralin during pregnancy have been reported.

No animal teratology studies of anthralin have been published.

Key References

None available.

ANTIHEMOPHILIC FACTOR

Synonyms

AHF, Factorate, Hemofil M, Humafac, Humate-P, Koate-HP, Monoclate, Profilate

Summary

Antihemophilic factor is a preparation of partially purified factor VIII obtained from human plasma. Antihemophilic factor is used in the treatment of hemophilia and von Willebrand disease.

Magnitude of Teratogenic Risk

Undetermined

Quality and Quantity of Data

None

Comment

A small risk cannot be excluded, but a high risk of congenital anomalies in the children of women treated with antihemophilic factor during pregnancy is unlikely.

No epidemiological studies of congenital anomalies among infants born to women treated with antihemophilic factor during pregnancy have been reported.

No animal teratology studies of antihemophilic factor have been published.

Key References

None available.

ANTI-INHIBITOR COAGULANT COMPLEX

Synonyms

Autoplex, Feiba VH Immuno

Summary

Anti-inhibitor coagulant complex, a preparation of human plasma proteins, is used to treat bleeding in patients with hemophilia who have antibodies to factor VIII.

Magnitude of Teratogenic Risk

Undetermined

Quality and Quantity of Data

None

Comment

A small risk cannot be excluded, but a high risk of congenital anomalies in the children of women treated with anti-inhibitor coagulant complex during pregnancy is unlikely.

No epidemiological studies of congenital anomalies among infants born to women treated with anti-inhibitor coagulant complex during pregnancy have been reported.

No animal teratology studies of anti-inhibitor coagulant complex have been published.

Key References

None available.

ANTIPYRINE

Synonyms

Analgesine, Antipyrin Salicylate, Azophenum, Breezeazy, Callyrium Eye Lotion, Felsol, Fenazona, Lanceotic, Migrenin, Phenazone

Summary

Antipyrine is used as an oral analgesic and antipyretic, and topically, as an anesthetic.

Magnitude of Teratogenic Risk

Undetermined

Quality and Quantity of Data

None

Comment

None

No adequate epidemiological studies of congenital anomalies in infants born to women who took antipyrine during pregnancy have been reported.

No animal teratology studies of antipyrine have been published.

Key References

None available.

ANTIVENIN (CROTALIDAE) POLYVALENT

Synonyms

Moccasin Antitoxic Serum, Polyvalent Antivenin, Snake Antivenin, Snake Antivenom

Summary

Antivenin (Crotalidae) polyvalent is a globulin preparation obtained from the sera of horses immunized to the venom of four species of American poisonous snakes. Antivenin is administered intravenously in the treatment of poisonous snake bites.

Magnitude of Teratogenic Risk

Undetermined

Quality and Quantity of Data

None

Comment

A small risk cannot be excluded, but a high risk of congenital anomalies in the children of women treated with antivenin (crotalidae) polyvalent during pregnancy is unlikely.

No epidemiological studies of congenital anomalies among infants born to women treated with antivenin (Crotalidae) polyvalent during pregnancy have been reported.

No animal teratology studies of antivenin (Crotalidae) polyvalent have been published.

Key References

None available.

ANTIVENIN (MICRURUS FULVIUS)

Synonyms

North American Coral Snake Antivenin

Summary

Antivenin (Micrurus fulvius) is an equine immunoglobulin preparation that is administered intravenously to treat bites of the Eastern coral snake.

Magnitude of Teratogenic Risk

Undetermined

Quality and Quantity of Data

None

Comment

None

No epidemiological studies of congenital anomalies among infants born to women treated with antivenin (Micrurus fulvius) during pregnancy have been reported.

No animal teratology studies of antivenin (Micrurus fulvius) have been published.

Key References

None available.

APROBARBITAL

Synonyms

Allylisopropylmalonylurea, Allypropymal, Alurate, Apronal, Aprozal, Isopropylallylbarbituric, Numal, Sodium Aprobarbital

Summary

Aprobarbital is a barbiturate that is used as a sedative-hypnotic agent.

Magnitude of Teratogenic Risk

Undetermined

Quality and Quantity of Data

None

Comment

None

No epidemiological studies of congenital anomalies in infants born to women treated with aprobarbital during pregnancy have been reported.

No animal teratology studies of aprobarbital have been published.

Please see agent summary on phenobarbital for information on a related drug that has been studied.

Key References

None available.

APTOCAINE

Synonyms

2-Pyrrolidin-1-ylpropiono-o-toluidide

Summary

Aptocaine is a local anesthetic that has vasoconstrictor activity.

Magnitude of Teratogenic Risk

Undetermined

Quality and Quantity of Data

None

Comment

None

No epidemiological studies of congenital anomalies in children born to women exposed to aptocaine during pregnancy have been reported.

No investigations of teratologic effects of aptocaine in experimental animals have been published.

Please see agent summary on procaine for information on a related agent that has been studied.

Key References

None available.

ARGININE

Synonyms

Arginina, Argininum

Summary

Arginine is an amino acid that is administered intravenously in the treatment of hyperammonemia. It is also taken as a dietary supplement.

Magnitude of Teratogenic Risk

Undetermined

Quality and Quantity of Data

None To Poor

Comment

None

No epidemiological studies of congenital anomalies in infants born to women treated with large amounts of arginine during pregnancy have been reported.

An increased frequency of hind limb malformations was found among the offspring of rats treated with arginine during pregnancy in a dose 1/25 that used in the therapy of hyperammonemia in humans (Naidu, 1973). The relevance of this observation to the clinical use of arginine in human pregnancy is unknown.

Key References

Naidu RC: The effect of L.arginine hydrochloride on the development of rat embryos. Aust J Exp Biol Med Sci 51:553-555, 1973. [A]

ARTICAINE

Synonyms

Carticaine, Ultracain

Summary

Articaine is a local anesthetic of the amide class that is used in dentistry.

Magnitude of Teratogenic Risk

Undetermined

Quality and Quantity of Data

None

Comment

A small risk cannot be excluded, but there is no indication that the risk of congenital anomalies in the children of women treated with articaine during pregnancy is likely to be great.

No epidemiological studies of congenital anomalies in children born to women exposed to articaine during pregnancy have been reported.

No investigations of teratologic effects of articaine in experimental animals have been published.

Please see agent summary on lidocaine for information on a related agent that has been studied.

Key References

None available.

ASCORBIC ACID

Synonyms

Cecon, Cemill, Cetane, Cevalin, Cevi-Bid, C-Span, Redoxon, Sodium Ascorbate, Vita Ce, Vitamin C

Summary

Ascorbic acid is vitamin C, an essential nutrient. The U.S. Recommended Dietary Allowance of ascorbic acid during pregnancy is 70 mg/d (NRC, 1989).

Magnitude of Teratogenic Risk

None

Quality and Quantity of Data

Poor

Comment

None

The frequency of supplemental ascorbic acid treatment during the first trimester of pregnancy was no greater than expected among the mothers of 175 infants with major malformations or of 283 women with minor anomalies in one case-control study (Nelson & Forfar, 1971). No epidemiological studies of malformations in infants born to women who took exceptionally large doses of ascorbic acid during pregnancy have been reported.

The frequency of malformations was no higher than expected among the offspring of mice or rats treated with ascorbic acid in doses respectively 36-4800 times and 537-4285 times the human recommended dietary allowance (Frohberg et al., 1973; Lavender & Fritz, 1975; Kola et al., 1989; Vogel & Spielmann, 1989; Pillans et al., 1990). Fetal deaths were increased in pregnant mice treated with 4800 times the human recommended dietary allowance (Pillans et al., 1990).

Increased ascorbic acid catabolism and consequently increased dietary requirements have been observed in newborn guinea pigs whose mothers were fed 100-200 times the guinea pig minimal daily requirement of ascorbic acid during pregnancy (Cochrane, 1965; Norkus & Rosso, 1975, 1981). A report of scurvy, despite documented adequate ascorbic acid intake in two children born to women who took about 8 times the recommended daily allowance of vitamin C during pregnancy, raises the possibility that a similar effect may occur in humans (Cochrane, 1965).

Key References

Cochrane WA: Overnutrition in prenatal and neonatal life: A problem? Can Med Assoc J 93:893-899, 1965. [R]

Frohberg VH, Gleich J, Kieser H: Reproduction toxicology studies on ascorbic acid in mice and rats. Arzneimittelforsch 23:1081-1082, 1973. [A]

Kola I, Vogel R, Spielmann H: Co-administration of ascorbic acid with cyclophosphamide (CPA) to pregnant mice inhibits the clastogenic activity of CPA in preimplantation murine blastocysts. Mutagenesis 4(4):297-301, 1989. [A]

Lavender LM, Fritz HI: Teratogenic effects of hypervitaminosis C on the developing rat fetus. Teratology 11:27A-28A, 1975. [A]

Nelson MM, Forfar JO: Associations between drugs administered during pregnancy and congenital abnormalities of the fetus. Br Med J 1:523-527, 1971. [E]

Norkus EP, Rosso P: Changes in ascorbic acid metabolism of the offspring following high maternal intake of this vitamin in the pregnant guinea pig. Ann NY Acad Sci 258:401-409, 1975. [A]

Norkus EP, Rosso P: Effects of maternal intake of ascorbic acid on the postnatal metabolism of this vitamin in the guinea pig. J Nutr 111:624-630, 1981. [A]

NRC (National Research Council): Recommended Dietary Allowances, 10th ed. Report of the Subcommittee on the Tenth Edition of the RDAs, Food and Nutrition Board, Commission on Life Sciences. Washington, D.C.: National Academy Press, 1989. [O]

Pillans PI, Ponzi SF, Parker MI: Effects of ascorbic acid on the mouse embryo and on cyclophosphamide-induced cephalic DNA strand breaks in vivo. Arch Toxicol 64:423-425, 1990. [A]

Vogel R, Spielmann H: Beneficial effects of ascorbic acid on preimplantation mouse embryos after exposure to cyclophosphamide in vivo. Teratogenesis Carcinog Mutagen 9:51-59, 1989. [A]

ASPARAGINASE

Synonyms

Colaspase, Crasnitin, Elspar, Erwinase, Glutaminase-Asparaginase, Kidrolase, Laspar, Leucogen, Leunase

Summary

Asparaginase is a bacterial enzyme that breaks down the amino acid l-asparagine. Asparaginase is administered intravenously in the treatment of leukemia.

Magnitude of Teratogenic Risk

Undetermined

Quality and Quantity of Data

Poor To Fair

Comment

The teratogenic risk of this agent, although undetermined, may be substantial because asparaginase has antineoplastic activity.

No epidemiological studies of congenital anomalies among the infants of women treated with asparaginase during pregnancy have been reported. The frequency of congenital anomalies did not appear to be unusually high among 16 children of parents who had been previously treated with asparaginase for pediatric malignancies (Green et al., 1991).

Dose-dependent increases in the frequencies of fetal death and skeletal, brain, and other malformations have been observed among the offspring of mice, rats, and rabbits treated respectively with 100-200, 75-500, or 2.5-5 times the usual human dose of asparaginase during pregnancy (Adamson & Fabro, 1968; Ohguro et al., 1969; Lorke & Tettenborn, 1970). Such doses produced maternal toxicity as well. Consistent teratogenic effects were not seen after the administration of lower doses of asparaginase to pregnant mice or rats (Ohguro et al., 1969; Adamson et al., 1970). The relevance of these observations to the therapeutic use of asparaginase in human pregnancy is unknown.

Key References

Adamson RH, Fabro S: Embryotoxic effects of L-asparaginase. Nature 218:1164-1165, 1968. [A]

Adamson RH, Fabro S, Hahn MA, Creech CE, et al.: Evaluation of the embryotoxic activity of L-asparaginase. Arch Int Pharmacodyn 186:310-320, 1970. [A]

Green DM, Zevon MA, Lowrie G, et al.: Congenital anomalies in children of patients who received chemotherapy for cancer in childhood and adolescence. N Engl J Med 325(3):141-146, 1991. [S]

Lorke D, Tettenborn D: Experimental studies on the toxicity of crasnitin in animals. Recent Results in Cancer Research 33:174-180, 1970. [A]

Ohguro Y, Imamura S, Koyama K, Hara T, et al.: Toxicological studies on L-asparaginase. Yamaguchi Igaku 18:271-292, 1969. [A]

ASPARTAME

Synonyms

APM, Canderel, Equal, Nutrasweet

Summary

Aspartame is a low-calorie sweetening agent that is widely used in beverages and foods. It is a dipeptide ester composed of phenylalanine and aspartic acid. The allowable daily intake of aspartame set by the United States Food and Drug Administration is 50 mg/kg/d, the equivalent of about a dozen 12-ounce cans of soda sweetened with aspartame (Sturtevant, 1985).

Magnitude of Teratogenic Risk

None To Minimal

Quality and Quantity of Data

Poor

Comment

None

No epidemiological studies of congenital anomalies in infants born to women who used aspartame during pregnancy have been reported.

No teratogenic effect was observed among the offspring of rats fed diets containing 1% aspartame during pregnancy (Lederer et al., 1985). Treatment of pregnant rabbits with aspartame in doses 40 times greater than the human allowable daily intake did not affect fetal weight or litter size in one study (Ranney et al., 1975). Behavioral alterations have been observed among the offspring of guinea pigs or mice treated respectively with 10 or 20-80 times the human allowable daily intake of aspartame during pregnancy (Mahalik & Gautieri, 1985; Dow-Edwards et al., 1989). The clinical relevance of these findings is unknown.

It has been suggested on theoretical grounds that use of aspartame by pregnant women who are heterozygous carriers of phenylketonuria may increase the risk of mental retardation in their offspring (Bhagavan, 1975), but available evidence suggests that this risk is unlikely to be of clinical significance (Sturtevant, 1985).

Key References

Bhagavan NV: Hazards in indiscriminate use of sweeteners containing phenylalanine. N Engl J Med 292:52-53, 1975. [O]

Dow-Edwards DL, Scribani LA, Riley EP: Impaired performance on odor-aversion testing following prenatal aspartame exposure in the guinea pig. Neurotoxicol Teratol 11:413-416, 1989. [A]

Lederer J, Bodin J, Colson A: Aspartame and its effect on gestation in rats. Journal de Toxicologie Clinique et Experimentale 5:7-14, 1985. [A]

Mahalik MP, Gautieri RF: Reflex responsiveness of CF-1 mouse neonates following maternal aspartame exposure. Res Commun Psychol Psych Behav 9:385-403, 1985. [A]

Ranney RE, Mares SE, Schroeder RE, Hutsell TC, et al.: The phenylalanine and tyrosine content of maternal and fetal body fluids from rabbits fed aspartame. Toxicol Appl Pharmacol 32:339-346, 1975. [A]

Sturtevant FM: Use of aspartame in pregnancy. Int J Fertil 30:85-87, 1985. [R]

ASPIRIN

Synonyms

Acetylsalicylic Acid, A.S.A., Bayer Aspirin, Claradin, Easprin, Ecotrin, Empirin, Encaprin, Entrophen, Measurin Tablets, Novasen, Salicylic Acid Acetate

Summary

Aspirin is a frequently used oral analgesic and antipyretic agent. Common occasional usage of aspirin for treatment of headache, muscle ache, fever, etc., is generally in "low" doses of 650-1300 mg/day. Much higher doses of aspirin (as much as 5000-6000 mg/day) are used to treat rheumatic disease.

Magnitude of Teratogenic Risk

None To Minimal

Quality and Quantity of Data

Fair To Good

Comment

1) This rating is based on maternal use of occasional low doses of aspirin. The risks associated with chronic high doses (such as those used to treat rheumatic diseases) and with toxic overdoses of aspirin are unknown.

2) Maternal aspirin use just prior to delivery may be associated with intracranial hemorrhage in premature infants (see discussion below).

Analysis of available data indicates that the risk of congenital anomalies is not substantially increased among children born to women who have taken occasional low doses of aspirin during pregnancy (Corby, 1978; Rudolph, 1981; Hertz-Picciotto et al., 1990). Although various malformations have been associated with maternal aspirin use early in gestation in case-control studies involving hundreds of affected patients (Nelson & Forfar, 1971; Richards 1972; Saxen, 1975; Rothman et al., 1979; Zierler & Rothman, 1985) and in a Tasmanian cohort study of 56,037 infants (Correy et al., 1991), the types of anomalies associated with maternal aspirin use have varied among the studies and the findings have not been consistently reproducible (Turner & Collins, 1975; Slone et al., 1976; Jick et al., 1981; Aselton et al., 1985; Winship et al., 1984; Werler et al., 1989; Hertz-Picciotto et al., 1990; Tikkanen & Heinonen, 1991). Data from the U.S. Collaborative Perinatal Project, a cohort study which included more than 5000 women who took aspirin for at least eight days during the first four lunar months of pregnancy, indicate that the risk of congenital anomalies among such babies is unlikely to be greater than that among the infants of untreated mothers (Slone et al., 1976). One infant with malformations was observed among 31 born to women who had taken overdoses of aspirin at various times during pregnancy in one series (McElhatton et al., 1991).

Anecdotal observations of various congenital anomalies in infants of women who took aspirin during pregnancy (McNiel, 1973; Benawra et al., 1980; Agapitos et al., 1986) cannot be interpreted as indicating a causal relationship because chance associations are very likely for an agent used as frequently as aspirin is.

Maternal aspirin use during the first half of pregnancy was associated with slightly lower IQ scores in 421 four-year-old children in one study (Streissguth et al., 1987), but no such effect was seen in a similar study of the children of more than 19,000 women from the Collaborative Perinatal Project (Klebanoff & Berendes, 1988).

Aspirin in doses two or more times greater than those used to treat rheumatic disease in humans is teratogenic in rats, mice, dogs, cats, and monkeys (Wilson et al., 1977; Klein ct al., 1981; Khera, 1984). Typical dose-response relationships are often observed, and a variety of anomalies may be produced, including neural tube defects, skeletal malformations, and facial clefts. Behavioral alterations have been found among the offspring of rats treated during pregnancy with aspirin in doses several times those used to treat rheumatic disease in humans (Vorhees et al., 1982).

Aspirin is an inhibitor of prostaglandin synthesis. More potent prostaglandin synthesis inhibitors are used therapeutically to produce closure of the ductus arteriosus and consequent changes in cardiovascular and pulmonary function in newborns with patent ductus arteriosus. There is anecdotal evidence of an association between maternal high-dose aspirin use and premature closure of the fetal ductus arteriosus (Levin et al., 1978), but a causal relationship is uncertain. If maternal high- dose aspirin use does cause premature closure of the fetal ductus arteriosus, it must do so infrequently. Premature closure of the ductus arteriosus has been produced in the fetuses of rats, rabbits, and sheep treated late in pregnancy with very high doses of aspirin (Heymann & Rudolph, 1976). Mild constriction of the ductus arteriosus was observed among the fetuses of rats treated shortly before delivery with aspirin in doses similar to those commonly used in humans (Momma & Takao, 1990).

The onset of labor may be delayed and its duration prolonged in women who take high-dose aspirin chronically in late pregnancy (Lewis & Schulman, 1973). Some studies suggest that babies born to such women have lower birth weights than expected (Turner & Collins, 1975), but other studies do not support this conclusion (Shapiro et al., 1976). Prolonged gestation and labor, decreased fetal weight, and increased fetal mortality have been observed in pregnant rats exposed to aspirin in doses as great or greater than those used to treat rheumatic disease in humans (Tuchmann-Duplessis et al., 1975; Lubawy & Garrett, 1977; Klein et al., 1981; Tagashira et al., 1981).

Maternal aspirin use within a week of delivery causes abnormalities of hemostasis in human newborns as well as their mothers (Stuart et al., 1982). These hemostatic defects usually produce very little, if any, clinical manifestation in the term infant but may be associated with an increased risk of intracranial hemorrhage in premature and low birth weight infants (Rumack et al., 1981).

Aspirin is metabolized more slowly and is less completely bonded to serum proteins in neonates than in adults (Levy & Garrettson, 1974; Levy et al., 1975). Thus, the serum concentration of aspirin in the fetus or immediate newborn is often higher than that in a mother who has taken the drug. Salicylate intoxication in the infant of a mother who took large doses of aspirin during pregnancy (Lynd et al., 1976) and fetal death associated with maternal toxic salicylism have been reported (Rejent & Baik, 1985).

Maternal treatment with very low doses (60-150 mg/d) of aspirin during the second and third trimesters of pregnancy has been used for the prevention of fetal growth retardation, pregnancy-induced hypertension, and stillbirth in high-risk pregnancies (Beaufils et al., 1985; Wallenburg et al., 1986; Wallenburg & Rotmans, 1987; Trudinger et al., 1988; Benigni et al., 1989; Schiff et al., 1989; McParland et al., 1990; Hertz-Picciotto et al., 1990; Barton & Sibai, 1991; Imperiale et al., 1991; Uzan et al., 1991). Adverse fetal effects of the aspirin have not been noted in these circumstances.

Key References

Agapitos M, Georgiou-Theodoropoulou M, Koutselinis A, Papacharalampus N: Cyclopia and maternal ingestion of salicylates. Pediatr Pathol 6:309-310, 1986. [C]

Aselton P, Jick H, Milunsky A, Hunter JR, et al.: First-trimester drug use and congenital disorders. Obstet Gynecol 65:451-455, 1985. [S]

Barton JR, Sibai BM: Low-dose aspirin to improve perinatal outcome. Clin Obstet Gynecol 34(2):251-261, 1991. [R]

Beaufils M, Uzan S, Donsimoni R, Colau JC: Prevention of pre-eclampsia by early antiplatelet therapy. Lancet 1:840-842, 1985. [E]

Benawra R, Mangurten HH, Duffell DR: Cyclopia and other anomalies following maternal ingestion of salicylates. J Pediatr 96:1069-1071, 1980. [C]

Benigni A, Gregorini G, Frusca T, Chiabrando C, et al.: Effect of low-dose aspirin on fetal and maternal generation of thromboxane by platelets in women at risk for pregnancy-induced hypertension. New Engl J Med 321:357-362, 1989. [E]

Corby DG: Aspirin in pregnancy: Maternal and fetal effects. Pediatrics 62:930-937, 1978. [R]

Correy JF, Newman NM, Collins JA, Burrows EA, et al.: Use of prescription drugs in the first trimester and congenital malformations. Aust NZ J Obstet Gynaecol 31(4):340-344, 1991. [E]

Hertz-Picciotto I, Hopenhayn-Rich C, Golub M, Hooper K: The risks and benefits of taking aspirin during pregnancy. Epidemiol Rev 12:108-148, 1990. [R]

Heymann MA, Rudolph AM: Effects of acetylsalicylic acid on the ductus arteriosus and circulation in fetal lambs in utero. Circ Res 38:418-422, 1976. [A]

Imperiale TF, Petrulis AS: A meta-analysis of low-dose aspirin for the prevention of pregnancy-induced hypertensive disease. JAMA 266:261-265, 1991. [E]

Jick H, Holmes LB, Hunter JR, Madsen S, et al.: First-trimester drug use and congenital disorders. JAMA 246:343-346, 1981. [S]

Khera KD: Adverse effects in humans and animals of prenatal exposure to selected therapeutic drugs and estimation of embryo-fetal sensitivity of animals for human risk assessment. Issues Rev Teratol 2:399-507, 1984. [R]

Klebanoff MA, Berendes HW: Aspirin exposure during the first 20 weeks of gestation and IQ at four years of age. Teratology 37:249-255, 1988. [E]

Klein KL, Scott WJ, Wilson JG: Aspirin-induced teratogenesis: A unique pattern of cell death and subsequent polydactyly in the rat. J Exp Zool 216:107-112, 1981. [A]

Levin DL, Fixler DE, Morriss FC, Tyson J: Morphologic analysis of the pulmonary vascular bed in infants exposed in utero to prostaglandin synthetase inhibitors. J Pediatr 92:478-483, 1978. [C]

Levy G, Garrettson LK: Kinetics of salicylate elimination by newborn infants of mothers who ingested aspirin before delivery. Pediatrics 53:201-210, 1974. [S]

Levy G, Procknal JA, Garrettson LK: Distribution of salicylate between neonatal and maternal serum at diffusion equilibrium. Clin Pharmacol Ther 18:210-214, 1975. [O]

Lewis RB, Schulman JD: Influence of acetylsalicylic acid, an inhibitor of prostaglandin synthesis, on the duration of human gestation and labor. Lancet 2:1159-1161, 1973. [E]

Lubawy WC, Garrett RJ: Effects of aspirin and acetaminophen on fetal and placental growth in rats. J Pharm Sci 66:111-113, 1977. [A]

Lynd PA, Andreasen AC, Wyatt RJ: Intrauterine salicylate intoxication in a newborn. Clin Pediatr 15:912-913, 1976. [C]

McElhatton PR, Sullivan FM, Walton L: Analgesic overdose during pregnancy. Teratology 44(3):17A, 1991. [S]

McNiel JR: The possible teratogenic effect of salicylates on the developing fetus: Brief summaries of eight suggestive cases. Clin Pediatr 12:347-350, 1973. [C]

McParland P, Pearce JM, Chamberlain GVP: Doppler ultrasound and aspirin in recognition and prevention of pregnancy-induced hypertension. Lancet 335:1552-1555, 1990. [E]

Momma K, Takao A: Transplacental cardiovascular effects of four popular analgesics in rats. Am J Obstet Gynecol 162(5):1304-1310, 1990. [A]

Nelson MM, Forfar JO: Associations between drugs administered during pregnancy and congenital abnormalities of the fetus. Brit Med J 1:523-527, 1971. [C]

Rejent TA, Baik S-O: Fatal in utero salicylism. J Forensic Sci 30:942-944, 1985. [C]

Richards ID: A retrospective inquiry into possible teratogenesis effect of drugs in pregnancy. Adv Exp Med Biol 27:441-455, 1972. [E]

Rothman KJ, Fyler DC, Goldblatt A, Kreidberg MB: Exogenous hormones and other drug exposures of children with congenital heart disease. Am J Epidemiol 109:433-439, 1979. [E]

Rudolph AM: Effects of aspirin and acetaminophen in pregnancy and in the newborn. Arch Intern Med 141:358-363, 1981. [R] & [A]

Rumack CM, Guggenheim MA, Rumack BH, Peterson RG, et al.: Neonatal intracranial hemorrhage and maternal use of aspirin. Obstet Gynecol 58:52s-56s, 1981. [E]

Saxen I: Associations between oral clefts and drugs taken during pregnancy. Int J Epidemiol 4:37-44, 1975. [E]

Schiff E, Peleg E, Goldenberg M, Rosenthal T, et al.: The use of aspirin to prevent pregnancy-induced hypertension and lower the ratio of thromboxane A2 to prostacyclin in relatively high risk pregnancies. N Engl J Med 321:351-356, 1989. [E]

Shapiro S, Siskind V, Monson RR, Heinonen OP, et al.: Perinatal mortality and birth-weight in relation to aspirin taken during pregnancy. Lancet 1:1375-1376, 1976. [R]

Slone D, Siskind V, Heinonen OP, Monson RR, et al.: Aspirin and congenital malformations. Lancet 1:1373-1375, 1976. [E]

Streissguth AP, Treder RP, Barr HM, Shepard TH et al.: Aspirin and acetaminophen use by pregnant women and subsequent child IQ and attention decrements. Teratology 35:211-219, 1987. [E]

Stuart MJ, Gross SJ, Elrad H, Graeber JE: Effects of acetylsalicylic-acid ingestion on maternal and neonatal hemostasis. N Engl J Med 307:909-912, 1982. [E]

Tagashira E, Nako K, Urano T, Ishikawa S, et al.: Correlation of teratogenicity of aspirin to the stagespecific distribution of salicylic acid in rats. Jpn J Pharmacol 31:563-571, 1981. [A]

Tikkanen J, Heinonen OP: Maternal hyperthermia during pregnancy and cardiovascular malformations in the offspring. Eur J Epidemiol 7(6):628-635, 1991. [E]

Trudinger BJ, Cook CM, Thompson RS, Giles WB, et al.: Low-dose aspirin therapy improves fetal weight in umbilical placental insufficiency. Am J Obstet Gynecol 159:681-685, 1988. [E]

Tuchmann-Duplessis H, Hiss D, Mottot G, Rosner I: Effects of prenatal administration of acetylsalicylic acid in rats. Toxicology 3:207-211, 1975. [A]

Turner G, Collins E: Fetal effects of regular salicylate ingestion in pregnancy. Lancet 2:338-339, 1975. [E]

Uzan S, Beaufils M, Breart G, Bazin B, et al.: Prevention of fetal growth retardation with low-dose aspirin: Findings of the EPREDA trial. Lancet 337:1427-1431, 1991. [E]

Vorhees CV, Klein KL, Scott WJ: Aspirin-induced psychoteratogenesis in rats as a function of embryonic age. Teratogenesis Carcinog Mutagen 2:77-84, 1982. [A]

Wallenburg HCS, Dekker GA, Makovitz JW, Rotmans P: Low-dose aspirin prevents pregnancy-induced hypertension and pre-eclampsia in angiotensin-sensitive primigravidae. Lancet 1:1-3, 1986. [E]

Wallenburg HCS, Rotmans N: Prevention of recurrent idiopathic fetal growth retardation by low-dose aspirin and dipyridamole. Am J Obstet Gynecol 157:1230-1235, 1987. [E]

Werler MM, Mitchell AA, Shapiro S: The relation of aspirin use during the first trimester of pregnancy to congenital cardiac defects. N Engl J Med 321:1639-1642, 1989. [E]

Wilson JG, Ritter EJ, Scott WJ, Fradkin R: Comparative distribution and embryotoxicity of acetylsalicylic acid in pregnant rats and rhesus monkeys. Toxicol Appl Pharmacol 41:67-78, 1977. [A]

Winship KA, Cahal DA, Weber JCP, Griffin JP: Maternal drug histories and central nervous system anomalies. Arch Dis Child 59:1052-1060, 1984. [E]

Zierler S, Rothman KJ: Congenital heart disease in relation to maternal use of Bendectin and other drugs in early pregnancy. N Engl J Med 313:347-352, 1985. [E]

ATENOLOL

Synonyms

Blokium, Tenormin

Summary

Atenolol is a cardioselective beta-adrenoreceptor blocking agent. It is used for treating hypertension, cardiac arrhythmias, and angina pectoris.

Magnitude of Teratogenic Risk

Undetermined

Quality and Quantity of Data

Poor

Comment

A small risk cannot be excluded, but there is no indication that the risk of congenital anomalies in the children of women treated with atenolol during pregnancy is likely to be great.

No epidemiological studies of congenital anomalies in infants born to women who had

48

been treated with atenolol during pregnancy have been published.

The frequency of malformations was not increased among the offspring of rats or rabbits treated during pregnancy with atenolol in doses 10-1000 or 10-200 times those usually employed in humans (Esaki & Imai, 1980; Esaki, 1980). Increased frequencies of fetal death were noted in the rats at 100-1000 times the usual human dose and in the rabbits at 200 times the usual human dose.

Atenolol is chemically related to other beta blockers such as propranolol. Maternal treatment with these agents during pregnancy has been associated with fetal growth retardation and difficulties in perinatal adaptation, although these effects may result from the maternal disease rather than from its treatment (Frishman & Chesner, 1988; *see also propranolol agent summary*). Fetal growth retardation and neonatal bradycardia have been associated with maternal atenolol therapy in controlled therapeutic trials in hypertensive women in the second and third trimester of pregnancy (Rubin et al., 1983; Butters et al., 1990; Marlettini et al., 1990). No abnormalities were found on follow-up physical and developmental examinations to one year of age in 55 infants of women who had been treated with atenolol for hypertension during pregnancy (Reynolds et al., 1984).

Key References

Butters L, Kennedy S, Rubin PC: Atenolol in essential hypertension during pregnancy. BMJ 301:587-589, 1990. [E]

Esaki K: Effects of oral administration of atenolol on the rabbit fetus. Preclin Rep Cent Inst Exper Anim 6:259-264, 1980. [A]

Esaki K, Imai K: Effects of oral administration of atenolol on reproduction in rats. II. Experiments on drug administration during the organogenesis period. Preclin Rep Cent Inst Exper Anim 6:247-252, 1980. [A]

Frishman WH, Chesner M: Beta-adrenergic blockers in pregnancy. Am Heart J 115(1):147-152, 1988. [R]

Marlettini MG, Crippa S, Morselli-Labate AM, et al.: Randomized comparison of calcium antagonists and beta-blockers in the treatment of pregnancy-induced hypertension. Curr Ther Res 48(4):684-694, 1990. [E]

Reynolds B, Butters L, Evans J, Adams T, et al.: First year of life after the use of atenolol in pregnancy associated with hypertension. Arch Dis Child 59:1061-1063, 1984. [E]

Rubin PC, Clark DM, Sumner DJ, Low RA, et al.: Placebo-controlled trial of atenolol in treatment of pregnancy-associated hypertension. Lancet 1:431-434, 1983. [E]

ATRACURIUM

Synonyms

Atracurium Besylate, Tracrium

Summary

Atracurium is a skeletal muscle relaxant that is used intravenously.

Magnitude of Teratogenic Risk

Undetermined

Quality and Quantity of Data

None To Poor

Comment

None

No epidemiological studies of congenital anomalies in infants born to women treated with atracurium during pregnancy have been reported.

No teratogenic effect is said to have been observed among the offspring of rats treated with less than the usual human dose of atracurium during pregnancy (Skarpa et al., 1983).

Administration of atracurium directly to the fetus has been used to reduce fetal movement during intrauterine diagnostic and therapeutic procedures (Bernstein et al., 1988; Fan et al., 1990).

49

Key References

Bernstein HH, Chitkara U, Plosker H, et al.: Use of atracurium besylate to arrest fetal activity during intrauterine intravascular transfusions. Obstet Gynecol 72(5):813-816, 1988. [S]

Fan S-Z, Huang F-Y, Lin S-Y, et al.: Intrauterine neuromuscular blockade in fetus. Anaesth Sinica (Ma Tsui Hsueh Tsa Chi)28:31-34, 1990. [S]

Skarpa M, Dayan AD, Follenfant M, James DA, et al.: Toxicity testing of atracurium. Br J Anaesth 55:27S-29S, 1983. [A]

ATROPINE

Synonyms

Atropin Minims, Atropt, Cicloplegyl, Methylatropine Bromide, Mydriasine, Ocean-A/S, Steropine

Summary

Atropine is an anticholinergic alkaloid that is often used as a preanesthetic medication to reduce airway secretions. It is also employed in the treatment of gastrointestinal disorders, bronchial asthma, bradycardia, Parkinsonism, and organophosphorous insecticide poisoning.

Magnitude of Teratogenic Risk

None To Minimal

Quality and Quantity of Data

Fair

Comment

None

The frequency of congenital anomalies was no greater than expected among the children of 401 women treated with atropine during the first four lunar months of pregnancy or the children of 1198 women treated with this drug anytime during pregnancy in the Collaborative Perinatal Project (Heinonen et al., 1977). Similarly, congenital anomalies were observed no more often than expected among the infants of more than 50 women who took atropine during the first trimester of pregnancy in the Boston Collaborative Drug Surveillance Program (Jick et al., 1981).

The frequency of skeletal variations, but not of brain or visceral malformations, was increased among the offspring of mice treated once during pregnancy with atropine in doses about 1500 times those used clinically (Arcuri & Gautieri, 1973). Behavioral alterations have been observed among the offspring of rats treated during pregnancy with about four times the usual human dose of atropine (Watanabe et al., 1985). The relevance, if any, of these observations to the risks associated with therapeutic use of atropine in humans is unclear.

Key References

Arcuri PA, Gautieri RF: Morphine-induced fetal malformations. III: Possible mechanisms of action. J Pharm Sci 62:1626-1634, 1973. [A]

Heinonen OP, Slone D, Shapiro S: Birth Defects and Drugs in Pregnancy. Littleton, Mass.: John Wright-PSG, 1977, pp 346, 439. [E]

Jick H, Holmes LB, Hunter JR, Madsen S, et al.: First-trimester drug use and congenital disorders. JAMA 246:343-346, 1981. [S]

Watanabe T, Matsuhashi K, Takayama S: Study on the postnatal neurobehavioral development in rats treated prenatally with drugs acting on the autonomic nervous systems. Folia Pharmacol Japon 85:79-90, 1985. [A]

AURANOFIN

Synonyms

Ridaura

Summary

Auranofin is an orally administered gold compound used in the treatment of rheumatoid arthritis.

Magnitude of Teratogenic Risk

Undetermined

Quality and Quantity of Data

Poor

Comment

None

No epidemiological studies of congenital anomalies in the children of women treated with auranofin during pregnancy have been reported.

No teratogenic effect was apparent among the offspring of rats treated with 4-42 times the human dose of auranofin during pregnancy, but larger doses were toxic to the mothers and produced fetal loss (Szabo et al., 1978b). Frequencies of congenital anomalies and fetal loss were increased among the offspring of rabbits treated with 33-270 times the human dose of auranofin during pregnancy, but maternal toxicity also occurred (Szabo et al., 1978a). The effect of doses that were smaller but still several times greater than those used clinically was unclear. The relevance of these observations to the therapeutic use of auranofin in pregnant women is unknown.

Key References

Szabo KT, Difebbo ME, Phelan DG: The effects of gold-containing compounds on pregnant rabbits and their fetuses. Vet Pathol 15:97-102, 1978a. [A]

Szabo KT, Guerriero FJ, Kang YJ: The effects of gold-containing compounds on pregnant rats and their fetuses. Vet Pathol 15:89-96, 1978b. [A]

AUROTHIOGLUCOSE

Synonyms

Solganal

Summary

Aurothioglucose is a gold compound that is administered intramuscularly for treatment of rheumatic disorders.

Magnitude of Teratogenic Risk

Minimal

Quality and Quantity of Data

Poor To Fair

Comment

None

The frequency of congenital anomalies did not appear unusually high in one series of 119 infants born to women treated with aurothioglucose or aurothiomalate (a closely-related compound) during the first trimester of pregnancy (Miyamoto et al., 1974).

No animal teratology studies of aurothioglucose have been published.

Please see agent summary on gold sodium thiomalate for information on a closely related agent that has been studied.

Key References

Miyamoto T, Miyaji S, Horiuchi Y, Hara M, Ishihara K: Gold therapy in bronchial asthma--special emphasis upon blood level of gold and its teratogenicity. J Japan Soc Int Med 63:1190-1197, 1974. [S]

AUROTHIOGLYCANIDE

Summary

Aurothioglycanide is a gold compound used to treat rheumatoid arthritis.

Comment

None

Magnitude of Teratogenic Risk

Undetermined

Quality and Quantity of Data

None

Comment

None

No epidemiological studies of malformations in infants whose mothers took aurothioglycanide during embryonic development have been reported.

No animal teratology studies of aurothioglycanide have been published.

Please see agent summary on gold sodium thiomalate for information on a closely related drug which has been more thoroughly studied.

Key References

None available.

AZACITIDINE

Synonyms

AZA-CR, 5-Azacytidine, 5-AZC, Ladakamycin, Mylosar, NSC-102816

Summary

Azacitidine is an antineoplastic agent that inhibits pyrimidine synthesis. Azacytidine is given intravenously in the treatment of leukemia.

Magnitude of Teratogenic Risk

Undetermined

Quality and Quantity of Data

Poor To Fair

Comment

Studies in experimental animals and the pharmacological nature of this agent suggest that maternal treatment with azacitidine during early pregnancy is likely to pose a substantial teratogenic risk in humans.

No epidemiological studies of congenital anomalies among infants born to women treated with azacitidine during pregnancy have been reported.

Central nervous system, skeletal, and other malformations as well as fetal death occur with increased frequency among the offspring of mice and rats treated with azacitidine during pregnancy in doses well below those used therapeutically in humans (Seifertova et al., 1968; Schmahl et al., 1984; Takeuchi & Takeuchi, 1985; Matsuda, 1990; Rosen et al., 1990). The teratogenic effect shows typical dependency on dose and gestational age (Schmahl et al., 1984; Rosen et al., 1990). Behavioral alterations and an increased frequency of leukemia and other malignant neoplasms have been observed among the offspring of pregnant mice treated with azacitidine in doses lower than those used therapeutically in humans (Rodier et al., 1979; Schmahl et al., 1985).

Key References

Matsuda M: Comparison of the incidence of 5-azacytidine-induced exencephaly between MT/Hokldr and Slc:ICR mice. Teratology 41:147-154, 1990. [A]

Rodier PM, Reynolds SS, Roberts WN: Behavioral consequences of interference with CNS development in the early fetal period. Teratology 19:327-336, 1979. [A]

Rosen MB, House HS, Francis BM, Chernoff N: Teratogenicity of 5-azacytidine in the Sprague-Dawley rat. J Toxicol Environ Health 29:201-210, 1990. [A]

Schmahl W, Geber E, Lehmacher W: Diaplacental, carcinogenic effects of 5-azacytidine in NMRI-mice. Cancer Lett 27:81-90, 1985. [A]

Schmahl W, Torok P, Kriegel H: Embryotoxicity of 5-azacytidine in mice. Phase- and dose-specificity studies. Arch Toxicol 55:143-147, 1984. [A]

Seifertova M, Vesely J, Sorm F: Effect of 5-azacytidine on developing mouse embryo. Experientia 24:487-488, 1968. [A]

Takeuchi IK, Takeuchi YK: 5-Azacytidine-induced exencephaly in mice. J Anat 140(3):403-412, 1985. [A]

AZACONAZOLE

Synonyms

Madurox

Summary

Azaconazole is an antifungal agent.

Magnitude of Teratogenic Risk

Undetermined

Quality and Quantity of Data

None

Comment

None

No epidemiological studies of congenital anomalies in infants born to women who used azaconazole during pregnancy have been reported.

No animal teratology studies of azaconazole have been published.

Key References

None available.

AZATADINE

Synonyms

Azatadine Maleate, Optimine

Summary

Azatadine is an antihistamine used to treat allergic disorders.

Magnitude of Teratogenic Risk

Undetermined

Quality and Quantity of Data

None

Comment

None

No epidemiological studies of congenital anomalies in children born to women who took azatadine during pregnancy have been reported.

No animal teratology studies of azatadine have been published.

Key References

None available.

AZATHIOPRINE

Synonyms

Imuran

Summary

Azathioprine is a purine antimetabolite. It is used as an immunosuppressant in treatment of autoimmune diseases and in prevention of transplant rejection.

Magnitude of Teratogenic Risk

Minimal To Small

Quality and Quantity of Data

Poor To Fair

Comment

Serious or even fatal neonatal anemia, thrombocytopenia, and lymphopenia have been observed among the children of women treated with azathioprine during pregnancy (see below).

No controlled epidemiological studies of congenital anomalies in infants born to women treated with azathioprine during pregnancy have been reported. In two series of infants born to renal transplant recipients who had been treated with azathioprine and prednisone throughout pregnancy, the frequency of congenital anomalies was 4/44 (9%) and 7/110 (6.4%), respectively (Penn et al., 1980; Registration Committee of the European Dialysis and Transplant Association, 1980). No specificity was seen in the kinds of anomalies that occurred. It is difficult to know whether or not this rate of congenital anomalies is higher than expected because these mothers took other drugs besides azathioprine and often had azotemia. In more recent series of renal transplant recipients who were treated with azathioprine during pregnancy, none of 23 liveborn children in one group and none of 24 liveborn children in another had congenital anomalies (Brown et al., 1991). No congenital anomalies occurred among 14 infants of women treated with azathioprine during the first trimester of pregnancy for inflammatory bowel disease (Alstead et al., 1990).

The frequencies of prematurity and fetal growth retardation appear to be increased in pregnancies of renal transplant recipients treated with azathioprine, especially if the woman has reduced renal function, previous rejection, or requires high-dose immunosuppressive therapy (Penn et al., 1980; Registration Committee of the European Dialysis and

Transplant Association, 1980; Pirson et al., 1985; Marushak et al., 1986; Brown et al., 1991).

Increased frequencies of limb malformations, ocular anomalies, and cleft palate were observed among the offspring of rabbits treated with azathioprine in doses 1-2 times those used in humans (Tuchmann-Duplessis & Mercier-Parot, 1964). Similar anomalies were observed among the offspring of mice treated with azathioprine at 4-6 times the human therapeutic dose in one study (Rosenkrantz et al., 1967), but not another (Tuchmann-Duplessis & Mercier-Parot, 1964). The rate of malformations was not increased among the offspring of mice or rats treated during pregnancy with azathioprine in doses within the human therapeutic range or twice as great, but increased frequencies of fetal loss and growth retardation were regularly seen (Tuchmann-Duplessis & Mercier-Parot, 1964; Rosenkrantz et al., 1967; Scott, 1977; Fein et al., 1983).

Fatal neonatal anemia, thrombocytopenia, and lymphopenia have been reported in an infant born to a renal transplant recipient treated with azathioprine and prednisone during pregnancy (DeWitte et al., 1984). Neonatal lymphopenia and thrombocytopenia have been observed in several other children born to women who received similar therapy (Lower et al., 1971; Price et al., 1976; Rudolph et al., 1979; Penn, 1980; Davison et al., 1985). It seems likely that these hematologic abnormalities resulted from a toxic effect of azathioprine on the fetus similar to that which occasionally occurs with the drug in adults. This interpretation is supported by the fact that thymic hypoplasia and hematopoietic depression can be induced in the offspring of mice treated during pregnancy with azathioprine in doses that do not cause anemia in the mothers but are 2-6 times those used in humans (Rosenkrantz et al., 1967).

Increased frequencies of acquired chromosomal breaks and rearrangements have been observed in blood cells of renal transplant recipients receiving azathioprine therapy and, transiently, in the infants of women who were given such treatment during pregnancy (Sharon et al., 1974; Price et al., 1976). One case has also been reported of a child with two separate de novo constitutional chromosomal anomalies who was born to a woman treated before and during pregnancy with azathioprine and prednisone (Ostrer et al., 1984). These observations raise the possibility, but do not prove, that parental azathioprine treatment during gametogenesis may predispose to constitutional cytogenetic abnormalities in subsequently conceived children. If this does occur, it must be infrequent (Penn et al., 1980; Registration Committee of the European Dialysis and Transplant Association, 1980; Pirson et al., 1985).

Key References

Alstead EM, Ritchie JK, Lennard-Jones JE, et al.: Safety of azathioprine in pregnancy in inflammatory bowel disease. Gastroenterology 99:443-446, 1990. [S]

Brown JH, Maxwell AP, McGeown MG: Outcome of pregnancy following renal transplantation. Ir J Med Sci 160(8):255-256, 1991. [S]

Davison JM, Dellagrammatikas H, Parkin JM: Maternal azathioprine therapy and depressed haemopoiesis in the babies of renal allograft patients. Br J Obstet Gynaecol 92:233-239, 1985. [S]

DeWitte DB, Buick MK, Cyran SE, Maisels MJ: Neonatal pancytopenia and severe combined immunodeficiency associated with antenatal administration of azathioprine and prednisone. J Pediatr 105:625-628, 1984. [C]

Fein A, Gross A, Serr DM, Nebel L: Effect of Imuran on placental and fetal development in rats. Isr J Med Sci 19:73-75, 1983. [A]

Lower GD, Stevens LE, Najarian JS, Reemtsma K: Problems from immunosuppressives during pregnancy. Am J Obstet Gynecol 111:1120-1121, 1971. [C]

Marushak A, Weber T, Bock J, et al.: Pregnancy following kidney transplantation. Acta Obstet Gynecol Scand 65:557-559, 1986. [S]

Ostrer H, Stamberg J, Perinchief P: Two chromosome aberrations in the child of a woman with systemic lupus erythematosus treated with azathioprine and prednisone. Am J Med Genet 17:627-632, 1984. [C]

Penn I, Makowski EL, Harris P: Parenthood following renal transplantation. Kidney Int 18:221-233, 1980. [S]

Pirson Y, Van Lierde M, Ghysen J, Squifflet JP, et al.: Retardation of fetal growth in patients receiving immunosuppressive therapy. N Eng J Med 313:328, 1985. [O]

Price HV, Salaman JR, Laurence KM, Langmaid H: Immunosuppressive drugs and the foetus. Transplantation 21:294-298, 1976. [C]

Registration Committee of the European Dialysis and Transplant Association, 1980: Successful pregnancies in women treated by dialysis and kidney transplantation. Br J Obstet Gynaecol 87:839-845, 1980. [S]

Rosenkrantz JG, Githens JH, Cox SM, Kellum DL: Azathioprine (Imuran) and pregnancy. Am J Obstet Gynecol 97:387-394, 1967. [A]

Rudolph JE, Schweizer RT, Bartus SA: Pregnancy in renal transplant patients. Transplantation 27:26-29, 1979. [R]

Scott JR: Fetal growth retardation associated with maternal administration of immunosuppressive drugs. Am J Obstet Gynecol 128:668-676, 1977. [A]

Sharon E, Jones J, Diamond H, Kaplan D: Pregnancy and azathioprine in systemic lupus erythematosus. Am J Obstet Gyn 118:25-28, 1974. [C]

Tuchmann-Duplessis H, Mercier-Parot L: [Teratogenic tests. Difference of reaction of three animal species to an antitumoral agent.] C R Soc Biol 158:1984-1990, 1964. [A]

AZLOCILLIN

Synonyms

Azlin, Monosodium Azlocillin, Securopen, Sodium Azlocillin

Summary

Azlocillin is a semisynthetic derivative of penicillin. It is used parenterally as a broad-spectrum antibiotic.

Magnitude of Teratogenic Risk

Undetermined

Quality and Quantity of Data

None

Comment

A small risk cannot be excluded, but a high risk of congenital anomalies in the children of women treated with azlocillin during pregnancy is unlikely.

No epidemiological studies of congenital anomalies among infants born to women treated with azlocillin during pregnancy have been reported.

No animal teratology studies of azlocillin have been published.

Please see agent summary on penicillin for information on a related agent that has been more thoroughly studied.

Key References

None available.

BACAMPICILLIN

Synonyms

Albaxin, Ambacamp, Ambaxin, Ambaxino, Amplibac, Bacacil, Carampicillin, Penglobe, Spectrobid, Velbacil

Summary

Bacampicillin is an antibiotic used orally in the treatment of bacterial infections. Bacampicillin is rapidly converted to ampicillin in the body.

Magnitude of Teratogenic Risk

Undetermined

Quality and Quantity of Data

None To Poor

Comment

A small risk cannot be excluded, but a high risk of congenital anomalies in the children of women treated with bacampicillin during pregnancy is unlikely.

No epidemiological studies of congenital anomalies among infants born to women treated with bacampicillin during pregnancy have been reported.

No teratogenic effect was observed among the offspring of rats treated during pregnancy with bacampicillin in doses 1-62 times those used in humans (Noguchi & Ohwaki, 1979). The frequency of malformations was not increased among the offspring of pregnant rabbits treated with 1-5 times the human dose of bacampicillin, but fetal death occurred at 2-5 times the human dose and maternal death at 5 times the human dose (Noguchi & Ohwaki, 1979).

Please see agent summary on ampicillin for information on a closely related agent that has been more thoroughly studied.

Key References

Noguchi Y, Ohwaki Y: Reproductive and teratologic studies of bacampicillin hydrochloride in rats and rabbits. Chemotherapy (Tokyo) (Nippon Kagaku Ryoho Gakkai Zasshyi) 27(Suppl 4):30-35, 1979. [A]

BACITRACIN

Synonyms

Baciguent, Bacitin

Summary

Bacitracin is a polypeptide produced by a lichenform Bacillus subtilis. It is used topically on skin or in the eye to treat susceptible infections.

Magnitude of Teratogenic Risk

Undetermined

Quality and Quantity of Data

None

Comment

None

No epidemiological studies of infants born after maternal bacitracin exposure during pregnancy have been published.

There is no published information regarding the offspring of experimental animals treated with bacitracin during pregnancy.

Key References

None available.

BARIUM

Synonyms

Barii Sulphidum, Baryta Sulphureta, Sulphurated Baryta

Summary

Barium is used as a contrast medium in diagnostic radiographic procedures involving the alimentary tract. It is not absorbed from the gastrointestinal tract. Soluble barium salts and elemental barium are toxic.

Magnitude of Teratogenic Risk

Undetermined

Quality and Quantity of Data

None

Comment

None

No epidemiological studies of congenital anomalies in infants whose mothers either took barium for a radiographic investigation or exhibited barium toxicity during pregnancy have been reported.

No animal teratology studies of barium have been published.

Key References

None available.

BCG VACCINE

Synonyms

Antigen Alpha, Antigen MbaA, Bacillus Calmette-Guerin, BCG, Bromcresol Green, Thera-Cys, Tice

Summary

BCG vaccine contains living Mycobacteria bovis. It is given percutaneously to elicit immunity to tuberculosis.

Magnitude of Teratogenic Risk

Undetermined

Quality and Quantity of Data

None

Comment

A small risk cannot be excluded, but a high risk of congenital anomalies in the children of women treated with BCG vaccine during pregnancy is unlikely.

No epidemiological studies of congenital anomalies among infants born to women immunized with BCG vaccine during pregnancy have been reported.

No animal teratology studies of BCG vaccine have been published.

Key References

None available.

BECLOMETHASONE

Synonyms

Aldecin, Becloforte, Beclovent, Beconase, Becotide, Propaderm

Summary

Beclomethasone is a synthetic glucocorticoid used topically to treat skin disorders and by inhalation in the prevention and therapy of asthma.

Magnitude of Teratogenic Risk

None To Minimal

Quality and Quantity of Data

Poor To Fair

Comment

None

The frequency of malformations was not obviously increased among a series of 42 children born to women who used beclomethasone throughout pregnancy or beginning in the first trimester for treatment of asthma (Greenberger & Patterson, 1983).

Beclomethasone, when administered to pregnant mice in doses 7 or more times greater than those used in humans, produces an increased frequency of cleft palate in the offspring (Nomura et al., 1977; Tamagawa et al., 1982). No such effect was seen with lower doses, but a typical dose-dependent response occurred with higher doses (Esaki et al., 1976; Furuhashi et al., 1977). Similar results have been observed in rabbits (Furuhashi et al., 1977). No malformations were observed among the offspring of seven rhesus monkeys treated with 4-17 times the usual human dose of beclomethasone during pregnancy, although severe growth retardation was seen in one animal and fetal demise in another (Tanioka, 1976). The relevance of these findings to the therapeutic use of beclomethasone in human pregnancy is unknown.

Key References

Esaki K, Izumiyama K, Yasuda Y: [Effects of the inhalant administration of beclomethasone dipropionate on reproduction in mice. 2. Administration during the fetal organogenesis stage]. Jitchuken Zenrinsho Kenkyuho 2:213-222, 1976. [A]

Furuhashi T, Nomura A, Hasegawa T, Nakazawa M: [Teratological studies on beclomethasone dipropionate. 1. Teratogenicity in rabbits by oral administration]. Oyo Yakuri (Pharmacometrics) 13:71-77, 1977. [A]

Greenberger PA, Patterson R: Beclomethasone diproprionate for severe asthma during pregnancy. Ann Intern Med 98:478-480, 1983. [S]

Nomura A, Furuhashi T, Nakazawa M: [Teratological studies on beclomethasone dipropionate. IV. Teratogenicity in mice by inhalation]. Oyo Yakuri (Pharmacometrics) 13:195-204, 1977. [A]

Tamagawa M, Hatori M, Ooi A, Nishioeda R, et al.: [Comparative teratological study of flunisolide in mice]. Oyo Yakuri (Pharmacometrics) 24:741-750, 1982. [A]

Tanioka Y: [Teratogenicity test on beclomethasone dipropionate by inhalation in rhesus monkeys]. Jitchuken Zenrinsho Kenkyuho 2:155-164, 1976. [A]

BELLADONNA

Synonyms

Atrobel, Bellafit, Bellafolin, Deadly Nightshade, Death's Herb, Locus Purgat, Tremoforat

Summary

Belladonna is a mixture of plant alkaloids with anticholinergic actions. It is used to prevent smooth muscle spasm, especially in intestinal and biliary colic.

Magnitude of Teratogenic Risk

Minimal

Quality and Quantity of Data

Poor To Fair

Comment

None

A very weak but statistically significant association was observed between congenital anomalies and maternal use of belladonna among the infants of 554 women who took this drug during the first four lunar months of pregnancy in the Collaborative Perinatal Project (Heinonen et al., 1977). This association was almost entirely due to minor anomalies. The frequency of congenital anomalies was no greater than expected among the children of 1355 women who took belladonna anytime during pregnancy. If maternal belladonna use early in pregnancy does increase the risk of congenital aberrations in an infant, the added risk (primarily for minor anomalies) is unlikely to be more than 3%.

No teratology studies of belladonna in experimental animals have been published.

Key References

Heinonen OP, Slone D, Shapiro S: Birth Defects and Drugs in Pregnancy. Littleton, Mass.: John Wright-PSG, 1977, pp 439, 477, 492. [E]

BENDECTIN

Summary

Bendectin is a fixed combination of doxylamine (an antihistamine) and pyridoxine used in the treatment of nausea and vomiting of pregnancy. Bendectin is no longer available in the United States, although its components can be purchased without a prescription.

Magnitude of Teratogenic Risk

None

Quality and Quantity of Data

Excellent

Comment

None

Extensive epidemiological studies provide no evidence that maternal Bendectin use during pregnancy measurably alters the risk of congenital anomalies in an infant (MacMahon, 1982; Cordero & Oakley, 1983; Holmes, 1983; Sheffield & Batagol, 1985). Several cohort studies, each involving several hundred to more than 2700 babies born to women treated with Bendectin during the first trimester of pregnancy, have not shown any consistent association with major congenital malformations (Milkovich & van den Berg, 1976, Shapiro et al., 1977; Fleming et al., 1981; Gibson et al., 1981; Jick et al., 1981; Morelock et al., 1982; Michaelis et al., 1983; Aselton et al., 1985; Shiono & Klebanoff, 1989). Case-control studies involving hundreds of affected infants provide no consistent indication that maternal use of Bendectin during the first trimester of pregnancy increases the risk of congenital heart disease, oral clefts, limb reduction defects, or pyloric stenosis (Rothman et al., 1979; Cordero et al., 1981; Mitchell et al., 1981, 1983; Eskenazi

& Bracken, 1982; Aselton et al., 1984; McCredie et al., 1984; Elbourne et al., 1985; Zierler & Rothman, 1985; Adams et al., 1989). The data indicate, with high likelihood, that if maternal use of Bendectin early in pregnancy does cause birth defects in the offspring, the risk is much less than 1% and is small compared to the "background" risk of birth defects which accompanies every pregnancy.

The frequency of malformations was no greater than expected among the offspring of cynomolgus monkeys, rhesus monkeys, or baboons treated with Bendectin during pregnancy in doses respectively 2-40, 10-40, and 1-10 times those used in humans (Hendrickx et al., 1985a, b). Transiently delayed closure of the muscular ventricular septum was seen in midgestation in all three species, but this effect was not dose-related, and these anomalies were not apparent at term. The frequency of malformations was no greater than expected among the offspring of rats treated during pregnancy with 125-310 times the usual human dose of Bendectin; a slight increase in the frequency of skeletal malformations was observed among the offspring of pregnant rats treated with 500 times the human dose, but this also caused substantial maternal toxicity and mortality (Tyl et al., 1988). No significant teratogenic effect was observed among the offspring of rats or rabbits treated with Bendectin in doses 8-80 times those used clinically (Gibson et al., 1968). In light of the extensive epidemiological and whole animal teratology research that has been done on Bendectin, the demonstration of effects with this drug in some in vitro teratology and mutagenicity studies is irrelevant to the estimation of teratogenic risks in humans.

Key References

Adams MM, Mulinare J, Dooley K: Risk factors for conotruncal cardiac defects in Atlanta. J Am Coll Cardiol 14(2):432-442, 1989. [E]

Aselton P, Jick H, Milunsky A, Hunter JR, et al.: First-trimester drug use and congenital disorders. Obstet Gynecol 65:451-455, 1985. [S]

Aselton P, Jick H, Chentow SJ, Perera DR, et al.: Pyloric stenosis and maternal Bendectin exposure. Am J Epidemiol 120:251-256, 1984. [E]

Cordero JF, Oakley GP: Drug exposure during pregnancy: Some epidemiologic considerations. Clin Obstet Gynecol 26:418-428, 1983. [R]

Cordero JF, Oakley GP, Greenberg F, James LM: Is Bendectin a teratogen? JAMA 245:2307-2310, 1981. [E]

Elbourne D, Mutch L: Debendox revisited. Br J Obstet Gynecol 92:780-785, 1985. [E]

Eskenazi B, Bracken MB: Bendectin (debendox) as a risk factor for pyloric stenosis. Am J Obstet Gynecol 144:919-924, 1982. [E]

Fleming DM, Knox JDE, Crombie DL: Debendox in early pregnancy and fetal malformation. Br Med J 283:99-101, 1981. [E]

Gibson GT, Colley DP, McMichael AJ, Hartshorne JM: Congenital anomalies in relation to the use of doxylamine/dicyclomine and other antenatal factors. An ongoing prospective study. Med J Aust 1:410-414, 1981. [E]

Gibson JP, Staples RE, Larson EJ, Kuhn WL, et al.: Teratology and reproduction studies with an antinauseant. Toxicol Appl Pharmacol 13:439-447, 1968. [A]

Hendrickx AG, Cukierski M, Prahalada S, Janos G, et al.: Evaluation of Bendectin embryotoxicity in nonhuman primates: I. Ventricular septal defects in prenatal macaques and baboon. Teratology 32:179-189, 1985a. [A]

Hendrickx AG, Cukierski M, Prahalada S, Janos G, et al.: Evaluation of Bendectin embryotoxicity in nonhuman primates: II. Double-blind study in term cynomolgus monkeys. Teratology 32:191-194, 1985b. [A]

Holmes LB: Teratogen update: Bendectin. Teratology 27:277-281, 1983. [R]

Jick H, Holmes LB, Hunter JR, Madsen S, et al.: First-trimester drug use and congenital disorders. JAMA 246:343-346, 1981. [S]

MacMahon B: More on Bendectin. JAMA 246:371-372, 1982. [R]

McCredie J, Kricker A, Elliott J, Forrest J: The innocent bystander: Doxylamine/dicyclomine/pyridoxine and congenital limb defects. Med J Aust 141:546-547, 1984. [E]

Michaelis J, Michaelis H, Gluck E, Koller S: Prospective study of suspected associations between certain drugs administered during early pregnancy and congenital malformations. Teratology 27:57-64, 1983. [E]

Milkovich L, van den Berg BJ: An evaluation of the teratogenicity of certain antinauseant drugs. Am J Obstet Gynecol 125:244-248, 1976. [E]

Mitchell AA, Rosenberg L, Shapiro S, Slone D: Birth defects related to Bendectin use in pregnancy. JAMA 245:2311-2314, 1981. [E]

Mitchell AA, Schwingle PJ, Rosenberg L, Louik C, et al.: Birth defects in relation to Bendectin use in pregnancy. Am J Obstet Gynecol 147:737-742, 1983. [E]

Morelock S, Hingson R, Kayne H, Dooling E, et al.: Bendectin and fetal development. Am J Obstet Gynecol 142:209-213, 1982. [E]

Rothman KJ, Fyler DC, Goldblatt A, Kreidberg MB: Exogenous hormones and other drug exposures of children with congenital heart disease. Am J Epidemiol 109:433-439, 1979. [E]

Shapiro S, Heinonen OP, Siskind V, Kaufman DW, et al.: Antenatal exposure to doxylamine succinate and dicyclomine hydrochloride (Bendectin) in relation to congenital malformations, perinatal mortality rate, birth weight, and intelligence quotient score. Am J Obstet Gynecol 128:480-485, 1977. [E]

Sheffield LJ, Batagol R: The creation of therapeutic orphans--or, what have we learnt from the debendox fiasco? Med J Aust 143:143-147, 1985. [R]

Shiono PH, Klebanoff MA: Bendectin and human congenital malformations. Teratology 40:151-155, 1989. [E]

Tyl RW, Price CJ, Marr MC, Kimmel CA: Developmental toxicity evaluation of Bendectin in CD rats. Teratology 37:539-552, 1988. [A]

Zierler S, Rothman KJ: Congenital heart disease in relation to maternal use of Bendectin and other drugs in early pregnancy. N Engl J Med 313:347-352, 1985. [E]

BENDROFLUMETH-IAZIDE

Synonyms

Aprinox, Berkozide, Centyl, Naturetin, Nco-NaClex

Summary

Bendroflumethiazide is an oral thiazide diuretic used to treat hypertension and edema.

Magnitude of Teratogenic Risk

Undetermined

Quality and Quantity of Data

Poor

Comment

None

The frequency of congenital anomalies was not increased among the infants of 1156 women treated with bendroflumethiazide anytime during pregnancy in the Collaborative Perinatal Project (Heinonen et al., 1977). Only 13 of these women were treated during the first four lunar months of pregnancy. The frequencies of congenital anomalies, stillbirths, and neonatal deaths were no greater than expected among the children of 1011 women treated with bendroflumethiazide after the thirtieth week of pregnancy in a controlled trial of diuretic therapy in the prevention of preeclampsia (Cuadros & Tatum, 1964). This study is difficult to interpret, however, because the incidence of congenital anomalies was <1% in both the treated and untreated groups, suggesting substantial underascertainment of anomalies.

No teratogenic effect was observed among the offspring of rats treated with 310 times the human therapeutic dose of bendroflumethiazide during pregnancy (Stevens et al., 1984).

Please see agent summary on chlorothiazide for information on a closely related agent that has been more thoroughly studied.

Key References

Cuadros A, Tatum HJ: The prophylactic and therapeutic use of bendroflumethiazide in pregnancy. Am J Obstet Gynecol 89:891-897, 1964. [E]

Heinonen OP, Slonc D, Shapiro S: Birth Defects and Drugs in Pregnancy. Littleton, Mass.: John Wright-PSG, 1977, pp 372, 441, 495. [E]

Stevens AC, Keysser CH, Kulesza JS, et al.: Preclinical safety evaluation of the nadolol/bendroflumethiazide combination in mice, rats, and dogs. Fundam Appl Toxicol 4:360-369, 1984. [A]

BENOMYL

Synonyms

Benlate, Methyl-1-(Butylcarbamoyl)

Summary

Benomyl is a benzimidazole carbamate that is widely used in agriculture and home gardening as a fungicide. Benomyl is also used as an antihelmintic in veterinary medicine. The Threshold Limit Value for occupational exposure to benomyl is 10 mg/cu m as an 8-hour time-weighted average (Hathaway et al., 1991).

Magnitude of Teratogenic Risk

Undetermined

Quality and Quantity of Data

Poor

Comment

A small risk cannot be excluded, but a high risk of congenital anomalies in the children of women with usual exposures to benomyl during pregnancy is unlikely.

No epidemiological studies of congenital anomalies among infants born to women treated with benomyl during pregnancy have been reported.

Increased frequencies of fetal death and congenital anomalies were observed among the offspring of rats and mice treated during pregnancy with benomyl in doses of 31.2-250 mg/kg/d or 200 mg/kg/d (Shtenberg & Torchinskii, 1977; Kavlock et al., 1982; Zeman et al., 1986; Ellis et al., 1987, 1988;

Hoogenboom et al., 1991). Central nervous system, ocular, and facial anomalies were frequently seen, and the teratogenic effect exhibited typical dose dependence.

Key References

Ellis WG, De Roos F, Kavlock RJ, Zeman FJ: Relationship of periventricular overgrowth to hydrocephalus in brains of fetal rats exposed to benomyl. Teratogenesis Carcinog Mutagen 8:377-391, 1988. [A]

Ellis WG, Semple JL, Hoogenboom ER, et al.: Benomyl-induced craniocerebral anomalies in fetuses of adequately nourished and protein-deprived rats. Teratog Carcinog Mutagen 7:357-375, 1987. [A]

Hathaway GJ, Proctor NH, Hughes JP, Fischman ML (eds): Proctor and Hughes' Chemical Hazards of the Workplace, 3rd ed. New York: Van Nostrand Reinhold, 1991, pp 102-103. [R]

Hoogenboom ER, Ransdell JF, Ellis WG, et al.: Effects on the fetal rat eye of maternal benomyl exposure and protein malnutrition. Curr Eye Res 10:601-612, 1991. [A]

Kavlock RJ, Chernoff N, Gray LE, et al.: Teratogenic effects of benomyl in the Wistar rat and CD-1 mouse, with emphasis on the route of administration. Toxicol Appl Pharmacol 62:44-54, 1982. [A]

Shtenberg AI, Torchinskii AM: Adaptation to the action of some teratogens following administration of pesticides during pregnancy. Bull Exp Biol Med 83:247-249, 1977. [A]

Zeman FJ, Hoogenboom ER, Kavlock RJ, et al.: Effects on the fetus of maternal benomyl exposure in the protein-deprived rat. J Toxicol Environ Health 17:405-417, 1986. [A]

BENOXINATE

Synonyms

Alcon Opulets Benoxinate, Dorsacaine, Oxibuprocaine Chloride, Oxibuprokain Minims

Summary

Benoxinate is a surface anesthetic of the ester class that is used in ophthalmology.

Magnitude of Teratogenic Risk

Undetermined

Quality and Quantity of Data

None

Comment

A small risk cannot be excluded, but there is no indication that the risk of congenital anomalies in the children of women treated with benoxinate during pregnancy is likely to be great.

No epidemiological studies of congenital anomalies in children born to women exposed to benoxinate during pregnancy have been reported.

No investigations of teratologic effects of benoxinate in experimental animals have been published.

Please see agent summary on procaine for information on a related agent that has been studied.

Key References

None available.

BENZALKONIUM SALTS

Synonyms

Germitol, Pentalcol, Roccal, Sabol, Zephiran

Summary

Benzalkonium salts are quaternary ammonium cationic surfactants widely used as disinfectants. Benzalkonium salts are employed in cleaning wounds, skin, and mucous membranes, in shampoos for seborrheic dermatitis, in throat lozenges, and in creams for diaper rash. Creams containing benzalkonium salts are also used as vaginal spermicides.

Magnitude of Teratogenic Risk

None To Minimal

Quality and Quantity of Data

Poor To Fair

Comment

None

The frequency of congenital anomalies was not increased among the children of 50 women treated topically with benzalkonium salts during the first four lunar months of pregnancy in the Collaborative Perinatal Project (Heinonen et al., 1977).

A dose-related increase in the frequency of embryonic or fetal death was observed among pregnant rats treated vaginally with 50-200 mg/kg of benzalkonium salts prior to implantation (Buttar, 1985); the effective dose was estimated to be about 143 times that used for vaginal contraception in women. No such effect was noted after treatment with 25 mg/kg. The frequency of malformations among the offspring was not increased at any of the doses tested. The frequency of malformations was no greater than expected among the offspring of pregnant mice fed 0.001-0.05 mg/kg/d of benzalkonium throughout pregnancy or 3-30 mg/kg/d prior to and during implantation (Momma et al., 1987).

Key References

Buttar HS: Embryotoxicity of benzalkonium chloride in vaginally treated rats. J Appl Toxicol 5:398-401, 1985. [A]

Heinonen OP, Slone D, Shapiro S: Birth Defects and Drugs in Pregnancy. Littleton, Mass.: John Wright-PSG, 1977, pp 300, 302. [E]

Momma J, Takada K, Aida Y, et al.: Effects of benzalkonium chloride on pregnant mice. Eisei Shikenjo Hokoku 105:20-25, 1987. [A]

BENZAMINE

Synonyms

Betacaine, Beta-Eucaine, Eucaine

Summary

Benzamine is a local anesthetic that has been used topically.

Magnitude of Teratogenic Risk

Undetermined

Quality and Quantity of Data

None

Comment

None

No epidemiological studies of congenital anomalies in children born to women exposed to benzamine during pregnancy have been reported.

No investigations of teratologic effects of benzamine in experimental animals have been published.

Key References

None available.

BENZENE

Synonyms

Benzol, Cyclohexatriene, Phenyl Hydride

Summary

Benzene is a hydrocarbon used widely as an industrial solvent (Marcus, 1987). Benzene has also been employed medicinally as a pediculicide. Benzene is readily absorbed through the skin, gastrointestinal tract, and lungs. The 8-hour time-weighted average occupational exposure limit for benzene in air is 0.1 ppm (Hathaway et al., 1991).

Magnitude of Teratogenic Risk

None To Minimal

Quality and Quantity of Data

Poor

Comment

None

Epidemiological studies of congenital anomalies and maternal occupational or environmental exposures to agents such as benzene are difficult to interpret (Taskinen, 1990; Kallen, 1988). Case-control studies generally depend on inferences about past exposures made on the basis of occupation or questionnaire. Cohort studies usually define "exposed" and "unexposed" groups on the basis of occupation or residence without evidence regarding whether, to what extent, or at what time in pregnancy the mothers of affected infants actually were exposed to the agent. Both kinds of studies may be confounded by exposure to other agents in the same occupational or environmental setting as well as by the usual demographic, socioeconomic, and personal factors that may affect any reproductive epidemiology investigation. Thus, both "positive" and "negative" studies need to be interpreted very cautiously.

In a cohort study of university laboratory employees, the frequency of miscarriage among 41 pregnancies in women exposed to benzene during the first trimester was no greater than expected (Axelsson et al., 1984). A slightly increased rate of employment during pregnancy in occupations associated with benzene exposure was observed among the mothers of 2096 stillborn infants (OR=1.3, 95% CI 1.0-1.8) in one case-control study (Savitz et al., 1989). No association with prematurity or low birth weight was seen.

The teratogenicity of benzene has been well studied in mice, rats, and rabbits

(Chatburn et al., 1981; Ungvary & Tatrai, 1985; Schreiner, 1983; ATSDR, 1987). Fetal death and delayed ossification have consistently been demonstrated after maternal exposure to benzene fumes in doses that are maternally toxic and many times greater than the maximum permissible level of human exposure. There is no convincing evidence of an increased frequency of malformations even at such high exposure levels. Increased frequencies of jaw and palatal defects have been observed among the offspring of mice injected once with 3 ml/kg of benzene during pregnancy; this treatment also produced depression of the white blood cell counts in the mothers (Watanabe & Yoshida, 1970). Alterations of hematopoiesis have been observed among the offspring of pregnant mice exposed to 5-20 ppm of benzene in air (Keller & Snyder, 1988).

Several studies have demonstrated an increased frequency of acquired chromosomal abnormalities in the white blood cells of people who have suffered benzene toxicity or were exposed occupationally for many years to high levels (in excess of the current maximum permissible level of exposure) (Barlow & Sullivan, 1982; Haas & Schottenfeld, 1979; Sasiadek, 1992). In one study, an increased frequency of acquired lymphocyte cytogenetic abnormalities was seen in a group of 14 children whose mothers had been chronically exposed to benzene and other organic solvents (Funes-Cravioto et al., 1977). The relevance of acquired somatic cytogenetic aberrations to the risk of malformations or any other disease is unknown.

Key References

ATSDR (Agency for Toxic Substances and Disease Registry): Toxicological Profile for Benzene. Oak Ridge: Oak Ridge National Laboratory, 1987. [R]

Axelsson G, Lutz C, Rylander R: Exposure to solvents and outcome of pregnancy in university laboratory employees. Br J Ind Med 41:305-312, 1984. [E]

Barlow SM, Sullivan FM: Reproductive Hazards of Industrial Chemicals. New York: Academic Press, 1982, pp 83-103. [R]

Chatburn G, Sharratt M, Wickramaratne GA: Chemical industries association/institute of petroleum joint committee on benzene: Reports of task forces on toxicology and teratology of benzene. II. Reproductive effects, embryotoxicity, and teratology of benzene. Regul Toxicol Pharmacol 1:205-210, 1981. [R]

Funes-Cravioto F, Kolmodin-Hedman B, Lindsten J, Nordenskjold M, et al.: Chromosome aberrations and sister-chromatid exchange in workers in chemical laboratories and a rotoprinting factory and in children of women laboratory workers. Lancet 2:322-325, 1977. [E]

Haas JF, Schottenfeld D: Risks to the offspring from parental occupational exposures. J Occup Med 21:607-613, 1979. [R]

Hathaway GJ, Proctor NH, Hughes JP, Fischman ML (eds): Proctor and Hughes' Chemical Hazards of the Workplace, 3rd ed. New York: Van Nostrand Reinhold, 1991, p 103. [R]

Kallen B: Epidemiology of Human Reproduction. Boca Raton: CRC Press, 1988, pp 157-170. [R]

Keller KA, Snyder CA: Mice exposed in utero to 20 ppm benzene exhibit altered numbers of recognizable hematopoietic cells up to seven weeks after exposure. Fundam Appl Toxicol 10:224-232, 1988. [A]

Marcus WL: Chemical of current interest--benzene. Toxicol Ind Health 3:205-266, 1987. [R]

Sasiadek M: Nonrandom distribution of breakpoints in the karyotypes of workers occupationally exposed to benzene. Environ Health Perspect 97:255-257, 1992. [E]

Savitz DA, Whelan EA, Kleckner RC: Effect of parents' occupational exposures on risk of stillbirth, preterm delivery, and small-for-gestational-age infants. Am J Epidemiol 129(6):1201-1218, 1989. [E]

Schreiner CA: Petroleum and petroleum products: A brief review of studies to evaluate reproductive effects. Adv Mod Environ Toxicol 3:29-45, 1983. [R]

Taskinen HK: Effects of parental occupational exposures on spontaneous abortion and congenital malformation. Scand J Work Environ Health 16:297-314, 1990. [R]

Ungvary G, Tatrai E: On the embryotoxic effects of benzene and its alkyl derivatives in mice, rats and rabbits. Arch Toxicol 8(Suppl):425-430, 1985. [A]

Watanabe G-I, Yoshida S: The teratogenic effect of benzene in pregnant mice. Acta Medica et Biologica 17(4):285-291, 1970. [A]

BENZOCAINE

Synonyms

Americaine, Anaesthesin, Anaesthesinum, Baby Anbesol, Hurricaine, Orajel Mouth-Aid, Topicaine

Summary

Benzocaine is a topical anesthetic of the amide class.

Magnitude of Teratogenic Risk

None To Minimal

Quality and Quantity of Data

Poor

Comment

A small risk cannot be excluded, but there is no indication that the risk of congenital anomalies in the children of women treated with benzocaine during pregnancy is likely to be great.

The frequency of congenital anomalies was not significantly greater than expected among the children of 47 women treated with benzocaine during the first four lunar months of pregnancy or among the children of 238 women treated any time during pregnancy in the Collaborative Perinatal Project (Heinonen et al., 1977).

No investigations of teratologic effects of benzocaine in experimental animals have been published.

Please see agent summary on lidocaine for information on a related agent that has been more thoroughly studied.

Key References

Heinonen OP, Slone D, Shapiro S: Birth Defects and Drugs in Pregnancy. Littleton, Mass.: John Wright-PSG, 1977, pp 358, 360, 440. [E]

BENZONATATE

Synonyms

Exangit, Tesalon, Tessalin, Tessalon, Ventussin

Summary

Benzonatate is used as a cough suppressant.

Magnitude of Teratogenic Risk

Undetermined

Quality and Quantity of Data

None

Comment

None

No epidemiological studies of congenital anomalies in infants born to women treated with benzonatate during pregnancy have been reported.

No animal teratology studies of benzonatate have been published.

Key References

None available.

BENZOYL PEROXIDE

Synonyms

Acetoxyl, Acnegel, Benoxyl, Benzagel, Clearasil Acne Treatment, Dry and Clear, Fostex BPO, Lucidol, Teen, Theraderm, Topex

Summary

Benzoyl peroxide is a keratolytic agent used topically in the treatment of acne. Benzoyl peroxide is absorbed by the skin which metabolizes the drug to benzoate. Benzoyl peroxide is also used in the food and plastics industries. The eight-hour time-weighted average occupational exposure limit for benzoyl peroxide is 5 mg/cu m (ACGIH, 1991).

Magnitude of Teratogenic Risk

Undetermined

Quality and Quantity of Data

None

Comment

A small risk cannot be excluded, but a high risk of congenital anomalies in the children of women treated with benzoyl peroxide during pregnancy is unlikely.

No epidemiological studies of congenital anomalies among infants born to women who used benzoyl peroxide during pregnancy have been reported.

No animal teratology studies of benzoyl peroxide have been published.

Key References

ACGIH: 1991-1992 Threshold Limit Values for Chemical Substances and Physical Agents and Biological Exposure Indices. Cincinnati, Ohio: Am Conference Govt Ind Hyg, 1991, p 13. [O]

BENZPHETAMINE

Synonyms

Benzfetamine, Benzofetamina, Didrex, Inapetyl

Summary

Benzphetamine is a sympathomimetic amine that is used as an appetite suppressant.

Magnitude of Teratogenic Risk

Undetermined

Quality and Quantity of Data

None

Comment

None

No epidemiological studies of congenital anomalies in infants born to women treated with benzphetamine during pregnancy have been reported.

No animal teratology studies of benzphetamine have been published.

Please see dextroamphetamine agent summary for information on a related agent that has been studied.

Key References

None available.

BENZTHIAZIDE

Synonyms

Aquatag, Diucene, Edemex, Exna, Exosalt, Fovane, Freeuril, Proaqua, Regulon

Summary

Benzthiazide is a thiazide diuretic. It is used orally in the treatment of edema and hypertension.

Magnitude of Teratogenic Risk

Undetermined

Quality and Quantity of Data

None

Comment

A small risk cannot be excluded, but a high risk of congenital anomalies in the children of women treated with benzthiazide during pregnancy is unlikely.

No epidemiological studies of congenital anomalies in infants born to women treated with benzthiazide during pregnancy have been reported.

No animal teratology studies of benzthiazide have been published.

Please see agent summaries on chlorothiazide and hydrochlorothiazide for information on related agents that have been studied.

Key References

None available.

BENZTROPINE

Synonyms

Bensylate, Benzatropine Mesylate, Cogentin

Summary

Benztropine is an anticholinergic with antihistaminic, local anesthetic, and sedative properties. It is used to treat Parkinsonism and similar neurological disorders.

Magnitude of Teratogenic Risk

Undetermined

Quality and Quantity of Data

None To Poor

Comment

None

No epidemiological studies of malformations in infants born to women treated with benztropine during pregnancy have been reported.

No animal teratology studies of benztropine have been published.

The "small left colon syndrome" (decreased intestinal motility, abdominal distension, vomiting, and failure to pass meconium) has been reported in two newborn infants whose mothers had been treated late in pregnancy with benztropine and other psychotropic drugs (Falterman & Richardson, 1980). Both children did well after the meconium obstruction was relieved by enema.

Key References

Falterman CG, Richardson CJ: Small left colon syndrome associated with maternal ingestion of psychotropic drugs. J Pediatr 92:308-310, 1980. [C]

BENZYL BENZOATE

Synonyms

Ascabiol, Benzemul, Scabanca

Summary

Benzyl benzoate is used topically as an insect repellent and as an insecticide to treat mite and lice infestations. Benzyl benzoate is also used as a solubilizing agent in foods and injectable medications.

Magnitude of Teratogenic Risk

Undetermined

Quality and Quantity of Data

None To Poor

Comment

A small risk cannot be excluded, but there is no indication that the risk of congenital anomalies in the children of women treated with benzyl benzoate during pregnancy is likely to be great.

No epidemiological studies of congenital anomalies in infants whose mothers were exposed to benzyl benzoate during pregnancy have been reported.

No teratogenic effect was observed in the offspring of pregnant rats or mice that had been given 5-130 or 60 times the World Health Organization acceptable daily intake of benzyl benzoate for humans (Morita et al., 1981; Eibs et al., 1982).

Key References

Eibs HG, Spielmann H, Hagele M: Teratogenic effects of cyproterone acetate and medroxyprogesterone treatment during the pre- and postimplantation period of mouse embryos. I. Teratology 25:27-36, 1982. [A]

Morita S, Yamada A, Ohgaki S, Noda T, et al.: Safety evaluation of chemicals for use in household products (II). Teratological studies on benzyl benzoate and 2-(Morpholinothio)-benzothiazole in rats. Annu Rep Osaka City Inst Publ Health Environ Sci 43:90-97, 1981. [A]

BETAMETHASONE

Synonyms

Alphatrex, Beben, Benisone, Betacort, Betaderm, Betatrex, Betnovate, Celestoderm, Diprolene, Diprosone, Ectosone, Metaderm, Novobetamet, Valisone

Summary

Betamethasone is a synthetic glucocorticoid used to treat inflammatory and allergic disorders.

Magnitude of Teratogenic Risk

Undetermined

Quality and Quantity of Data

Poor

Comment

None

No epidemiological studies of congenital anomalies among infants born to women treated with betamethasone during pregnancy have been reported.

The frequency of cleft palate was substantially increased in the offspring of pregnant rats, mice, and rabbits treated during pregnancy with betamethasone in doses similar to or greater than those used in humans (Walker, 1971; Ishimura et al., 1975; Yamada et al., 1981; Mosier et al., 1982). In some cases, a typical dose-response relationship was observed (Walker, 1971; Yamada et al., 1981). An increased frequency of omphalocele or umbilical hernia was also seen in the offspring of exposed rats (Mosier et al., 1982; Yamada et al., 1981). Similar results have been observed with other corticosteroids in experimental animal studies, but not in humans.

Betamethasone caused constriction of the fetal ductus arteriosus when administered to pregnant rats near term (Momma et al., 1981; Momma & Takao, 1989). This effect was dose-dependent and occurred with doses equivalent to those used in humans. Although constriction of the ductus arteriosus can sometimes be demonstrated by echocardiography in human fetuses after maternal betamethosone therapy to promote fetal lung maturation, the effect does not appear to be of clinical significance (Wasserstrum et al., 1989).

Decreased fetal body and organ weights were observed in the offspring of rabbits and rats treated with betamethasone during late pregnancy in doses <1-3 or more times those employed clinically (Barrada et al., 1980; Mosier et al., 1982; Dearden et al., 1986; Tabor et al., 1991). Similar effects were observed in rhesus monkeys after treatment for 2 days in the last third of pregnancy (Epstein et al., 1977; Johnson et al., 1979, 1981).

Maternal betamethasone treatment late in pregnancy accelerates maturation of the fetal lungs and other organs in experimental animals (Epstein et al., 1977; Hallman et al., 1985; Rider et al., 1990; Snyder et al., 1992). Short-term betamethasone therapy has been used in humans to accelerate fetal pulmonary development in women with premature labor (Cosmi & Di Renzo, 1989; Roberts & Morrison, 1991). No consistent abnormalities of growth or intellectual function have been observed among children born after such treatment and followed through childhood (MacArthur et al., 1982; Smolders-de Haas et al., 1990; Schmand et al., 1990).

Please see agent summary on prednisone for information on a related agent that has been more thoroughly studied.

Key References

Barrada MI, Blomquist CH, Kotts C: The effects of betamethasone on fetal development in the rabbit. Am J Obstet Gynecol 136:234-238, 1980. [A]

Cosmi EV, Di Renzo GC: Prevention and treatment of fetal lung immaturity. Fetal Ther 4(Suppl 1):52-62, 1989. [R]

Dearden LC, Mosier HD Jr, Brundage M, et al.: The effects of different steroids on costal and epiphyseal cartilage of fetal and adult rats. Cell Tissue Res 246:401-412, 1986. [A]

Epstein MF, Farrell PM, Sparks JW, Pepe G, et al.: Maternal betamethasone and fetal growth and development in the monkey. Am J Obstet Gynecol 127:261-263, 1977. [A]

Hallman M, Teramo K, Sipinen S, Raivio K: Effects of betamethasone and ritodrine on the fetal secretion of lung surfactant. J Perinat Med 13:23-29, 1985. [S]

Ishimura K, Honda Y, Neda K, Ishikawa I, et al.: Teratological studies on betamethasone 17-Benzoate (MS-1112) II. Teratogenicity test in rabbits. Oyo Yakuri 10:685-694, 1975. [A]

Johnson JWC, Mitzner W, Beck JC, London WT, et al.: Long-term effects of betamethasone on fetal development. Am J Obstet Gynecol 141:1053-1064, 1981. [A]

Johnson JWC, Mitzner W, London WT, Palmer AE, et al.: Betamethasone and the rhesus fetus: Multisystemic effects. Am J Obstet Gynecol 133:677-684, 1979. [A]

MacArthur BA, Howie RN, Dezoete JA, Elkins J: School progress and cognitive development of 6-year-old children whose mothers were treated antenatally with betamethasone. Pediatrics 70:99-105, 1982. [S]

Momma K, Nishihara S, Ota Y: Constriction of the fetal ductus arteriosus by glucocorticoid hormones. Pediatr Res 15:19-21, 1981. [A]

Momma K, Takao A: Increased constriction of the ductus arteriosus with combined administration of indomethacin and betamethasone in fetal rats. Pediatr Res 25(1):69-75, 1989. [A]

Mosier HD, Dearden LC, Jansons RA, Roberts RC, et al.: Disproportionate growth of organs and body weight following glucocorticoid treatment of the rat fetus. Dev Pharmacol Ther 4:89-105, 1982. [A]

Rider ED, Jobe AH, Ikegami M, et al.: Antenatal betamethasone dose effects in preterm rabbits studied at 27 days gestation. J Appl Physiol 68(3):1134-1141, 1990. [A]

Roberts WE, Morrison JC: Pharmacologic induction of fetal lung maturity. Clin Obstet Gynecol 34(2):319-327, 1991. [R]

Schmand B, Neuvel J, Smolders-de Haas H, et al.: Psychological development of children who were treated antenatally with corticosteroids to prevent respiratory distress syndrome. Pediatrics 86(1):58-64, 1990. [E]

Smolders-de Haas H, Neuvel J, Schmand B, et al.: Physical development and medical history of children who were treated antenatally with corticosteroids to prevent respiratory distress syndrome: A 10- to 12-year follow-up. Pediatrics 85:65-70, 1990. [E]

Snyder JM, Rodgers HF, O'Brien JA, et al.: Glucocorticoid effects on rabbit fetal lung maturation in vivo: An ultrastructural morphometric study. Anat Rec 232:133-140, 1992. [A]

Tabor BL, Rider ED, Ikegami M, et al.: Dose effects of antenatal corticosteroids for induction of lung maturation in preterm rabbits. Am J Obstet Gynecol 164:675-681, 1991. [A]

Walker BE: Induction of cleft palate in rats with antiinflammatory drugs. Teratology 4:39-42, 1971. [A]

Wasserstrum N, Huhta JC, Mari G, et al.: Betamethasone and the human fetal ductus arteriosus. Obstet Gynecol 74:897-900, 1989. [E]

Yamada T, Nakano M, Ichihashi T, et al.: Fetal concentration after topical application of betamethasone 17, 21-dipropionate (S-3440) ointment and teratogenesis in mice and rabbits. Oyo Yakuri (Pharmacometrics) 21:645-655, 1981. [A]

BETAXOLOL

Synonyms

Betoptic, Betoptima, Kerlone

Summary

Betaxolol is a cardioselective beta-1-adrenergic receptor blocking agent. It is used orally to treat hypertension and as an ophthalmic solution to treat glaucoma. Systemic absorption of the ophthalmic preparation may occur.

Magnitude of Teratogenic Risk

Undetermined

Quality and Quantity of Data

Poor

Comment

A small risk cannot be excluded, but a high risk of congenital anomalies in the children of women treated with betaxolol as an ophthalmic solution during pregnancy is unlikely.

No epidemiological studies of congenital anomalies among infants born to women treated with betaxolol during pregnancy have been reported.

The frequency of malformations was not increased among the offspring of pregnant rats or rabbits treated respectively with 10-250 times or 1-45 times the human dose of betaxolol (Tateda et al., 1990; Tesh et al., 1990).

No adverse effects attributable to the medication were observed among the infants of 28 women who were treated with betaxolol for hypertension in the second or third trimester of pregnancy (Morselli et al., 1990; Boutroy et al., 1990).

Please see agent summary on propranolol for information on a related agent that has been more thoroughly studied.

Key References

Boutroy MJ, Morselli PL, Bianchetti G, et al.: Betaxolol: A pilot study of its pharmacological and therapeutic properties in pregnancy. Eur J Clin Pharmacol 38:535-539, 1990. [S]

Morselli PL, Boutroy MJ, Bianchetti G, et al.: Placental transfer and perinatal pharmacokinetics of betaxolol. Eur J Clin Pharmacol 38:477-483, 1990. [S]

Tateda C, Ichikawa K, Ono C, et al.: [Reproduction study of betaxolol (2) -- teratogenicity study in rats]. Yakuri To Chiryo 18(Suppl 7):107-127, 1990. [A]

Tesh JM, Ross FW, Tesh SA, et al.: [Reproduction study of betaxolol (4) -- teratogenicity study in rabbits]. Yakuri To Chiryo 18(Suppl 7):129-140, 1990. [A]

BETHANECHOL

Synonyms

Duvoid, Mechothane, Muscaran, Myo Hermes, Myocholine, Myotonachol, Myotonine, Urecholine, Vesicholine

Summary

Bethanechol is a parasympathomimetic agent that is used in the treatment of gastric and urinary retention and abdominal distention. It is administered orally or subcutaneously.

Magnitude of Teratogenic Risk

Undetermined

Quality and Quantity of Data

None

Comment

None

No epidemiological studies of congenital anomalies among infants born to women treated with bethanechol during pregnancy have been reported.

No in vivo teratology studies of bethanechol in mammals have been published.

Key References

None available.

BIFONAZOLE

Synonyms

Amycor, Azolmen, Bifazol, Bifonazolum, Mycospor, Trifonazole

Summary

Bifonazole is a topical antifungal agent that is poorly absorbed from the skin.

Magnitude of Teratogenic Risk

None

Quality and Quantity of Data

None To Poor

Comment

None

No epidemiological studies of congenital anomalies in infants born to women treated with bifonazole during pregnancy have been reported.

The frequency of malformations was not increased among the offspring of rabbits or rats given 3-10 and 10-100 times the usual human dose of bifonazole intragastrically during pregnancy, but loss of almost all of the embryos occurred in pregnant rabbits treated with 30 times the human dose (Schluter, 1983).

Key References

Schluter G: The toxicology of bifonazole. Arzneimittelforsch 33:739-745, 1983. [A]

BIPHENAMINE

Synonyms

Alvinine Shampoo, Xenylsalate

Summary

Biphenamine is a topical anesthetic.

Magnitude of Teratogenic Risk

Undetermined

Quality and Quantity of Data

None

Comment

None

No epidemiological studies of congenital anomalies in children born to women exposed to biphenamine during pregnancy have been reported.

No investigations of teratologic effects of biphenamine in experimental animals have been published.

Key References

None available.

BISACODYL

Synonyms

Bisacolax, Deficol, Dulcolax, Spirolax, Theralax

Summary

Bisacodyl is a cathartic agent that is administered orally or rectally. It is poorly absorbed when used rectally.

Magnitude of Teratogenic Risk

Undetermined

Quality and Quantity of Data

None

Comment

None

No epidemiological studies of congenital anomalies in infants whose mothers were treated with bisacodyl during pregnancy have been reported.

No animal teratology studies of bisacodyl have been published.

Key References

None available.

BISMUTH

Synonyms

Anusol Cream, Pepto Bismol, Ulcerone, Vismut

Summary

Bismuth is a heavy metal that is toxic to humans. As a salt or metal it has been given by injection to treat syphillis and yaws. Insoluble preparations have been used topically as protective agents and orally as antacids and to treat diarrhea.

Magnitude of Teratogenic Risk

Undetermined

Quality and Quantity of Data

Poor

Comment

None

The frequency of congenital anomalies was no greater than expected among the children of 144 women treated with bismuth subgallate (an insoluble salt) anytime during pregnancy in the Collaborative Perinatal Project (Heinonen et al., 1977). Only 13 of these women used bismuth during the first four lunar months of gestation.

In one study in which four ewes were given bismuth tartrate during pregnancy in doses similar to those used in humans, one of the lambs had multiple congenital anomalies, onc was spontaneously aborted, and two were normal (James et al., 1966). Bismuth was not detectable by X-ray spectography in either maternal or fetal tissues at parturition. The relevance of this observation to the risks associated with bismuth exposure in human pregnancy is unknown.

Key References

Heinonen OP, Slone D, Shapiro S: Birth Defects and Drugs in Pregnancy. Littleton, Mass.: John Wright-PSG, 1977, pp 385, 497. [E]

James LF, Lazar VA, Binns W: Effects of sublethal doses of certain minerals on pregnant ewes and fetal development. Am J Vet Res 27:132-135, 1966. [A]

BISOPROLOL

Synonyms

Concor, Emcor, Monocor

Summary

Bisoprolol is a cardioselective beta-adrenergic receptor blocking agent. It is administered orally in the treatment of hypertension and angina pectoris.

Magnitude of Teratogenic Risk

Undetermined

Quality and Quantity of Data

Poor

Comment

None

No epidemiological studies of congenital anomalies among infants born to women treated with bisoprolol during pregnancy have been reported.

The frequency of malformations was not increased among the offspring of pregnant rats or rabbits treated with 25-250 or 5-125 the human therapeutic dose of bisoprolol (Suzuki et al., 1989). Increased fetal death was seen at high doses in both species, and fetal growth retardation was noted at high doses in rats.

Please see agent summary on propranolol for information on a related agent that has been more thoroughly studied.

Key References

Suzuki T, Naito Y, Narama T, et al.: [Reproduction studies of bisoprolol fumarate in rats and rabbits]. Kiso To Rinsho 23(3):46-56, 1989. [A]

BLEOMYCIN

Synonyms

Blenoxane, Bleo Oil, Blexane

Summary

Bleomycin is a glycopeptide antibiotic used to treat malignant neoplasms.

Magnitude of Teratogenic Risk

Undetermined

Quality and Quantity of Data

Poor

Comment

Although the teratogenic risk of this agent is undetermined, it may be substantial because bleomycin has antineoplastic activity.

No epidemiological studies of congenital anomalies among the infants of women treated with bleomycin during pregnancy have been reported. No congenital anomalies were observed among 22 children born to women who had been treated with cancer chemotherapeutic regimens that included bleomycin in one series (Aviles et al., 1991). Eleven of these women were treated during the first trimester.

The frequency of malformations was no greater than expected among the offspring of rats treated with daily doses of bleomycin 2-8 times those used once a week in humans (Thompson et al., 1976). Fetal death and skeletal variants, as well as maternal toxicity, were seen with increased frequency at the higher doses. The frequency of malformations was not increased among the offspring of rabbits treated with bleomycin in daily doses 1.2-5 times those used weekly in humans, but fetal death occurred with the higher doses (Thompson et al., 1976).

Transient neonatal leukopenia and neutropenia were observed in a premature infant born to a woman who had been treated with bleomycin, etoposide, and cisplatin 7-10 days prior to delivery (Raffles et al., 1989).

Key References

Aviles A, Diaz-Maqueo JC, Talavera A, et al.: Growth and development of children of mothers treated with chemotherapy during pregnancy: Current status of 43 children. Am J Hematol 36:243-248, 1991. [S]

Raffles A, Williams J, Costeloe K, Clark P: Transplacental effects of maternal cancer chemotherapy. Case Report. Br J Obstet Gynaecol 96:1099-1100, 1989. [C]

Thompson DJ, Strabing RJ, Dyke IL, et al.: Effects of bleomycin (NSC-125066) on reproduction, pre- and postnatal development in the rat and on prenatal development in the rabbit. NTIS (National Technical Information Service) Report/PB-261972, 1976. [A]

BORATE

Synonyms

Borax, Boric Acid

Summary

Borate is an alkalizing agent with weak bacteriostatic action. It is used as a mild astringent in lotions and mouthwashes, as an emulsifying agent, and as a stain remover.

Magnitude of Teratogenic Risk

None

Quality and Quantity of Data

Poor To Fair

Comment

None

The frequencies of congenital anomalies in general, of major malformations, and of minor anomalies were no greater than expected among the infants of 253 women who used boric acid topically during the first four lunar months of pregnancy in the Collaborative Perinatal Project (Heinonen et al., 1977). Similarly, the frequency of congenital anomalies was not significantly increased among the children of 463 women in this study who used topical boric acid anytime in pregnancy.

No mammalian teratology studies of borate have been published.

Key References

Heinonen OP, Slone D, Shapiro S: Birth Defects and Drugs in Pregnancy. Littleton, Mass.: John Wright-PSG, 1977, p 300. [E]

BROMODIPHENHYDRA-MINE

Synonyms

Ambodryl, Bromazine

Summary

Bromodiphenhydramine is an ethanolamine antihistaminic agent that is administered orally for the treatment of upper respiratory symptoms.

Magnitude of Teratogenic Risk

Undetermined

Quality and Quantity of Data

None

Comment

A small risk cannot be excluded, but a high risk of congenital anomalies in the children of women treated with bromodiphenhydramine during pregnancy is unlikely.

No epidemiological studies of congenital anomalies in infants whose mothers used bromodiphenhydramine during pregnancy have been reported.

No animal teratology studies of bromodiphenhydramine have been published.

Please see agent summary on diphenhydramine for information on a related agent that has been studied.

Key References

None available.

BROMPERIDOL

Synonyms

Azuren, Bromidol, Impromen, Tesoprel

Summary

Bromperidol is a neuroleptic agent used in treating psychoses.

Magnitude of Teratogenic Risk

Undetermined

Quality and Quantity of Data

None To Poor

Comment

None

No epidemiological studies of congenital anomalies in infants born to women treated with bromperidol during pregnancy have been reported.

The frequency of malformations was not increased and no behavioral abnormalities were noted in the offspring of rats treated during pregnancy with bromperidol in doses 1-50 times those used clinically (Imai et al., 1984).

Please see agent summary on haloperidol for information on a closely related drug that has been more thoroughly studied.

Key References

Imai S, Tauchi K, Huamg KJ, Takeshima T, et al.: Teratogenicity study on bromperidol in rats. J Toxicol Sci 9:109-126, 1984. [A]

BROMPHENIRAMINE

Synonyms

Bromfeniramina, Dimetane, Dimetane Tablets, Drauxin, Ebalin, Gammistin, Veltane

Summary

Brompheniramine is an antihistamine. It is used, often in combination with other drugs, to treat allergies and colds.

Magnitude of Teratogenic Risk

None

Quality and Quantity of Data

Fair

Comment

None

The frequency of congenital anomalies was not increased among the infants of more than 270 women who took brompheniramine during the first trimester of pregnancy in two cohorts of the Boston Collaborative Drug Surveillance Program (Jick et al., 1981; Aselton et al., 1985). A slightly increased frequency of congenital anomalies was found among the children of 65 women who took brompheniramine during the first four lunar months of pregnancy in the Collaborative Perinatal Project, but this increase was due entirely to mild defects that occurred with widely varying rates at participating institutions (Heinonen et al., 1977). The association is of doubtful clinical significance. The frequency of congenital anomalies was not increased among the children of 412 women who took brompheniramine anytime during pregnancy in this study (Heinonen et al., 1977).

No animal teratology studies of brompheniramine have been published.

Key References

Aselton P, Jick H, Milunsky A, Hunter JR, Stergachis A: First-trimester drug use and congenital disorders. Obstet Gynecol 65:451-455, 1985. [S]

Heinonen OP, Slone D, Shapiro S: Birth Defects and Drugs in Pregnancy. Littleton, Mass.: John Wright-PSG, 1977, pp 323-325, 437. [E]

Jick H, Holmes LB, Hunter JR, Madsen S, Stergachis A: First-trimester drug use and congenital disorders. JAMA 246:343-346, 1981. [S]

BUCLIZINE

Synonyms

Aphilan R, Bucladin-S, Longifene

Summary

Buclizine is a piperazine antihistamine that is administered orally to prevent nausea.

Magnitude of Teratogenic Risk

Undetermined

Quality and Quantity of Data

Poor

Comment

A small risk cannot be excluded, but a high risk of congenital anomalies in the children of women treated with buclizine during pregnancy is unlikely.

No epidemiological studies of congenital anomalies among infants born to women who took buclizine during pregnancy have been reported.

An increased frequency of cleft palate, skeletal malformations, and other congenital anomalies was observed among the offspring of rats treated with buclizine in doses 13-67 times those used in humans (King & Howell, 1966). No teratogenic effect was noted after maternal treatment with 10 times the usual human dose of buclizine during pregnancy. The relevance of these findings to the therapeutic use of buclizine in human pregnancy is unknown.

Please see agent summary on hydroxyzine for information on a related agent that has been more thoroughly studied.

Key References

King CTG, Howell J: Teratogenic Effect of buclizine and hydroxyzine in the rat and chlorcyclizine in the mouse. Am J Obstet Gynecol 95:109-111, 1966. [A]

BUFEXAMAC

Synonyms

Droxaryl, Parfenac

Summary

Bufexamac is a nonsteroidal anti-inflammatory agent. It is used orally in the treatment of arthritis and topically to treat dermatoses.

Magnitude of Teratogenic Risk

Undetermined

Quality and Quantity of Data

None To Poor

Comment

A small risk cannot be excluded, but a high risk of congenital anomalies in the children of women treated with bufexamac during pregnancy is unlikely.

No epidemiological studies of congenital anomalies among infants born to women treated with bufexamac during pregnancy have been reported.

No teratogenic effect was observed among the offspring of rats or rabbits treated with bufexamac during pregnancy in doses twice those used in humans (Roba et al., 1970). Decreased fetal weight gain occurred at higher doses, but these were toxic to the mothers.

Please see agent summary on ibuprofen for information on a related agent that has been more thoroughly studied.

Key References

Roba J, Lambelin G, Buu-Hoi NP: Teratological studies of p- butoxphenylacethydroxamic acid (CP 1044 J3) in rats and rabbits. Arzneimittelforsch 20:565-569, 1970. [A]

BUMETANIDE

Synonyms

Bumex

Summary

Bumetanide is a loop diuretic that may be administered orally or parenterally.

Magnitude of Teratogenic Risk

Undetermined

Quality and Quantity of Data

None To Poor

Comment

None

No epidemiological studies of congenital anomalies in infants whose mothers were treated with bumetanide during pregnancy have been reported.

The frequency of malformations was no greater than expected among the offspring of rats, mice, rabbits, or hamsters treated during pregnancy with bumetanide in doses, respectively, 2-5000, 2-5000, 1.5-15, and 2-20 times the usual oral therapeutic dose in humans (McClain & Dammers, 1981).

Key References

McClain RM, Dammers KD: Toxicologic evaluation of bumetanide, a potent diuretic agent. J Clin Pharmacol 21: 543-554, 1981. [A]

BUPIVACAINE

Synonyms

Marcain

Summary

Bupivacaine is a long-acting local anesthetic of the amide class.

Magnitude of Teratogenic Risk

Undetermined

Quality and Quantity of Data

None

Comment

None

No epidemiological studies of congenital anomalies in children born to women exposed to bupivacaine during pregnancy have been reported.

No investigations of teratogenic effects of bupivacaine in experimental animals have been published.

Transient fetal bradycardia and increased fetal heart rate variability have been observed in some studies of women who had epidural or regional anesthesia with bupivacaine during labor (Teramo, 1971; Abboud et al., 1982; Lavin et al., 1981; Puolakka et al., 1984; Stavrou et al., 1990). The neurobehavioral status of infants born of such pregnancies is usually normal (Lieberman et al., 1979; Merkow et al., 1980; Abboud et al., 1982; Harrison & Cullen, 1986), although alterations of neonatal behavior are sometimes observed (Rosenblatt et al., 1981; Morikawa et al., 1990).

Please see agent summary on lidocaine for information on a related agent that has been more thoroughly studied.

Key References

Abboud TK, Khoo SS, Miller F, Doan R, et al.: Maternal, fetal, and neonatal responses after epidural anesthesia with bupivacaine, 2-chloroprocaine, or lidocaine. Anesth Analg 61:638-644, 1982. [E]

Harrison RF, Cullen R: A comparative study of the behaviour of the neonate following various forms of maternal intrapartum analgesia and anaesthesia. Ir J Med Sci 155:12-18, 1986. [E]

Lavin JP, Samuels SV, Miodovnik M, et al.: The effects of bupivacaine and chloroprocaine as local anesthetics for epidural anesthesia on fetal heart

rate monitoring parameters. Am J Obstet Gynecol 141(6):717-722, 1981. [S]

Lieberman BA, Rosenblatt DB, Belsey E, Packer M, et al.: The effects of maternally administered pethidine or epidural bupivacaine on the fetus and newborn. Br J Obstet Gynaecol 86:598-606, 1979. [E]

Merkow AJ, McGuinness GA, Erenberg A, Kennedy RL: The neonatal neurobehavioral effects of bupivacaine, mepivacaine, and 2-chloroproxaine used for pudendal block. Anesthesiology 52:309-312, 1980. [S]

Morikawa S, Ishikawa J, Kamatsuki H, et al.: Neurobehavior and mental development of newborn infants delivered under epidural analgesia with bupivacaine. Nippon Sanka Fujinka Gakkai Zasshi 42(11):1495-1502, 1990. [E]

Puolakka J, Jouppila R, Jouppila P, Puukka M: Maternal and fetal effects of low-dosage bupivacaine paracervical block. J Perinat Med 12:75-84, 1984. [S]

Rosenblatt DB, Belsey EM, Lieberman BA, et al.: The influence of maternal analgesia on neonatal behaviour: II. Epidural bupivacaine. Br J Obstet Gynecol 88:407-413, 1981. [S]

Stavrou C, Hofmeyr GJ, Boezaart AP: Prolonged fetal bradycardia during epidural analgesia. Incidence, timing and significance. S Afr Med J 77:66-68, 1990. [S]

Teramo K: Effects of obstetrical paracervical blockade on the fetus. Acta Obstet Gynecol Scand Suppl 16:1-55, 1971. [R]

BUPROPION

Synonyms

Amfebutamone, Wellbatrin, Wellbutrin

Summary

Bupropion is an aminoketone antidepressant that is used orally.

Magnitude of Teratogenic Risk

Undetermined

Quality and Quantity of Data

None To Poor

Comment

None

No epidemiological studies of congenital anomalies among infants born to women treated with bupropion during pregnancy have been reported.

The frequency of malformations was not increased among the offspring of rats or rabbits treated during pregnancy with 17-50 or 3-17 times the maximum human therapeutic dose of bupropion (Tucker, 1983).

Key References

Tucker WE: Preclinical toxicology of bupropion: An overview. J Clin Psychiatry 44:60-62, 1983. [A]

BUSPIRONE

Synonyms

Buspar

Summary

Buspirone is an oral antianxiety agent, chemically unrelated to those used more commonly.

Magnitude of Teratogenic Risk

Undetermined

Quality and Quantity of Data

None To Poor

Comment

None

No epidemiological studies of congenital anomalies in infants whose mothers were treated with buspirone during pregnancy have been reported.

The frequency of malformations was not increased among the offspring of rats treated with 2-62 times the human therapeutic dose of busipirone during pregnancy (Kai et al., 1990).

Key References

Kai S, Kohmura H, Ishikawa K, et al.: Reproductive and developmental toxicity studies of buspirone hydrochloride. (I). Oral administration to rats during the period of fetal organogenesis. J Toxicol Sci 15(Suppl 1):31-60, 1990. [A]

BUTABARBITAL

Synonyms

Buticaps, Butisol

Summary

Butabarbital is a barbiturate that is administered orally as a sedative and hypnotic.

Magnitude of Teratogenic Risk

None To Minimal

Quality and Quantity of Data

Poor To Fair

Comment

None

In the Collaborative Perinatal Project, an increased frequency of congenital anomalies was observed among the infants of 109 women who took butabarbital during the first four lunar months of pregnancy when defects with non-uniform rates among participating hospitals were included (Heinonen et al., 1977). However, this association is of doubtful clinical importance because no statistically significant association was seen when only congenital anomalies with uniform rates among participating hospitals were considered. The frequency of congenital anomalies was no greater than expected among the infants of 305 women who took butabarbital anytime during pregnancy in this study.

No animal teratology studies of butabarbital have been published.

Please see agent summary on phenobarbital for information on a related agent that has been more thoroughly studied.

Key References

Heinonen OP, Slone D, Shapiro S: Birth Defects and Drugs in Pregnancy. Littleton, Mass.: John Wright-PSG, 1977, pp 335-337, 438. [E]

BUTACAINE

Synonyms

Butacaine Sulphate

Summary

Butacaine is a surface anesthetic of the ester class.

Magnitude of Teratogenic Risk

Undetermined

Quality and Quantity of Data

None

Comment

None

No epidemiological studies of congenital anomalies in children born to women exposed to butacaine during pregnancy have been reported.

No investigations of teratologic effects of butacaine in experimental animals have been published.

Please see agent summary on procaine for information on a related agent that has been studied.

Key References

None available.

BUTALBITAL

Synonyms

Alisobumalum, Allylbarbital, Allylbarbituric Acid, Itobarbital, Tetrallobarbital

Summary

Butalbital is a short-acting barbiturate with hypnotic and sedative actions.

Magnitude of Teratogenic Risk

None To Minimal

Quality and Quantity of Data

Fair

Comment

None

The Collaborative Perinatal Project included 112 pregnancies exposed to butalbital during the first trimester; the frequency of malformations was no greater than expected among the offspring of these pregnancies (Heinonen et al., 1977).

No animal teratology studies of butalbital have been published.

Transient neonatal withdrawal symptoms similar to those which occur with phenobarbital have been reported after chronic maternal use of butalbital in therapeutic doses late in pregnancy (Ostrea, 1982).

Key References

Heinonen OP, Slone D, Shapiro S: Birth Defects and Drugs in Pregnancy. Littleton, Mass.: John Wright-PSG, 1977, p 336. [E]

Ostrea EM: Neonatal withdrawal from intrauterine exposure to butalbital. Am J Obstet Gynecol 143:597-599, 1982. [C]

BUTAMBEN

Synonyms

Butesin Picrate, Butyl Aminobenzoate

Summary

Butamben is a local anesthetic of the ester class that has been used topically.

Magnitude of Teratogenic Risk

Undetermined

Quality and Quantity of Data

None

Comment

None

No epidemiological studies of congenital anomalies in children born to women exposed to butamben during pregnancy have been reported.

No investigations of teratologic effects of butamben in experimental animals have been published.

Please see agent summary on procaine for information on a related agent that has been studied.

Key References

None available.

BUTANILICAINE

Synonyms

Hostacain

Summary

Butanilicaine is an injectable local anesthetic of the amide class.

Magnitude of Teratogenic Risk

Undetermined

Quality and Quantity of Data

None

Comment

None

No epidemiological studies of congenital anomalies in children born to women exposed to butanilicaine during pregnancy have been reported.

No investigations of teratologic effects of butanilicaine in experimental animals have been published.

Please see agent summary on lidocaine for information on a related agent that has been studied.

Key References

None available.

BUTETHAMINE

Synonyms

Ibylcaine Chloride, Ibylcaine Hydrochloride, Monocaine

Summary

Butethamine is a local anesthetic of the ester class that has been used in dentistry.

Magnitude of Teratogenic Risk

Undetermined

Quality and Quantity of Data

None

Comment

None

No epidemiological studies of congenital anomalies in children born to women exposed to butethamine during pregnancy have been reported.

No investigations of teratologic effects of butethamine in experimental animals have been published.

Please see agent summary on procaine for information on a related agent that has been studied.

Key References

None available.

BUTOCONAZOLE

Synonyms

Butoconazole Nitrate, Femstat

Summary

Butoconazole is an antifungal agent.

Magnitude of Teratogenic Risk

Undetermined

Quality and Quantity of Data

None

Comment

None

No epidemiological studies of congenital anomalies in infants born to women who used butoconazole during pregnancy have been reported.

No animal teratology studies of butoconazole have been published.

Key References

None available.

BUTOPAMINE

Synonyms

Compound LY 131126

Summary

Butopamine is a cardiotonic drug.

Magnitude of Teratogenic Risk

Undetermined

Quality and Quantity of Data

None

Comment

None

No epidemiological studies of congenital anomalies in infants born to women treated with butopamine during pregnancy have been reported.

No animal teratology studies of butopamine have been published.

Key References

None available.

CAFFEINE

Synonyms

Coffee, Efed 11 Black, Methyltheobromine, No Doz

Summary

Caffeine is a methylated xanthine that acts as a central nervous system stimulant. Caffeine is contained in many commonly used beverages including coffee, tea, and colas. Many over-the-counter and prescription medicines include caffeine, usually in combination with other agents.

Magnitude of Teratogenic Risk

Malformations: None

Spontaneous Abortions: None To Minimal

Quality and Quantity of Data

Malformations: Good

Spontaneous Abortion: Fair To Good

Comment

1) Risk assessment is for usual caffeine intake as occurs with moderate drinking of coffee, tea, or colas.

2) The available data are inadequate to determine the risk related to very high doses of caffeine.

The frequency of congenital anomalies was not increased among the children of 595 women who drank four or more cups of coffee per day during the first trimester of pregnancy in a well-controlled cohort study (Linn et al., 1982). Similarly, the frequency of congenital anomalies was no greater than expected among the infants of 5378 women who took medicines containing caffeine during the first four lunar months of pregnancy or among the infants of 12,696 women who took such medicines anytime during pregnancy in the Collabortive Peri-

natal Project (Heinonen et al., 1977). The frequency of heavy maternal consumption of caffeinated beverages or maternal use of caffeine-containing medications during pregnancy was no more frequent than expected in case-control studies involving 2030, 706, 458 children with a variety of congenital anomalies (Rosenberg et al., 1982; Kurppa et al., 1983; Nelson & Forfar, 1971). In two other case-control studies, statistically significant associations were observed with consumption of caffeinated beverages during pregnancy among mothers of 464 anencephalic infants and 190 children with various malformations (Fedrick, 1974; Borlee et al., 1978). The association was weak in both instances, however, and both studies have serious methodological limitations (Pieters, 1985; James & Paull, 1985).

Associations between maternal coffee drinking during pregnancy and miscarriage or poor fetal growth have been repeatedly observed in epidemiological studies (van den Berg, 1977; Weathersbee et al., 1977; Hogue, 1981; Linn et al., 1982; Kuzma & Sokol, 1982; Watkinson & Fried, 1985; Srisuphan & Bracken, 1986; Martin & Bracken, 1987; Beaulac-Baillargeon & Desrosiers, 1987; Brooke et al., 1989; Caan & Goldhaber, 1989; Wilcox et al., 1990), but in many instances these associations are largely attributable to confounding effects of maternal cigarette smoking or other factors. Some of these studies have very serious methodological limitations (Heller, 1987; Leviton, 1988; Berger, 1988), and there may be an interaction between the effects of maternal cigarette smoking and coffee drinking (Beaulac-Baillargeon & Desrosiers, 1987). If maternal consumption of caffeine-containing beverages in conventional amounts during pregnancy does have an adverse effect on the rate of miscarriage or fetal growth retardation, the effect appears to be relatively small.

Fetal and neonatal cardiac arrhythmias have been reported among the infants of women who drank unusually large amounts of caffeine-containing beverages during pregnancy; these arrhythmias resolved after elimination of the caffeine intake (Oei et al., 1989).

Stillbirths and miscarriages were observed with increased frequency among the offspring

84

of macaque monkeys treated during pregnancy with caffeine in a dose equivalent to 5-7 or 12-17 cups of coffee per day (Gilbert et al., 1988). The cause for the stillbirths was not apparent on necropsy; no malformations were seen. An increased frequency of malformations, especially of the limbs and palate, has been observed among the offspring of rats or mice treated with caffeine during pregnancy in doses equivalent to human consumption of 40 or more cups of coffee daily (Collins et al., 1981; Scott, 1983; Smith et al., 1987; Muther, 1988). Fetal death, growth retardation, and skeletal variations are often seen in these experiments after maternal treatment with very high doses of caffeine during pregnancy.

In one study an increased frequency of cleft palate was observed among the offspring of rats given the equivalent of 5-19 cups of coffee a day during pregnancy (Palm et al., 1978). An increased rate of cardiac defects was observed among the offspring of rats treated during pregnancy with the equivalent of 15 or more cups of coffee per day in another study (Matsuoka et al., 1987). Most investigations do not show an increased frequency of malformations among the offspring of rodents treated during pregnancy with caffeine in similar or somewhat greater doses (Nolen, 1982; Elmazar et al., 1982; Collins et al., 1983, 1987; Kavlock et al., 1985; Smith et al., 1987).

Persistent behavioral alterations have been observed among the offspring of rats and mice treated during pregnancy with caffeine in doses equivalent to 10-60 cups of coffee a day (Sinton et al., 1981; Groisser et al., 1982; Concannon et al., 1983; Hughes & Beveridge, 1986, 1990; Sobotka, 1989). Behavioral alterations have also been observed among the offspring of monkeys born to mothers treated with an unspecified dose of caffeine during pregnancy (Rice & Gilbert, 1990). The relevance of these observations to the risks in infants born to women who drink large amounts of caffeinated beverages during pregnancy is unknown.

Key References

Beaulac-Baillargeon L, Desrosiers C: Caffeine-cigarette interaction on fetal growth. Am J Obstet Gynecol 157:1236-1240, 1987. [E]

Berger A: Effects of caffeine consumption on pregnancy outcome: A review. J Reprod Med 33:945-956, 1988. [R]

Borlee I, Lecht MF, Bouckaert A, Misson C: Le cafe, facteur de risque pendant la grossesse? Louvain Med 97:279-284, 1978. [E]

Brooke OG, Anderson HR, Bland JM, et al.: Effects on birth weight of smoking, alcohol, caffeine, socioeconomic factors, and psychosocial stress. BMJ 298:795-801, 1989. [E]

Caan BJ, Goldhaber MK: Caffeinated beverages and low birthweight: A case-control study. Am J Public Health 79(9):1299-1300, 1989. [E]

Collins TFX, Welsh JJ, Black TN, Collins EV: A study of the teratogenic potential of caffeine given by oral intubation to rats. Regulatory Toxicol Pharmacol 1:355-378, 1981. [A]

Collins TFX, Welsh JJ, Black TN, Ruggles DI: A study of the teratogenic potential of caffeine ingested in drinking-water. Food Chem Toxicol 21:763-777, 1983. [A]

Collins TFX, Welsh JJ, Black TN, Whitby KE, O'Donnell MW: Potential reversibility of skeletal effects in rats exposed in utero to caffeine. Food Chem Toxicol 25(9):647-662, 1987. [A]

Concannon JT, Braughler JM, Schechter MD: Pre- and postnatal effects of caffeine on brain biogenic amines, cyclic nucleotides and behavior in developing rats. J Pharmacol Exp Ther 226:673-679, 1983. [A]

Elmazar MMA, McElhatton PR, Sullivan FM: Studies on the teratogenic effects of different oral preparations of caffeine in mice. Toxicology 23:57-71, 1982. [A]

Fedrick J: Anencephalus and maternal tea drinking: Evidence for a possible association. Proc R Soc Med 67:356-360, 1974. [E]

Gilbert SG, Rice DC, Reuhl KR, Stavric B: Adverse pregnancy outcome in the monkey (Macaca fascicularis) after chronic caffeine exposure. J Pharmacol Exp Ther 245(3):1048-1053, 1988. [A]

Groisser DS, Rosso P, Winick M: Coffee consumption during pregnancy: Subsequent behavioral abnormalities of the offspring. J Nutr 112:829-832, 1982. [A]

Heinonen OP, Slone D, Shapiro S: Birth Defects and Drugs in Pregnancy. Littleton: Mass.: John Wright-PSG, 1977, pp 11, 366-370, 436, 440, 477, 493. [E]

Heller J: What do we know about the risks of caffeine consumption in pregnancy? Br J Addict 82:885-889, 1987. [R]

Hogue CJ: Coffee in pregnancy. Lancet 1:554, 1981. [E]

Hughes RN, Beveridge IJ: Behavioral effects of prenatal exposure to caffeine in rats. Life Sci 38:861-868, 1986. [A]

Hughes RN, Beveridge IJ: Sex- and age-dependent effects of prenatal exposure to caffeine on open-field behavior, emergence latency and adrenal weights in rats. Life Sci 47:2075-2088, 1990. [A]

James JE, Paull I: Caffeine and human reproduction. Rev Environ Health 5:151-167, 1985. [R]

Kavlock RJ, Chernoff N, Rogers EH: The effect of acute maternal toxicity on fetal development in the mouse. Teratogenesis Carcinog Mutagen 5:3-13, 1985. [A]

Kurppa K, Holmberg PC, Kuosma E, Saxen L: Coffee consumption during pregnancy and selected congenital malformations: A nationwide case-control study. Am J Publ Health 73:1397-1399, 1983. [E]

Kuzma JW, Sokol RJ: Maternal drinking behavior and decreased intrauterine growth. Alcohol Clin Exp Res 6:396-402, 1982. [E]

Leviton A: Caffeine consumption and the risk of reproductive hazards. J Reprod Med 33:175-178, 1988. [R]

Linn S, Schoenbaum SC, Monson RR, Rosner B, et al.: No association between coffee consumption and adverse outcomes of pregnancy. N Engl J Med 306:141-145, 1982. [E]

Martin TR, Bracken MB: The association between low birth weight and caffeine consumption during pregnancy. Am J Epidemiol 126(5):813-821, 1987. [E]

Matsuoka R, Uno H, Tanaka H, et al.: Caffeine induces cardiac and other malformations in the rat. Am J Med Genet (Suppl 3):433-443, 1987. [A]

Muther TF: Caffeine and reduction of fetal ossification in the rat: Fact or artifact? Teratology 37:239-247, 1988. [A]

Nelson MM, Forfar JO: Associations between drugs administered during pregnancy and congenital abnormalities of the fetus. Br Med J 1:523- 527, 1971. [E]

Nolen GA: A reproduction/teratology study of brewed and instant decaffeinated coffees. J Toxicol Environ Health 10:769-783, 1982. [A]

Oei SG, Vosters RPL, van der Hagen NLJ: Fetal arrhythmia caused by excessive intake of caffeine by pregnant women. BMJ 298:568, 1989. [C]

Palm PE, Arnold EP, Rachwall PC, Leyczek JC, et al.: Evaluation of the teratogenic potential of fresh-brewed coffee and caffeine in the rat. Toxicol Appl Pharmacol 44:1-16, 1978. [A]

Pieters JJL: Nutritional teratogens: A survey of epidemiological literature. Prog Clin Biol Res 163B:419-429, 1985. [R]

Rice DC, Gilbert SG: Automated behavioral procedures for infant monkeys. Neurotoxicol Teratol 12:429-439, 1990. [A]

Rosenberg L, Mitchell AA, Shapiro S, Slone D: Selected birth defects in relation to caffeine-containing beverages. JAMA 247:1429-1432, 1982. [E]

Scott WJ: Caffeine-induced limb malformations: Description of malformations and quantitation of placental transfer. Teratology 28:427-435, 1983. [A]

Sinton CM, Valatx JL, Jouvet M: Gestational caffeine modifies offspring behavior in mice. Psychopharmacology 75:69-74, 1981. [A]

Smith SE, McElhatton PR, Sullivan FM: Effects of administering caffeine to pregnant rats either as a single daily dose or as divided doses four times a day. Food Chem Toxicol 25(2):125-133, 1987. [A]

Sobotka TJ: Neurobehavioral effects of prenatal caffeine. Ann NY Acad Sci 562:327-339, 1989. [R]

Srisuphan W, Bracken MB: Caffeine consumption during pregnancy and association with late spontaneous abortion. Am J Obstet Gynecol 154(1):14-20, 1986. [E]

van den Berg BJ: Epidemiologic observations of prematurity: Effects of tobacco, coffee and alcohol. In: Reed DM, Stanley FJ (eds). The Epidemiology of Prematurity. Baltimore: Urban and Schweartzenberg, 1977, pp 157-176. [E]

Watkinson B, Fried PA: Maternal caffeine use before, during, and after pregnancy and effects upon offspring. Neurobehav Toxicol Teratol 7:9-17, 1985. [E]

Weathersbee PS, Olsen LK, Lodge JR: Caffeine and pregnancy. Postgrad Med 62:64-69, 1977. [E]

Wilcox AJ, Weinberg CR, Baird DD: Risk factors for early pregnancy loss. Epidemiology 1:382-385, 1990. [E]

CALAMINE

Synonyms

Hemimorphite, Hydrozincite

Summary

Calamine, which is composed of zinc oxide and a small amount of ferric oxide, has astringent and mild antiseptic actions and is used topically in the treatment of a variety of skin conditions.

Magnitude of Teratogenic Risk

Undetermined

Quality and Quantity of Data

None

Comment

A small risk cannot be excluded, but a substantial risk of congenital anomalies in the children of women treated with calamine during pregnancy is unlikely.

No epidemiological studies of congenital anomalies in infants whose mothers were treated with calamine during pregnancy have been reported.

No animal teratology studies of calamine have been published.

Key References

None available.

CALCIUM SALTS

Synonyms

Calcipur, Calphosan, Dragocal, Ebucin, Efical, Glucal, Hydroxyapatite, Ibercal, Kalpren, Neocalglucon

Summary

Calcium is an essential electrolyte; its concentration in the blood is regulated within narrow limits. Calcium ions are required for normal cardiac, muscle, nerve, and hemostatic function. The U.S. Recommended Dietary Allowance of calcium for pregnant women is 1200 mg/day (NRC, 1989).

Magnitude of Teratogenic Risk

None To Minimal

Quality and Quantity of Data

Fair

Comment

None

The frequencies of malformations in general, of major malformations, and of minor anomalies were no greater than expected among the children of 1007 women who took calcium supplements during the first four lunar months of pregnancy in the Collaborative Perinatal Project (Heinonen et al., 1977). The frequencies of most major classes of congenital anomalies were also no greater than expected among the children of these women, but the frequency of central nervous system malformations were slightly, but significantly, increased. No specific anomaly accounted for this association. Congenital anomalies were not found more often than expected among the infants of 3739 women who took calcium salts anytime during pregnancy in this study. If maternal use of calcium salts early in gestation does increase the risk of malformations in the offspring, this increase is small compared to the background risk of congenital anomalies that attends every pregnancy.

No teratogenic effect was observed among the offspring of mice, rats, or rabbits treated during pregnancy with calcium sulfate in doses of 16-1600 mg/kg/d (Anonymous, 1974). Similarly, the frequency of malformations was not increased among the offspring of rats fed a diet containing 1.7 times the usual amount of calcium during pregnancy in one study (McCormack et al., 1979). In another study in which pregnant rats were given about 1600 mg/kg/d of calcium chloride in their drinking water, fetal death and growth retardation were increased, but maternal toxicity also occurred (Hayasaka et al., 1990).

Key References

Anonymous: Teratologic evaluation of FDA 71-86 (calcium sulfate) in mice, rats and rabbits. NTIS (National Technical Information Service) Report/PB-234 873, 1974. [A]

Hayasaka I, Murakami K, Kato Z, Tamaki F, et al.: Preventive effects of maternal electrolyte supplementation on azosemide-induced skeletal malformations in rats. Environ Med 34:61-67, 1990. [A]

Heinonen OP, Slone D, Shapiro S: Birth Defects and Drugs in Pregnancy. Littleton, Mass,: John Wright-PSG, 1977, pp 444, 479, 498. [E]

McCormack KM, Ottosen LD, Sanger VL, Spraque S, et al.: Effect of prenatal administration of aluminum and parathyroid hormone on fetal development in the rat (40493). Proc Soc Exp Biol Med 161:74-77, 1979. [A]

NRC (National Research Council): Recommended Dietary Allowances, 10th ed. Report of the Subcommittee on the Tenth Edition of the RDAs, Food and Nutrition Board, Commission on Life Sciences. Washington, D.C.: National Academy Press, 1989. [O]

CAMPHOR

Synonyms

Alcanfor, Bornan-2-one, Canfora, Kampfer

Summary

Camphor is a cyclic ketone that is used topically as a rubefacient and mild analgesic.

Magnitude of Teratogenic Risk

None To Minimal

Quality and Quantity of Data

Poor To Fair

Comment

This risk assessment is for topical use only.

The frequency of congenital anomalies was no greater than expected among the children of 168 women treated with camphor topically during the first four lunar months of pregnancy or among the children of 763 women who received such treatment anytime during pregnancy in the Collaborative Perinatal Project (Heinonen et al., 1977).

No animal teratology studies of camphor have been published.

Neonatal death occurred in an infant born to a woman who had ingested a toxic dose of camphor shortly before delivery (Riggs et al., 1965).

Key References

Heinonen OP, Slone D, Shapiro S: Birth Defects and Drugs in Pregnancy. Littleton, Mass.: John Wright-PSG, 1977, pp 410, 411, 444, 499. [E]

Riggs J, Hamilton R, Homel S, McCabe J: Camphorated oil intoxication in pregnancy. Obstet Gynecol 25(2):255-258, 1965. [C]

CANTHARIDIN

Synonyms

Canthacur, Cantharone, Kantaridin, Kantharidin, Verr-Canth

Summary

Cantharidin is a topical irritant prepared from dried beetles. It is used for the removal of warts and is considered an aphrodisiac in some cultures.

Magnitude of Teratogenic Risk

Undetermined

Quality and Quantity of Data

None

Comment

None

No epidemiological studies of congenital anomalies in infants born to women treated with cantharidin during pregnancy have been reported.

No animal teratology studies of cantharidin have been published.

Key References

None available.

CAPREOMYCIN

Synonyms

Capastat, Caprocin

Summary

Capreomycin is a natural mixture of polypeptide antibiotics that is given intramuscularly in the treatment of tuberculosis.

Magnitude of Teratogenic Risk

Undetermined

Quality and Quantity of Data

None

Comment

None

No epidemiological studies of congenital anomalies among infants born to women treated with capreomycin during pregnancy have been reported.

No animal teratology studies of capreomycin have been published.

Key References

None available.

CAPTAN

Synonyms

Amercide, Captex, Hexacap, Malipur, Merpan, Neracid, Orthocide, Osocide, Trimegol

Summary

Captan is an antifungal agent used in agriculture. The Threshold Limit Value for occupational exposure to captan in the air as an 8-hour time-weighted average is 5 mg/cu m (ACGIH, 1990).

Magnitude of Teratogenic Risk

Minimal

Quality and Quantity of Data

Poor To Fair

Comment

This rating is for occupational exposure within accepted limits. There may be a substantial risk to a pregnant woman with exposures that are toxic.

Increased frequencies of miscarriage, premature delivery, and infants with congenital anomalies were observed in an interview study of 10,481 pregnancies of female floriculture workers and 3503 pregnancies of wives of male floriculture workers (Restrepo et al., 1990a). Captan was the pesticide used most frequently by these workers. Examination of the children reported to have birth defects revealed that this could be confirmed in only 38%; 8% of the children reported to be normal were found to have a birth defect (Restrepo et al., 1990b). Analysis of 222 cases with confirmed birth defects showed a weak association with suspected maternal exposure to pesticides during pregnancy (RR=1.8, 95% confidence interval 1.2-2.7); this association was largely attributable to birthmarks.

No congenital anomalies were observed among the offspring of 21 monkeys given oral doses of 10-75 mg/kg/d of captan during pregnancy (Vondruska et al., 1971). No teratogenic effect was seen among the offspring of pregnant dogs fed 30-60 mg/kg/d of captan (Kennedy et al., 1975). The frequency of malformations was no greater than expected but fetal death was increased among the offspring of rats or rabbits fed captan during pregnancy in doses of 50-2000 or 19-150 mg/kg/d (Fabro et al., 1966; Kennedy et al., 1968; Anonymous, 1989). Microphthalmia and death were found more often than expected among the fetuses of pregnant mice given captan in doses of 100-464 mg/kg/d (Anonymous, 1989); maternal toxicity was also seen. Increased frequencies of a variety of fetal anomalies and of fetal death have been observed in pregnant hamsters fed 500-2500 mg/kg/d of captan (Robens, 1970; Kennedy et al., 1968); considerable maternal toxicity was also seen with this treatment.

Key References

ACGIH: 1990-1991 Threshold Limit Values for Chemical Substances and Physical Agents and Biological Exposure Indices. Cincinnati, Ohio: Am Conference Govt Ind Hyg, 1990. [O]

Anonymous: Final report on the safety assessment of captan. J Am Coll Toxicol 8(4):643-680. [R]

Kennedy G, Fancher OE, Calandra JC: An investigation of the teratogenic potential of captan, flopet and difolatan. Toxicol Appl Pharmacol 13:420-430, 1968. [A]

Kennedy GL Jr, Fancher OE, Calandra JC: Nonteratogenicity of captan in beagles. Teratology 11:223-226, 1975. [A]

Restrepo M, Munoz N, Day N, et al.: Birth defects among children born to a population occupationally exposed to pesticides in Colombia. Scand J Work Environ Health 16:239-246, 1990. [E]

Restrepo M, Munoz N, Day N, et al.: Prevalence of adverse reproductive outcomes in a population occupationally exposed to pesticides in Colombia. Scand J Work Environ Health 16:232-238, 1990. [E]

Robens JF: Teratologic activity of several phthalimide derivatives in the golden hamster. Toxicol Appl Pharmacol 16:24-34, 1970. [A]

Vondruska JF, Fancher OE, Calandra JC: An investigation into the teratogenic potential of captan, folpet, and difolatan in nonhuman primates. Toxicol Appl Pharmacol 18:619-624, 1971. [A]

CAPTOPRIL

Synonyms

Acepril, Alopresin, Capoten, Captolane, Cesplon, Dilabar, Garranil, Lopirin, Lopril, Tensoprel

Summary

Captopril is an inhibitor of angiotensin converting enzyme (ACE). It is given orally in the treatment of hypertension.

Magnitude of Teratogenic Risk

First-Trimester Use: Undetermined

Use Later In Pregnancy: Moderate

Quality and Quantity of Data

First-Trimester Use: Poor

Use Later In Pregnancy: Fair To Good

Comment

1) A small risk cannot be excluded, but a high risk of congenital anomalies in the children of women treated with captopril during the first trimester is unlikely.

2) There is a substantial risk of oligohydramnios and fetal distress or death in hypertensive women treated with captopril in the latter part of pregnancy. The effect may be related to the pharmacological action of this drug on the fetus (see below).

No epidemiological studies of congenital anomalies in infants born to women treated with captopril during pregnancy have been reported. In one clinical series, no malformations were observed among 14 infants born to women who were treated with captopril during the first trimester of pregnancy (Kreft-Jais & Boutroy, 1988).

Oligohydramnios and fetal anuria and neonatal pulmonary hypoplasia, renal failure, joint contractures, and death have been repeatedly observed after maternal treatment with captopril or related drugs during pregnancy (Rothberg & Lorenz, 1984; Anonymous, 1989; Rosa et al., 1989; Boutroy, 1989; Brent & Beckman, 1991; Hanssens et al., 1991). Women who require such treatment have hypertension which may be severe, and hypertension per se is known to be associated with similar fetal and neonatal complications. Although no epidemiological studies are available to permit apportionment of risk, it appears that these complications are unusually common in the pregnancies of hypertensive women who are treated with ACE inhibitors (Boutroy et al., 1984; Fiocchi et al., 1984; Anonymous, 1989; Rosa et al., 1989; Boutroy, 1989; Brent & Beckman, 1991; Hanssens et al., 1991). It is important to note that these effects do not appear to reflect abnormal embryogenesis but rather a pharmacologic response of the fetus to captopril during the second half of gestation (Brent & Beckman, 1991).

Three cases have been reported in which hypocalvaria, an unusual underdevelopment of the skull bones, and other skeletal anomalies occurred in the infant or fetus of women treated with captopril throughout pregnancy (Duminy & Berger, 1981; Rothberg & Lorenz, 1984; Barr & Cohen, 1991). Three infants with similar unusual skull defects have been observed after maternal treatment throughout pregnancy with other ACE inhibitors (Mehta & Modi, 1989; Cunniff et al., 1990; Barr & Cohen, 1991).

No increase in malformations but increased frequencies of fetal growth retardation and death were observed among the offspring of rats treated during pregnancy with 1.5-5 times the human therapeutic dose of captopril (Al-Shabanah et al., 1991). Decreased ossification of the skull and other bones was observed at the higher dose. Pregnant rabbits and sheep given captopril late in gestation in doses similar to those used in humans had an unexpectedly high frequency of fetal deaths (Broughton Pipkin et al., 1982; Keith et al., 1982; Ferris & Weir, 1983). Fetal hypotension was demonstrated in sheep after such treatment (Broughton Pipkin et al., 1982; Robillard et al., 1983; Lumbers et al., 1992).

Please see agent summary on enalapril for information on a related agent.

Key References

Al-Shabanah OA, Al-Harbi MM, AlGharably NMA, Islam MW: The effect of maternal administration of captopril on fetal development in rat. Res Commun Chem Pathol Pharmacol 73:221-230, 1991. [A]

Anonymous: Are ACE inhibitors safe in pregnancy? Lancet 2:482-483, 1989. [O]

Barr M Jr, Cohen MM Jr: ACE inhibitor fetopathy and hypocalvaria: The kidney-skull connection. Teratology 44:485-495, 1991. [S]

Boutroy MJ: Fetal effects of maternally administered clonidine and angiotensin-converting enzyme inhibitors. Dev Pharmacol Ther 13:199-204, 1989. [R]

Boutroy MJ, Vert P, de Ligny BH, Miton A: Captopril administration in pregnancy impairs fetal angiotensin converting enzyme activity and neonatal adaptation. Lancet 2:935-936, 1984. [C]

Brent RL, Beckman DA: Angiotensin-converting enzyme inhibitors, and embryopathic class of drugs with unique properties: Information for clinical teratology counselors. Teratology 43:543-546, 1991. [O]

Broughton Pipkin F, Symonds EM, Turner SR: The effect of captopril (SQ14,225) upon mother and fetus in the chronically cannulated ewe and in the pregnant rabbit. J Physiol 323:415-422, 1982. [A]

Cunniff C, Jones KL, Phillipson J, et al.: Oligohydramnios sequence and renal tubular malformation associated with maternal enalapril use. Am J Obstet Gynecol 162:187-189, 1990. [C]

Duminy PC, Burger P du T: Fetal abnormality associated with the use of captopril during pregnancy. S Afr Med J 60:805, 1981. [C]

Ferris FF, Weir EK: Effect of captopril on uterine blood flow and prostaglandin E synthesis in the pregnant rabbit. J Clin Invest 71:809-815, 1983. [A]

Fiocchi R, Lijnen P, Fagard R, Staessen J, et al.: Captopril during pregnancy. Lancet 2:1153, 1984. [C]

Hanssens M, Keirse MJNC, Vankelecom F, Van Assche FA: Fetal and neonatal effects of treatment with angiotensin-converting enzyme inhibitors in pregnancy. Obstet Gynecol 78(1):128-135, 1991. [R]

Keith IM, Will JA, Weir EK: Captopril: Association with fetal death and pulmonary vascular changes in the rabbit (41446). Proc Soc Exp Biol Med 170:378-383, 1982. [A]

Kreft-Jais C, Boutroy M-J: Angiotensin-converting enzyme inhibitors during pregnancy: A survey of 22 patients given captopril and nine given enalapril. Br J Obstet Gynecol 95:420-422, 1988. [S]

Lumbers ER, Kingsford NM, Menzies RI, Stevens AD: Acute effects of captopril, an angiotensin-converting enzyme inhibitor, on the pregnant ewe and fetus. Am J Physiol 262(5, Pt. 2):R754-760, 1992. [A]

Mehta N, Modi N: ACE inhibitors in pregnancy. Lancet 2:96-97, 1989. [C]

Robillard JE, Weismann DN, Gomez RA, Ayres NA: Renal and adrenal responses to converting-enzyme inhibition in fetal and newborn life. Am J Physiol 244:R249-R256, 1983. [A]

Rosa FW, Bosco LA, Graham CF, et al.: Neonatal anuria with maternal angiotensin-converting enzyme inhibition. Obstet Gynecol 74:371-374, 1989. [S]

Rothberg AD, Lorenz R: Can captopril cause fetal and neonatal renal failure? Pediatr Pharmacol 4:189-192, 1984. [C]

CARAMIPHEN

Synonyms

2-Diethylaminoethyl 1-phenylcyclopentane-1-carboxylate

Summary

Caramiphen is an anticholinergic that is used in cough medicines and to treat parkinsonism and related disorders.

Magnitude of Teratogenic Risk

None To Minimal

Quality and Quantity of Data

Poor To Fair

Comment

None

The Collaborative Perinatal Project reported that the frequency of congenital anomalies was not significantly greater than expected among 38 infants whose mothers took caramiphen during the first trimester of pregnancy or among 236 infants born to women who took the drug anytime during pregnancy (Heinonen et al., 1977).

No animal teratology studies of caramiphen have been published.

Key References

Heinonen OP, Slone D, Shapiro S: Birth Defects and Drugs in Pregnancy. Littleton, Mass.: John Wright-PSG, 1977, pp 378, 442. [E]

CARBAMAZEPINE

Synonyms

Amizepin, Biston, Epitol, Hermolepsin, Mazepine, Neurotol, Nordotol, Sirtal, Tegretal, Timonil

Summary

Carbamazepine is an anticonvulsant agent used to prevent grand mal, psychomotor, and partial seizures.

Magnitude of Teratogenic Risk

Small

Quality and Quantity of Data

Fair To Good

Comment

1) Teratogenic risks associated with polydrug therapy that includes carbamazepine may be greater than those associated with carbamazepine monotherapy.

2) It has been suggested that the frequency of congenital anomalies among the children of epileptic women treated with carbamazepine during pregnancy might be reduced by administering folate supplements to them before and in the first few months after conception (Kaneko, 1991; Dansky et al., 1992; Delgado-Escueta & Janz, 1992; Hiilesmaa, 1992), but the value of such therapy has not yet been demonstrated.

3) Prenatal diagnosis by high-resolution ultrasound examination and alpha-fetoprotein measurement is available for some of the serious malformations that are seen among infants of epileptic women treated with carbamazepine during pregnancy (Delgado-Escueta & Janz, 1992; Hiilesmaa, 1992; Gladstone et al., 1992).

Epidemiological studies of malformations in infants born to women who took carbamazepine during pregnancy are difficult to interpret because assessment of the effects of anticonvulsant drug exposure is confounded by many other factors (Kelly, 1984; Schardein, 1985; Hanson, 1986; Friis, 1989; Dansky & Finnell, 1991). Among these confounders are the facts that most women with seizures are treated with some anticonvulsant drug, that many women are treated with more than one anticonvulsant at a time, that women who are not treated or are treated with a single agent probably have milder disease, and that carbamazepine treatment is unusual in women without seizures.

In several cohort studies, each of which involved fewer than 100 epileptic women treated with carbamazepine during the first trimester of pregnancy, the frequency of malformations in the infants, although 2-3 times as great as that generally seen among normal populations, was similar to that in children born to epileptic women who had been treated with other anticonvulsants (Starreveld-Zimmerman, et al., 1973; Nakane et al., 1980; Lindhout et al., 1982, 1992a; Kaneko et al., 1988; Battino et al., 1992). Higher frequencies of anomalies have been observed among infants born to mothers treated with carbamazepine in combination with other anticonvulsant agents, especially valproic acid (Lindhout et al., 1984; Kaneko et al., 1988; Shakir et al., 1991; Kaneko et al., 1992).

No association with maternal carbamazepine use during pregnancy was observed in an Hungarian population-based case-control study of 10,698 infants with congenital anomalies (OR=2.8, 95% confidence interval 0.1-10.1) (Czeizel et al., 1992). There did appear to be an association with maternal use of multiple anticonvulsant agents including carbamazepine during pregnancy, however. No association with maternal carbamazepine treatment during pregnancy was observed in another case-control study of 7607 infants with congenital anomalies identified through the Italian Multicentric Registry of Birth Defects (Bertollini et al., 1985).

In one study of 20 children born to mothers who had been treated with carbamazepine alone during pregnancy, the average head circumference (but not the weight or length) was significantly decreased both at birth and at 18 months of age (Hiilesmaa et al., 1981). The head circumference among these children was not significantly decreased at 5.5 years of age, however, and both of the carbamazepine-exposed 5.5-year-old children whose head circumferences were two or more standard deviations below the mean in this study had normal intellectual function (Gaily et al., 1990a). The average IQ of 34 5.5-year-old children whose mothers had taken carbamazepine during pregnancy was no different from controls; one other child in this study who was exposed was severely retarded, apparently for a different reason (Gaily et al., 1988). The frequency of specific cognitive dysfunction was no greater than expected among 30 of these children who were tested (Gaily et al., 1990b). Similarly, the frequencies of neurological dysfunction and school problems were no greater than expected among 23 six- to 13-year-old children of epileptic women who had been treated with carbamazepine during pregnancy (van der Pol et al., 1991).

An increased frequency of neural tube defects among the children of women treated with carbamazepine during pregnancy has been suggested on the basis of clinical observations and data from Michigan Medicaid recipients (Bod, 1989; Jones et al., 1989a; Rosa, 1991; Gladstone et al., 1992; Lindhout et al., 1992b). Cases of spina bifida have been observed in several epidemiological studies of infants born to women treated with carbamazepine during pregnancy, but this putative association has not been confirmed statistically (Bertollini et al., 1985; Kallen et al., 1989; Czeizel et al., 1992; Omtzig et al., 1992).

The existence of a fetal carbamazepine syndrome of growth and developmental delay associated with minor facial and other anomalies similar to those seen in association with maternal use of some other anticonvulsants has been suggested (Jones et al., 1989b; van Allen et al., 1988). Features of this syndrome were seen in most of 35 children born to women treated with carbamazepine monotherapy in one study (Jones et al., 1989b). It is unclear whether these features are a result of the population evaluated or method of study or due to the medication, the maternal epilepsy, or some

related factor (Scialli & Lione, 1989; Dow & Riopelle, 1989).

Central nervous system and other anomalies have been observed among the offspring of mice treated with carbamazepine in doses 5-100 times those used clinically, but no clear dose-response relationship was apparent (Paulson et al., 1979; Finnell et al., 1986; Finnell & Dansky, 1991). Although maternal toxicity occurred at the higher dose levels, drug concentration in the animals' blood was within or below the range that would be considered therapeutic in humans. Results of mouse teratology studies involving doses 2-10 times those used in humans have been inconsistent (Fritz et al., 1976; Sullivan & McElhatten, 1977; Wray et al., 1982; Finnell & Dansky, 1991). In rats, dose-dependent increased frequencies of congenital anomalies were observed among the offspring of pregnant animals treated with carbamazepine in doses 17-25 times those used in humans (Vorhees et al., 1990). Such doses produced maternal toxicity and blood levels 2-3 times greater than those considered to be therapeutic in humans. The relevance of these findings to the risks associated with therapeutic use of carbamazepine in human pregnancy is unknown.

Key References

Battino D, Binelli S, Caccamo ML, Canevini MP, et al.: Malformations in offspring of 305 epileptic women: A prospective study. Acta Neurol Scand 85(3):204-207, 1992. [E]

Bertollini R, Mastroiacovo P, Segni G: Maternal epilepsy and birth defects: A case-control study in the Italian Multicentric Registry of Birth Defects (IPIMC). Eur J Epidemiol 1(1):67-72, 1985. [E]

Bod M: Teratogenic evaluation of anticonvulsants in a population-based Hungarian material. Teratology 40(3):277, 1989. [E]

Czeizel AE, Bod M, Halasz P: Evaluation of anticonvulsant drugs during pregnancy in a population-based Hungarian study. Eur J Epidemiol 8(1):122-127, 1992. [E]

Dansky LV, Finnell RH: Parental epilespy, anticonvulsant drugs, and reproductive outcome: Epidemiologic and experimental findings spanning three decades; 2: Human studies. Reprod Toxicol 5(4):301-335, 1991. [R]

Dansky LV, Rosenblatt DS, Andermann E: Mechanisms of teratogenesis: Folic acid and antiepileptic therapy. Neurology 42(Suppl 5):32-42, 1992. [R]

Delgado-Escueta AV, Janz D: Consensus guidelines: Preconception counseling, management, and care of the pregnant woman with epilepsy. Neurology 42(Suppl 5):149-160, 1992. [R]

Dow KE, Riopelle RJ: Teratogenic effects of carbamazepine [letter]. N Engl J Med 321:1480-1481, 1989. [O]

Finnell RH, Dansky LV: Parental epilepsy, anticonvulsant drugs and reproductive outcome: Epidemiologic and experimental findings spanning three decades; 1: Animal studies. Reprod Toxicol 5(4):281-299, 1991. [A]

Finnell RH, Mohl VK, Bennet GD, Taylor SM: Failure of epoxide formation to influence carbamazepine-induced teratogenesis in a mouse model. Teratogenesis Carcinog Mutagen 6:393-401, 1986. [A]

Friis ML: Facial clefts and congenital heart defects in children of parents with epilepsy: Genetic and environmental etiologic factors. Acta Neurol Scand 79:433-459, 1989. [R]

Fritz H, Muller D, Hess R: Comparative study of the teratogenicity of phenobarbitone, diphenylhydantoin and carbamazepine in mice. Toxicology 6:323-330. 1976. [A]

Gaily EK, Granstrom M-L, Hiilesmaa VK, et al.: Head circumference in children of epileptic mothers: Contributions of drug exposure and genetic background. Epilepsy Res 5:217-222, 1990a. [E]

Gaily EK, Kantola-Sorsa E, Granstrom M-L: Intelligence of children of epileptic mothers. J Pediatr 113:677-684, 1988. [E]

Gaily EK, Kantola-Sorsa E, Granstrom M-L: Specific cognitive dysfunction in children with epileptic mothers. Dev Med Child Neurol 32:403-414, 1990b. [E]

Gladstone DJ, Bologa M, Maguire C, Pastuszak A, et al.: Course of pregnancy and fetal outcome following maternal exposure to carbamazepine and phenytoin: A prospective study. Reprod Toxicol 6:257-261, 1992. [E]

Hanson JW: Teratogen update: Fetal hydantoin effects. Teratology 33:349-353, 1986. [R]

Hiilesmaa VK: Pregnancy and birth in women with epilepsy. Neurology 42(Suppl 5):8-11, 1992. [R]

Hiilesmaa VK, Teramo K, Granstrom ML, Bardy AH: Fetal head growth retardation associated with maternal antiepileptic drugs. Lancet 2:165-167, 1981. [S]

Jones KL, Johnson KA, Adams J, Lacro RV: Teratogenic effects of carbamazepine [Letter]. N Engl J Med 321:1480-1481, 1989a. [O]

Jones KL, Lacro RV, Johnson KA, Adams J: Pattern of malformations in the children of women treated with carbamazepine during pregnancy. N Engl J Med 320:1661-1666, 1989b. [E]

Kallen B, Robert E, Mastroiacovo P, et al.: Anticonvulsant drugs and malformations. Is there a drug specificity? Eur J Epidemiol 5(1):31-36, 1989. [E]

Kaneko S: Antiepileptic drug therapy and reproductive consequences: Functional and morphologic effects. Reprod Toxicol 5:179-198, 1991. [R]

Kaneko S, Otani K, Fukushima Y, et al.: Teratogenicity of antiepileptic drugs: Analysis of possible risk factors. Epilepsia 29(4):459-467, 1988. [E]

Kaneko S, Otani K, Kondo T, Fukushima Y, et al.: Malformation in infants of mothers with epilepsy receiving antiepileptic drugs. Neurology 42(suppl 5):68-74, 1992. [E]

Kelly TE: Teratogenicity of anticonvulsant drugs. I: Review of the literature. Am J Med Genet 19:413-434, 1984. [R]

Lindhout D, Hoppener RJ, Meinardi H: Teratogenicity of antiepileptic drug combinations with special emphasis on epoxidation (of carbamazepine). Epilepsia 25:77-83, 1984. [A]

Lindhout D, Meinardi H, Barth PG: Hazards of fetal exposure to drug combinations. In: Jantz D et al. (eds). Epilepsy, Pregnancy and the Child. New York: Raven Press, 1982, pp 275-281. [S]

Lindhout D, Meinardi H, Meijer JWA, Nau H: Antiepileptic drugs and teratogenesis in two consecutive cohorts: Changes in prescription policy paralleled by changes in pattern of malformations. Neurology 42(Suppl 5):94-110, 1992a. [E]

Lindhout D, Omtzigt JGC, Cornel MC: Spectrum of neural-tube defects in 34 infants prenatally exposed to antiepileptic drugs. Neurology 42(Suppl 5):111-118, 1992b. [S]

Nakane Y, Okuma T, Takahashi R, Sato Y, et al.: Multi-institutional study on the teratogenicity and fetal toxicity of antiepileptic drugs: A report of a collaborative study group in Japan. Epilepsia 21:663-680, 1980. [E]

Omtzigt JGC, Los FJ, Grobbee DE, Pijpers L, et al.: The risk of spina bifida aperta after first-trimester exposure to valproate in a prenatal cohort. Neurology 42(Suppl 5):118-125, 1992. [E]

Paulson RB, Paulson GW, Jreissaty S: Phenytoin and carbamazepine in production of cleft palates in mice. Comparison of teratogenic effects. Arch Neurol 36:832-836, 1979. [A]

Rosa FW: Spina bifida in infants of women treated with carbamazepine during pregnancy. N Engl J Med 324(10):674-677, 1991. [S]

Schardein JL: Chemically Induced Birth Defects. New York: Marcel Dekker, 1985, pp. 142-189. [R]

Scialli AR, Lione A: Teratogenic effects of carbamazepine [letter]. N Engl J Med 321:1480-1481, 1989. [O]

Shakir RA, Abdulwahab B: Congenital malformations before and after the onset of maternal epilepsy. Acta Neurol Scand 84:153-156, 1991. [E]

Starreveld-Zimmerman AA, van der Kolk WJ, Meinardi H, Elshove J: Are anticonvulsants teratogenic? Lancet 2:48-49, 1973. [E]

Sullivan FM, McElhatton PR: A comparison of the teratogenic activity of the antiepileptic drugs carbamazepine, clonazepam, ethosuximide, phenobarbital, phenytoin, and primidone in mice. Toxicol Appl Pharmacol 40:365-378, 1977. [A]

van Allen MJ, Yerby M, Leavitt A, McCormick KB, et al.: Increased major and minor malformations in infants of epileptic mothers: Preliminary results of the pregnancy and epilepsy study. Am J Hum Gen 43(Suppl):A73, 1988. [E]

van der Pol MC, Hadders-Algra M, Huisjes HJ, Touwen BCL: Antiepileptic medication in pregnancy: Late effects on the children's central nervous system development. Am J Obstet Gynecol 164:121-128, 1991. [E]

Vorhees CV, Acuff KD, Weisenburger WP, et al.: Teratogenicity of carbamazepine in rats. Teratology 41:311-317, 1990. [A]

Wray SD, Hassell TM, Phillips C, Johnston MC: Preliminary study of the effects of carbamazepine on congenital orofacial defects in offspring of A/J mice. Epilepsia 23:101-110, 1982. [A]

CARBAZERAN

Synonyms

Carbazeranum

Summary

Carbazeran is a cardiotonic drug.

Magnitude of Teratogenic Risk

Undetermined

Quality and Quantity of Data

None

Comment

None

No epidemiological studies of congenital anomalies in infants born to women who were treated with carbazeran during pregnancy have been reported.

No animal teratology studies of carbazeran have been published.

Key References

None available.

CARBENICILLIN

Synonyms

Anabactyl, Carfecillin, Carindapen, Fugacillin, Geocillin, Geopen, Gripenin, Microcillin, Pyocianil, Pyopen

Summary

Carbenicillin is a semisynthetic penicillin used in the treatment of serious infections.

Magnitude of Teratogenic Risk

Undetermined

Quality and Quantity of Data

None To Poor

Comment

A small risk cannot be excluded, but a high risk of congenital anomalies in the children of women treated with carbenicillin during pregnancy is unlikely.

No epidemiological studies of congenital anomalies among the infants of women treated with carbenicillin during pregnancy have been reported.

No teratogenic effect was noted among the offspring of pregnant rats or mice treated with carbenicillin in doses similar to those used in humans in one study that has not been reported in detail (Anonymous, 1970).

Please see agent summary on penicillin for information on a related agent that has been more thoroughly studied.

Key References

Anonymous: Carbenicillin (Monograph). Rx Bull 1:9-14, 1970. [A]

CARBIDOPA

Synonyms

Lodosyn

Summary

Carbidopa is an inhibitor of peripheral decarboxylation of levodopa to dopamine. It is usually used in combination with levodopa in the treatment of Parkinson's disease and other dyskinetic disorders.

Magnitude of Teratogenic Risk

Undetermined

Quality and Quantity of Data

None

Comment

None

No epidemiological studies of congenital anomalies in infants born to mothers who were treated with carbidopa during pregnancy have been published.

Pregnant rats given about 50 times the usual human dose of carbidopa throughout gestation had offspring with an increased frequency of hemorrhage in their brown adipose tissue (Kitchin & DiStefano, 1976). Brown adipose tissue is thought to be important in temperature control, but the relevance, if any, of this observation to the clinical use of carbidopa in pregnant women is unknown.

Key References

Kitchin KT, DiStefano V: L-Dopa and brown fat hemorrhage in the rat pup. Toxicol Pharmacol 38:251-263, 1976. [A]

CARBINOXAMINE

Synonyms

Allergefon, Clistin, Davenol, Histex, Lergefin, Polistine, Ziriton

Summary

Carbinoxamine is an antihistiminic agent of the ethanolamine class. It is used to treat allergic conditions.

Magnitude of Teratogenic Risk

Undetermined

Quality and Quantity of Data

None To Poor

Comment

None

No epidemiologic studies of malformations in the infants of women who took carbinoxamine during pregnancy have been published.

In one study, the frequency of malformations was not increased among the offspring of rats or mice treated, respectively, with 3-130 and 3-170 times the usual human dose of carbinoxamine during pregnancy (Maruyama & Yoshida, 1968).

Please see agent summary on diphenhydramine for information on a related drug that has been more thoroughly studied.

Key References

Maruyama H, Yoshida S: [Pharmacology of a new antihistamine, carbinoxamine diphenyldisulfonate. (2) Toxicity and influence on fetuses]. J Med Soc Toho Univ (Jpn) 15:367-374, 1968. [A]

CARBOXYMETHYL-CELLULOSE

Synonyms

Carmellose Sodium, Relatin, Serogel

Summary

Carboxymethylcellulose is used as a suspending and emulsifying agent in the pharmaceutical and food industries. It is also used as a protective agent for ostomies and for oral and perioral lesions and for the treatment of dry mouth.

Magnitude of Teratogenic Risk

Undetermined

Quality and Quantity of Data

None To Poor

Comment

A small risk cannot be excluded, but a substantial risk of congenital anomalies in the children of women treated with carboxymethylcellulose during pregnancy is unlikely.

No epidemiological studies of congenital anomalies among infants born to women who ingested very large amounts of carboxymethylcellulose during pregnancy have been reported.

No teratogenic effect was observed among the offspring of hamsters treated with carboxymethylcellulose during pregnancy in doses of 50 mg/kg/d (Robens, 1969).

Key References

Robens JF: Teratologic studies of carbaryl, diazinon, norea, disulfiram, and thiram in small laboratory animals. Toxicol Appl Pharmacol 15:152-163, 1969. [A]

CARBUTAMIDE

Synonyms

Aminophenurobutane, Bucarban, Bucrol, Glucidoral, Glucofren, Invenol, Nadisan, Oranil

Summary

Carbutamide is an orally active hypoglycemic medication used to treat diabetes.

Magnitude of Teratogenic Risk

Undetermined

Quality and Quantity of Data

Poor

Comment

A small risk cannot be excluded, but there is no indication that the risk of congenital anomalies in the children of women treated with carbutamide during pregnancy is likely to be great.

No epidemiological studies of congenital anomalies in infants born to women treated with carbutamide during pregnancy have been reported.

The frequency of malformations was increased among the offspring of mice and rats treated with carbutamide during pregnancy in doses respectively 20-40 and 7-60 times those used therapeutically in humans (Anonymous, 1971; Tuchmann-Duplessis & Mercier-Parot, 1959, 1963; Anonymous, 1966). A variety of malformations including eye and neural tube defects were seen, and typical dose-dependence of the effect was demonstrated. The frequency of malformations was also increased among the offspring of rabbits treated during pregnancy with carbutamide in doses 40, but not 10-30, times those used in humans (Tuchmann-Duplessis & Mercier-Parot, 1963; Somers, 1969). The relevance of these observations to the risks associated with clinical use of carbutamide in human pregnancy is unknown.

Key References

Anonymous: The evaluation of drugs for foetal toxicity and teratogenicity in the rat. Proc Eur Soc Study Drug Toxic 7:216-228, 1966. [A]

Anonymous: Recherches des effets teratogenes etude methodologique chez la souris. Proc Eur Soc Study Drug Toxic 12:307-331, 1971. [A]

Somers GF: The evaluation of drugs for foetal toxicity and teratogenicity in the rabbit. Proc Eur Soc Study Drug Toxic 10:227-234, 1969. [A]

Tuchmann-Duplessis H, Mercier-Parot L: Sur l'action teratogen d'un sulfamide hypoglycemiant etude experimentale chez la ratte. J Physiologie 51:65-83, 1959. [A]

Tuchmann-Duplessis H, Mercier-Parot: Production de malformations chez la souris et le lapin par administration d'un sulfamide hypoglycemiant, la carbutamide. CR Soc Biol 157:1193-1197, 1963. [A]

CARISOPRODOL

Synonyms

Caprodat, Carisoma, Flexartal, Mioxom, Rela, Releaxo-Powel, Sanoma, Soma, Somadril, Soprodol

Summary

Carisoprodol is used orally as a skeletal muscle relaxant. One of its metabolites is meprobamate.

Magnitude of Teratogenic Risk

Undetermined

Quality and Quantity of Data

None To Poor

Comment

None

No epidemiological studies of congenital anomalies in infants whose mothers were treated with carisoprodol during pregnancy have been reported.

Decreased litter size and fetal weight were observed among the offspring of mice treated with 43 times the human dose of carisoprodol during pregnancy (Grizzle et al., 1992). This dose also produced generalized toxicity in adult animals. No such effect was seen with doses 11-34 times those used in humans.

Please see agent summary on mepro-bamate for information on this metabolite of carisoprodol.

Key References

Grizzle TB, George JD, Fail PA, Heindel JJ: Reproductive toxicity of carisoprodol (CARI) as evaluated by the continous breeding protocol. Toxicologist 12(1):197, 1992. [A]

CARMUSTINE

Synonyms

BCNU, BiCNU

Summary

Carmustine is an alkylating agent of the nitrosourea class that is administered intravenously in the treatment of malignant neoplasms.

Magnitude of Teratogenic Risk

Undetermined

Quality and Quantity of Data

Poor

Comment

Because this agent is an antimetabolite, it must be suspected of having teratogenic activity, although this has not been demonstrated in humans.

No epidemiological studies of congenital anomalies in infants of women treated with carmustine during pregnancy have been reported.

Increased frequencies of malformations were observed among the offspring of rats treated during pregnancy with carmustine in doses smaller than those used in humans, but maternal toxicity regularly occurred in these experiments (Thompson et al., 1974). A variety of malformations were seen in the offspring;

abdominal wall defects, eye malformations, and central nervous system anomalies were most common. The frequency of malformations was not consistently increased among the offspring of rabbits after similar treatment, although maternal toxicity also occurred in this species. Increased frequencies of fetal and neonatal death, growth retardation, and malformations of the palate, face, limbs, and tail were found among the offspring of pregnant mice treated with 4-8 but not 1-2 times the human dose of carmustine (Wong & Wells, 1989).

Increased frequencies of chromosomal breaks and rearrangements have been observed in human lymphocyte cultures after in vivo or in vitro treatment with carmustine (Harrod & Cortner, 1968). The relevance of these observations to the risks associated with maternal carmustine therapy in human pregnancy is unknown.

Key References

Harrod EK, Cortner JA: Prolonged survival of lymphocytes with chromosomal defects in children treated with 1,3-Bis(2-Chloroethyl)-1-Nitrosourea. J Natl Cancer Inst 40:269-282, 1968. [S]

Thompson DJ, Molello JA, Strebing RJ, Dyke IL, et al.: Reproduction and teratology studies with oncolytic agents in the rat and rabbit. I. I,3-bis(2-Chloroethyl)-I-Nitrosourea (BCNU). Toxicol Appl Pharmacol 30:422-439, 1974. [A]

Wong M, Wells PG: Modulation of embryonic glutathione reductase and phenytoin teratogenicity by 1,3-bis(2-chloroethyl)-1-nitrosourea (BCNU). J Pharmacol Exp Ther 250(1):336-342, 1989. [A]

CASCARA SAGRADA

Synonyms

Brevilax, Cascara Evacuant, Cascara-Salax, Cascararinde, Cas-Evac, Chittem Bark, Peristaltine, Rhamni Purshianae Cortex, Sacred Bark

Summary

Cascara sagrada, the dried bark of Rhamnus purshiana, is administered orally as a laxative. Some systemic absorption of the anthraquinones contained in cascara sagrada occurs.

Magnitude of Teratogenic Risk

None To Minimal

Quality and Quantity of Data

Poor To Fair

Comment

None

The frequency of congenital anomalies was not significantly increased among the children of 53 women who took cascara sagrada during the first four lunar months of pregnancy in the Collaborative Perinatal Project (Heinonen et al., 1977). Similarly, the frequency of congenital anomalies was not significantly greater than expected among the children of 188 women who took cascara sagrada anytime during pregnancy (Heinonen et al., 1977).

No animal teratology studies of cascara sagrada have been published.

Key References

Heinonen OP, Slone D, Shapiro S: Birth Defects and Drugs in Pregnancy. Littleton, Mass.: John Wright-PSG, 1977, pp 385, 438, 442, 497. [E]

CEFACLOR

Synonyms

Alfatil, Ceclor, Cefaclorum, Dista, Distaclor, Kefolor, Panacef, Panoral

Summary

Cefaclor is a cephalosporin antibiotic.

Magnitude of Teratogenic Risk

Undetermined

Quality and Quantity of Data

None To Poor

Comment

None

No epidemiological studies of infants of women treated with cefaclor during pregnancy have been reported.

No teratogenic effect was observed in the offspring of mice, rats, rabbits, or ferrets treated with cefaclor during pregnancy (Markham et al., 1978; Furuhashi et al., 1979; Nomura et al., 1979). Doses used were 8-60 times (mice and rats), <1-2.5 times (rats), and 1-4 times (ferrets) those used in humans.

Key References

Furuhashi T, Nomura A, Uehara, Komuro E, et al.: Reproduction studies on cefaclor (CCL). 2. Fertility study and perinatal-postnatal study in rats. Chemotherapy 27:865-880, 1979. [A]

Markham JK, Hanasono GK, Adams ER, Owen NV: Reproduction studies on cefaclor. Toxicol Appl Pharmacol 45:292, 1978. [A]

Nomura A, Furuhashi T, Ikeya E, Sawaki A, et al.: Reproduction study of cefaclor (CCL). 1. Teratological study in mice, rats and rabbits. Chemotherapy 27:846-864, 1979. [A]

CEFADROXIL

Synonyms

Baxan, Bidocef, Cefadril, Cefamox, Cephos, Duracef, Kefroxil, Longacef, Oracefal, Ultracef

Summary

Cefadroxil is a cephalosporin antibiotic.

Magnitude of Teratogenic Risk

Undetermined

Quality and Quantity of Data

None To Poor

Comment

None

No epidemiological studies of congenital anomalies in infants born to women treated with cefadroxil during pregnancy have been reported.

The frequency of malformations was no greater than expected among the offspring of rats, mice, and rabbits treated during pregnancy with cefadroxil in doses, respectively, 3-75, 3-15, and 0.5-3 times those used in humans (Hickey et al., 1978; Tauchi et al., 1980a, b).

Key References

Hickey TE, Botta JA, Clemento AJ: Cefadroxil - A new antibiotic with low toxicity potential. Infection (Suppl 5):S549-S553, 1980. [A]

Tauchi K, Kawanishi H, Igarashi N, Maeda Y, et al.: Studies on the toxicity of cefadroxil (S-578). VI. Teratogenic study in rats. Jpn J Antibiot 33:487-496, 1980a. [A]

Tauchi K, Kawanishi H, Igarashi N, Maeda Y, et al.: Studies on the toxicity of cefadroxil (S-578). VII. Teratogenic study in rabbits. Jpn J Antibiot 33:497-502, 1980b. [A]

CEFAZOLIN

Synonyms

Acef, Caricef, Elzogram, Kefzol, Lampocef, Neofazol, Recef, Sicef, Zolicef, Zolival

Summary

Cefazolin is a semisynthetic cephalosporin antibiotic that is given parenterally for treatment of serious infections.

Magnitude of Teratogenic Risk

Undetermined

Quality and Quantity of Data

None To Poor

Comment

A small risk cannot be excluded, but a high risk of congenital anomalies in the children of women treated with cefazolin during pregnancy is unlikely.

No epidemiological studies of congenital anomalies among infants born to women treated with cefazolin during pregnancy have been reported.

The frequency of malformations was not increased but fetal growth retardation was observed among the offspring of rats treated during pregnancy with cefazolin in 2-4 times the human therapeutic dose (Hasegawa & Yoshida, 1980; Hasegawa et al., 1987).

Key References

Hasegawa Y, Takegawa Y, Yoshida Y: Reproduction of rats under 6351S (Flomoxef). 2. Intravenous administration during fetal organogenesis. Chemotherapy (Tokyo) (Nippon Kagaku Ryoho Gakkai Zasshi) 35(Suppl 1):370-403, 1987. [A]

Hasegawa Y, Yoshida T: A teratology study on 6059-S in rats. Chemotherapy (Tokyo) (Nippon Kagaku Ryoho Gakkai Zasshi) 28(Suppl 7):1119-1141, 1980. [A]

CEFOTAXIME

Synonyms

Cefacron, Claforan, Primafen, Zariviz

Summary

Cefotaxime is a cephalosporin antibiotic used parenterally to treat serious infections.

Magnitude of Teratogenic Risk

Undetermined

Quality and Quantity of Data

Poor

Comment

A small risk cannot be excluded, but there is no indication that the risk of congenital anomalies in the children of women treated with cefotaxime during pregnancy is likely to be great.

No epidemiological studies of congenital anomalies in infants born to women treated with cefotaxime during pregnancy have been reported.

The frequency of malformations was no greater than expected among the offspring of mice or rabbits treated during pregnancy with <1-25 and <1 times the human dose of cefotaxime (Sugisaki et al., 1981a, b; Doerr et al., 1982); maternal toxicity occurred with higher doses in rabbits.

Key References

Doerr BI, Glomot R, Kief H, Kramer M, et al.: Cefotaxime toxicity studies: A review of preclinical studies and some clinical reports. Rev Infect Dis 4(Suppl):S354-S359, 1982. [R]

Sugisaki T, Akaike M, Hayashi S: [Teratological study of cefotaxome given intravenously in rabbits.] Oyo Yakuri (Pharmacometrics) 21:375-384, 1981a. [A]

Sugisaki T, Kitatani T, Takagi S, Akaike M, et al.: [Reproduction studies of cefotaxime in mice.] Oyo Yakuri (Pharmacometrics) 21:351-373, 1981b. [A]

CELLULOSE, MICROCRYSTALLINE

Synonyms

Avicel, Crystalline Cellulose, Emcocel, Microcrystalline Cellulose

Summary

Microcrystalline cellulose is used as a suspending agent for pharmaceutical preparations. It is neither digested nor absorbed by humans.

Magnitude of Teratogenic Risk

Undetermined

Quality and Quantity of Data

Poor

Comment

A small risk cannot be excluded, but there is no indication that the risk of congenital anomalies in the children of women treated with microcrystalline cellulose during pregnancy is likely to be great.

No epidemiological studies of congenital anomalies in infants born to women who took microcrystalline cellulose during pregnancy have been reported.

The frequency of malformations was no greater than expected among the offspring of pregnant mice in which one-third of the dietary intake was microcrystalline cellulose (Yasuda et al., 1974).

Key References

Yasuda Y, Kihara T, Nishimura H: Embryotoxic effects of feeding bracken fern (Pteridium aquilinum) to pregnant mice. Toxicol Appl Pharmacol 28:264-268, 1974. [A]

CEPHALEXIN

Synonyms

Acaxina, Ceporex, Keflex, Keforal, Latoral, Neolexina, Oroxin, Palitrex, Sencephalin, Ultralexin

Summary

Cephalexin is a cephalosporin antibiotic.

Magnitude of Teratogenic Risk

Undetermined

Quality and Quantity of Data

Poor

Comment

None

No epidemiological studies of congenital anomalies among infants born to women treated with cephalexin during pregnancy have been reported.

No consistent teratogenic effect was observed among the offspring of pregnant mice or rats treated with 3-10 or 3-50 times the human dose of cephalexin during pregnancy (Welles et al., 1969; Aoyama et al., 1969).

Key References

Aoyama T, Furuoka R, Hasegawa N, Nemoto K: Teratologic studies of cephalexin in mice and rats. Oyo Yakuri 3:249-263, 1969. [A]

Welles JS, Froman RO, Gibson WR, Owen NV, et al.: Toxicology and pharmacology of cephalexin in laboratory animals. Antimicrob Agents Chemother (1968):489-496, 1969. [A]

CEPHRADINE

Synonyms

Cefamid, Cefradex, Dicefalin, Eskacef, Lisacef, Megacef, Sefril, Velosef

Summary

Cephradine is a cephalosporin antibiotic.

Magnitude of Teratogenic Risk

None To Minimal

Quality and Quantity of Data

Poor To Fair

Comment

None

The frequency of congenital anomalies was not increased among 54 infants born to women treated with cephradine during the first trimester of pregnancy in the Boston Collaborative Drug Surveillance Program (Aselton et al., 1985).

No teratogenic effects were observed among the offspring of rats or mice treated with 1-4 times the usual human therapeutic doses of cephradine during pregnancy (Hassert et al., 1973).

Key References

Aselton P, Jick H, Milunsky A, Hunter JR, et al.: First-trimester drug use and congenital disorders. Obstet Gynecol 65(4):451-455, 1985. [S]

Hassert GL, DeBaecke PJ, Kulesza JS, Traina VM, et al.: Toxicological, pathological, and teratological studies in animals with cephradine. Antimicrobial Agents and Chemotherapy 3(6):682-685, 1973. [A]

CETIRIZINE

Synonyms

Zirtek, Zyrtec

Summary

Cetirizine is an oral H1 antihistamine that is used to treat allergies.

Magnitude of Teratogenic Risk

Undetermined

Quality and Quantity of Data

None

Comment

A small risk cannot be excluded, but a high risk of congenital anomalies in the children of women treated with cetirizine during pregnancy is unlikely.

No epidemiological studies of congenital anomalies among the children of women who were treated with cetirizine during pregnancy have been reported.

No animal teratology studies of cetirizine have been published.

Please see agent summary on hydroxyzine for information on a similarly-used agent that has been studied.

Key References

None available.

CETYL ALCOHOL

Synonyms

Cetanol, Cetylol, Crodacol C, 1-Hexadecanol, Hexadecyl Alcohol, Laurex 16, Palmityl Alcohol

Summary

Cetyl alcohol is used as a solvent in ointments and creams.

Magnitude of Teratogenic Risk

Undetermined

Quality and Quantity of Data

None

Comment

None

No epidemiological studies of congenital anomalies in infants whose mothers used cetyl alcohol during pregnancy have been reported.

No animal teratology studies of cetyl alcohol have been published.

Key References

None available.

CETYLPYRIDINIUM

Synonyms

Aktivex, Biosept, Cetasol, Nitrogenol, Pristacin, Pyrisept, Seprisan, Sterogenol

Summary

Cetylpyridinium is a quaternary ammonium compound used in mouth washes, lozenges, and as a topical disinfectant.

Magnitude of Teratogenic Risk

None To Minimal

Quality and Quantity of Data

Poor To Fair

The frequencies of congenital anomalies in general, of major malformations, and of minor anomalies were no greater than expected among the children of 326 women who used cetylpyridinium during the first four lunar months of pregnancy in the Collaborative Perinatal Project (Heinonen et al., 1977). The frequency of congenital anomalies was also not increased among the children of 490 women who used cetylpyridinium anytime during pregnancy in this same study. A marginally increased risk (relative risk=2.0, 95% confidence interval 1.0-3.8) of congenital anomalies was observed among the children of 292 women who used cetylpyridinium during the first trimester of pregnancy in one cohort of the Boston Collaborative Surveillance Program (Aselton et al., 1985). In contrast, risk of congenital anomalies was not increased among the children of 314 women who used this agent in the first trimester in an earlier cohort of this same study (Jick et al., 1981).

Oral administration of cetylpyridinium during pregnancy in a dose of 27 mg/kg/d was associated with decreased fetal weight in rats (Gilman & De Salva, 1979). The relevance of this observation to the topical use of cetylpyridinium in human pregnancy is unknown.

Key References

Aselton P, Jick H, Milunsky A, et al.: First-trimester drug use and congenital disorders. Obstet Gynecol 65:451-455, 1985. [S]

Gilman MR, De Salva SJ: Teratology studies of benzethonium chloride, cetyl pyridinium chloride and chlorhexidine in rats. Toxicol Appl Pharmacol 48:A35, 1979. [A]

Heinonen OP, Slone D, Shapiro S: Birth Defects and Drugs in Pregnancy. Littleton, Mass.: John Wright-PSG, 1977, pp 300, 302, 309, 311, 434-435, 473. [E]

Jick H, Holmes LB, Hunter JR, et al.: First-trimester drug use and congenital disorders. JAMA 246:343-346, 1981. [S]

CHARCOAL, ACTIVATED

Synonyms

Actidose-Aqua, Actisorb, Arm-A-Char, Carbomix, Carbonet, Charcocaps, Haemocol, Medicoal, Norit, Swine Fly Ash

Summary

Activated charcoal is an insoluble agent used medically to remove drugs from the gastrointestinal tract in the treatment of acute poisoning. It is also used as an adsorbant to purify gases and liquids.

Magnitude of Teratogenic Risk

Undetermined

Quality and Quantity of Data

None

Comment

A small risk cannot be excluded, but a high risk of congenital anomalies in the children of women treated with activated charcoal during pregnancy is unlikely.

No epidemiological studies of congenital anomalies in infants whose mothers were treated with activated charcoal during pregnancy have been reported.

No animal teratology studies of activated charcoal have been published.

Key References

None available.

CHLORAL HYDRATE

Synonyms

Aquachloral, Chloradorm, Chloralex, Dormel, Elix-Nocte, Medianox, Noctec, Novochlorhydrate, Rectules, Somnox

Summary

Chloral hydrate is a hypnotic and sedative.

Magnitude of Teratogenic Risk

None To Minimal

Quality and Quantity of Data

Poor To Fair

Comment

None

The frequency of congenital anomalies was not significantly greater than expected among the infants born to 71 women who took chloral hydrate during the first four lunar months of pregnancy or to 358 women who took the drug anytime during pregnancy in the Collaborative Perinatal Project (Heinonen et al., 1977).

No gross external malformations were observed among the offspring of mice treated with <1-5 times the human dose of chloral hydrate during pregnancy (Kallman et al., 1984).

Key References

Heinonen OP, Slone D, Shapiro S: Birth Defects and Drugs in Pregnancy. Littleton, Mass.: John Wright-PSG, 1977, pp 336-337, 438. [E]

Kallman MJ, Kaempf GL, Balster RL: Behavioral toxicity of chloral in mice: An approach to evaluation. Neurobehav Teratol Toxicol 6:137-146, 1984. [A]

CHLORAMPHENICOL

Synonyms

Antibiopto, Chloromycetin, Chloroptic, Econochlor, Fenicol, Isopto Fenicol, Mychel, Novochlorocap, Ophthochlor, Pentamycetin

Summary

Chloramphenicol is an antibiotic used topically and systemically to treat serious infections.

Magnitude of Teratogenic Risk

None To Minimal

Quality and Quantity of Data

Poor To Fair

Comment

None

The frequency of congenital anomalies was no greater than expected among the children of 98 women treated with chloramphenicol during the first four lunar months or among the children of 348 women treated with the drug anytime in pregnancy in the Collaborative Perinatal Project (Heinonen et al., 1977).

The frequency of congenital anomalies was not increased among the offspring of mice or rabbits treated with chloramphenicol during pregnancy in doses 10-40 times those used in humans (Fritz & Hess, 1971). Similarly, no teratogenic effect was observed in rats after maternal treatment with 2-4 times the usual human dose (Prochazka et al., 1964), although various fetal anomalies were induced by maternal treatment with 10-40 times the human dose of chloramphenicol (Takaya, 1965; Fritz & Hess, 1971). Typical dose and gestational age dependency of this effect was demonstrated. An increased frequency of fetal death and decreased fetal weight were seen after such treatment in all three species. Behavioral alterations have been reported among adult rats born to dams treated during pregnancy with chloramphenicol in doses similar to those used in human therapy (Bertolini et al., 1980). The relevance of these observations to the risks associated with therapeutic use of chloramphenicol in human pregnancy is unknown.

Indirect evidence and one human case report (Oberheuser, 1971) suggest that maternal chloramphenicol treatment late in pregnancy may produce vascular collapse ("the grey baby syndrome") in the newborn infant. Grey baby syndrome is a well-known complication of chloramphenicol therapy in neonates (Sutherland, 1959; Weiss et al., 1960), and the drug freely crosses the placenta at term (Scott & Warner, 1950). Thus, it is reasonable to suspect that this condition could occur after maternal chloramphenicol treatment shortly before delivery.

Key References

Bertolini A, Poggioli R, Bernardi M, Genedani S, et al.: Pharmacological interferences in the protein synthesis during the fetal or neonatal period, in the rat: Behavioral outcomes in the adulthood. Pharmacol Res Commun 12:227-232, 1980. [A]

Fritz H, Hess R: The effect of chloramphenicol on the prenatal development of rats, mice, and rabbits. Toxicol Appl Pharmacol 19:667-674, 1971. [A]

Heinonen OP, Slone D, Shapiro S: Birth Defects and Drugs in Pregnancy. Littleton, Mass.: John Wright-PSG, 1977, pp 297, 301, 435. [E]

Oberheuser F: Praktische erfahrungen mit medikamenten in der schwangerschaft. Therapiewoche 31:2198-2202, 1971. [C]

Prochazka J, Simkova V, Havelka J, Hejzlar M, et al.: [Concerning the penetration of the placenta by chloramphenicol.] Pediatriia 19:311-314, 1964. [A]

Scott WC, Warner RF: Placental transfer of chloramphenicol (chloromycetin). JAMA 142:1331-1332, 1950. [S]

Sutherland JM: Fatal cardiovascular collapse of infants receiving large amounts of chloramphenicol. Am J Dis Child 97:761-767, 1959. [C]

Takaya M: [Teratogenic effects of antibiotics]. J Osaka City Med Cent 14:107-115, 1965. [A]

Weiss CF, Glazko AJ, Weston JK: Chloramphenicol in the newborn infant. A physiologic explanation of its toxicity when given in excessive doses. N Engl J Med 262:787-794, 1960. [R]

CHLORDANE

Synonyms

Belt, Chlordan, Corodane, Niran, Octachlor, Ortho-Klor, Sydane, Synklor, Toxichlor, Velsicol 1068

Summary

Chlordane is a chlorinated hydrocarbon insecticide that is used to control termites and infestations of citrus and vegetable crops. The threshold limit value for occupational exposure to chlordane is 0.5 mg/cu m of air as a time-weighted average (Hathaway et al., 1991); dermal exposure can lead to substantial absorption of this chemical. The acceptable daily dose for oral ingestion is 0.001 mg/kg (WHO/FAO, 1968).

Magnitude of Teratogenic Risk

Undetermined

Quality and Quantity of Data

Poor

Comment

None

No epidemiological studies of congenital anomalies among infants born to women exposed to chlordane during pregnancy have been reported.

No effect on neonatal weight or viability was observed among the offspring of mice treated during pregnancy with 50 mg/kg/d of chlordane (Chernoff & Kavlock, 1982). Similarly, no teratogenic effect was observed among the offspring of rats treated with 20-80 mg/kg/d of chlordane despite the occurrence of substantial maternal toxicity at the highest dose

(Usami et al., 1986). Behavioral alterations have been observed among the offspring of mice treated with 1-2.5 mg/kg/d chlordane during pregnancy (Al- Hachim & Al-Baker, 1973). Various alterations of granulocyte and macrophage function have been found among the offspring of mice treated with 4-16 mg/kg/d of chlordane during pregnancy (Barnett et al., 1985, 1990a, b; Theus et al., 1992a, b). The relevance of these observations to chlordane exposure in human pregnancy is unknown.

A history of prenatal exposure to chlordane was recorded in two children with neuroblastoma (Infante et al., 1978), but such isolated anecdotes do not indicate whether the association is causal or just fortuitious.

Key References

Al-Hachim GM, Al-Baker A: Effects of chlordane on conditioned avoidance response, brain seizure threshold and open-field performance of prenatally-treated mice. Br J Pharmacol 49:311-315, 1973. [A]

Barnett JB, Blaylock BL, Gandy J, Menna JH, et al.: Alteration of fetal liver colony formation by prenatal chlordane exposure. Fundam App Toxicol 15:820-822, 1990b. [A]

Barnett JB, Blaylock BL, Gandy J, Menna JH, et al.: Long-term alteration of adult bone marrow colony formation by prenatal chlordane exposure. Fundam Appl Toxicol 14:688-695, 1990a. [A]

Barnett JB, Soderberg LSF, Menna JH: The effect of prenatal chlordane exposure on the delayed hypersensitivity response of balb/c mice. Toxicol Lett 25:173-183, 1985. [A]

Chernoff N, Kavlock RJ: An in vivo teratology screen utilizing pregnant mice. J Toxicol Environ Health 10:541-550, 1982. [A]

Hathaway GJ, Proctor NH, Hughes JP, Fischman ML (eds): Proctor and Hughes' Chemical Hazards of the Workplace, 3rd ed. New York: Van Nostrand Reinhold, 1991, pp 149-151. [R]

Infante PF, Epstein SS, Newton WA: Blood dyscrasias and childhood tumors and exposure to chlordane and heptachlor. Scand J Work Env Health 4:137-150, 1978. [S]

Theus SA, Lau KA, Tabor DR, Soderberg LSF, et al.: In vivo prenatal chlordane exposure induces development of endogenous inflammatory macrophages. J Leukoc Biol 51(4);366-372, 1992b. [A]

Theus SA, Tabor DR, Soderberg LSF, Barnett JB: Macrophage tumoricidal mechanisms are selectively altered by prenatal chlordane exposure. Agents Actions 37(1-2):140-146, 1992a. [A]

Usami M, Kawashima K, Nakaura S, Yamaguchi M, et al.: Effect of chlordane on prenatal developments of rats. Bull Natl Inst Hyg Sci (Tokyo) 0:68-73, 1986. [A]

WHO/FAO (World Health Organization, Food and Agricultural Organization of the United Nations). 1967 Evaluation of Some Pesticide Residues in Food. WHO/Food Add./68.30. Joint Meeting of the FAO Working Party of Experts and the WHO Expert Committee on Pesticide Residues, December 4-11, 1967. Geneva: World Health Organization, 1968. [R]

CHLORDANTOIN

Synonyms

Clodantoin, Sporostacin

Summary

Chlordantoin is an antifungal agent used topically to treat candidiasis infections.

Magnitude of Teratogenic Risk

None

Quality and Quantity of Data

Poor

Comment

A small risk cannot be excluded, but there is no indication that the risk of congenital anomalies in the children of women treated with chlordantoin during pregnancy is likely to be great.

The Collaborative Perinatal Project reported no increased frequency of malformations in 24 infants born to women who used chlordantoin during the first four lunar months of pregnancy (Heinonen et al., 1977).

No animal teratology studies of chlordantoin have been published.

Key References

Heinonen OP, Slone D, Sharpio S: Birth Defects and Drugs in Pregnancy. Littleton, Mass.: John Wright-PSG, 1977, pp 300, 302. [E]

CHLORDIAZEPOXIDE

Synonyms

Calmoden, Libritabs Tablets, Librium, Menrium Tablets, Methaminodiazepoxide, SK-Lygen Capsules, Tropium

Summary

Chlordiazepoxide is a widely used benzodiazepine tranquilizer. It also has sedative, anticonvulsant, and muscle relaxant properties.

Magnitude of Teratogenic Risk

None To Minimal

Quality and Quantity of Data

Fair To Good

Comment

This risk estimate is for therapeutic doses; the risk with maternally toxic doses is unknown but likely to be greater.

The frequency of malformations was no greater than expected among the children of women who took chlordiazepoxide during the first trimester of pregnancy in four cohort studies involving respectively 38, 98, 89, and 257 infants (Crombie et al., 1975; Kullander & Kallen, 1976; Heinonen et al., 1977). An association between congenital anomalies (loosely defined) in children and maternal use of chlordiazepoxide early in pregnancy was suggested in a cohort study that included 35 women who were prescribed this medication in the first 42 days following their last menstrual period (Milkovich & van den Berg, 1974). No specificity of the anomalies present in the affected children was apparent. No association was found between maternal use of chlordiazepoxide during the first trimester of pregnancy and congenital anomalies in a case-control study of 1427 affected infants (Bracken & Holford, 1981). Similarly, no association was observed between maternal treatment with chlordiazepoxide early in pregnancy and cardiac malformations in a case-control study of 390 affected children (Rothman et al., 1979) or between such treatment and cleft lip and/or palate in a case-control study involving 1201 affected infants (Czeizel, 1988).

The frequency of congenital anomalies was no greater than expected among the children of 175 and 740 women who took chlordiazepoxide anytime in pregnancy in two cohort studies (Milkovich & van den Berg, 1974; Heinonen et al., 1977). In the Collaborative Perinatal Project, mental and motor status scores at 8 months of age and IQ scores at 4 years of age did not differ between children born to mothers who had taken chlordiazepoxide during pregnancy and those who did not (Hartz et al., 1975).

A dose-dependent increase in the frequency of central nervous system malformations was observed among the offspring of hamsters treated with chlordiazepoxide in doses 45-500 times those used clinically (Guram et al., 1982). Dose-dependent maternal toxicity was also seen with this treatment. The frequency of malformations was not increased among the offspring of rats treated during pregnancy with chlordiazepoxide in doses 1.5-16 times those used in humans, although skeletal variants, growth retardation, and fetal death were more common at the higher doses (Buttar, 1980; Saito et al., 1984). Decreased postnatal weight gain has been observed among the offspring of pregnant mice and rats treated respectively with 2-5 or <1-3 times the human dose of chlordiazepoxide (Buttar, 1980; Adams, 1982; Pankaj & Brain, 1991; Kurishingal et al., 1992). Both neonatal and long-lasting behavioral alterations are seen among the offspring of rats and mice treated respectively with <1-7 and 2-5 times the human dose of chlordiazepoxide during pregnancy (Harris & Case, 1979; Buttar, 1980; Adams, 1982; Avinmelech-Gigus et al., 1986; Pankaj et al., 1991; Kurishingal et al., 1992). The relevance of these observations to the risks associated with therapeutic use of chlordiazepoxide in human pregnancy is unknown.

Key References

Adams PM: Effects of perinatal chlordiazepoxide exposure on rat preweaning and postweaning behavior. Neurobehav Toxicol Teratol 4:279-282, 1982. [A]

Avnimelech-Gigus N, Feldon J, Tanne Z, et al.: The effects of prenatal chlordiazepoxide administration on avoidance behavior and benzodiazepine receptor density in adult albino rats. Eur J Pharmacol 129:185-188, 1986. [A]

Bracken MB, Holford TR: Exposure to prescribed drugs in pregnancy and association with congenital malformations. Obstet Gynecol 58:336-344, 1981. [E]

Buttar HS: Effects of chlordiazepoxide on the pre- and postnatal development of rats. Toxicology 17:311-321, 1980. [A]

Crombie DL, Pinsent RJ, Fleming DM, Rumeau-Rouquette C, et al.: Fetal effects of tranquilizers in pregnancy. N Engl J Med 293:198-199, 1975. [E]

Czeizel A: Lack of evidence of teratogenicity of benzodiazepine drugs in Hungary. Reprod Toxicol 1(3):183-188, 1988. [E]

Guram MS, Gill TS, Geber WF: Comparative teratogenicity of chlordiazepoxide, amitriptyline, and combination of the two compounds in the fetal hamster. Neurotoxicology 3:83-90, 1982. [A]

Harris RA, Case J: Effects of maternal consumption of ethanol, barbital, or chlordiazepoxide on the behavior of the offspring. Behav Neural Biol 26:234-247, 1979. [A]

Hartz SC, Heinonen OP, Shapiro S, Siskind V, et al.: Antenatal exposure to meprobamate and chlordiazepoxide in relation to malformations, mental development, and childhood mortality. N Engl J Med 292:726-728, 1975. [E]

Heinonen OP, Slone D, Shapiro S: Birth Defects and Drugs in Pregnancy. Littleton, Mass.: John Wright-PSG, 1977, p 491. [E]

Kullander S, Kallen B: A prospective study of drugs and pregnancy. Acta Obstet Gynecol Scand 55:25-33, 1976. [E]

Kurishingal H, Palanza P, Brain PF: Effects of exposure of pregnant mice to chlordiazepoxide (CDP) on the development and ultrasound production of their offspring. Gen Pharmacol 23(1):49-53, 1992. [A]

Milkovich L, van den Berg BJ: Effects of prenatal meprobamate and chlordiazepoxide hydrochloride on human embryonic and fetal development. N Engl J Med 291:1268-1271, 1974. [E]

Pankaj V, Brain PF: Effects of prenatal exposure to benzodiazepine-related drugs on early development and adult social behaviour in Swiss mice--I. Agonists. Gen Pharmacol 22(1):33-41, 1991. [A]

Rothman KJ, Fyler DC, Goldblatt A, Kreidberg MB: Exogenous hormones and other drug exposures of children with congenital heart disease. Am J Epidemiol 109:433-439, 1979. [E]

Saito H, Kobayashi H, Takeno S, Sakai T: Fetal toxicity of benzodiazepines in rats. Res Commun Chem Pathol Pharmacol 46:437-447, 1984. [A]

CHLORMEZANONE

Synonyms

Chlomedinon, Chlormethazanone, Chlormezanonum, Muskel Trancopal, Myolespen, Relizon, Rexan, Rilaquil, Supotran, Tanafol

Summary

Clormezanone is a tranquilizer used to treat anxiety.

Magnitude of Teratogenic Risk

Undetermined

Quality and Quantity of Data

Poor

Comment

None

The frequency of congenital anomalies was significantly greater than expected among the children of 26 women treated with chlormezanone anytime during pregnancy in the Collaborative Perinatal Project (Heinonen et al., 1977). Only five of these women took the medication during the first four lunar months of gestation, and the association is based on only three affected children whose anomalies are not described. The clinical importance of this observation is uncertain.

No animal teratology studies of chlormezanone have been published.

Key References

Heinonen OP, Slone D, Shapiro S: Birth Defects and Drugs in Pregnancy. Littleton, Mass.: John-Wright-PSG, 1977, p 438. [E]

CHLOROFORM

Synonyms

Formyl Trichloride, Methane Trichloride, Methenyl Trichloride, Methyl Trichloride, Trichlormethan, Trichloroform, Trichloromethane, Triclorometano

Summary

Chloroform is a widely used industrial and laboratory solvent. It has been employed as an inhalant anesthetic. Chloroform is also used topically as a rubefacient and in consumables as a flavoring and preservative. The U.S. OSHA Permissible Exposure Limit for occupational exposure to chloroform vapors as a time-weighted average is 2 ppm (approximately 10 mg/cu m) (ACGIH, 1990).

Magnitude of Teratogenic Risk

Undetermined

Quality and Quantity of Data

None To Poor

Comment

None

The frequency of congenital anomalies was no greater than expected among 492 children of laboratory workers exposed to organic solvents during the first trimester of pregnancy (Axelsson et al., 1984). One hundred and twenty-eight of these mothers reported first trimester exposure to chloroform.

The frequency of cleft palate was increased among the offspring of mice exposed chronically during pregnancy to chloroform vapors in a concentration of 100 ppm (about 1/100 the anesthetic dose) (Murray et al., 1979). Anal atresia was observed with increased frequency among the offspring of pregnant rats after similar exposure, but not after exposure to 30 ppm (Schwetz et al., 1974). In both studies, considerable maternal toxicity occurred. In contrast, the frequency of malformations was no greater than expected among the offspring of rats or rabbits given chloroform orally during pregnancy in doses as great as 400 mg/kg/d or 50 mg/kg/d, respectively (Thompson et al., 1974; Ruddick et al., 1983).

Significantly higher frequencies of acquired chromosomal aberrations were noted in the lymphocytes of women occupationally exposed to chloroform and other organic solvents (Funes-Cravioto et al., 1977). Similar findings were observed in the children of these women. This study has not been independently confirmed, and the relevance of acquired somatic chromosomal aberrations to the risk of malformations or any other disease in the offspring is unknown.

Key References

ACGIH: 1990-1991 Threshold Limit Values for Chemical Substances and Physical Agents and Biological Exposure Indices. Cincinnati, Ohio: Am Conference Govt Ind Hyg, 1990. [O]

Axelsson G, Lutz C, Rylander R: Exposure to solvents and outcome of pregnancy in university laboratory employees. Br J Ind Med 41:305-312, 1984. [E]

Funes-Cravioto F, Kolmodin-Hedman B, Lindsten J, Nordenskjold M, et al.: Chromosome aberrations and sister-chromatid exchange in workers in chemical laboratories and a rotoprinting factory and in children of women laboratory workers. Lancet 2:322-325, 1977. [E]

Murray FJ, Schwetz BA, McBride JG, Staples RE: Toxicity of inhaled chloroform in pregnant mice and their offspring. Toxicol Appl Pharmacol 50:515-522, 1979. [A]

Ruddick JA, Villeneuve DC, Chu I: A teratological assessment of four trihalomethanes. J Environ Sci Health:B18(3), 333-349, 1983. [A]

Schwetz BA, Leong BKJ, Gehring PJ: Embryo- and fetotoxicity of inhaled chloroform in rats. Toxicol Appl Pharmacol 28:442-451, 1974. [A]

Thompson DJ, Warner SD, Robinson VB: Teratology studies on orally administered chloroform in the rat and rabbit. Toxicol Appl Pharmacol 29:348-357, 1974. [A]

CHLOROPROCAINE

Synonyms

Nesacaine

Summary

Chloroprocaine is an injectable local anesthetic of the ester class that is used for infiltration and regional nerve block.

Magnitude of Teratogenic Risk

Undetermined

Quality and Quantity of Data

None

Comment

None

No epidemiological studies of congenital anomalies among infants born to women given chloroprocaine during pregnancy have been reported.

No animal teratology studies of chloroprocaine have been published.

Episodes of fetal heart rate deceleration have occasionally been reported during epidural anesthesia with chloroprocaine for labor (Clark, 1985). Subtle behavioral alterations at three days of age (but not at one day) have been observed among infants delivered to women who received epidural anesthesia with chloroprocaine (Abboud et al., 1984; Kuhnert & Linn, 1985). The clinical significance of these findings is unknown.

Please see agent summary on procaine for information on a related agent that has been more thoroughly studied.

Key References

Abboud TK, Afrasiabi A, Sarkis F, Daftarian F, et al.: Continuous infusion epidural analgesia in parturients receiving bupivacaine, chloroprocaine, or lidocaine--Maternal, fetal, and neonatal effects. Anesth Analg 63:421-428, 1984. [E]

Clark RB: Fetal and neonatal effects of epidural anesthesia. Obstet Gynecol Ann 14:240-252, 1985. [R]

Kuhnert BR, Linn PL: The effect of chloroprocaine on neonatal neurobehavior. Anesth Analg 64:1223-1224, 1985. [E]

CHLOROQUINE

Synonyms

Aralen, Avloclor, Delagil, Lagaquin, Malarivon, Nivaquine, Resochin, Trochin

Summary

Chloroquine is a quinine derivative used to treat malarial and amoebic infections and inflammatory diseases.

Magnitude of Teratogenic Risk

Daily Dose: Minimal

113

Quality and Quantity of Data

Poor To Fair

Comment

None

The frequency of major malformations was no greater than expected among a cohort of 169 infants born to women who took low dose chloroquine weekly for malaria prophylaxis (Wolfe & Cordero, 1985). No malformations were observed among four children born to women treated daily with chloroquine for systemic lupus erythematosus in one series (Parke, 1988); these women miscarried or had stillbirths in four other pregnancies while on this treatment, but such outcomes are a recognized complication of lupus. In another series of pregnancies in women who were treated with chloroquine during the first trimester, there were 14 liveborn infants, none of whom had congenital anomalies (Levy et al., 1991).

Anecdotal observations have suggested an association between maternal use of chloroquine during pregnancy and auditory, vestibular, retinal, or other neurologic dysfunction in children (Hart & Naunton, 1964; Matz & Naunton, 1968; Paufique & Magnard, 1969; Roubenoff et al., 1988; Cook, 1992). Although such problems appear to be uncommon among children born to women treated with chloroquine during pregnancy (Klumpp, 1965; Anonymous, 1983; Roubenoff et al., 1988; Levy et al., 1991), a causal relationship seems possible. Chloroquine treatment occasionally produces similar toxic manifestations in adults (Tanenbaum & Tuffanelli, 1980), and a radio-labelled chloroquine analog administered to the mother has been shown to concentrate in the uveal tract of the eye and in the cochlea and ampulla of the inner ear in a macaque fetus (Dencker et al., 1975).

No difference in birth weight was seen between the infants of women who were treated weekly with chloroquine during pregnancy and the infants of untreated women in an area in which malaria is hyperendemic (Cot et al., 1992).

When administered to pregnant rats, chloroquine in doses 100 times greater than those used in humans produces embryonic death and ocular malformations (Udalova, 1967). Fetal growth retardation and skeletal anomalies were noted with increased frequency among the offspring of pregnant rats treated with 70 times the human therapeutic dose of chloroquine (Sharma & Rawat, 1989). No teratogenic effect was observed in mice after treatment with an unspecified, but probably greater than therapeutic, dose of chloroquine (Yielding et al., 1976)

Key References

Anonymous: Malaria in pregnancy. Lancet 2:84-85, 1983. [O]

Cook GC: Use of antiprotozoan and anthelmintic drugs during pregnancy: Side-effects and contra-indications (editorial). J Infect 25:1-9, 1992. [R]

Cot M, Roisin A, Barro D, Yada A, et al.: Effect of chloroquine chemoprophylaxis during pregnancy on birth weight: Results of a randomized trial. Am J Trop Med Hyg 46(1):21-27, 1992. [E]

Dencker L, Lindquist NG, Ullberg S: Distribution of an 125 I-Labelled chloroquine analogue in a pregnant macaca monkey. Toxicology 5:255-264, 1975. [A]

Hart CW, Naunton RF: The ototoxicity of chloroquine phosphate. Arch Otolaryngol 80:407-412, 1964. [C]

Klumpp TG: Safety of chloroquine in pregnancy. JAMA 191:765, 1965. [O]

Levy M, Buskila D, Gladman DD, Urowitz MB, et al.: Pregnancy outcome following first trimester exposure to chloroquine. Am J Perinatol 8(3):174-178, 1991. [S]

Matz GJ, Naunton RF: Ototoxicity of chloroquine. Arch Otolaryngol 88:370-372, 1968. [C]

Parke A: Antimalarial drugs and pregnancy. Am J Med 85(Suppl 4A): 30-33, 1988. [S]

Paufique L, Magnard P: [Retinal degeneration in two children following preventive antimalarial treatment of the mother during pregnancy.] Bull Soc Ophtalmol Fr 69:466-467, 1969. [C]

Roubenoff R, Hoyt J, Petri M, Hochberg MC, et al.: Effects of antiinflammatory and immunosuppressive drugs on pregnancy and fertility. Semin Arthritis Rheum 18(2):88-110, 1988. [R]

Sharma A, Rawat AK: Toxicological consequences of chloroquine and ethanol on the developing fetus. Pharmacol Biochem Behav 34:77-82, 1989. [A]

Tanenbaum L, Tuffanelli DL: Antimalarial agents: Chloroquine, hydroxychloroquine, and quinacrine. Arch Dermatol 116:587-591, 1980. [R]

Udalova LD: [The effect of chloroquine on the embryonal development of rats.] Pharmacol Toxical (Russian) 2:226-228, 1967. [A]

Wolfe MS, Cordero JF: Safety of chloroquine in chemosuppression of malaria during pregnancy. Br Med J 290:1466-1467, 1985. [E]

Yielding LW, Riley TL, Yielding KL: Preliminary study of caffeine and chloroquine enhancement of x-ray induced birth defects. Biochem Biophys Res Commun 68:1356-1361, 1976. [A]

CHLOROTHIAZIDE

Synonyms

Azide, Chlotride, Clotride, Diuret, Diuril, Diurilix, Diurone, Saluretil, Saluric, SK-Chlorothiazide

Summary

Chlorothiazide is a thiazide diuretic used in the treatment of edema and hypertension.

Magnitude of Teratogenic Risk

None To Minimal

Quality and Quantity of Data

Poor To Fair

Comment

None

In the Collaborative Perinatal Project, the frequency of congenital anomalies was no greater than expected among the children of 63 women who took chlorothiazide during the first four lunar months of pregnancy or among the children of 5283 women who took the drug anytime in pregnancy (Heinonen et al., 1977). Similarly, the frequency of congenital anomalies was no greater than expected among the children of 506 women treated with chlorothiazide during the second and third trimester of pregnancy (Kraus et al., 1966).

No increase in the frequency of malformations was observed among the offspring of rats treated with chlorothiazide in a dose 12 times that used in humans (Maren & Ellison, 1972). In another study, treatment of rats with about 30 times the human therapeutic dose of chlorothiazide during pregnancy produced chronic hypertension in the offspring (Grollman & Grollman, 1962). This effect has not been investigated in humans.

Neonatal thrombocytopenic purpura has been reported in several children whose mothers received treatment with chlorothiazide late in pregnancy (Rodriguez et al., 1964). The possibility that this association is causal is supported by the fact that thrombocytopenia is known to be a rare complication of thiazide therapy in adults. The frequency of symptomatic neonatal thrombocytopenia in the offspring of women who take chlorothiazide late in pregnancy is unknown but probably very small (Finnerty & Assali, 1964; Kraus et al., 1966).

Key References

Finnerty FA, Assali NS: Thiazide and neonatal thrombocytopenia. N Engl J Med 271:160-161, 1964. [O]

Grollman A, Grollman EF: The teratogenic induction of hypertension. J Clin Invest 41:710-714, 1962. [A]

Heinonen OP, Slone D, Shapiro S: Birth Defects and Drugs in Pregnancy. Littleton, Mass.: John Wright-PSG, 1977, pp 372, 441, 495. [E]

Kraus GW, Marchese JR, Yen SSC: Prophylactic use of hydrochlorothiazide in pregnancy. JAMA 198:1150-1154, 1966. [E]

Maren TH, Ellison AC: The teratological effect of certain thiadiazoles related to acetazolamide, with a note on sulfanilamide and thiazide diuretics. Johns Hopkins Med J 130:95-104, 1972. [A]

Rodriguez SU, Leikin SL, Hiller MC: Neonatal thrombocytopenia associated with ante-partum administration of thiazide drugs. N Engl J Med 270:881-884, 1964. [C]

CHLOROXINE

Synonyms

Capitrol, Chlofucid, Chlorhydroxyquinoline, Chloroxyquinoline, Chlorquinol, Clofuzid, Halquinol, Quesyl, Quinolor, Quixaline

Summary

Chloroxine is a synthetic antibacterial agent that is used topically to treat dandruff and seborrheic dermatitis.

Magnitude of Teratogenic Risk

Undetermined

Quality and Quantity of Data

None

Comment

None

No epidemiological studies of congenital anomalies in infants whose mothers were treated with chloroxine during pregnancy have been reported.

No animal teratology studies of chloroxine have been published.

Key References

None available.

CHLOROXYLENOL

Synonyms

Anti-Sept, Benzytol, Bristol Pine Disinfectant, Camel, Espadol Quirurgico, Ibcol, Jeypine, Metasep, Parachlorometaxylenol, Pynol

Summary

Chloroxylenol is a disinfectant. It is used in topical antiseptics and to clean instruments.

Magnitude of Teratogenic Risk

Undetermined

Quality and Quantity of Data

None

Comment

A small risk cannot be excluded, but a high risk of congenital anomalies in the children of women treated with chloroxylenol during pregnancy is unlikely.

No epidemiological studies of congenital anomalies in infants born to women treated with chloroxylenol during pregnancy have been reported.

No animal teratology studies of chloroxylenol have been published.

Key References

None available.

CHLORPHENIRAMINE

Synonyms

Chlor-100, Chloramin, Chlor-Mal, Chlorspan, Chlortab, Chlortrimeton, Novopheniram, Teledrin, Trimeton

Summary

Chlorpheniramine is an antihistamine commonly used to treat rhinitis and allergic disorders.

Magnitude of Teratogenic Risk

None To Minimal

Quality and Quantity of Data

Fair To Good

Comment

None

The frequencies of major malformations, minor anomalies, and congenital anomalies in general were no greater than expected among the infants of 1070 women who took chlorpheniramine during the first four lunar months of pregnancy in the Collaborative Perinatal Project (Heinonen et al., 1977). Small but statistically significant associations were seen between maternal use of chlorpheniramine during the first four lunar months of pregnancy and inguinal hernia (RR=1.53, 95% confidence interval 1.09-2.14) and eye or ear anomalies (RR=2.89, 95% confidence interval 1.16-5.92) among the children. No increase in the frequency of congenital anomalies was observed among more than 275 infants born to women who took chlorpheniramine during the first trimester of pregnancy in two sequential cohorts of the Boston Colloabarative Drug Surveillance Program (Jick et al., 1981; Aselton et al., 1985). The frequency of congenital anomalies was no greater than expected among the children of 3931 women who took chlorpheniramine anytime during pregnancy in the Collaborative Perinatal Project (Heinonen et al., 1977).

Increased frequencies of embryonic, fetal, and neonatal death were reported among the offspring of mice treated with 65-650 times the usual human dose of chlorpheniramine during pregnancy in one study (Naranjo & de Naranjo, 1968). The relevance of this observation to the therapeutic use of chlorpheniramine in human pregnancy is unknown.

Key References

Aselton P, Jick H, Milunsky A, Hunter JR, et al: First-trimester drug use and congenital disorders. Obstet Gynecol 65:451-455, 1985. [S]

Heinonen OP, Slone D, Shapiro S: Birth Defects and Drugs in Pregnancy. Littleton, Mass.: John Wright-PSG, 1977, pp 323-324, 437. [E]

Jick H, Holmes LB, Hunter JR, Madsen S, et al.: First-trimester drug use and congenital disorders. JAMA 246: 343-346, 1981. [S]

Naranjo P, de Naranjo E: Embryotoxic effects of antihistamines. Arzneimittelforsch 18:188-195, 1968. [A]

CHLORPROMAZINE

Synonyms

Chlorazine, Chlor-Promanyl, Largactil, Novochlorpromazine, Promapar, Promazin, Thorazine

Summary

Chlorpromazine is a widely used phenothiazine. It is employed as a tranquilizer and sedative in the treatment of psychoses and as a premedication for operations and diagnostic procedures. Chlorpromazine is also used as an anti-emetic.

Magnitude of Teratogenic Risk

None To Minimal

Quality and Quantity of Data

Fair To Good

Comment

Transient neurological dysfunction may occur among newborn infants born to women treated with chlorpromazine late in pregnancy.

The frequency of congenital anomalies was no greater than expected among the children of 142 women treated with chlorpromazine during the first four lunar months of pregnancy or the children of 284 women treated with this drug anytime during pregnancy in the Collaborative Perinatal Project (Heinonen et al., 1977). Similarly, the frequency of congenital anomalies was not increased among the infants of 264 women treated with a low dose of chlorpromazine for hyperemesis gravidarum in the first trimester of pregnancy in another cohort study (Farkas & Farkas, 1971).

In most investigations, the frequency of malformations was no greater than expected among the offspring of rats treated with chlorpromazine during pregnancy in doses 1 to 6 times those used in humans (Brock & von Kreybig, 1964; Jelinek et al., 1967; Beall, 1972; Robertson et al., 1980; Jones-Price et al., 1983a). Increased fetal loss, decreased fetal weight gain, and maternal toxicity were often observed, especially at the higher doses. Increased frequencies of skeletal, central nervous system, and other anomalies have been reported in other studies among the offspring of pregnant rats treated with chlorpromazine in doses 2-10 times those used in humans (Brock & von Kreybig, 1964; Singh & Padmanabhan, 1978). In mice, increased frequencies of eye, palate, skeletal, and other anomalies as well as of fetal death have been observed among the offspring of animals treated with chlorpromazine in doses <1-2 times those used in humans (Jones-Price et al., 1983b; Yu et al., 1988). These doses also produce maternal toxicity in mice.

Many behavioral studies in the offspring of mice and rats treated with chlorpromazine during pregnancy have been published. A variety of long-lasting alterations of behavior and neurological function have been observed in the offspring with maternal treatment using <1-3 times the usual human dose of chlorpromazine (Robertson et al., 1980; Saillenfait & Vannier, 1988). The design and results of these studies vary, and their relevance to the therapeutic use of chlorpromazine in human pregnancy is unknown.

Neurological dysfunction with extrapyramidal signs has been reported in several infants born to women treated with chlorpromazine during pregnancy (Hill et al., 1966; Tamer et al., 1969; Hammond & Toseland, 1970; Levy & Wisniewski, 1974). The muscle rigidity, hypertonia, and tremor seen in these children is quite unusual among newborns. Although the abnormalities appear to be transient, they may last for months. It seems likely that the neurological dysfunction in these infants is related to their mothers' drug therapy because similar signs of extrapyramidal dysfunction may occur as a side effect of chlorpromazine administration in adults. The frequency of this complication among infants born to women treated with chlorpromazine during pregnancy is unknown but probably low.

Key References

Beall JR: A teratogenic study of chlorpromazine, orphenadrine, perphenazine, and LSD-25 in rats. Toxicol Appl Pharmacol 21:230-236, 1972. [A]

Brock N, von Kreybig T: [Experimental contribution to the testing of the teratogenic effect of drugs on the laboratory rat.] Naunyn Schmiedebergs Arch Exp Pathol Pharmakol 249:117-145, 1964. [A]

Farkas VG, Farkas G: [Teratogenic action of hyperemesis in pregnancy and of medication used to treat it.] Zentralbl Gynakol 10:325-330, 1971. [S]

Hammond JE, Toseland PA: Placental transfer of chlorpromazine. A case report. Arch Dis Childhood 45:139, 1970. [C]

Heinonen OP, Slone D, Shapiro S: Birth Defects and Drugs in Pregnancy. Littleton, Mass.: John Wright-PSG, 1977, pp 323, 437. [E]

Hill RM, Desmond MM, Kay JL: Extrapyramidal dysfunction in an infant of a schizophrenic mother. J Pediatr 69:589-595, 1966. [C]

Jelinek V, Zikmund E, Reichlova R: [The influence of some psychotropic drugs on the development of the rat fetus.] Therapie 22:1429-1433, 1967. [A]

Jones-Price C, Wolkowski-Tyl R, Marr MC: Teratologic evaluation of chlorpromazine hydrochloride (CAS No. 69-09-0) administered to Fischer

344 rats on gestational days 6 through 15. NTIS (National Technical Information Service) Report/ PB83-191080, 1983a. [A]

Jones-Price C, Wolkowski-Tyl R, Marr MC: Teratologic evaluation of chlorpromazine hydrochloride (CAS No. 69-09-0) administered to CD-1 mice on gestational days 6 through 15. NTIS (National Technical Information Service) Report/ PB83-179846, 1983b. [A]

Levy W, Wiseniewski K: Chlorpromazine causing extrapyramidal dysfunction in newborn infant of psychotic mother. NY State J Med 74:684-685, 1974. [C]

Robertson RT, Majka JA, Peter CP, Bokelman DL: Effects of prenatal exposure to chlorpromazine on postnatal development and behavior of rats. Toxicol Appl Pharmacol 53:541-549, 1980. [A]

Saillenfait AM, Vannier B: Methodological proposal in behavioural teratogenicity testing: Assessment of propoxyphene, chlorpromazine, and vitamin A as positive controls. Teratology 37:185-199, 1988. [A]

Singh S, Padmanabhan R: Teratogenic effects of chlorpromazine hydrochloride in rat foetuses. Indian J Med Res 67:300-309, 1978. [A]

Tamer A, McKey R, Arias D, Worley L, et al.: Phenothiazine-induced extrapyramidal dysfunction in the neonate. J Pediatr 75:479-480, 1969. [C]

Yu J-F, Yang Y-S, Wang W-Y, Xiong G-X, et al.: Mutagenicity and teratogenicity of chlorpromazine and scopalamine. Chin Med J 101:339-345, 1988. [A]

CHLORPROPAMIDE

Synonyms

Catanil, Chloromide, Chloronase, Diabinese, Glucamide, Glymese, Insulase, Novopropamide, Promide, Stabinol

Summary

Chlorpropamide is an oral hypoglycemic agent.

Magnitude of Teratogenic Risk

Minimal To Small

Quality and Quantity of Data

Poor To Fair

Comment

Interpretation of available data on this agent is difficult because all women who took this medication had diabetes, which itself can alter embryonic and fetal development.

Ten of 20 infants born to women who had non-insulin dependent diabetes mellitus and were treated with oral hypoglycemic agents, usually chlorpropamide, during the first trimester had minor or major congenital anomalies in one study; this frequency was greater than that observed in a comparison group of infants born to women with non-insulin dependent diabetes who were untreated in early pregnancy (Piacquadio et al., 1991). Two of the infants whose mothers took chlorpropamide early in pregnancy had cardiac and vertebral malformations; both of these children and three others born to women who took chlorpropamide early in pregnancy had auricular malformations. In contrast, only one infant with congenital anomalies was observed in a clinical series of 41 born to women with non-insulin dependent diabetes mellitus treated with chlorpropamide during the first trimester of pregnancy; this child had multiple malformations including sacral agenesis (Coetzee & Jackson, 1984).

Chronic maternal chlorpropamide therapy late in pregnancy was associated with very high perinatal mortality rates in some early studies (Jackson et al., 1962), but this association appears to have been due to poor control of the maternal diabetes rather than to the drug (Notelovitz, 1971; Sutherland et al., 1973, 1974; Anonymous, 1974; Fraser, 1982). Neonatal hypoglycemia may occur in infants born to diabetic mothers who took chlorpropamide late in pregnancy (Zucker & Simon, 1968), but it is difficult to determine if this is an effect of the drug, the disease, or both. Prolonged neonatal hypoglycemia has also been observed with greater than expected frequency among the children of women with non-insulin dependent diabetes mellitus who were treated with oral hypoglycemic agents, often chlorpropamide, during the first trimester but not in later pregnancy (Piacquadio et al., 1991).

No congenital anomalies were observed among the offspring of rats treated during pregnancy with chlorpropamide in doses 200-300 times those usually employed in humans (Tuchmann-Duplessis & Mercier-Parot, 1959), but malformations were noted among embryos of one strain of pregnant rats treated with a single high therapeutic dose of chlorpropamide prior to implantation (Brock & von Kreybig, 1964).

An increased frequency of chromosomal breaks and acquired rearrangements was observed in peripheral blood specimens from diabetic patients treated with oral hypoglycemic agents, usually chlorpropamide (Watson et al., 1976). The relevance of this finding to the occurrence of congenital anomalies among the children of women treated with chlorpropamide during pregnancy is unknown.

Please see agent summary on tolbutamide for information on a related agent that has been studied.

Key References

Anonymous: Chlorpropamide in diabetic pregnancy. Lancet 2:32, 1974. [R]

Brock N, Von Kreybig TH: Experiments regarding the testing of teratogenic drugs in the laboratory rat. Naunyn-Schmiedebergs Arch Pathol Pharmacol 249:117-145, 1964. [A]

Coetzee EJ, Jackson WPU: Oral hypoglycaemics in the first trimester and fetal outcome. S Afr Med J 65:635-637, 1984. [S]

Fraser RB: The fate of the pregnant diabetic in a developing country: Kenya. Diabetologia 22:21-24, 1982. [E]

Jackson WPU, Campbell GD, Notelovitz M, Blumsohn D: Tolbutamide and chlorpropamide during pregnancy in human diabetics. Diabetes 2(Suppl):98-101, 1962. [S]

Notelovitz M: Sulphonylurea therapy in the treatment of the pregnant diabetic. S Afr Med J 45:226-229, 1971. [E]

Piacquadio K, Hollingsworth DR, Murphy H: Effects of in-utero exposure to oral hypoglycaemic drugs. Lancet 338:866-869, 1991. [E]

Sutherland HW, Bewsher PD, Cormack JD, Hughes CRT, et al.: Effect of moderate dosage of chlorpropamide in pregnancy on fetal outcome. Arch Dis Child 49:283-291, 1974. [S]

Sutherland HW, Stowers JM, Cormack JD, Bewsher PD: Evaluation of chlorpropamide in chemical diabetes diagnosed during pregnancy. Br Med J 3:9-13, 1973. [S]

Tuchmann-Duplessis MH, Mercier-Parot L: Action of chlorpropamide on gestation and fetal development of the rat. C R Acad Sci (Paris) 249:1160-1162, 1959. [A]

Watson WAF, Petrie JC, Galloway DB, et al.: In vivo cytogenetic activity of sulphonylurea drugs in man. Mutat Res 38:71-80, 1976. [E]

Zucker P, Simon G: Prolonged symptomatic neonatal hypoglycemia associated with maternal chlorpropamide therapy. Pediatrics 42:824-825, 1968. [C]

CHLORPYRIFOS

Synonyms

Brodan, Dursban, EF121, Fospirate, Killmaster, Piridane, Pyrinex, Reldan, Spannit, Torelle

Summary

Chlorpyrifos is an organophosphorus compound that acts as a potent inhibitor of cholinesterase. It is used as an insecticide.

Magnitude of Teratogenic Risk

Undetermined

Quality and Quantity of Data

None To Poor

Comment

The risk of damage to the embryo or fetus is related to the amount of exposure and degree of maternal toxicity. Since exposure to insecticides such as chlorpyrifos cannot be controlled, a careful assessment of maternal exposure must be made

through documentation of maternal history and toxic responses, and measurements of serum cholinesterase.

No epidemiological studies of congenital anomalies among infants born to women treated with chlorpyrifos during pregnancy have been reported.

The frequency of malformations was not consistently increased among the offspring of mice fed 0.1-25 mg/kg/d of chlorpyrifos during pregnancy (Deacon et al., 1980). Maternal symptoms of organophosphate toxicity were seen at doses of 10 mg/kg/d and above and biochemical evidence of cholinesterase inhibition was seen at 1 mg/kg/d and above in these experiments.

Key References

Deacon MM, Murray JS, Pilny MK, et al.: Embryotoxicity and fetotoxicity of orally administered chlorpyrifos in mice. Toxicol Appl Pharmacol 54:31-40, 1980. [A]

CHLORTHALIDONE

Synonyms

Axamin, Higrotona, Hygroton, Igrolina, Igroton, Natriuran, Novothalidone, Oxodolin, Renidone, Uridon

Summary

Chlorthalidone is a diuretic used in the treatment of hypertension and edema.

Magnitude of Teratogenic Risk

None To Minimal

Quality and Quantity of Data

Fair

Comment

None

The Collaborative Perinatal Project, a large cohort study, included only 20 pregnancies exposed to chlorthalidone in the first trimester, but 1310 exposed anytime during pregnancy (Heinonen et al., 1977). In the latter group, a slightly increased frequency of congenital anomalies, mostly congenital dislocation of the hip, was seen. In a randomized controlled trial, the average weight and length of 108 infants born to mothers who took chlorthalidone from 16 weeks of pregnancy through term to prevent toxemia was slightly, but significantly, greater than controls (Tervila & Vartianen, 1971). No other differences in the exposed and unexposed newborns were noted.

No teratogenic effect was observed in the offspring of hamsters, rabbits, mice, or rats treated with chlorthalidone during pregnancy (Fratta et al., 1965). Doses used were about 150 times (hamsters), 50-150 times (rabbits), 200 times (mice), and 100-2000 times (rats) greater than those used in humans.

Key References

Fratta I, Harper KH, Stenger EG, Sigg EB: Effect of chlorthalidone on embryonic development. Med Pharmacol Exp 12:245-253, 1965. [A]

Heinonen OP, Slone D, Shapiro S: Birth Defects and Drugs in Pregnancy. Littleton, Mass.: John Wright-PSG, 1977, pp 372-373, 441. [E]

Tervila L, Vartianen E: The effects and side effects of diuretics in the prophylaxis of toxaemia of pregnancy. Acta Obstet Gynecol Scand 50:351-356, 1971. [E]

CHLORZOXAZONE

Synonyms

Biomioran, Chlorobenzoxazolinone, Chloroxazone, Escoflex, Flexazone, Myoflexine, Paraflex, Parafon Forte DSC, Solaxin

Summary

Chlorzoxazone is a centrally acting muscle relaxant.

Magnitude of Teratogenic Risk

Undetermined

Quality and Quantity of Data

None

Comment

None

No epidemiological studies of malformations in children born to women who used chlorzoxazone during pregnancy have been reported.

No animal teratology studies of chlorzoxazone have been published.

Please see agent summary for mephenesin for information on a related drug that has been more thoroughly studied.

Key References

None available.

CHOLERA VACCINE

Synonyms

Vibriomune

Summary

Cholera vaccine is made from killed bacteria. It is given by injection for protection against cholera.

Magnitude of Teratogenic Risk

Undetermined

Quality and Quantity of Data

None

Comment

A small risk cannot be excluded, but a high risk of congenital anomalies in the children of women treated with cholera vaccine during pregnancy is unlikely.

No epidemiological studies of congenital anomalies among infants born to women immunized with cholera vaccine during pregnancy have been reported.

No animal teratology studies of cholera vaccine have been published.

Key References

None available.

CHORIONIC GONADOTROPIN

Synonyms

A.P.L., Chorigon, Choron 10, Follutein, Gonabion, Pregnyl, Profasi

Summary

Chorionic gonadotropin is a glycoprotein hormone produced by the human placenta. Chorionic gonadotropin, which has actions very similar to those of pituitary luteinizing hormone, is given intramuscularly to induce ovulation after follicular stimulation in women with infertility or who are undergoing in vitro fertilization.

Magnitude of Teratogenic Risk

None

Quality and Quantity of Data

Poor To Fair

Comment

1) The altered sex ratio and increased frequency of spontaneous abortion reported in some studies of pregnancies in which chorionic gonadotropin was used to induce ovulation may be related to the underlying infertility and altered hormonal state rather than to chorionic gonadotropin per se.

2) The increased rate of twinning and associated fetal anomalies in pregnancies in which chorionic gonadotropin is used to induce ovulation may be related to the underlying infertility and altered hormonal state rather than to chorionic gonadotropin per se.

The frequency of malformations was no greater than expected among a cohort of 213 infants born to women in whom ovulation had been induced by treatment with menotropins and chorionic gonadotropin for infertility (Kurachi et al., 1983). However, the frequencies of congenital anomalies in both the study and control groups were unusually low in this investigation, suggesting underascertainment of anomalies. The frequency of major malformations did not appear to differ from expected rates in uncontrolled series of 100-200 infants born to women in whom ovulation had been induced with menotropins and chorionic gonadotropin (Hack et al., 1970; Caspi et al., 1976). Increased frequencies of spontaneous abortion and altered sex ratios with increased proportions of female infants were observed in these studies.

Greatly increased frequencies of multifetal gestations, often with triplets or higher multiples, have consistently been observed in the pregnancies of women whose ovulation was induced with menotropins and chorionic gonadotropin (Tyler, 1968; Hack et al., 1970; Spadoni et al., 1974; Caspi et al., 1976; Oelsner et al., 1978). The reported rates of multifetal pregnancy have varied somewhat, but are usually in the range of 20-40%. As expected, late gestational fetal death, perinatal death, premature delivery, and fetal deformations are often observed among these pregnancies.

Altered sex ratio, fetal death, and malformations, especially of the palate, eyelids, and limbs, have been observed among the offspring of mice in which ovulation was induced by chorionic gonadotropin (Elbling, 1973, 1975; Sakai et al., 1986; Sakai & Endo, 1987; Elmazar et al., 1989). Increased frequencies of fetal death occurred in pregnant rats, hamsters, mice, and sheep treated with chorionic gonadotropin during pregnancy in doses similar to or a few times greater than those used to induce ovulation in humans (Yang & Chang, 1968; Moor et al., 1969; Banik, 1975; Hoshino, 1977; Basu & Chatterjee, 1978).

Please see agent summary on clomiphene for information on a drug that is often used in combination with chorionic gonadotropin to induce ovulation.

Key References

Banik UK: Pregnancy-terminating effect of human chorionic gonadotrophin in rats. J Reprod Fert 42:67-76, 1975. [A]

Basu R, Chatterjee A: Pregnant mare's serum gonadotropin. IV. Induction of premature labor by pregnant mare's serum gonadotropin and its prevention by using clomiphene or indomethacin. Fertil Steril 29: 640-642, 1978. [A]

Caspi E, Ronen J, Schreyer P, Goldberg MD: The outcome of pregnancy after gonadotrophin therapy. Br J Obstet Gynaecol 83:967-973, 1976. [S]

Elbling L: Congenital malformations in mice after gonadotropin-induced ovulation. Proc Soc Exp Biol Med 149:376-379, 1975. [A]

Elbling L: Does gonadotrophin-induced ovulation in mice cause malformations in the offspring? Nature 246:37-39, 1973. [A]

Elmazar MMA, Vogel R, Spielmann H: Maternal factors influencing development of embryos from mice superovulated with gonadotropins. Reprod Toxicol 3(2):135-138, 1989. [A]

Hack M, Brish M, Serr M, Insler V, et al.: Outcome of pregnancy after induced ovulation. Follow-up of pregnancies and children born after gonadotropin therapy. JAMA 211(5):791-797, 1970. [S]

Hoshino K: Transplacental hormonal carcinogenesis and teratogenesis. Adv Obstet Gynecol (Sanfujinka No Shimpo) 30:499-511, 1977. [A]

Kurachi K, Aono T, Minagawa J, Miyake Λ: Congenital malformations of newborn infants after

123

clomiphene-induced ovulation. Fertil Steril 40(2):187-189, 1983. [E]

Moor RM, Rowson LEA, Hay MF, Caldwell BV: The effect of exogenous gonadotrophins on the conceptus and corpus luteum in pregnant sheep. J Endocrinol 44:495-499, 1969. [A]

Oelsner G, Serr DM, Mashiach S, Blankstein J, et al.: The study of induction of ovulation with menotropins: Analysis of results of 1897 treatment cycles. Fertil Steril:538-544, 1978. [S]

Sakai N, Endo A: Potential teratogenicity of gonadotropin treatment for ovulation induction in the mouse offspring. Teratology 36:229-233, 1987. [A]

Sakai N, Endo A: Teratogenic effects of ovulation induction by PMS/HCG in mouse fetuses. Teratology 34(3):447, 1986. [A]

Spadoni LR, Cox DW, Smith DC: Use of human menopausal gonadotropin for the induction of ovulation. Amer J Obstet Gynecol 120:988-993, 1974. [S]

Tyler ET: Treatment of anovulation with menotropins. JAMA 205 (1):16-22, 1968. [S]

Yang WH, Chang MC: Interruption of pregnancy in the rat and hamster by administration of PMS or HCG. Endocrinology 83:217-224, 1968. [A]

CHROMIUM SALTS

Synonyms

Chrome Alum, Chrometrace, Chromic Potassium Sulfate, Chromium Chloride, Chromium Trichloride, Chromium Trioxide, Dichromate, Hexaaquachromium Chloride, Scleremo, Trichlorochromium

Summary

Chromium forms salts as both a trivalent and hexavalent ion. $CrCl_3$ and Cr_2O_3, a green pigment, are examples of the former and CrO_2, a powerful oxidizing agent, is an example of the latter. Chromium is considered to be an essential dietary trace element with recommended intake of 0.05-0.2 mg/d.

Magnitude of Teratogenic Risk

Undetermined

Quality and Quantity of Data

Poor

Comment

None

No epidemiological studies of congenital anomalies among infants born to women exposed to large amounts of chromium salts during pregnancy have been reported.

No malformations were noted among the offspring of rats fed diets containing 2-5% Cr_2O_3 during pregnancy (Ivankovick & Preussmann, 1975). Increased frequencies of fetal death, cleft palate, and other malformations were observed among the offspring of hamsters treated with 5-15 mg/kg of CrO_3 during pregnancy (Gale, 1978; Gale & Bunch, 1979). This teratogenic effect exhibited typical dose and time of gestation dependence. Similarly, increased frequencies of malformations including cleft palates and neural tube defects were observed among the offspring of pregnant mice treated with 100 mg/kg/d of $CrCl_3$ or 20 mg/kg/d of CrO_3 (Iijima et al., 1975, 1979). The relevance of these observations to exposures to chromium salts that occur in humans is unknown.

Key References

Gale TF: Embryotoxic effects of chromium trioxide in hamsters. Environ Res 16:101-109, 1978. [A]

Gale TF, Bunch JD: The effect of the time of administration of chromium trioxide on the embryotoxic response in hamsters. Teratology 19:81-86, 1979. [A]

Iijima S, Mansumoto N, Lu CC, Katsunuma H: Placental transfer of $CrCl_3$ and its effects of fetal growth and development in mice. Teratology 12:198, 1975. [A]

Iijima S, Shimizu M, Matsumoto, N: Embryotoxic and fetotoxic effects of chromium trioxide in mice. Teratology 20:152, 1979. [A]

Ivankovic S, Preussmann R: Absence of toxic and carcinogenic effects after administration of high doses of chromic oxide pigment in subacute and long-term feeding experiments in rats. Fd Cosmet Toxicol 13:347-351, 1975. [A]

CICLOPIROX

Synonyms

Batrafen, Hoe 296, Loprox

Summary

Ciclopirox is an antifungal agent that is used topically to treat dermal mycotic infections. Absorption from skin is poor.

Magnitude of Teratogenic Risk

Undetermined

Quality and Quantity of Data

Poor

Comment

A small risk cannot be excluded, but a high risk of congenital anomalies in the children of women treated with ciclopirox during pregnancy is unlikely.

No epidemiological studies of congenital anomalies in infants born to women who used ciclopirox during pregnancy have been reported.

No teratogenic effects were observed among the offspring of pregnant rats of mice treated subcutaneously with ciclopirox in doses up to 10 mg/kg/d or orally in doses up to 100 mg/kg/d during pregnancy (Miyamoto et al., 1975).

Key References

Miyamoto M, Ohtsu M, Sugisaki T, Takayama K: Teratological studies of 6-cyclo-hexyl-1-hydroxy-4-methyl-2(1h)-pyridone ethanolamine salt (HOE 296) in mice and rats. Oyo Yakuri 9:97-108, 1975. [A]

CIGARETTE SMOKING (Tobacco)

Synonyms

Smoking, Snuff, Tobacco

Summary

Tobacco is the leaf of the plant Nicotiana tabacum. It is widely used by smoking, chewing, or dipping. Cigarette smoke contains several hundred different chemicals; nicotine and carbon monoxide are among the most abundant. Many studies of the reproductive effects of cigarette smoking have been performed. Extensive reviews are available on this subject (Stillman et al., 1986; Rosenberg, 1986; McIntosh, 1984a, b).

Magnitude of Teratogenic Risk

Malformations: None To Minimal

Fetal Growth Retardation: Moderate To High

Intrauterine Death: Small To Moderate

Quality and Quantity of Data

Malformations: Good

Fetal Growth Retardation: Good To Excellent

Intrauterine Death: Good

Comment

These risks are greatest for heavy smokers and may be less in women who stop smoking during pregnancy.

Congenital Anomalies: The relationship of maternal smoking and congenital anomalies has been examined in many epidemiological studies involving thousands of children (McIntosh, 1984a; Stillman et al., 1986). In general, no association between the frequency of major congenital anomalies and maternal smoking has been observed (Kullander & Kallen, 1971; Andrews & McGarry, 1972; Heinonen et al., 1977; Evans et al., 1979; Christianson, 1980; Hemminki et al., 1983; Shino et al., 1986; Malloy et al., 1989; Seidman et al., 1990; Werler et al., 1990; Van Den Eeden, et al., 1990; Tikkanen & Heinonen, 1991; Erickson, 1991; Werler et al., 1992). A few studies have found associations between maternal smoking and various congenital anomalies (Fedrick, et al., 1971; Himmelberger et al., 1978; Christianson, 1980; Aro, 1983; Goldbaum et al., 1990), but such associations have generally been weak and not reproducible in other investigations. A weak association between maternal smoking and facial clefts has been reported in several studies (Andrews & McGarry, 1972; Ericson et al., 1979; Khoury et al., 1989), but remains controversial.

Spontaneous Abortion: Well-controlled studies involving thousands of women have generally shown that the frequency of spontaneous abortion is 20-80% higher than expected among women who smoke cigarettes during pregnancy (McIntosh, 1984b; Stillman et al., 1986). The risks appear to be greater for heavy smokers than for light smokers. Some studies, but not others, suggest that perinatal mortality and other complications of pregnancy may also be increased among the infants of women who smoke cigarettes during pregnancy.

Fetal Growth Retardation: Dozens of studies involving hundreds of thousands of pregnancies have examined the association between maternal cigarette smoking and infant birth weight (McIntosh, 1984a; Stillman et al., 1986; Cnattingius, 1989; Hjortdal et al., 1989). Low birth weight is unequivocally associated with maternal smoking in a dose-related fashion. This effect seems to be due primarily to fetal growth retardation rather than to prematurity. Controversy exists regarding whether the fetal growth retardation seen among the infants of women who smoke is caused by the smoking or due to other correlated factors. The preponderance of evidence favors the former view. Persistent mild reduction of growth and intellectual performance has been observed among the children of women who smoked during pregnancy (Rush & Callahan, 1989). Some studies suggest that birth weight is also decreased slightly among the children of non-smoking women exposed to tobacco smoke in their environment (Haddow et al., 1989; Seidman & Mashiach, 1991; Ogawa et al., 1991).

Intellectual Development And Behavior: An association between maternal cigarette smoking during pregnancy and slightly lower than expected measured intelligence levels has been observed in some studies (Davie et al., 1972; Dunn et al., 1977; Fried, 1989; Rush & Callahan, 1989). Behavioral abnormalities have also been found more often than expected among the children of women who smoked cigarettes during pregnancy (Dunn et al., 1977; Naeye & Tafari, 1983; Rush & Callahan, 1989). The effects of postnatal factors as well as other prenatal factors confound such investigations so that a causal inference is not possible (Rush & Callahan, 1989).

Childhood Cancer: A few epidemiological studies suggest that maternal smoking during pregnancy slightly increases the risk of subsequent development of childhood cancer among the offspring (Stjernfeldt et al., 1986; Golding et al., 1990; John et al., 1991), but other studies do not show this effect (Pershagen et al., 1989). These investigations may be confounded by a variety of other factors that correlate with maternal smoking during pregnancy.

Animal Studies: Experimental teratology studies of simulated tobacco use in experimental animals are of questionable relevance to interpreting the risks of cigarette smoking in humans (Abel, 1980; Mactutus, 1989). Congenital arthrogryposis occurs in the offspring of pigs fed tobacco stems during pregnancy (Menges et al., 1970; Crowe & Swerczek, 1974).

Key References

Abel EL: Smoking during pregnancy: A review of effects on growth and development of offspring. Hum Biol 52:593-626, 1980. [R]

Andrews J, McGarry JM: A community study of smoking in pregnancy. J Obstet Gynaecol Br Commonw 79 (12):1057-1073, 1972. [E]

Aro T: Maternal diseases, alcohol consumption and smoking during pregnancy associated with reduction limb defects. Early Hum Dev 9:49-57, 1983. [E]

Christianson RE: The relationship between maternal smoking and the incidence of congenital anomalies. Am J Epidemiol 112 (5):684-695, 1980. [E]

Cnattingius S: Does age potentiate the smoking-related risk of fetal growth retardation? Early Hum Dev 20:203-211, 1989. [E]

Crowe MW, Swerczek TW: Congenital arthrogryposis in offspring of sows fed tobacco (Nicotiana tabacum). Am J Vet Res 35:1071-1073, 1974. [A]

Davie R, Butler N, Goldstein H: From Birth to Seven: A report of the National Child Development Study. London: Longman and the National Children's Bureau, 1972, pp 175-177. [R] & [E]

Dunn HG, Karaa A, Ingram S, Hunter CM: Maternal cigarette smoking during pregnancy and the child's subsequent development. II. Neurological and intellectual maturation to the age of six and one-half years. Can J Public Health 68:43-49, 1977. [E]

Erickson JD: Risk factors for birth defects: Data from the Atlanta Birth Defects Case-Control Study. Teratology 43:41-51, 1991. [E]

Ericson A, Kallen B, Westerholm P: Cigarette smoking as an etiologic factor in cleft lip and palate. Am J Obstet Gynecol 135:348-351, 1979. [E]

Evans DR, Newcombe RG, Campbell H: Maternal smoking habits and congenital malformations: A population study. Br Med J 2:171-173, 1979. [E]

Fedrick J, Alberman ED, Goldstein H: Possible teratogenic effect of cigarette smoking. Nature 231:529-530, 1971. [E]

Freid PA: Cigarettes and marijuana: Are there measurable long-term neurobehavioral teratogenic effects? Neurotoxicology 10:577-584, 1989. [E]

Goldbaum G, Daling J, Milham S: Risk factors for gastroschisis. Teratology 42:397-403, 1990. [E]

Golding J, Paterson M, Kinlen LJ: Factors associated with childhood cancer in a national cohort study. Br J Cancer 62:304-308, 1990. [E]

Haddow JE, Knight GJ, Palomaki GE, et al.: Serum cotinine levels in pregnant nonsmokers in relation to birthweight. Ann NY Acad Sci 562:370-371, 1989. [E]

Heinonen OP, Slone D, Shapiro S: Birth Defects and Drugs in Pregnancy. Littleton, Mass.: John Wright-PSG, 1977, pp 2, 14, 27. [E]

Hemminki K, Mutanen P, Saloniemi I: Smoking and the occurrence of congenital malformations and spontaneous abortions: Multivariate analysis. Am J Obstet Gynecol 145:61-66, 1983. [E]

Himmelberger DU, Brown Jr BW, Cohen EN: Cigarette smoking during pregnancy and the occurrence of spontaneous abortion and congenital abnormality. Am J Epidemiol 108:470-479, 1978. [E]

Hjortdal JO, Hjortdal VE, Foldspang A: Tobacco smoking and fetal growth. A review. Scand J Soc Med (Suppl 0) 45:I-II, 1-22, 1989. [R]

John EM, Savitz DA, Sandler DP: Prenatal exposure to parents' smoking and childhood cancer. Am J Epidemiol 133(2):123-132, 1991. [E]

Khoury MJ, Gomez-Farias M, Mulinare J: Does maternal cigarette smoking during pregnancy cause cleft lip and palate in offspring? Am J Dis Child 143:333-337, 1989. [E]

Kullander S, Kallen B: A prospective study of smoking and pregnancy. Acta Obstet Gynec Scand 50:83-94, 1971. [E]

Mactutus CF: Developmental neurotoxicity of nicotine, carbon monoxide, and other tobacco smoke constituents. Ann NY Acad Sci 562:105-122, 1989. [R]

Malloy MH, Kleinman JC, Bakewell JM, et al.: Maternal smoking during pregnancy: No association with congenital malformations in Missouri 1980-83. Am J Public Health 79:1243-1246, 1989. [E]

McIntosh ID: Smoking and pregnancy: I. Maternal and placental risks. Public Health Rev 12:1-28, 1984b. [O]

McIntosh ID: Smoking and pregnancy: II. Offspring risks. Public Health Rev 12:29-63, 1984a. [O]

Menges RW, Selby LA, Marienfeld CJJ, Aue WA, et al.: A tobacco related epidemic of congenital limb deformities in swine. Environ Res 3:285-302, 1970. [A]

Naeye RL, Tafari N: Risk Factors in Pregnancy and Diseases of the Fetus and Newborn. Baltimore: Williams & Wilkins, 1983, pp 180-183. [R]

Ogawa H, Tominaga S, Hori K, et al.: Passive smoking by pregnant women and fetal growth. J Epidemiol Community Health 45:164-168, 1991. [E]

Pershagen G: Childhood cancer and malignancies other than lung cancer related to passive smoking. Mutat Res 222:129-135, 1989. [R]

Rosenberg MJ: Smoking and Reproductive Health. Littleton, Mass.: Publishing Science Group, 1986. [R]

Rush D, Callahan KR: Exposure to passive cigarette smoking and child development. A critical review. Ann NY Acad Sci 562:74-100, 1989. [R]

Seidman DS, Ever-Hadani P, Gale R: Effect of maternal smoking and age on congenital anomalies. Obstet Gynecol 76(6):1046-1050, 1990. [E]

Seidman DS, Mashiach S: Involuntary smoking and pregnancy. Eur J Obstet Gynecol Reprod Biol 41:105-116, 1991. [R]

Shiono PH, Klebanoff MA, Berendes HW: Congenital malformations and maternal smoking during pregnancy. Teratology 34:65-71, 1986. [E]

Stillman RJ, Rosenberg MJ, Sachs BP: Smoking and reproduction. Fertil Steril 46 (4):545-566, 1986. [R]

Stjernfeldt M, Berglund K, Lindsten J, Ludvigsson J: Maternal smoking during pregnancy and risk of childhood cancer. Lancet 1(8494):1350-1352, 1986. [E]

Tikkanen J, Heinonen OP: Maternal exposure to chemical and physical factors during pregnancy and cardiovascular malformations in the offspring. Teratology 43:591-600, 1991. [E]

Van Den Eeden SK, Karagas MR, Daling JR, Vaughan TL: A case-control study of maternal smoking and congenital malformations. Paediatr Perinat Epidemiol 4(2):147-155, 1990. [E]

Werler MM, Lammer EJ, Rosenberg L, Mitchell AA: Maternal cigarette smoking during pregnancy in relation to oral clefts. Am J Epidemiol 132(5):926-932, 1990. [E]

Werler MM, Mitchell AA, Shapiro S: Demographic, reproductive, medical, and environmental factors in relation to gastroschisis. Teratology 45:353-360, 1992. [E]

CILASTATIN

Summary

Cilastatin is an inhibitor of the renal enzyme dehydropeptidase I. It is administered parenterally with the antibiotic imipenem to prevent metabolism of imipenem to an inactive form.

Magnitude of Teratogenic Risk

Undetermined

Quality and Quantity of Data

None

Comment

None

No epidemiological studies of congenital anomalies in infants born to women who took cilastatin during pregnancy have been reported.

An increased frequency of embryonic death was observed among pregnant cynomolgus monkeys treated with imipenem/cilastatin in doses that, although similar to those used in humans, were maternally toxic (Cukierski et al., 1990). No malformations were seen among surviving offspring. The frequency of malformations was not increased among the offspring of rats treated during pregnancy with <1-6 times the maximum human dose of imipenem/cilastatin (Clark et al., 1985).

Key References

Clark RL, Robertson RT, MacDonald JS et al.: Imipenem/cilastatin sodium: Teratogenicity study in rats pre- and postnatal observation. Chemotherapy (Tokyo) (Nippon Kagaku Ryoho Gakkai Zasshi) 33(Suppl 4):227-241, 1985. [A]

Cukierski MA, Wise LD, Korte R, et al.: Developmental toxicity studies of imipenem/cilastatin sodium in monkeys. Teratology 41(5):546-547, 1990. [A]

CIMETIDINE

Synonyms

Acinil, Brumetidina, Cimal, Duogastril, Dyspamet, Histodil, Novocimetine, Peptol, Tagamet, Ulcedine

Summary

Cimetidine is a histamine receptor antagonist that raises gastric pH. It is widely used in the treatment of peptic ulcer disease.

Magnitude of Teratogenic Risk

Undetermined

Quality and Quantity of Data

None To Poor

Comment

None

No epidemiological studies of congenital anomalies among infants born to women treated with cimetidine during pregnancy have been reported. No malformations were observed in one series of eight infants born to women who had been treated with cimetidine during the first trimester of pregnancy (Koren & Zemlickis, 1991).

The frequency of malformations was not increased among the offspring of pregnant rats, mice, or rabbits treated with cimetidine in doses respectively <1-42, up to 20, and <1-20 times those used in humans (Leslie & Walker, 1977; Hirakawa et al., 1980; Kitao et al., 1983; Brimblecombe et al., 1985). Increased frequencies of fetal growth retardation and death were often seen at high doses.

Male offspring of rats treated with <1-3 times the usual human dose of cimetidine during pregnancy have been noted to have decreased virilization in some studies (Anand & Van Thiel, 1982; Parker et al., 1984). Other investigators have not observed such effects despite administration of even larger doses of the drug (Leslie & Walker, 1977; Walker et al., 1987; Shapiro et al., 1988). Sexual development has not been studied in boys born to women treated with cimetidine during pregnancy, and the clinical relevance of the animal studies is unknown.

No neonatal complications attributable to maternal cimetidine therapy prior to delivery were observed in infants born by elective or emergency Caesarean section (Johnston et al., 1982a, b).

Key References

Anand S, Van Thiel DH: Prenatal and neonatal exposure to cimetidine results in gonadal and sexual dysfunction in adult males. Science 218:493-494, 1982. [A]

Brimblecombe RW, Leslie GB, Walker TF: Toxicology of cimetidine. Hum Toxicol 4:13-25, 1985. [A]

Hirakawa T, Suzuki T, Hayashizaki A, Nishimura N, et al.: Reproduction studies of cimetidine. Clin Rep 14:2819-2831, 1980. [A]

Johnston JR, McCaughey W, Moore J, Dundee JW: Cimetidine as an oral antacid before elective Caesarean section. Anaesthesia 37:26-32, 1982b. [E]

Johnston JR, McCaughey W, Moore J, Dundee JW: A field trial of cimetidine as the sole oral antacid in obstetric anaesthesia. Anaesthesia 37:33-38, 1982a. [E]

Kitao T, Yamamoto M, Morimoto T, Ueshita S: Reproduction studies of FPF 1002 (cimetidine) 2.

Teratogenicity study in rats. Yakuri to Chiryo (Basic Pharm Ther) 11:1727-1741, 1983. [A]

Koren G, Zemlickis M: Outcome of pregnancy after first trimester exposure to H2 receptor antagonists. Am J Perinatol 8(1):37-38, 1991. [S]

Leslie GB, Walker TF: A toxicological profile of cimetidine. Int Congr Ser Excerpta Med 416:24-37, 1977. [A]

Parker S, Schade RR, Pohl CR, Gavaler JS, et al.: Prenatal and neonatal exposure of male rat pups to cimetidine but not ranitidine adversely affects subsequent adult sexual functioning. Gastroenterology 86:675-680, 1984. [A]

Shapiro BH, Hirst SA, Babalola GO, et al.: Prospective study on the sexual development of male and female rats perinatally exposed to maternally administered cimetidine. Toxicol Lett 44:315-329, 1988. [A]

Walker TF, Bott JH, Bond BC: Cimetidine does not demasculinize male rat offspring exposed in utero. Fund Appl Toxicol 8:188-197, 1987. [A]

CINOXACIN

Synonyms

Cinobac, Cinobactin, Nossacin, Uronorm, Uroxacin

Summary

Cinoxacin is a 4-quinolone antibacterial agent used primarily to treat urinary tract infections.

Magnitude of Teratogenic Risk

Undetermined

Quality and Quantity of Data

Poor

Comment

A small risk cannot be excluded, but a high risk of congenital anomalies in the children of women treated with cinoxacin during pregnancy is unlikely.

No epidemiological studies of congenital anomalies in infants whose mothers took cinoxacin during pregnancy have been reported.

The frequency of malformations was no greater than expected among the offspring of rats or rabbits treated during pregnancy with 2.5-15 or 5-40 times the usual human dose of cinoxacin (Sato et al., 1980; Sato & Kobayashi, 1980).

Please see agent summary on nalidixic acid for information on a related agent that has been studied.

Key References

Sato T, Kaneko Y, Saegusa T: Reproduction studies of cinoxacin in rats. Chemotherapy 28:484-506, 1980. [A]

Sato T, Kobayashi F: Teratological study on cinoxacin in rabbits. Chemotherapy 28:508-515, 1980. [A]

CIPROFLOXACIN

Synonyms

Ciflox, Cipro, Cipro IV, Ciprobay, Ciproxin

Summary

Ciprofloxacin is a quinoline derivative with antimicrobial activity. It is administered orally in the treatment of urinary tract infections.

Magnitude of Teratogenic Risk

Undetermined

Quality and Quantity of Data

None

Comment

None

No epidemiological studies of congenital anomalies in infants whose mothers were treated with ciprofloxacin during pregnancy have been reported.

No animal teratology studies of ciprofloxacin have been published.

Key References

None available.

CITRATE

Synonyms

Citric Acid

Summary

Citrate is an organic anion involved in normal intermediary metabolism. It is contained in a variety of beverages, mouth washes, effervescing mixtures, and eye lotions. Citrate is also used as a urinary irrigation solution.

Magnitude of Teratogenic Risk

Undetermined

Quality and Quantity of Data

None To Poor

Comment

A small risk cannot be excluded, but a substantial risk of congenital anomalies in the children of women treated with citrate during pregnancy is unlikely.

No epidemiological studies of malformations in infants born to women who ingested excessive amounts of citrate during pregnancy have been reported.

No teratogenic effect was observed among the offspring of mice, rats, hamsters, or rabbits treated with citrate during pregnancy in doses of 2.4-241, 3.0-295, 2.7-272, and 4.2-425

mg/kg/d, respectively (Food and Drug Research Labs, 1973).

Key References

Food and Drug Research Labs: Teratologic evaluation of FDA 71-54 (citric acid). NTIS (National Technical Information Services) Report/PB-223 814, 1973. [A]

CLARITHROMYCIN

Synonyms

Biaxin, CLA

Summary

Clarithromycin is an antibacterial agent administered orally to treat respiratory tract infections.

Magnitude of Teratogenic Risk

Undetermined

Quality and Quantity of Data

None

Comment

A small risk cannot be excluded, but a high risk of congenital anomalies in the children of women treated with clarithromycin during pregnancy is unlikely.

No epidemiological studies of congenital anomalies in infants whose mothers were treated with clarithromycin during pregnancy have been reported.

No animal teratology studies of clarithromycin have been published.

Please see agent summary on erythromycin for information on a related agent that has been more thoroughly studied.

Key References

None available.

CLEMASTINE

Synonyms

Aller-eze, Clemanil, Clemastine Fumarate, Histamedine, Tavegil, Tavist

Summary

Clemastine is an antihistaminic agent used orally to treat allergic rhinitis, urticaria, and angioedema.

Magnitude of Teratogenic Risk

Undetermined

Quality and Quantity of Data

None

Comment

None

No epidemiological studies of congenital anomalies among infants born to women treated with clemastine during pregnancy have been reported.

No animal teratology studies of clemastine have been published.

Please see agent summary on diphenhydramine for information on a related agent that has been studied.

Key References

None available.

CLIDINIUM BROMIDE

Synonyms

Bromure de Clidinium, Bromuro de Clidinio, Quarzan, Quarzan Bromide

Summary

Clidinium bromide is an anticholinergic agent used in the treatment of peptic ulcer disease and other gastro-intestinal disorders.

Magnitude of Teratogenic Risk

Undetermined

Quality and Quantity of Data

None

Comment

None

No epidemiological studies of malformations in infants born to women treated with clidinium bromide during pregnancy have been reported.

No animal teratology studies of clidinium bromide have been published.

Please see agent summary on atropine for information on a related drug that has been more thoroughly studied.

Key References

None available.

CLINDAMYCIN

Synonyms

Chlolincocin, Chlorodeoxylincomycin, Chlorolincomycin, Cleocin, Clindamicina, Dalacin C, Sobelin

Summary

Clindamycin is an antibiotic used to treat anaerobic infections.

Magnitude of Teratogenic Risk

Undetermined

Quality and Quantity of Data

Poor

Comment

A small risk cannot be excluded, but there is no indication that the risk of congenital anomalies in the children of women treated with clindamycin during pregnancy is likely to be great.

No epidemiological studies of congenital anomalies in infants born to women who were treated with clindamycin early in pregnancy have been reported. The frequency of congenital anomalies was no greater than expected among the infants of 104 women treated with clindamycin in the second or third trimester of pregnancy as part of a controlled trial of therapy to prevent low birth weight (McCormack et al., 1987).

The frequency of malformations was no greater than expected among the offspring of mice or rats given <1-12 or 1-12 times the human therapeutic dose of clindamycin during pregnancy (Gray et al., 1972; Bollert et al., 1972).

Key References

Bollert JA, Gray JE, Highstrete JD, Moran J, et al.: Teratogenicity and neonatal toxicity of clindamycin 2-phosphate in laboratory animals. Toxicol Appl Pharm 27:322-329, 1972. [A]

Gray JE, Weaver RN, Bollert JA, Feenstra ES: The oral toxicity of clindamycin in laboratory animals. Toxicol Appl Pharm 21:516-531, 1972. [A]

McCormack WM, Rosner B, Lee YH, Munoz A, et al.: Effect on birth weight of erythromycin treatment of pregnant women. Obstet Gynecol 69:202-207, 1987. [E]

CLIOQUINOL

Synonyms

Alchloquin, Amoenol, Bactol, Barquinol, Budoform, Chinoform, Chloroiodoquine, Entero-Vioform, Vioform

Summary

Clioquinol is an antifungal and antibacterial agent that is administered orally in the treatment of intestinal amebiasis and used topically to treat skin infections and dermatoses. Absorption from the skin is variable.

Magnitude of Teratogenic Risk

Undetermined

Quality and Quantity of Data

None

Comment

None

No epidemiological studies of congenital anomalies among infants born to women treated with clioquinol during pregnancy have been reported.

No mammalian teratology studies of clioquinol have been published.

Key References

None available.

CLOFAZIMINE

Synonyms

Chlofazimine, Hansepran, Lampren, Lamprene

Summary

Clofazimine is a dye that is used to treat leprosy. The drug has an extremely long half-life (about 70 days) after oral administration (Levy, 1974).

Magnitude of Teratogenic Risk

Minimal

Quality and Quantity of Data

Poor To Fair

Comment

Skin discoloration, a recognized side effect of clofazimine treatment in adults, has been noted in infants born to women who took this medication during pregnancy (Farb et al., 1982).

No epidemiological studies of congenital anomalies among the infants of women treated with clofazimine during pregnancy have been reported. Three neonatal deaths have been observed among 15 published cases in which the mother was treated with clofazimine for leprosy during pregnancy (Farb et al., 1982; Holdiness, 1989). The cause of the infant's death appeared to be different in each instance, and no association between this event and the mother's treatment is obvious.

No teratogenic effect was observed among the offspring of rats or rabbits treated during pregnancy with clofazimine in doses 2.5-25 or 2.5-7.5 times those usually employed in humans (Stenger et al., 1970). Increased frequencies of fetal death occurred in pregnant mice treated with 12-25 times the usual human dose of clofazimine (Stenger et al., 1970). The relevance of this observation to the therapeutic use of clofazimine in human pregnancy is uncertain.

Key References

Farb H, West DP, Pedvis-Leftick A: Clofazimine in pregnancy complicated by leprosy. Obstet Gynecol 59:122-123, 1982. [C]

Holdiness MR: Clofazimine in pregnancy [letter]. Early Hum Dev 18:297-298, 1989. [R]

Levy L: Pharmacologic studies of clofazimine. Amer J Trop Med Hyg 23:1097-1109, 1974. [A] & [O]

Stenger VEG, Aeppli L, Peheim E, Thomann PE: A contribution to the toxicology of the leprostatic drug 3-(p-chloranilino)-10-(p-chlorphenyl)-2,10-dihydro-2(isopropylimino)-phenazin (G 30320). Arzneimittelforsch 20:794-799, 1970. [A]

CLOMIPHENE

Synonyms

Clomid, Clomiphene Citrate, Dyneric, Enclomid, Enclomiphene, Fertyl, Omifin, Pergotime, Serophene

Summary

Clomiphene is a non-steroidal triphenylethylene derivative with both estrogenic and anti-estrogenic activity. It is administered orally to induce ovulation and is, therefore, intended to be used prior to conception.

Magnitude of Teratogenic Risk

Ovulation Induction: None To Minimal

Exposure During Embryogenesis: Undetermined

Quality and Quantity of Data

Ovulation Induction: Fair

Exposure During Embryogenesis: Poor

Comment

1) The above risks refer to malformations not to deformations or other complications related to multifetal gestation.

2) Induction of ovulation in infertile women is associated with an increased rate of multifetal gestations and related pregnancy complications including deformations (see below).

The frequency of congenital anomalies was no greater than expected among infants of women who had been treated with clomiphene to induce ovulation in three cohort studies involving respectively 225, 340, and 935 children (Harlap, 1976; Barrat & Leger, 1979; Kurachi et al., 1983) or in a case-control study of 4904 infants with major congenital anomalies (Mili et al., 1991). In contrast, Czeizel (1989) observed an apparent association with maternal ovulation induction among 10,990 infants with various congenital anomalies in the Hungarian registry (OR=3.6 based on an exposure rate of 0.1% among controls).

An association with maternal ovulation induction was observed among 825 infants with neural tube defects in this study (Czeizel, 1989), and a similar association was seen in another case-control study involving 94 cases with neural tube defects (Cornel et al., 1989; Vollset., 1990). This finding was not confirmed in three other case-control studies involving respectively 107, 345, and 571 cases (Cuckle & Wald, 1989; Mills et al., 1990; Mills, 1991; Mili et al., 1991) or in a cohort study of 438 women who used clomiphene during the three months prior to conception (Milunsky et al., 1990). Several large clinical series of pregnancies among patients who conceived after ovulation induction, usually with clomiphene, suggest that the frequency of neural tube defects among the offspring is similar to or slightly greater than exected (Rosa, 1990; Cornel et al., 1990). If the risk for neural tube defects among children born of pregnancies conceived after clomiphene-induced ovulation is increased, this risk appears to be no greater than 0.5% in most populations. Maternal serum alpha- fetoprotein determination and high-resolution ultrasound examination can be used for prenatal diagnosis of neural tube defects in such pregnancies.

Multifetal gestation, usually twinning, occurs in 8-13% of pregnancies conceived by women treated with clomiphene (Asch & Greenblatt, 1976; Lamont, 1982; Scialli, 1986). Premature delivery and other complications of multifetal gestation may occur in such pregnancies. Miscarriage is seen somewhat more often in clomiphene-induced pregnancy than in spontaneous pregnancy, but this appears to be related to the underlying reproductive problems that lead to clomiphene therapy (Asch & Greenblatt, 1976; Scialli, 1986; Lev-Gur et al., 1990). Ectopic gestation has been observed with increased frequency in pregnancies conceived during clomiphene treatment (Weiss & Aboulafia, 1975; Marchbanks et al., 1985; Cohen et al., 1986; Raccuia et al., 1989; Kauppi-Sahla et al., 1990; Asher & Ben-Shlomo, 1990), but this may also be related more closely to the underlying infertility than to its treatment (Dickey et al., 1989).

Neuroectodermal tumors (including neuroblastoma) were observed unexpectedly often among children born after ovulation induction and in vitro fertilization in one clinical series (White et al., 1989). Ovulation induction was reported more often than expected among the mothers of 887 children with neuroblastoma identified through the Japan Children's Cancer Register (Kobayashi et al., 1991). No causal inference can be made on the basis of these observations, for which it is difficult to envision a biological basis.

No malformations were observed among the offspring of 18 rhesus monkeys treated with 1-2 times the usual human dose of clomiphene during embryogenesis, although two of the infant animals were stillborn (Courtney & Valerio, 1968). The frequencies of embryonic loss, fetal death, hydrops, renal anomalies and cataracts were increased among the offspring of rats treated with clomiphene during embryogenesis in doses <1-100 times those used in humans (Diener & Hsu, 1967; Eneroth et al., 1971; Marois & Marois, 1974; Cummings et al., 1991). In contrast, no increase in malformations was apparent among the offspring of rats treated with clomiphene around the time of conception in doses similar to those used in humans (Staples, 1966) or among the offspring of rabbits treated with clomiphene during embryogenesis in doses 2-7 times greater than those used in humans (Morris et al., 1967).

Epithelial abnormalities of the female genital tract similar to those seen after maternal treatment with diethylstilbesterol have been noted among the offspring of rats treated during embryogenesis with clomiphene in doses similar to those used in humans (Clark & McCormack, 1980). Epithelial hyperplasia has also been observed in human fetal genital tract tissue grown in nude mice injected with clomiphene pellets (Cunha et al., 1987). Studies of vaginal cytology in girls and women born after clomiphene-induced ovulation have not yet been reported.

Key References

Asch RH, Greenblatt RB: Update on the safety and efficacy of clomiphene citrate as a therapeutic agent. J Reprod Med 17:175-180, 1976. [R]

Asher UA, Ben-Shlomo I: Bilateral simultaneous tubal pregnancies following clomiphene citrate: A case report. Isr J Med Sci 26:222-224, 1990. [C]

Barrat J, Leger D: Avenir des grossesses obtenues apres stimulation de l'ovulation. J Gynecol Obstet Biol Reprod 8:333-342, 1979. [E]

Clark JH, McCormack SA: The effect of clomid and other triphenylethylene derivatives during pregnancy and the neonatal period. J Steroid Biochem 12:47-53, 1980. [A]

Cohen J, Mayaux M-J, Guihard-Moscato M-L, Schwartz D: In-vitro fertilization and embryo transfer: A collaborative study of 1163 pregnancies on the incidence and risk factors of ectopic pregnancies. Hum Reprod 1(4):255-258, 1986. [S]

Cornel MC, ten Kate LP, Dukes MNG, de Jong-v d Berg LTW, et al.: Ovulation induction and neural tube defects. Lancet 1:1386, 1989. [E]

Cornel MC, ten Kate LP, te Meerman GJ: Association between ovulation stimulation, in vitro fertilsation, and neural tube defects? Teratology 42:201-203, 1990. [R] & [O]

Courtney KD, Valerio DA: Teratology in Macaca mulatta. Teratology 1:163-172, 1968. [A]

Cuckle H, Wald N: Ovulation induction and neural tube defects. Lancet 2:1281, 1989. [E]

Cummings AM, Perreault SD, Harris ST: Validation of protocols for assessing early pregnancy failure in the rat: Clomiphene citrate. Fundam Appl Toxicol 16:506-516, 1991. [A]

Cunha GR, Taguchi O, Namikawa R, Nishizuka Y, et al.: Teratogenic effects of clomiphene, tamoxifen, and diethylstilbesterol on the developing human female genital tract. Human Pathol 18:1132-1143, 1987. [A]

Czeizel A: Ovulation induction and neural tube defects. Lancet 2:167, 1989. [E]

Dickey RP, Matis R, Olar TT, et al.: The occurrence of ectopic pregnancy with and without clomiphene citrate use in assisted and nonassisted reproductive technology. J In Vitro Fert Embryo Transf 6:294-297, 1989. [E]

Diener Rm, Hsu BYD: Effects of certain basic phenolic ethers on the rat fetus. Toxicol Appl Pharmacol 10:565-576, 1967. [A]

Eneroth G, Forsberg U, Grant CA: Hydramnios and congenital cataracts induced in rats by clomiphene. Proc Eur Soc Study Drug Toxic 12:299-306, 1971. [A]

Harlap S: Ovulation induction and congenital malformations. Lancet 2:961, 1976. [E]

Kauppi-Sahla M, Rintala H, Makinen J: Bilateral tubal pregnancy: A case report and review of the literature. Eur J Obstet Gynecol Reprod Biol 90:145-147, 1990. [R] & [C]

Kobayashi N, Matsui I, Tanimura M, et al.: Childhood neuroectodermal tumours and malignant lymphoma after maternal ovulation induction. Lancet 338(8772):955, 1991. [E]

Kurachi K, Aono T, Minagawa J, Miyake A: Congenital malformations of newborn infants after clomiphene-induced ovulation. Fertil Steril 40:187-189, 1983. [E]

Lamont JA: Twin pregnancies following induction of ovulation. Acta Genet Med Gemellol 31:247-253, 1982. [R]

Lev-Gur M, Rodriguez LJ, Smith KD, Steinberger E: Risk factors for pregnancy loss apparent at conception in infertile couples. Int J Fertil 35(1):51-57, 1990. [E]

Marchbanks PA, Coulam CB, Annegers JF: An association between clomiphene citrate and ectopic pregnancy: A preliminary report. Fertil Steril 44:268-270, 1985. [E]

Marois M, Marois G: Clomifene, nidation et survie des foetus. C R Soc Biol (Paris) 168(4-5):405-410, 1974. [A]

Mili F, Khoury MJ, Lu X: Clomiphene citrate use and the risk of birth defects: A population-based case-control study. Teratology 43(5):422-423, 1991. [E]

Mills JL: Clomiphene and neural-tube defects. Lancet 337(8745):853, 1991. [O]

Mills JL, Simpson JL, Rhoads GG, et al.: Risk of neural tube defects in relation to maternal fertility and fertility drug use. Lancet 336:103-104, 1990. [E]

Milunsky A, Derby LE, Jick H: Ovulation induction and neural tube defects. Teratology 42:467, 1990. [O]

Morris JM, van Wagenen G, McCann T, Jacob D: Compounds interfering with ovum implantation and development: II. Synthetic estrogens and anti-estrogens. Fertil Steril 18:18-34, 1967. [A]

Raccuia JS, Neckles S, Butler D, Kahn M, et al.: Synchronous intrauterine and ectopic pregnancy associated with clomiphene citrate. Surg Gynecol Obstet 168:417-420, 1989. [C]

Rosa F: Ovulation induction and neural tube defects. Lancet 336(8726):1327, 1990. [O]

Scialli AR: The reproductive toxicity of ovulation induction. Fertil Steril 45:315-323, 1986. [R]

Staples RE: Effect of clomiphene on blastocyst nidation in the rat. Endocrinol 78:82-86, 1966. [A]

Vollset SE: Ovulation induction and neural tube defects. Lancet 335:178, 1990. [E]

Weiss DB, Aboulafia Y: Ectopic gestation and hydatidiform mole in clomiphene-induced pregnancies. Lancet 2:1094-1095, 1975. [S]

White L, Giri N, Vowels MR, Lancaster PAL: Neuroectodermal tumours in children born after assisted conception. Lancet 336:1577, 1989. [S]

CLOMIPRAMINE

Synonyms

Anafranil, Anaphranil, Chlorimipramine, Clomipramina, Clomipraminum

Summary

Clomipramine is a tricyclic antidepressant.

Magnitude of Teratogenic Risk

Undetermined

Quality and Quantity of Data

Poor

Comment

Transient behavioral and physiological abnormalities have been observed in infants of women who were treated with clomipramine late in pregnancy (see below).

No epidemiological studies of congenital anomalies among the infants of women treated with clomipramine during pregnancy have been reported.

Increased frequencies of central nervous system and other malformations have been observed among the offspring of mice treated with 36 times the human therapeutic dose of clomipramine during pregnancy (Jurand, 1980). Persistent alterations of behavior occur in the offspring of pregnant rats treated with clomipramine in doses equivalent to or greater than those used therapeutically in humans (File & Tucker, 1983; de Ceballos et al., 1985; Drago et al., 1985).

Abnormalities of perinatal adaptation and seizures have been reported among infants of women treated with clomipramine prior to delivery (Musa & Smith, 1979; Ostergaard and Pedersen, 1982; Cowe et al., 1982; Singh et al., 1990).

Please see agent summary on amitriptyline for information on a related agent that has been more thoroughly studied.

Key References

de Ceballos ML, Benedi A, de Felipe C, del Rio J: Prenatal exposure of rats to antidepressants enhances agonist affinity of brain dopamine receptors and dopamine-mediated behaviour. Eur J Pharmacol 116:257-262, 1985. [A]

Cowe L, Lloyd DJ, Dawling S: Neonatal convulsions caused by withdrawal from maternal clomipramine. Br Med J 284:1837-1838, 1982. [C]

Drago F, Continella G, Alloro MC, Scapagnini U: Behavioral effects of perinatal administration of antidepressant drugs in the rat. Neurobehav Toxicol Teratol 7:493-497, 1985. [A]

File SE, Tucker JC: Neonatal clomipramine treatment in the rat does not effect social, sexual and exploratory behaviors in adulthood. Neurobehav Toxicol Teratol 5(1):3-8, 1983. [A]

Jurand A: Malformations of the central nervous system induced by neurotropic drugs in mouse embryos. Dev Growth Differ 22:61-78, 1980. [A]

Musa AB: Neonatal effects of maternal clomipramine therapy [letter]. Arch Dis Child 54(5):405, 1979. [C]

Ostergaard GZ, Pedersen SE: Neonatal effects of maternal clomipramine treatment. Pediatrics 69(2):233-234, 1982. [C]

Singh S, Gulati S, Narang A, Bhakoo ON: Non-narcotic withdrawal syndrome in a neonate due to maternal clomipramine therapy [Letter]. J Paediatr Child Health 26(2):110, 1990. [C]

CLONAZEPAM

Synonyms

Cloazepam, Clonazepamum, Clonopin, Iktorivil, Klonopin, Rivotril

Summary

Clonazepam is a benzodiazepine that is used as an anticonvulsant.

Magnitude of Teratogenic Risk

None To Minimal

Quality and Quantity of Data

Poor To Fair

Comment

The frequency of congenital anomalies may be increased among the children of women with epilepsy, regardless of anticonvulsant medication (Shapiro et al., 1976; Dieterich et al., 1980; Kelly, 1984; Kelly et al., 1984a, b; Koch et al., 1992).

Maternal use of clonazepam during pregnancy was not signficantly more frequent than expected in a population-based Hungarian case-control study of 10,698 infants with congenital anomalies (Czeizel et al., 1992). Only two of the case infants were born to women who took clonazepam during gestation. Congenital anomalies have been reported among the children of epileptic women who took clonazepam during pregnancy, but the features have not been described sufficiently to determine if these represent a pattern of anomalies similar to that seen with other anticonvulsants (Dieterich et al., 1980; Robert & Guibaud, 1982; Pardi et al., 1982; Lander & Eadie, 1990; Czeizel et al., 1992).

The frequency of malformations was not significantly increased among the offspring of rats, mice, or rabbits treated respectively with 150-625, 2-50, or 6-250 times the usual therapeutic dose of clonazepam during pregnancy (Blum et al., 1973; Saito et al., 1974; Sullivan & McElhatton, 1977; Takeuchi et al., 1977; Jurand, 1980). Altered T-lymphocyte responsiveness has been observed among the offspring of rats treated with 8 times the human dose of clonazepam during pregnancy (Schlumph et al., 1990).

Please see agent summary on diazepam for information on a related drug that has been more thoroughly studied.

Key References

Blum VJE, Haefely W, Jalfre M, Polc P, et al.: [Pharmacology and toxicology of the antiepileptic drug clonazepam.] Arzneimittelforsch 23:377-389, 1973. [A]

Czeizel AE, Bod M, Halasz P: Evaluation of anticonvulsant drugs during pregnancy in a population-based Hungarian study. Eur J Epidemiol 8(1):122-127, 1992. [E]

Dieterich E, Steveling A, Lukas A, Seyfeddinipur N, et al.: Congenital anomalies in children of epileptic mothers and fathers. Neuopediatrics 11:274-283, 1980. [S]

Jurand A: Malformations of the central nervous system induced by neurotropic drugs in mouse embryos. Dev Growth Differ 22:61-78, 1980. [A]

Kelly TE: Teratogenicity of anticonvulsant drugs. I: Review of the literature. Am J Med Genet 19:413-434, 1984. [R]

Kelly TE, Edwards P, Rein M, Miller JQ, et al.: Teratogenicity of anticonvulsant drugs. II: A prospective study. Am J Med Genet 19:435-443, 1984a. [S]

Kelly TE, Rein M, Edwards P: Teratogenicity of anticonvulsant drugs. IV: The association of clefting and epilepsy. Am J Med Genet 19:451-458, 1984b. [S]

Koch S, Losche G, Jager-Roman E, Jakob S, et al.: Major and minor birth malformations and antiepileptic drugs. Neurology 42(suppl 5):83-88, 1992. [E]

Lander CM, Eadie MJ: Antiepileptic drug intake during pregnancy and malformed offspring. Epilepsy Res 7:77-82, 1990. [E]

Pardi G, Como ML, De Giambattista M, Oldrini A et al.: [Epilessia e gravidanza: Aspetti ostetrici di uno studio prospettico multidisciplinare.] Ann Ost Gin Med Perin 103:254- 263, 1982. [S]

Robert E, Guibaud P: Maternal valproic acid and congenital neural tube defects. Lancet 2:937, 1982. [E]

Saito H, Kobayashi H, Takeno S, Sakai T: Fetal toxicity of benzodiazepines in rats. Res Commun Chem Pathol Pharmacol 46:437-447, 1984. [A]

Schlumpf M, Parmar R, Ramseier HR, Lichtenstieger W: Prenatal benzodiazepine immunosuppression: Possible involvement of peripheral benzodiazepine site. Dev Pharmacol Ther 15:178-185, 1990. [A]

Shapiro S, Slone D, Hartz SC, Rosenberg L, et al.: Anticonvulsants and parental epilepsy in the development of birth defects. Lancet 1:272-275, 1976. [E]

Sullivan FM, McElhatton PR: A comparison of the teratogenic activity of the antiepileptic drugs carbamazepine, clonazepam, ethosuximide, phenobarbital, phenytoin, and primidone in mice. Toxicol Appl Pharmacol 40:365-378, 1977. [A]

Takeuchi Y, Shiozaki U, Noda A, Shimizu M, et al.: [Studies on the toxicity of clonazepam. Part 3. Teratogenicity tests in rabbits.] Yakuri to Chiryo 5:2457-2466, 1977. [A]

CLONIDINE

Synonyms

Catapres, Catapresan, Chlophazolin, Dixarit, Drylon, Hemiton, Hyposyn, Ipotensium, Katapresan, Tensinova

Summary

Clonidine is an alpha-2 adrenergic agonist used to treat hypertension.

Magnitude of Teratogenic Risk

Undetermined

Quality and Quantity of Data

Poor

Comment

A small risk cannot be excluded, but there is no indication that the risk of congenital anomalies in children of women treated with clonidine during pregnancy is likely to be great.

No adverse effect of maternal clonidine therapy was apparent among the infants of 47 hypertensive women treated during the last half of pregnancy in a double-blind controlled trial (Horvath et al., 1985). No difference in head size, neurological examination or school performance compared to matched controls was found among 22 three- to nine-year-old children of women who had been treated with clonidine in pregnancy, usually after the end of the first trimester (Huisjes et al., 1986). Sleep disturbances were reported more often among the exposed children, but no other behavioral abnormalities were noted. The clinical importance of this observation is uncertain.

The frequency of malformations was not increased among the offspring of rats, mice, or rabbits treated during pregnancy with clonidine in doses 1-40 or more times that used in humans (von Delbruck, 1966; Angelova et al., 1975). Inconsistent reductions of weight have been observed among the offspring of rats treated during pregnancy with clonidine in doses 2.5-16 times those used in humans (Pizzi et al., 1988; Ryan & Pappas, 1990).

Transient neonatal hypertension has been reported among the infants of women treated with clonidine late in pregnancy (Boutroy et al., 1988), but this complication appears to be uncommon (Horvath et al., 1985).

Key References

Angelova O, Gendzhev Z, Ilieva J, Ivanov K: Investigations on the reproductive function of rats treated with high doses of clonidine. Zentralbl Pharmakother Laboratoriumsdiagn 114:251-255, 1975. [A]

Boutroy MJ, Gisonna CR, Legagneur M: Clonidine: Placental transfer and neonatal adaption. Early Hum Dev 17:275-286, 1988. [E]

Horvath JS, Phippard A, Korda A, et al.: Clonidine hydrochloride--A safe and effective antihypertensive agent in pregnancy. Obstet Gynecol 66(5):634-638, 1985. [E]

Huisjes HJ, Hadders-Algra M, Touwen BCL: Is clonidine a behavioral teratogen in the human? Early Hum Dev 17:399-407, 1986. [O]

Pizzi WJ, Ali SF, Holson RR: Behavioral evaluation of rats prenatally exposed to the adrenergic agonists clonidine and lofexidine. Neurotoxicology 9(3):559-566, 1988. [A]

Ryan CL, Pappas BA: Prenatal exposure to antiadrenergic antihypertensive drugs: Effects on neurobehavioral development and the behavioral consequences of enriched rearing. Neurotoxicol Teratol 12:359-366, 1990. [A]

von Delbruck VO: The results of toxicologic and teratologic animal trials with 2-(2,6-dichlorophenylamino)-2-imidazoline-hydrochloride. Arzneimittelforsch 16:1053-1055, 1966. [A]

CLORAZEPATE

Synonyms

Azene, Chlorazepate Dipotassium, Dipotassium Chlorazepate, Nansius, Transene, Tranxene, Tranxilium

Summary

Clorazepate is a benzodiazepine used to treat anxiety.

Magnitude of Teratogenic Risk

Undetermined

Quality and Quantity of Data

None To Poor

Comment

None

No epidemiological studies of congenital anomalies in infants born to women who took clorazepate during pregnancy have been published. There is one report of an infant with multiple congenital anomalies whose mother took clorazepate early in pregnancy, but a cause and effect relationship seems unlikely (Patel & Patel, 1980).

The frequency of malformations was not increased among the offspring of mice, rats or rabbits treated with 25-100 times the usual human dose of clorazepate during pregnancy in one briefly reported study (Brunaud et al., 1970). No increase in malformation rate was observed among the offspring of pregnant rats treated with 60 times the usual human dose of clorazepate in another investigation, but behavioral alterations were noted among the pups (Corwin & DeMeyer, 1980; Jackson et al., 1980). The relevance of this finding to therapeutic use of clorazepate in human pregnancy is unknown.

Transient neonatal neurological depression has been observed among children born to women who took clorazepate late in pregnancy (Bavoux et al., 1981).

Key References

Bavoux F, Lanfranchi C, Olive G, et al.: Adverse effects on newborns from intra uterine exposure to benzodiazepines and other psychotropic agents. Therapie 36:305-312, 1981. [S]

Brunaud M, Navarro J, Salle J, Siou G: Pharmacological, toxicological, and teratological studies on dipotassium-7-chloro-3-carboxy-1,3-dihydro-2,2-dihydroxy-5-phenyl-2H-1,4-benzodiazepine-tranquilizer. Arzneimittelforsch 20:123-125, 1970. [A]

Corwin H, DeMyer W: Failure of clorazepate to cause malformations or fetal wastage in the rat. Arch Neurol 37:347-349, 1980. [A]

Jackson VP, DeMyer W, Hingtgen J: Delayed maze-learning in rats after prenatal exposure to clorazepate. Arch Neurol 37:350-351, 1980. [A]

Patel DA, Patel AR: Clorazepate and congenital malformations. JAMA 244:135-136, 1980. [C]

CLOTRIMAZOLE

Synonyms

Canastene, Canesten, Chlortritylimidazol, Empecid, Eparol, Gyne-Lotremin, Lotrimin, Mycelex, Panmicol, Trimysten

Summary

Clotrimazole is an antifungal agent that is used in topical preparations that are absorbed poorly, if at all, through skin or mucous membranes (Tettenborn, 1974). Clotrimazole is also used orally for treatment of candidiasis; systemic absorption does occur with this route of administration.

Magnitude of Teratogenic Risk

None To Minimal

Quality and Quantity of Data

Poor To Fair

Comment

None

The frequency of maternal use of vaginal clotrimazole early in pregnancy was no greater than expected among 6564 infants diagnosed as having a "birth defect" in a record linkage study of Michigan Medicaid data (Rosa et al., 1987). Similar negative results were obtained in subgroups with oral clefts, cardiovascular defects, and spina bifida. A weak but statistically significant association was observed between maternal vaginal treatment with clotrimazole and spontaneous abortion in this study, but the association was only seen in compari-

son with one of two control groups and may have resulted from confounding factors (Rosa et al., 1987).

No teratogenic effects were reportedly observed among the offspring of mice, rats, or rabbits treated with clotrimazole in oral doses up to 200 times that used in humans (Tettenborn, 1974), but this study has not been published in sufficient detail to permit independent assessment of the data.

Key References

Rosa FW, Baum C, Shaw M: Pregnancy outcomes after first-trimester vaginitis drug therapy. Obstet Gynecol 69:751-755, 1987. [E]

Tettenborn D: Toxicity of clotrimazole. Postgrad Med J (July Suppl):17-20, 1974. [R]

CLOXACILLIN

Synonyms

Apo-Cloxi, Bactopen, Cloxapen, Novocloxin, Orbenin, Sodium Cloxacillin, Tegopen

Summary

Cloxacillin is a penicillin derivative used to treat infections by penicillinase-resistant bacteria.

Magnitude of Teratogenic Risk

Undetermined

Quality and Quantity of Data

None To Poor

Comment

A small risk cannot be excluded, but a substantial risk of congenital anomalies in the children of women treated with cloxacillin during pregnancy is unlikely.

No epidemiological studies of congenital anomalies among infants born to women treated with cloxacillin during pregnancy have been reported.

No teratogenic effect is said to have occurred in rabbits treated with cloxacillin in doses similar to those used in humans in a study reported only as an abstract (Brown et al., 1968).

Please see agent summary on penicillin for information on a related drug that has been more thoroughly studied.

Key References

Brown DM, Harper KH, Palmer AK, Tesh SA: Effect of antibiotics upon pregnancy in the rabbit. Toxicol Appl Pharmacol 12:295, 1968. [A]

COAL TAR

Synonyms

Alcatrao Mineral, Carbocort, Pentrax, Psoriderm, Psorox, Sebutone, Steinkohlenteer, Tar (Coal), Waxtar, Zetar

Summary

Coal tar, a product of the destructive distillation of coal, is comprised of a mixture of organic compounds. It is used topically to treat a variety of dermatoses.

Magnitude of Teratogenic Risk

Undetermined

Quality and Quantity of Data

None

Comment

1) A small risk cannot be excluded, but a high risk of congenital anomalies in the children of women treated with coal tar during pregnancy is unlikely.

2) The risk assessment pertains to the dermal use of coal tar and not to industrial exposures which may

be greater and therefore have a different risk associated with them.

No epidemiological studies of congenital anomalies among infants born to women treated with coal tar during pregnancy have been reported.

No mammalian teratology studies of coal tar have been published.

Key References

None available.

COAL TAR NAPHTHA

Synonyms

Benzine, Heavy Naphtha, Hi-Flash Naphtha, Naphtha Coal Tar, Naphtha Solvents, Petroleum Solvents, Refined Naphtha

Summary

Coal tar naphthas are various mixtures of toluene, xylene, benzene, and other aromatic hydrocarbons. They are used as solvents. Coal tar naphthas are volatile and may be absorbed by inhalation. They act as a central nervous system depressant.

Magnitude of Teratogenic Risk

Undetermined

Quality and Quantity of Data

None To Poor

Comment

Adverse effects are expected to be dose-related.

No epidemiological studies of congenital anomalies among infants born to women exposed to coal tar naphtha during pregnancy have been reported.

No teratogenic effect was observed among the offspring of pregnant rats exposed by inhalation for six hours daily to 0.2, 1.0, or 5.0 g/cu m of EDS hydrotreated naphtha, a coal-derived liquid (McKee et al., 1986).

Please see agent summaries on components listed above for more information on these specific agents and guidelines for permissible exposure levels.

Key References

McKee RH, Hinz JP, Traul KA: Evaluation of the teratogenic potential and reproductive toxicity of coal-derived naphtha. Toxicol Appl Pharmacol 84:149-158, 1986. [A]

COCAINE

Synonyms

Base, Baseball, BCA Eye Drops, Benzoylmethylecgonine, Blow, "C" Carrie, Coke, Crack, Freebase, Lady, Methyl Benzoylecgonine

Summary

Cocaine is a topical anesthetic, local vasoconstrictor, and central nervous system (CNS) stimulant that is widely abused recreationally (Gay, 1981; Farrar & Kearns, 1989; Johanson & Fischman, 1989).

Magnitude of Teratogenic Risk

Placental Abruption And Other Serious Pregnancy Complications: Moderate

Congenital Anomalies: Small To Moderate

Quality and Quantity of Data

Placental Abruption And Other Serious Pregnancy Complications: Fair To Good

Congenital Anomalies: Fair To Good

Comment

Vascular disruption in the fetus appears to be associated with maternal cocaine use and may be a particular hazard in the second or third trimester of pregnancy.

The extensive medical literature on the effects of maternal cocaine use in pregnancy must be interpreted with great caution. Confounding factors are present in human studies that often make it difficult to attribute abnormalities observed directly to a teratogenic effect of cocaine (Bandstra & Burkett, 1991; Chasnoff, 1991, 1992; Lutiger et al., 1991; Richardson & Day, 1991; Singer et al., 1991; Plessinger & Woods, 1991; Mayes et al., 1992; Volpe, 1992; Slutsker, 1992; Kain et al., 1992; Gingras et al., 1992). Documentation of the frequency, timing, and dosage of the mothers' use of cocaine, other illicit drugs, and alcohol is usually poor. Moreover, there appears to be a systematic publication bias in favor of studies that show an association between maternal cocaine use and untoward pregnancy outcomes and against studies that do not (Koren et al., 1989).

Thirteen of 32 full-term infants born to women with documented cocaine use during pregnancy were found to have disruptive brain anomalies on cranial ultrasound examination in one study (Dixon & Bejar, 1989). Increased frequencies of CNS infarction and congenital anomalies were observed by ultrasound, CT, or MR imaging in another study of 43 premature infants who had been born to women who abused cocaine during pregnancy (Heier et al., 1991). Similar brain lesions have been noted among infants of women who used cocaine during pregnancy in other series (Chasnoff et al., 1986; Sims & Walther, 1989; Kramer et al., 1990; Dominguez et al., 1991; Kapur et al., 1991; Volpe, 1992). Such defects may represent residua of cocaine-induced CNS hemorrhage or ischemia at various gestational ages (Volpe, 1992). Cerebral infarction is a recognized complication of cocaine use in children and adults (Jacobs et al., 1989; Brown et al., 1992).

Other congenital anomalies thought to be due to vascular disruption have been reported among children of mothers who abused cocaine during pregnancy. These abnormalities include segmental intestinal atresia in at least six infants, gastroschisis in at least three, sirenomelia in at least two, limb-body wall complex in at least two, and limb reduction defects in more than a dozen (MacGregor et al., 1987; Chasnoff et al, 1988; Hoyme et al., 1990; Drongowski et al., 1991; Hannig & Phillips, 1991; van den Anker et al., 1991; Sarpong & Headings, 1992; Sheinbaum & Badell, 1992; Spinazzola et al., 1992; Viscarello et al., 1992). The occurrence of neonatal necrotizing enterocolitis also seems to be associated with maternal cocaine use during pregnancy (Czyrko et al., 1991; Porat & Brodsky, 1991; Sehgal et al., 1993). Such anomalies may be caused by the vasoconstrictive and hypertensive actions of cocaine. However, no significant change in the prevalence of cases with multiple vascular disruption defects was seen in the Metropolitan Atlanta Congenital Defects Program between 1968 and 1989, a period during which cocaine abuse increased substantially (Martin et al., 1992). This suggests that cocaine abuse did not produce a major increase in the overall frequency of such birth defects in this population.

Data suggesting an association between maternal cocaine use during pregnancy and the occurrence of congenital anomalies of the genitourinary system in infants have been reported. Several infants with the rare prune belly anomaly have been born to women who used cocaine during pregnancy (Chasnoff et al., 1985, 1989a; Bingol et al., 1986). A small but statistically significant increase in the frequency of congenital anomalies of the urinary, but not of the genital, tract was found in one case-control study (Chavez et al., 1989). Nine of 52 infants born to women who chronically abused cocaine had genitourinary tract anomalies in another study (Chasnoff et al., 1988, 1989a). In contrast, congenital urogenital anomalies were no more frequent than expected in a cohort of 1324 children of women who abused cocaine during pregnancy (Rajegowda et al., 1991). Several other investigations also have found no increase in the frequency of urinary tract anomalies among the children of women who used cocaine during pregnancy (Bingol et al., 1987; Little et al., 1989; Neerhof et al., 1989; Rosenstein et al., 1990), but the sample sizes involved (50 to 100 exposed infants) are too small to rule out even a substantial increase in the rate.

An increased frequency of cardiovascular malformations was observed among 214 infants with neonatal toxicology screens showing the presence of cocaine in one study (Lipshultz et al., 1991), but meta-analysis of six other epidemiological studies revealed no significant association between maternal cocaine use in pregnancy and fetal cardiovascular malformations (Lutiger et al., 1991).

Significantly increased frequencies of congenital anomalies in general have been reported in studies of 138, 53, and 50 infants of women who abused cocaine during pregnancy (Bingol et al., 1987; Little et al., 1989; Neerhof et al., 1989), but not in other studies of similar or larger size (Hadeed & Siegel, 1989; Gillogley et al., 1990; Handler et al., 1991; Slutsker, 1992).

Growth retardation involving weight, length, and head circumference has consistently been noted among infants born to women who abused cocaine during pregnancy (Doering et al., 1989; Zuckerman et al., 1989; Rosenak et al., 1990; Gillogley et al., 1990; Little & Snell, 1991; Dombrowski et al., 1991; Eisen et al., 1991; Handler et al., 1991; Young et al., 1992; Harris et al., 1992; Koren & Graham, 1992; Slutsker, 1992; Bateman et al., 1993). Data on subsequent growth and development of these children are limited, but few differences were observed by two years of age between 106 infants whose mothers used cocaine and a group of infants whose mothers did not use cocaine but had similar use of alcohol, cigarettes, and marijuana during pregnancy (Chasnoff et al., 1992). Development at about 20 months of age was similar to controls in a group of 30 children born to women who used cocaine "socially" during the first trimester of pregnancy in another study (Graham et al., 1992).

Abnormalities of neonatal cardiorespiratory and neurological function have been observed among infants born to women who used cocaine during pregnancy (Chasnoff et al.,

144

1985, 1989a, b; Cherukuri et al., 1988; Doberczak et al., 1988; Anday et al., 1989; Kramer et al., 1990; van de Bor et al., 1990; Eisen et al., 1991; Neuspiel & Hamel, 1991; Scanlon, 1991; Plessinger & Woods, 1991; Silvestri et al., 1991; Singer et al., 1991; Young et al., 1992; Coles et al., 1992; Corwin et al., 1992; McCann & Lewis, 1992; Schneider & Chasnoff, 1992; Singer et al., 1992; Mayes et al., 1993; Dusick et al., 1993). Persistent arterial hypertension may be relatively frequent among children born to women who abuse cocaine during pregnancy (Horn, 1992).

An increased frequency of SIDS was observed in a cohort study of almost 1000 infants whose mothers had used cocaine during pregnancy (Durand et al., 1990). Very high frequencies of SIDS (10/66 and 4/71) have also been reported in two series of infants born to women who chronically abused cocaine during pregnancy (Chasnoff et al., 1988; Cordero & Custard, 1990) but not in most other investigations (Bauchner et al., 1988; Silvestri et al., 1991).

Abruptio placentae, often with fetal death, has been associated with cocaine use during pregnancy (Acker et al., 1983; Chasnoff et al., 1985; Bingol et al., 1987; Keith et al., 1989; Cohen et al., 1991; Dombrowski et al., 1991; Handler et al., 1991; Slutsker, 1992; Dusick et al., 1993). The occurrence of abruption in these cases is probably due to the vasoconstrictive and hypertensive effects of the drug.

A dose-dependent increase in the frequency of limb and tail reduction defects was observed among the offspring of pregnant rats treated with 2.5-4 times the usual human dose of cocaine (Webster & Brown-Woodman, 1990). Susceptibility was greatest at the completion of the organogenic period; two sequential doses produced a greater effect than a single dose. Some of the fetuses with limb defects were also found to have CNS anomalies of a type associated with vascular disruption (Webster et al., 1991). In another study, urinary tract anomalies were observed with increased frequency among the offspring of rats injected with cocaine in doses similar to those used recreationally in humans (El-Bizri et al., 1991). Increased frequencies of congenital anomalies, including brain, eye, urinary tract, and cardiovascular defects, have been observed among the offspring of mice given <1-3 times the usual human recreational dose of cocaine during pregnancy (Mahalik et al., 1980, 1982; Finnell et al., 1990; Gressens et al., 1992). This was not seen in other studies using similar doses in mice, rats, or rabbits (Fantel and MacPhail, 1982; Church et al., 1988; Henderson & McMillen, 1990; Weese-Mayer et al., 1991). Various behavioral abnormalities have been noted among the offspring of rats treated with cocaine during pregnancy (Hutchings et al., 1989; Smith et al., 1989; Spear et al., 1989; Henderson & McMillen, 1990; Sobrian et al., 1990; Church et al., 1991; Bilitzke & Church, 1992; Goodwin et al., 1992; Heyser et al., 1992a, b; Johns et al., 1992a, b; Maone et al., 1992).

Key References

Acker D, Sachs BP, Tracey KJ, Wise WE: Abruptio placentae associated with cocaine use. Am J Obstet Gynecol 146:220-221, 1983. [C]

Anday EK, Cohen ME, Kelley NE, Leitner DS: Effect of in utero cocaine exposure on startle and its modification. Dev Pharmacol Ther 12:137-145, 1989. [E]

Bandstra ES, Burkett G: Maternal-fetal and neonatal effects of in utero cocaine exposure. Semin Perinatol 15(4):288-301, 1991. [R]

Bateman DA, Ng SKC, Hansen CA, Heagarty MC: The effects of intrauterine cocaine exposure in newborns. Am J Public Health 83(2):190-193, 1993. [E]

Bauchner H, Zuckerman B, McClain M, Frank D, et al.: Risk of sudden infant death syndrome among infants with in utero exposure to cocaine. J Pediatr 113:831-834, 1988. [E]

Bilitzke PJ, Church MW: Prenatal cocaine and alcohol exposures affect rat behavior in a stress test (The Porsolt Swim Test). Neurotoxicol Teratol 14(5):359-364, 1992. [A]

Bingol N, Fuchs M, Diaz V, Stone RK, Gromisch DS: Teratogenicity of cocaine in humans. J Pediatr 110:93-96, 1987. [E]

Bingol N, Fuchs M, Holipas N, Henriquez R, et al.: Prune belly syndrome associated with maternal cocaine abuse. Am J Hum Gen 39:A51(147), 1986. [C]

Brown E, Prager J, Lee H-Y, Ramsey RG: CNS complications of cocaine abuse: Prevalence, pathophysiology, and neuroradiology. Am J Roentgenol 159:137-147, 1992. [R]

Chasnoff IJ: Cocaine and pregnancy: Clinical and methodologic issues. Clin Perinatol 18(1):113-123, 1991. [R]

Chasnoff IJ: Cocaine, pregnancy and the growing child. Curr Probl Pediatr 22(7):302-321, 1992. [R]

Chasnoff IJ, Burns WJ, Schnoll SH, Burns KA: Cocaine use in pregnancy. N Engl J Med 313:666-669, 1985. [E]

Chasnoff IJ, Bussey ME, Savich R, Stack CM: Perinatal cerebral infarction and maternal cocaine use. J Pediatr 108:456-459, 1986. [C]

Chasnoff IJ, Chisum GM, Kaplan WE: Maternal cocaine use and genitourinary tract malformations. Teratology 37:201-204, 1988. [S]

Chasnoff IJ, Griffith DR, MacGregor S, Dirkes K, et al.: Temporal patterns of cocaine use in pregnancy. JAMA 261:1741-1744, 1989a. [E]

Chasnoff IJ, Hunt CE, Kletter R, Kaplan D: Prenatal cocaine exposure is associated with respiratory pattern abnormalities. Am J Dis Child 143:583-587, 1989b. [E]

Chavez GF, Mulinare J, Cordero J: Maternal cocaine use during early pregnancy as a risk factor for congenital urogenital anomalies. JAMA 262:795-798, 1989. [E]

Cherukuri R, Minkoff H, Feldman J, Parekh A, et al.: A cohort study of alkaloidal cocaine ("crack") in pregnancy. Obstet Gynecol 72:147-151, 1988. [E]

Church MW, Dintcheff BA, Gessner PK: Dose-dependent consequences of cocaine on pregnancy outcome in the Long-Evans rat. Neurotoxicol Teratol 10:51-58, 1988. [A]

Church MW, Holmes PA, Overbeck GW, et al.: Interactive effects of prenatal alcohol and cocaine exposures on postnatal mortality, development and behavior in the Long-Evans rat. Neurotoxicol Teratol 13:377-386, 1991. [A]

Cohen HR, Green JR, Crombleholme WR: Peripartum cocaine use: Estimating risk of adverse pregnancy outcome. Int J Gynecol Obstet 35:51-54, 1991. [E]

Coles CD, Platzman KA, Smith I, et al.: Effects of cocaine and alcohol use in pregnancy on neonatal growth and neurobehavioral status. Neurotoxicol Teratol 14(1):23-33, 1992. [E]

Cordero L, Custard M: Effects of maternal cocaine abuse on perinatal and infant outcome. Ohio Med 86(5):410-412, 1990. [S]

Corwin MJ, Lester BM, Sepkoski C, et al.: Effects of in utero cocaine exposure on newborn acoustical cry characteristics. Pediatrics 89:1199-1203, 1992. [E]

Czyrko C, Del Pin CA, O'Neill JA, et al.: Maternal cocaine abuse and necrotizing enterocolitis: Outcome and survival. J Pediatr Surg 26(4):414-421, 1991. [E]

Dixon SD, Bejar R: Echoencephalographic findings in neonates associated with maternal cocaine and methamphetamine use: Incidence and clinical correlates. J Pediatr 115:770-778, 1989. [E]

Doberczak TM, Shanzer S, Senie RT, Kandall SR: Neonatal neurologic and electroencephalographic effects of intrauterine cocaine exposure. J Pediatr 113(2):354-358, 1988. [S]

Doering PL, Davidson CL, LaFauce L, et al.: Effects of cocaine on the human fetus: A review of clinical studies. DICP Ann Pharmacother 23:639-645, 1989. [R]

Dombrowski MP, Wolfe HM, Welch RA, et al.: Cocaine abuse is associated with abruptio placentae and decreased birth weight, but not shorter labor. Obstet Gynecol 77(1):139-141, 1991. [E]

Dominguez R, Vila-Coro AA, Slopis JM, et al.: Brain and ocular abnormalities in infants with in utero exposure to cocaine and other street drugs. Am J Dis Child 145:688-695, 1991. [S]

Drongowski RA, Smith RK Jr, Coran AG, Klein MD: Contribution of demographic and environmental factors to the etiology of gastroschisis: A hypothesis. Fetal Diagn Ther 6:14-27, 1991. [R] & [E]

Durand DJ, Espinoza AM, Nickerson BG: Association between prenatal cocaine exposure and sudden infant death syndrome. J Pediatr 117(6):909-911, 1990. [E]

Dusick AM, Covert RF, Schreiber MD, Yee GT, et al.: Risk of intracranial hemorrhage and other adverse outcomes after cocaine exposure in a cohort of 323 very low birth weight infants. J Pediatr 122:438-445, 1993. [E]

Eisen LN, Field TM, Bandstra ES, et al.: Perinatal cocaine effects on neonatal stress behavior and performance on the Brazelton Scale. Pediatrics 88(3):477-480, 1991. [E]

El-Bizri H, Guest I, Varma DR: Effects of cocaine on rat embryo development in vivo and in cultures. Pediatr Res 29(2):187-190, 1991. [A]

Fantel AG, MacPhail BJ: The teratogenicity of cocaine. Teratology 26:17-19, 1982. [A]

Farrar HC, Kearns GL: Cocaine: Clinical pharmacology and toxicology. J Pediatr 115:665-675, 1989. [R]

Finnell RH, Toloyan S, van Waes M, et al.: Preliminary evidence for a cocaine-induced embryopathy in mice. Toxicol Appl Pharmacol 103:228-237, 1990. [A]

Gay GR: You've come a long way, baby! Coke time for the new American lady of the eighties. J Psychoactive Drugs 13:297-318, 1981. [R]

Gillogley KM, Evans AT, Hansen RL, et al.: The perinatal impact of cocaine, amphetamine, and opiate use detected by universal intrapartum screening. Am J Obstet Gynecol 163(5):1535-1542, 1990. [E]

Gingras JL, Weese-Meyer DE, Hume RF Jr, O'Donnell KJ: Cocaine and development: Mechanisms of fetal toxicity and neonatal consequences of prenatal cocaine exposure. Early Hum Dev 31:1-24, 1992. [R]

Goodwin GA, Heyser CJ, Moody CA, Rajachandran L: A fostering study of the effects of prenatal cocaine exposure: II. Offspring behavioral measures. Neurotoxicol Teratol 14(6):423-432, 1992. [A]

Graham K, Feigenbaum A, Pastuszak A, Nulman I, et al.: Pregnancy outcome and infant development following gestational cocaine use by social cocaine users in Toronto, Canada. Clin Invest Med 15(4):384-394, 1992. [E]

Gressens P, Kosofsky BE, Evrard P: Cocaine-induced disturbances of corticogenesis in the developing murine brain. Neurosci Lett 140:113-116, 1992. [A]

Hadeed AJ, Siegel S: Maternal cocaine use during pregnancy: Effect on the newborn infant. Pediatrics 84:205-210, 1989. [E]

Handler A, Kistin N, Davis F, et al.: Cocaine use during pregnancy: Perinatal outcomes. Am J Epidemiol 133(8):818-825, 1991. [E]

Hannig VL, Phillips JA: Maternal cocaine abuse and fetal anomalies: Evidence for teratogenic effects of cocaine. South Med J 84(4):498-499, 1991. [C]

Harris EF, Friend GW, Tolley EA: Enhanced prevalence of ankyloglossia with maternal cocaine use. Cleft Palate Craniofac J 29(1):72-76, 1992. [E]

Heier LA, Carpanzano CR, Mast J, et al.: Maternal cocaine abuse: The spectrum of radiologic abnormalities in the neonatal CNS. AJNR 12(5):951-956, 1991. [E]

Henderson MG, McMillen BA: Effects of prenatal exposure to cocaine or related drugs on rat developmental and neurological indices. Brain Res Bull 24:207-212, 1990. [A]

Heyser CJ, Miller JS, Spear NE, Spear LP: Prenatal exposure to cocaine disrupts cocaine-induced conditioned place preference in rats. Neurotoxicol Teratol 14(1):57-64, 1992a. [A]

Heyser CJ, Spear NE, Spear LP: Effects of prenatal exposure to cocaine on conditional discrimination learning in adult rats. Behav Neurosci 106(5):837-845, 1992b. [A]

Horn PT: Persistent hypertension after prenatal cocaine exposure. J Pediatr 121:288-291, 1992. [S]

Hoyme HE, Jones KL, Dixon SD, Jewett T, et al.: Prenatal cocaine exposure and fetal vascular disruption. Pediatrics 85:743-747, 1990. [S]

Hutchings DE, Fico TA, Dow-Edwards DL: Prenatal cocaine: Maternal toxicity, fetal effects and locomotor activity in rat offspring. Neurotoxicol Teratol 11:65-69, 1989. [A]

Jacobs IG, Roszler MH, Kelley JK, Klein MA, et al.: Cocaine abuse: Neurovascular complications. Radiology 170:223-227, 1989. [S]

Johanson C-E, Fischman MW: The pharmacology of cocaine related to its abuse. Pharmacol Rev 41:3-52, 1989. [R]

Johns JM, Means LW, Means MJ, McMillen BA: Prenatal exposure to cocaine I: Effects on gestation, development, and activity in Sprague-Dawley rats. Neurotoxicol Teratol 14(5):337-342, 1992a. [A]

Johns JM, Means MJ, Anderson DR, Mean LW: Prenatal exposure to cocaine II: Effects on open-field activity and cognitive behavior in Sprague-Dawley rats. Neurotoxicol Teratol 14(5):343-349, 1992b. [A]

Kain ZN, Kain TS, Scarpelli EM: Cocaine exposure in utero: Perinatal development and neonatal manifestations--review. J Toxicol Clin Toxicol 30:607-636, 1992. [R]

Kapur RP, Shaw CM, Shepard TH: Brain hemorrhages in cocaine-exposed human fetuses. Teratology 44:11-18, 1991. [C]

Keith LG, MacGregor S, Friedell S, et al.: Substance abuse in pregnant women: Recent experience at the Perinatal Center for Chemical Dependence of Northwestern Memorial Hospital. Obstet Gynecol 73(5):715-720, 1989. [E]

Koren G, Graham K: Cocaine in pregnancy: Analysis of fetal risk. Vet Hum Toxicol 34(3):263-264, 1992. [E]

Koren G, Graham K, Shear H, Einarson T: Bias against the null hypothesis: The reproductive hazards of cocaine. Lancet 2:1440-1442, 1989. [O]

Kramer LD, Locke GE, Ogunyemi A, Nelson L: Neonatal cocaine-related seizures. J Child Neurol 5:60-64, 1990. [S]

Lipshultz SE, Frassica JJ, Orav EJ: Cardiovascular abnormalities in infants prenatally exposed to cocaine. J Pediatr 118(1):44-51, 1991. [E]

Little BB, Snell LM: Brain growth among fetuses exposed to cocaine in utero: Asymmetrical growth retardation. Obstet Gynecol 77(3):361-364, 1991. [E]

Little BB, Snell LM, Klein VR, Gilstrap LC: Cocaine abuse during pregnancy: Maternal and fetal implications. Obstet Gynecol 73:157-160, 1989. [E]

Lutiger B, Graham K, Einarson TR, Koren G: Relationship between gestational cocaine use and pregnancy outcome: A Meta-Analysis. Teratology 44:405-414, 1991. [R]

MacGregor SN, Keith LG, Chasnoff IJ, Rosner MA, et al.: Cocaine use during pregnancy: Adverse perinatal outcome. Am J Obstet Gynecol 157:686-690, 1987. [S]

Mahalik MP, Gautieri RF, Mann DE: Teratogenic potential of cocaine hydrochloride in CF-1 mice. J Pharm Sci 69:703-706, 1980. [A]

Mahalik MP, Hitner HW: Antagonism of cocaine-induced fetal anomalies by prazosin and diltiazem in mice. Reprod Toxicol 6:161-169, 1992. [A]

Maone TR, Mattes RD, Beauchamp GK: Cocaine-exposed newborns show an exaggerated sucking response to sucrose. Physiol Behav 51(3):487-491, 1992. [E]

Martin ML, Khoury MJ, Cordero JF, Waters GD: Trends in rates of multiple vascular disruption defects, Atlanta, 1968-1989: Is there evidence of a cocaine teratogenic epidemic? Teratology 45:647-653, 1992. [E]

Mayes LC, Granger RH, Bornstein MH, Zuckerman B: The problem of prenatal cocaine exposure. A rush to judgment. JAMA 267(3):406-408, 1992. [O]

Mayes LC, Granger RH, Frank MA, Schottenfeld R, et al.: Neurobehavioral profiles of neonates exposed to cocaine prenatally. Pediatrics 91(4):778-783, 1993. [E]

McCann EM, Lewis K: Control of breathing in babies of narcotic- and cocaine-abusing mothers. Early Hum Dev 27:175-186, 1991. [E]

Neerhof MG, MacGregor SN, Retzky SS, et al.: Cocaine abuse during pregnancy: Peripartum prevalence and perinatal outcome. Am J Obstet Gynecol 161(3):633-638, 1989. [E]

Neuspiel DR, Hamel SC: Cocaine and infant behavior. J Dev Behav Pediatr 12(1):55-64, 1991. [R]

Plessinger MA, Woods JR: The cardiovascular effects of cocaine use in pregnancy. Reprod Toxicol 5:99-113, 1991. [R]

Porat R, Brodsky N: Cocaine: A risk factor for necrotizing enterocolitis. J Perinatol 11 (1):30-32, 1991. [C]

Rajegowda B, Lala R, Nagaraj A, et al.: Does cocaine (CO) increase congenital urogenital abnormalities (CUGA) in newborns? Pediatr Res 29(4):71A, 1991. [E]

Richardson GA, Day NL: Maternal and neonatal effects of moderate cocaine use during pregnancy. Neurotoxicol Teratol 13:455-460, 1991. [E]

Rosenak D, Diamant YZ, Yaffe H, et al.: Cocaine: Maternal use during pregnancy and its effect on the mother, the fetus, and the infant. Obstet Gynecol Surv 45(6):348-359, 1990. [R]

Rosenstein BJ, Wheeler JS, Heid PL: Congenital renal abnormalities in infants with in utero cocaine exposure. J Urol 144:110-112, 1990. [S]

Sarpong S, Headings V: Sirenomelia accompanying exposure of the embryo to cocaine. South Med J 85:545-547, 1992. [C]

Scanlon JW: The neuroteratology of cocaine: Background, theory, and clinical implications. Reprod Toxicol 5:89-98, 1991. [R]

Schneider JW, Chasnoff IJ: Motor assessment of cocaine/polydrug exposed infants at age 4 months. Neurotoxicol Teratol 14(2):97-101, 1992. [E]

Seghal S, Ewing C, Waring P, Findlay R, et al.: Morbidity of low-birthweight infants with intrauterine cocaine exposure. J Natl Med Assoc 85(1):20-24, 1993. [E]

Sheinbaum KA, Badell A: Physiatric management of two neonates with limb deficiencies and prenatal cocaine exposure. Arch Phys Med Rehabil 73:385-388, 1992. [C]

Silvestri JM, Long JM, Weese-Mayer DE, Barkov GA: Effect of prenatal cocaine on respiration, heart rate, and sudden infant death syndrome. Pediatr Pulmonol 11:328-334, 1991. [E]

Sims ME, Walther FJ: Neonatal ultrasound casebook. J Perinatol 9:349-350, 1989. [C]

Singer L, Farkas K, Kliegman: Childhood medical and behavioral consequences of maternal cocaine use. J Pediatr Psychol 17(4):389-406, 1992. [R]

Singer LT, Garber R, Kliegman R: Neurobehavioral sequelae of fetal cocaine exposure. J Pediatr 119(4):667-672, 1991. [R]

Slutsker L: Risks associated with cocaine use during pregnancy. Obstet Gynecol 79:778-789, 1992. [R]

Smith RF, Mattran KM, Kurkjian MF, Kurtz SL: Alterations in offspring behavior induced by chronic prenatal cocaine dosing. Neurotoxicol Teratol 11:35-38, 1989. [A]

Sobrian SK, Burton LE, Robinson NL, et al.: Neurobehavioral and immunological effects of prenatal cocaine exposure in rat. Pharmacol Biochem Behav 35:617-629, 1990. [A]

Spear LP, Kirstein CL, Bell J, Yoottanasumpun V, et al.: Effects of prenatal cocaine exposure on behavior during the early postnatal period. Neurotoxicol Teratol 11:57-63, 1989. [A]

Spinazzola R, Kenigsberg K, Usmani SS, Harper RG: Neonatal gastrointestinal complications of maternal cocaine abuse. N Y State J Med 92(1):22-23, 1992. [C]

van de Bor M, Walther FJ, Ebrahimi M: Decreased cardiac output in infants of mothers who abused cocaine. Pediatrics 85:30-32, 1990. [E]

van den Anker JN, Cohen-Overbeek TE, Wladimiroff JW, Sauer PJJ: Prenatal diagnosis of limb-reduction defects due to maternal cocaine use. Lancet 338:1332, 1991. [C]

Viscarello RR, Ferguson DD, Nores J, Hobbins JC: Limb-body wall complex associated with cocaine abuse: Further evidence of cocaine's teratogenicity. Obstet Gynecol 80:523-526, 1992. [C]

Volpe JJ: Effect of cocaine use on the fetus. N Engl J Med 327(6):399-407, 1992. [R]

Webster WS, Brown-Woodman PDC: Cocaine as a cause of congenital malformations of vascular origin: Experimental evidence in the rat. Teratology 41:689-697, 1990. [A]

Webster WS, Brown-Woodman PDC, Lipson AH, Ritchie HE: Fetal brain damage in the rat following prenatal exposure to cocaine. Neurotoxicol Teratol 13:621-626, 1991. [A]

Weese-Mayer DE, Klemka-Walden LM, Chan MK, Gingras JL: Effects of prenatal cocaine exposure on perinatal morbidity and postnatal growth in the rabbit. Dev Pharmacol Ther 4:221-230, 1991. [A]

Young SL, Vosper HJ, Phillips SA: Cocaine: Its effects on maternal and child health. Pharmacotherapy 12(1):2-17, 1992. [R]

Zuckerman B, Frank DA, Hingson R, Amaro H, et al.: Effects of maternal marijuana and cocaine use on fetal growth. N Engl J Med 320:762-768, 1989. [E]

CODEINE

Synonyms

Actacode, Codate, Codipertussin, Codlin, Methylmorphine Phosphate, Metilmorfina, Schoolboy, Solcodein, Tricodein

Summary

Codeine is a commonly used narcotic analgesic often encountered as a constituent of multiple agent preparations. It is also widely used as an antitussive in a dose one-third to one-half as great.

Magnitude of Teratogenic Risk

None To Minimal

Quality and Quantity of Data

Fair To Good

Comment

None

The frequencies of congenital anomalies in general, of major malformations, and of minor anomalies were no greater than expected among the children of 563 women who took codeine during the first four lunar months of pregnancy in the Collaborative Perinatal Project (Heinonen et al., 1977). A slight but statistically significant excess of respiratory tract malformations was observed. The frequency of congenital anomalies was no greater than expected among the children of 2522 women who took codeine anytime during pregnancy in this study. No increase in congenital anomalies was observed among the children of more than 630 women who took medications containing codeine during the first trimester of pregnancy in two cohorts of the Boston Collaborative Drug Surveillance Program (Jick et al., 1981; Aselton et al., 1985).

In contrast, associations between first-trimester maternal use of codeine and various congenital anomalies have been observed in case-control studies. Bracken & Holford (1981) found an association with maternal codeine use in 1427 children with a variety of malformations. Saxen (1975a) reported an association with maternal use of narcotic analgesics (mostly codeine) among 599 children with cleft lip and/or palate, but no significant association was seen in a later study of 194 children with oral clefts (Saxen, 1975b). Three case-control studies involving respectively 390, 298, and 330 children with congenital heart disease have reported an association with maternal codeine use during the first trimester of pregnancy (Rothman et al., 1979; Zierler & Rothman, 1985; Bracken, 1986), but methodological limitations of these studies raise serious questions regarding the validity of this association. No association was observed with maternal codeine use during early pregnancy in another case-control study involving 141 infants with cardiac malformations (Shaw et al., 1990). No association with cardiovascular malformations was observed among the infants of 563 women who took codeine during the first four lunar months of pregnancy in the Collaborative Perinatal Project (Heinonen et al., 1977).

The frequency of malformations was not significantly increased among the offspring of mice, rats, or hamsters treated during pregnancy with codeine in doses equivalent to 15-125, 2-25, and 4-75 times those usually employed in humans (Geber & Schramm, 1975; Lehman, 1976; Ching & Tang, 1986; Price, 1987; Sleet et al., 1987; Williams et al., 1991). Fetal growth retardation was seen among the offspring of treated animals in each species. No teratogenic effect was observed among the offspring of rabbits treated during pregnancy with the equivalent of 1-6 times the usual human dose of codeine (Lehmann, 1976).

Narcotic withdrawal symptoms have been reported in neonates born to mothers who used codeine chronically late in pregnancy (Van Leeuwen, 1965; Mangurten & Benawra, 1980).

Please see agent summary on heroin for information regarding the chronic use and abuse of narcotics.

Key References

Aselton P, Jick H, Milunsky A, Hunter JR, et al.: First-trimester drug use and congenital disorders. Obstet Gynecol 65:451-455, 1985. [S]

Bracken MB: Drug use in pregnancy and congenital heart disease in offspring. N Engl J Med 314:1120, 1986. [C]

Bracken MG, Holford TR: Exposure to prescribed drugs in pregnancy and association with congenital malformations. Obstet Gynecol 58:336-344, 1981. [E]

Ching M, Tang L: Neuroleptic drug-induced alterations on neonatal growth and development. I. Prenatal exposure influences birth size, mortality rate, and the neuroendocrine system. Biol Neonate 49:261-269, 1986. [A]

Geber WF, Schramm LC: Congenital malformations of the central nervous system produced by narcotic analgesics in the hamster. Am J Obstet Gynecol 123:705-713, 1975. [A]

Heinonen OP, Slone D, Shapiro S: Birth Defects and Drugs in Pregnancy. Littleton, Mass.: John Wright-PSG, 1977, pp 287-288, 434. [E]

Jick H, Holmes LB, Hunter JR, Madsen S, et al.: First-trimester drug use and congenital disorders. JAMA 246:343-346, 1981. [S]

Lehmann VH: Teratologic studies in rabbits and rats with the morphine derivative codeine. Arzneimittelforsch 26:551-554, 1976. [A].

Mangurten HH, Benawra R: Neonatal codeine withdrawal in infants of nonaddicted mothers. Pediatrics 65:159-160, 1980. [C]

Price CJ: Teratologic evaluation of codeine (CAS No. 76-57-3) administered to CD-1 mice on gestational days 6 through 15. NTIS (National Technical Information Service) Report/PB87-209524, 1987. [A]

Rothman KJ, Fyler DC, Goldblatt A, Kreidberg MB: Exogenous hormones and other drug exposures of children with congenital heart disease. Am J Epidemiol 109:433-439, 1979. [E]

Saxen I: Associations between oral clefts and drugs taken during pregnancy. Int J Epidemiol 4:37-44, 1975a. [E]

Saxen I: Epidemiology of cleft lip and palate. Br J Prev Soc Med 29:103-110, 1975b. [E]

Shaw GM, Malcoe LH, Swan SH, et al.: Risks for congenital cardiac anomalies relative to selected maternal exposures during early pregnancy. Teratology 41(5):590, 1990. [E]

Sleet RB, Price CJ, George JD, Marr MC, et al.: Teratologic evaluation of codeine (CAS No. 76-57-3) administered to LVG hamsters on gestational days 5 through 13. NTIS (National Technical Information Service) Report/PB88-131040, 1987. [A]

Van Leeuwen G, Guthrie R, Stange F: Narcotic withdrawal reaction in a newborn infant due to codeine. Pediatrics 36:635-636, 1965. [C]

Williams J, Price CJ, Sleet RB, et al.: Codeine: Developmental toxicity in hamsters and mice. Fundam Appl Toxicol 16:401-413, 1991. [A]

Zierler S, Rothman KJ: Congenital heart disease in relation to maternal use of Bendectin and other drugs in early pregnancy. N Engl J Med 313:347-352, 1985. [E]

COLCHICINE

Synonyms

Colchineos, Colchisol, Colcin, Colgout, Colsaloid, Coluric, Condylon

Summary

Colchicine, an antimitotic agent, is an alkaloid obtained from plants of the genus Colchicum. Colchicine is used to treat gout, dermatitis herpetiformis, familial Mediterranean fever, and amyloidosis (Levy et al., 1991). Acute gout attacks may be treated with doses of colchicine ten times greater than those used chronically for prophylaxis.

Magnitude of Teratogenic Risk

Minimal

Quality and Quantity of Data

Poor To Fair

Comment

None

No epidemiological studies of congenital anomalies among infants born to women treated with colchicine during pregnancy have been reported. The frequency of malformations does not appear to be unusually high among more than 50 children born to women who were treated with colchicine during pregnancy in clinical series; most of these women conceived while on chronic colchicine therapy (Katsilambros, 1963; Nicholson, 1968; Zemer et al., 1976; Cohen et al., 1977; Ehrenfeld et al., 1987; Levy et al., 1991). Cytogenetic abnormalities do not appear to occur with unusual frequency among the children of women who are chronically treated with colchicine (Cohen et al., 1977; Rabinovitch et al., 1985). No causal inference can be made on the basis of anecdotal observations of individual children with vertebral defects or Down's syndrome whose mothers had taken colchicine early in pregnancy (Dudin et al., 1989; Rabinovitch et al., 1985).

Increased frequencies of fetal death and malformations were observed among the offspring of mice and hamsters treated during pregnancy with 50-100 times or 500-1000 times the maximum human dose of colchicine (Ferm, 1963; Ingalls et al., 1968; Sieber et al., 1978; Levy et al., 1991). Central nervous system, eye, facial, and skeletal malformations were seen most often; dependence of the effect on time of exposure and dose were noted. Abnormal brain development was found among the offspring of rats treated with 20 times the maximum human dose of colchicine late in pregnancy (Petit & Isaacson, 1976). Embryonic death can be produced by intrauterine injection of colchicine in cows, sheep, and ponies (Kastelic & Ginther, 1989). Increased frequencies of chromosomal abnormalities have been noted among the embryos of rodents treated with 25-50 times the maximum human dose of colchicine during pregnancy or at conception (Piko & Bonsel-Helmreich, 1960; McGaughey & Chang, 1969; Sieber et al., 1978). The relevance of these observations to the risks associated with use of therapeutic doses of colchicine in human pregnancy is unknown.

Key References

Cohen MM, Levy M, Eliakim M: A cytogenic evaluation of long-term colchicine therapy in the treatment of Familial Mediterranean Fever (FMF). Am J Med Sci 274:147-152, 1977. [S]

Dudin A, Rambaud-Cousson A, Shehatto M, Thalji A: Colchicine in the first trimester of pregnancy and vertebral malformations (Letter). Arch Fr Pediatr 46:627-628, 1989. [C]

Ehrenfeld M, Brzezinski A, Levy M, Eliakim M: Fertility and obstetric history in patients with familial Mediterranean fever on long-term colchicine therapy. Br J Obstet Gynaecol 94:1186-1191, 1987. [S]

Ferm VH: Colchicine teratogenesis in hamster embryos. Proc Soc Exp Biol Med 112:775-778, 1963. [A]

Ingalls TH, Curley FJ, Zapposodi P: Colchicine-induced craniofacial defects in the mouse embryo. Arch Environ Health 16:326-332, 1968. [A]

Kastelic JP, Ginther OJ: Fate of conceptus and corpus luteum after induced embryonic loss in heifers. J Am Vet Med Assoc 194(7):922-928, 1989. [A]

Katsilambros L: Colchicine in the preventive treatment of the rubella embryopathy. Arch Inst Pasteur Hellen 9:97-99, 1963. [S]

Levy M, Spino M, Read SE: Colchicine: A state-of-the-art review. Pharmacotherapy 11(3):196-211, 1991. [R]

McGaughey RW, Chang MC: Inhibition of fertilization and production of heteroploidy in eggs

of mice treated with colchicine. J Exp Zool 171:465-480, 1969. [A]

Nicholson HO: Cytotoxic drugs in pregnancy. J Obstet Gynaecol Br Commonw 75:307-312, 1968. [S]

Petit TL, Isaacson RL: Anatomical and behavioral effects of colchicine administration to rats late in utero. Dev Psychobiol 9:119-129, 1976. [A]

Piko L, Bomsel-Helmreich O: Triploid rat embryos and other chromosomal deviants after colchicine treatment and polyspermy. Nature 186:737-739, 1960. [A]

Rabinovitch O, Tugendreich D, Shaki R, Prass M, et al.: Colchicine therapy in F.M.F. suffering parents during the conception time: Possible effects on the fetus. Int Symp Fetus Patient Diagn Ther 2nd Israel: 136, 1985. [S]

Sieber SM, Whang-Peng J, Botkin C, Knutsen T: Teratogenic and cytogenetic effects of some plant-derived antitumor agents (vincristine, colchicine, maytansine, VP-16-213 and VM-26) in mice. Teratology 18:31-47, 1978. [A]

Zemer D, Pras M, Sohar E, Gafni J: Colchicine in familial Mediterranean fever. N Engl J Med 294:170-171, 1976. [S]

COLISTIMETHATE

Synonyms

Colimycin, Colimycin M, Colistin Sulfate, Colistin Sulphomethate, Colistinemethanesulfonate, Colomycin, Colymycin M, Polymixin E, Sodium Colistimethate

Summary

Colistimethate is a polypeptide antibiotic that is administered parenterally for treatment of systemic infections. The drug has also been used topically.

Magnitude of Teratogenic Risk

Undetermined

Quality and Quantity of Data

Poor

A small risk cannot be excluded, but a high risk of congenital anomalies in the children of women treated with colistimethate during pregnancy is unlikely.

No epidemiological studies of congenital anomalies among the infants of women treated with colistimethate during pregnancy have been reported.

The frequency of malformations was not increased among the offspring of mice, rats, or rabbits treated during pregnancy with colistimethate in doses respectively 150-5000, 50-400, and 500-800 times those used in humans (Tomizawa & Kamada, 1973; Saitoh et al., 1981; Tsuijtani et al., 1981a, b).

Key References

Saitoh T, Tsujitani M, Ohuchi M, Matsumoto T: Reproduction studies of sodium colistin methanesulfonate (CLM). II. Teratogenicity study in mice. Chemotherapy (Tokyo) 29(9):1051-1061, 1981. [A]

Tomizawa S, Kamada K: Effects of colistin sodium methanesulfonate on fetuses of mice and rats. Oyo Yakuri 7:1047-1060, 1973. [A]

Tsujitani M, Kawaguchi Y, Takada H: Reproduction studies of sodium colistin methanesulfonate. II. Teratogenicity study in rats. Chemotherapy (Toyko) 29(2):149-163, 1981a. [A]

Tsujitani M, Ohuchi M, Saitoh T, Matsumoto T: Reproduction studies of sodium colistin methanesulfonate. Teratogenicity study in rabbits. Chemotherapy (Toyko) 29(3):300-305, 1981b. [A]

COPPER DEFICIENCY

Summary

Copper is a trace metal that is essential for normal metabolism.

Magnitude of Teratogenic Risk

Undetermined

Quality and Quantity of Data

Poor

Comment

1) Data are inadequate to assess the teratogenic risk of copper deficiency in humans. However, animal studies suggest that a true maternal copper deficiency, which is rare in humans, may be associated with an increased risk of fetal anomalies.

2) Drugs that are chelating agents such as d-penicillamine and triethylenetramine may produce copper deficiency.

Dietary copper deficiency in humans is very uncommon without concomitant deficiency of other nutrients. A significantly lower mean serum copper concentration was observed among the mothers of nine anencephalic fetuses than among the mothers of normal infants in one study (Buamah et al., 1984), but no such association was seen in another study of equal size (Wald & Hambidge, 1977). Similarly, one study demonstrated a significant negative correlation between the frequency of anencephaly and the concentration of copper in local drinking water (Morton et al., 1976), but this was not found in another study (Elwood, 1977).

Dietary copper deficiency is teratogenic in lambs, goats, swine, guinea pigs, and rats, producing a neonatal ataxia that is often fatal (Hurley & Keen, 1979; Oster & Salgo, 1977; Keen et al., 1982). Fetal demise, hemorrhage, edema, growth retardation, and skeletal anomalies also occur with maternal copper deficiency in some species.

Key References

Buamah PK, Russell M, Millford-Ward A, Taylor P, et al.: Serum copper concentration significantly less in abnormal pregnancies. Clin Chem 30:1676-1677, 1984. [E]

Elwood M: Anencephalus and drinking water composition. Am J Epidemiol 105:460-468, 1977. [E]

Hurley LS, Keen CL: Teratogenic effects of copper. In: Nriagu JD (ed): Copper in the Environment, Part II, Health Effects. New York: John Wiley and Sons, 1979, pp 33-56. [R]

Keen CL, Lonnderdal B, Hurley LS: Teratogenic effects of copper deficiency and excess. Inflammatory Dis Copper (Proc Symp) 1981:109-121, 1982. [R]

Morton MS, Elwood PC, Abernathy M: Trace elements in water and congenital malformations of the central nervous system in South Wales. Brit J Prev Soc Med 30:36-39, 1976. [E]

Oster G, Salgo MP: Copper in mammalian reproduction. Adv Pharmacol Chemother 14:327-409, 1977. [R]

Wald N, Hambidge M: Maternal serum-copper concentration and neural-tube defects. Lancet 2:560, 1977. [E]

COPPER IUD's

Synonyms

Intrauterine Devices, IUDs

Summary

Copper is a trace metal that is essential for normal metabolism. Intrauterine devices containing copper are used for contraception.

Magnitude of Teratogenic Risk

None To Minimal

Quality and Quantity of Data

Poor

Comment

None

In one series of 167 children born to women who conceived while using copper-containing intrauterine devices, the frequency of malformations did not appear to be unusually high (Guillebaud, 1976). No malformations were observed among 11 embryos examined after induced abortion in women who had conceived while using a copper IUD (Barash et al., 1990).

The frequency of malformations was no greater than expected among the offspring of rats, mice, hamsters, or rabbits that had had copper wire inserted into their uterine cavities early in pregnancy (Chang & Tatum, 1973; Rasmussen & Christensen, 1979; Barlow et al., 1981).

Key References

Barash A, Shoham(Schwartz) Z, Borenstein R, Nebel L: Development of human embryos in the presence of a copper intrauterine device. Gynecol Obstet Invest 29:203-206, 1990. [S]

Barlow SM, Knight AF, House I: Intrauterine exposure to copper IUDs and prenatal development in the rat. J Reprod Fert 62:123-130, 1981. [A]

Chang CC, Tatum HJ: Absence of teratogenicity of intrauterine copper wire in rats, hamsters and rabbits. Contraception 7:413-434, 1973. [A]

Guillebaud J: IUD and congenital malformations. Br Med J 1:1016, 1976. [S]

Rasmussen BB, Christensen N: Teratogenicity of intrauterine copper wire in mice: A histopathological study. Acta Path Microbiol Scand Sect. A 87:261-264, 1979. [A]

CORTISONE

Synonyms

Acetisone, Cortelan, Cortistab, Cortisyl, Cortogen, Cortone, Kortison, Neosone, Ricortex, Sterop

Summary

Cortisone is a glucocorticoid normally excreted by the adrenal cortex. It is used for replacement therapy and to treat allergic and inflammatory diseases.

Magnitude of Teratogenic Risk

None To Minimal

Quality and Quantity of Data

Fair To Good

Comment

None

The frequency of congenital anomalies was no greater than expected among the children of women treated with cortisone during the first four lunar months of pregnancy in the Collaborative Perinatal Project (Heinonen et al., 1977). Four of 27 infants born to women treated with cortisone for hyperemesis gravidarum during the first half of pregnancy in another study had congenital anomalies, all of which were different from each other (Wells, 1953).

Cortisone in doses substantially greater than those usually employed in humans is definitely teratogenic in several animal species. Mice have been most extensively studied. A dose-dependent increase in the frequency of cleft palate is seen among the offspring of mice treated during pregnancy with cortisone in doses 30 to hundreds of times greater than those used clinically (Biddle & Fraser, 1976; Kalter, 1981). Similar effects are seen in hamsters treated in a similar dose range (Walker, 1971; Shah & Kilistoff, 1976; Mosier et al., 1982) and in rabbits with doses comparable to those used therapeutically in humans (Walker, 1967). A variety of malformations occurs in the offspring of beagle dogs treated with about 25 times the usual human dose of cortisone during pregnancy (Nakayama et al., 1978). The relevance, if any, of these observations to the therapeutic use of cortisone in human pregnancy is unknown.

Please see agent summary on prednisone for information on a related agent that has been more thoroughly studied .

Key References

Biddle FG, Fraser FC: Genetics of cortisone-induced cleft palate in the mouse--embryonic and maternal effects. Genetics 84:743-754, 1976. [A]

Heinonen OP, Slone D, Shapiro S: Birth Defects and Drugs in Pregnancy. Littleton, Mass.: John Wright-PSG, 1977, pp 389, 391. [E]

Kalter H: Dose-response studies with genetically homogeneous lines of mice as a teratology testing and risk-assessment procedure. Teratology 24:79-86, 1981. [A]

Mosier HD, Dearden LC, Jansons RA, Roberts RC, et al.: Disproportionate growth of organs and body weight following glucocorticoid treatment of the rat fetus. Dev Pharmacol Ther 4:89-105, 1982. [A]

Nakayama T, Hirayama M, Esaki K: Effects of cortisone acetate in the beagle fetus. Teratology 18:149, 1978. [A]

Shah RM, Kilistoff A: Cleft palate induction in hamster fetuses by glucocorticoid hormones and their synthetic analogues. J Embryol Exp Morphol 36:101-108, 1976. [A]

Walker BE: Induction of cleft palate in rabbits by several glucocorticoids. Proc Soc Exp Biol Med 125:1281-1284, 1967. [A]

Walker BE: Induction of cleft palate in rats with antiinflammatory drugs. Teratology 4:39-42, 1971. [A]

Wells CN: Treatment of hyperemesis gravidarum with cortisone. I. Fetal results. Am J Obstet Gynecol 66:598-601, 1953. [C]

COUMARIN

Synonyms

Cumarin, Kumarin, Rattex, Tonka Bean Camphor

Summary

Coumarin is a camphor found in tonka beans, sweet clover, and some other plants. Coumarin is used as a flavoring agent.

155

Magnitude of Teratogenic Risk

Undetermined

Quality and Quantity of Data

Poor

Comment

None

No epidemiological studies of congenital anomalies among infants born to women treated with coumarin during pregnancy have been reported.

No teratogenic effect was noted among the offspring of miniature pigs, rats, or rabbits treated during pregnancy with coumarin in combination with the flavonoid derivative troxerutin at doses respectively 100, 1-400, and 10-100 times the human therapeutic dose (Grote & Gunther, 1971; Grote & Weinmann, 1973; Grote et al., 1977; Preuss-Ueberschar et al., 1984). Similarly, no increase in malformations was observed among the offspring of mice fed diets containing 0.05-0.25% coumarin, although developmental delay was seen at the highest dose (Roll & Bar, 1967).

Although coumarin resembles warfarin chemically, it does not share similar pharmacological properties with warfarin. Its anticoagulant potential is 1/50,000th that of warfarin (Overman et al., 1944).

Key References

Grote W, Gunther R: Prufung einer Cumarin-Rutin-Kombination auf teratogenitat durch fetale skelettuntersuchungen. Arzneimittelforsch 21:2016-2022, 1971. [A]

Grote W, Schulz L-Cl, Uberschar S, et al.: Uberprufung einer kombination der wirkstoffe cumarin und troxerutin auf embryotoxische und teratogene nebenwirkungen an Gottinger miniaturschweinen. Arzneimittelforsch 27:613-617, 1977. [A]

Grote W, Weinmann I: Uberprufung der wirkstoffe cumarin und rutin im teratologischen versuch

and kaninchen. Arzneimittelforsch 23:1319-1320, 1973. [A]

Overman RS, Stahmann MA, Huebner CF, et al.: Studies on the hemorrhagic sweet clover disease. XIII. Anticoagulant activity and structure in the 4-hydroxycoumarin group. J Biol Chem 153:5-24, 1944. [A].

Preuss-Ueberschar C, Ueberschar S, Grote W: Reproduktionstoxikologische untersuchungen an ratten nach oraler verabreichung eines benzopyronpraparates. Arzneimittelforsch 34:1305-1313, 1984. [A]

Roll R, Bar F: Die Wirkung von cumarin (o-hydroxyzimtsaure-lacton) auf trachtige mauseweibchen. Arzneimittelforsch 17:97-100, 1967. [A]

CROMOLYN

Synonyms

Cromoglycate, Cromoptic, Intal, Lomupren, Lomusol, Nalcrom, Nasalcrom, Opticrom, Rynacrom, Sodium Cromoglycate

Summary

Cromolyn is used in the prevention of allergic diseases and related conditions.

Magnitude of Teratogenic Risk

None To Minimal

Quality and Quantity of Data

Poor To Fair

Comment

None

No epidemiological studies of congenital anomalies among infants born to women treated with cromolyn during pregnancy have been reported. The frequency of congenital anomalies did not appear to be increased in a series of 296 children of asthmatic women treated with cromolyn throughout pregnancy (Wilson, 1982).

The frequency of congenital anomalies was not increased among the offspring of rats, mice, or rabbits treated during pregnancy with cromolyn in doses respectively 56, up to 340, and 310 times those used in humans (Cox et al., 1970). Treatment of pregnant mice with cromolyn in doses more than 38 times that used in humans did increase the teratogenic effect produced by concurrent administration of isoproterenol (Cox et al., 1970). The clinical relevance of this observation is unknown.

Key References

Cox JSG, Beach JE, Blair AMJN, Clarke AJ, et al.: Disodium Cromoglycate (Ital). Adv Drug Res 5:115-196, 1970. [A]

Wilson J: Utilisation du cromoglycate de sodium au cours de la grossesse: Resultats sur 296 femmes asthmatiques. Acta Therap 8(Suppl):45-51, 1982. [S]

CROTAMITON

Synonyms

Bestloid, Crotalgin, Crotam, Crotamitex, Eurax, Euraxil, N-Ethyl-O-Crotonotoluide, Veteusan

Summary

Crotamiton is used topically to treat scabies and itching.

Magnitude of Teratogenic Risk

Undetermined

Quality and Quantity of Data

None

Comment

None

No epidemiological studies of congenital anomalies among infants born to women treated with crotamiton during pregnancy have been reported.

No animal teratology studies of crotamiton have been published.

Key References

None available.

CUPRIMYXIN

Synonyms

Copper Myxin, Unitop

Summary

Cuprimyxin is an antifungal agent.

Magnitude of Teratogenic Risk

Undetermined

Quality and Quantity of Data

None

Comment

None

No epidemiological studies of congenital anomalies in infants born to women who used cuprimyxin during pregnancy have been reported.

No animal teratology studies of cuprimyxin have been published.

Key References

None available.

CYANOCOBALAMIN

Synonyms

Berubigen, Betalin-12, Cabadon M, Cobamin, Crystamin, Cycobemin, Cyomin, Rubesol, Rubramin, Sytobex, Vitamin B_{12}

Summary

Cyanocobalamin is one form of vitamin B_{12}, a water-soluble vitamin. The U.S. Recommended Dietary Allowance of vitamin B_{12} is 2.2 mcg/d in pregnancy (NRC, 1989). Cyanocobalamin is administered in doses up to 450 times greater than this to treat vitamin B_{12} deficiency of pernicious anemia.

Magnitude of Teratogenic Risk

Undetermined

Quality and Quantity of Data

None To Poor

Comment

A small risk cannot be excluded, but a high risk of congenital anomalies in the children of women who took cyanocobalamin during pregnancy is unlikely.

No adequate epidemiological studies of congenital anomalies among infants born to women treated with large doses of cyanocobalamin during pregnancy have been reported.

The frequency of malformations was not increased among the offspring of mice treated during pregnancy with 5250-10,500 times the human therapeutic dose of cyanocobalamin (Mitala et al., 1978). Hydrocephalus, eye defects, and skeletal anomalies occurred with increased frequency among the offspring of pregnant rats fed a diet deficient in cyanocobalamin (Grainger et al., 1954; Woodard & Newberne, 1966).

Key References

Grainger RB, O'Dell BL, Hogan AG: Congenital malformations as related to deficiencies of ribo-flavin and vitamin B_{12} source of protein, calcium to phosphorus ratio and skeletal phosphorus metabolism. J Nutr 54:33-48, 1954. [A]

Mitala JJ, Mann DE, Gautieri RF: Influence of cobalt (dietary), cobalamins, and inorganic cobalt salts on phenytoin- and cortisone-induced teratogenesis in mice. J Pharm Sci 67:377-380, 1978. [A]

NRC (National Research Council): Recommended Dietary Allowances, 10th ed. Report of the Subcommittee on the Tenth Edition of the RDAs, Food and Nutrition Board, Commission on Life Sciences. Washington, D.C.: National Academy Press, 1989. [O]

Woodard JC, Newberne PM: Relation of vitamin B_{12} and one-carbon metabolism to hydrocephalus in the rat. J Nutri 88:375-381, 1966. [A]

CYCLACILLIN

Synonyms

Aminocyclohexylpenicillin, Calthor, Ciclacillin, Citocillin, Cyclapen-W, Orfilina, Ultracillin, Vastcillin, Vatracin, Wyvital

Summary

Cyclacillin is an oral antibiotic used to treat a variety of infections. It is closely related to ampicillin.

Magnitude of Teratogenic Risk

Undetermined

Quality and Quantity of Data

Poor

Comment

None

No epidemiological studies of congenital anomalies among the children of women treated with cyclacillin during pregnancy have been reported.

No teratogenic effect was observed among the offspring of rats or mice treated with cyclacillin in doses 2.5-5.0 times those used clinically in one study (Mizutani et al., 1970).

Please see agent summaries on penicillin and ampicillin agent for information on related agents that have been more thoroughly studied.

Key References

Mizutani M, Ihara T, Tanaka S, Kanamori H, et al.: Fetotoxic studies of amino-cyclohexyl penicillin in mice and rats. Takeda Kenkyusho HO (J Takeda Res Lab) 29:124-133, 1970. [A]

CYCLOBENZAPRINE

Synonyms

CBZ, Flexeril, MK-130, Proheptatriene Hydrochloride

Summary

Cyclobenzaprine is a centrally acting muscle relaxant used for relief of muscle spasms.

Magnitude of Teratogenic Risk

Undetermined

Quality and Quantity of Data

None

Comment

None

No epidemiological studies of congenital anomalies among infants born to women treated with cyclobenzaprine during pregnancy have been reported.

A child with a very unusual pattern of anomalies consisting of imperforate oropharynx, abnormal facies and vertebral defects, whose mother took cyclobenzaprine early in the first trimester of pregnancy, has been reported (Flannery, 1989). No causal relationship can be established on the basis of this anecdotal observation.

No animal teratology studies of cyclobenzaprine have been published.

Key References

Flannery DB: Syndrome of imperforate oropharynx with costovertebral and auricular anomalies. Am J Med Genet 32:189-191, 1989. [C]

CYCLOMETHYCAINE

Synonyms

Cainasurfa, Ciclometicaina, Cyclocaine, Surfacaine, Surfathesin, Topocaine

Summary

Cyclomethycaine is a local anesthetic that has been used topically.

Magnitude of Teratogenic Risk

Undetermined

Quality and Quantity of Data

None

Comment

None

No epidemiological studies of congenital anomalies in children born to women exposed to cyclomethycaine during pregnancy have been reported.

No investigations of teratologic effects of cyclomethycaine in experimental animals have been published.

Please see agent summary on procaine for information on a related agent that has been studied.

Key References

None available.

CYCLOPROPANE

Synonyms

Cyclopropane Carboxylate, Li-Ban Lice Control Spray, Trimethylene

Summary

Cyclopropane is a general anesthetic administered by inhalation.

Magnitude of Teratogenic Risk

Undetermined

Quality and Quantity of Data

None To Poor

Comment

None

No epidemiological studies of congenital anomalies in children born to women exposed to cyclopropane during pregnancy have been reported.

No studies of teratologic effects of cyclopropane in experimental animals have been published.

Key References

None available.

CYCLOSERINE

Synonyms

Cicloserina, Ciclovalidin, Closina, Cyclorin, Micoserina, Miroseryn, Novoserin, Oxamycin, Seromycin, Setavax

Summary

Cycloserine is an antibiotic that is given orally for treatment of tuberculous and other infections.

Magnitude of Teratogenic Risk

Undetermined

Quality and Quantity of Data

None

Comment

None

No epidemiological studies of congenital anomalies among children born to women treated with cycloserine during pregnancy have been reported.

No animal teratology studies of cycloserine have been published.

Key References

None available.

CYCLOSPORINE

Synonyms

Ciclosporine, Cyclosporin A, Sandimmune

Summary

Cyclosporine is a cyclic polypeptide of fungal origin. It is used as an immunosuppressant in the prevention and treatment of allograft rejection.

Magnitude of Teratogenic Risk

Minimal

Quality and Quantity of Data

Poor To Fair

Comment

Although fetal growth retardation has been observed in some studies (see below), it is unclear whether this effect is due to cyclosporine or to other medication used concurrently.

More than 50 pregnancies have been reported among women who had received organ transplants before conceiving and who were treated with cyclosporine, often in combination with other drugs, throughout gestation (Al-Khader et al., 1988; Kossoy et al., 1988; Niesert et al., 1988; Pickrell et al., 1988; Zeidan et al., 1991). Unfortunately, these cases are all anecdotal and no large prospective series or controlled epidemiological study has been published. Most of the children born to women treated with cyclosporine during pregnancy appear to be normal, but very few cases have been followed beyond infancy. Congenital anomalies have been reported in five cases but the defects reported are all different: bilateral cataracts and absence of the corpus callosum (Kossoy et al., 1988), hypospadias/clinodactyly (Niesert et al., 1988), hypoplasia of the legs (Pujals et al., 1989), and bilateral club foot (Zeidan et al., 1991). The frequency of infants with malformations does not appear to be excessive, given the anecdotal nature of the reports. Fetal growth retardation may be unusually frequent among the children of women treated with cyclosporine during pregnancy (Al-Khader et al., 1988; Niesert et al., 1988; Pickrell et al., 1988; Zeidan et al., 1991), but this is probably related, at least in part, to the mothers' underlying illnesses or other aspects of its treatment. The number of cases of twins described seems high (Burrows et al., 1988; Prieto et al., 1989; Grow et al., 1991), but this may well be a reporting bias. Transient neona-tal thrombocytopenia and neutropenia have occasionally been reported in the infants of women treated with cyclosporine during pregnancy (Grischke et al., 1986; Grow et al., 1991).

The frequency of malformations was not increased among the offspring of rats or rabbits treated with <1-1.5 or <1-5 times the usual human dose of cyclosporine (Ryffel et al., 1983; Brown et al., 1985). Fetal growth retardation and death were increased in both species at doses at or just above the maximum used therapeutically in humans, but such doses were also toxic to the mothers (Ryffel et al., 1983; Mason et al., 1985; Brown et al., 1985).

Key References

Al-Khader AA, Absy M, Al-Hasani MK, et al.: Successful pregnancy in renal transplant recipients treated with cyclosporine. Transplantation 45(5):987-988, 1988. [C]

Brown PAJ, Gray ES, Whiting PH, Simpson JG, et al.: Effects of cyclosporin A on fetal development in the rat. Bio Neonate 48:172-180, 1985. [A]

Burrows DA, O'Neil TJ, Sorrells TL: Successful twin pregnancy after renal transplant maintained on cyclosporine A immunosuppression. Obstet Gynecol 72(3):459-461, 1988. [C]

Grischke E, Kaufmann M, Dreikorn K, et al.: [Successful pregnancy with kidney transplant and cyclosporin A]. Geburtshilfe Frauenheilkd 46:176-179, 1986. [C]

Grow DR, Simon NV, Liss J, Delp WT: Twin pregnancy after orthotopic liver transplantation, with exacerbation of chronic graft rejection. Am J Perinatol 8(2):135-138, 1991. [C]

Kossoy LR, Herbert CM III, Wentz AC: Management of heart transplant recipients: Guidelines for the obstetrician-gynecologist. Am J Obstet Gynecol 159(2):490-499, 1988. [R]

Mason RJ, Thomson AW, Whiting PH, Gray ES, et al.: Cyclosporine-induced fetotoxicity in the rat. Transplantation 39(1):9-12, 1985. [A]

Niesert S, Gunter H, Grei U: Pregnancy after renal transplantation. Br Med J 296:1736, 1988. [S]

Pickrell MD, Sawer R, Michael J: Pregnancy after renal transplantation: Severe intrauterine growth retardation during treatment with cyclosporin A. Br Med J 296:825, 1988. [C]

Prieto C, Errasti P, Olaizola JI, et al.: Successful twin pregnancies in renal transplant recipients taking cyclosporine. Transplantation 48(6):1065-1067, 1989. [C]

Pujals JM, Figueras G, Puig JM, et al.: Osseous malformation in baby born to woman on cyclosporin. Lancet 1:667, 1989. [C]

Ryffel B, Donatsch P, Madorin M, Matter BE, et al.: Toxicological evaluation of cyclosporin A. Arch Toxicol 53:107-141, 1983. [A]

Zeidan BS, Waltzer WC, Monheit AG, Rapaport FT: Anemia associated with pregnancy in a cyclosporine-treated renal allograft recipient. Transplant Proc 23(4):2301-2303, 1991. [C]

CYPROHEPTADINE

Synonyms

Antegan, Cipractin, Dihexazine, Ifrasarl, Nuran, Periactin, Perideca, Peritol, Sigloton, Vimicon

Summary

Cyproheptadine is an antihistamine used orally to treat allergic disorders. It also has anticholinergic and antiserotoninergic activity.

Magnitude of Teratogenic Risk

Undetermined

Quality and Quantity of Data

Poor

Comment

A small risk cannot be excluded, but there is no indication that the risk of congenital anomalies in children of women treated with cyproheptadine during pregnancy is likely to be great.

No epidemiological studies of congenital anomalies in infants whose mothers took cyproheptadine during pregnancy have been reported.

The frequency of malformations was not increased among the offspring of rats treated with cyproheptadine in doses within the human therapeutic range or up to 15 times greater (Weinstein et al., 1975; Druga et al., 1988). An increased frequency of fetal death and anomalies occurred when the mothers were treated with 4-100 times the usual human dose in other investigations (de la Fuente & Alia, 1982; Rodriguez-Gonzalez et al., 1983; Druga et al., 1988). Glucose intolerance and increased pancreatic insulin levels have been observed among the offspring of rats treated with cyproheptadine during pregnancy in a dose 22 times that used in humans (Chow & Fischer, 1984). The relevance of these findings to the clinical use of cyproheptadine in human pregnancy is unknown.

Key References

Chow SA, Fischer LJ: Alterations in rat pancreatic B-cell function induced by prenatal exposure to cyproheptadine. Diabetes 33:572-575, 1984. [A]

de la Fuente M, Alia M: The teratogenicity of cyproheptadine in two generations of Wistar rats. Arch Int Pharmacodyn 257:168-176, 1982. [A]

Druga A, Nyritray M, Magyar B: Teratogenicity of cyproheptadine chlorhydrate and possible mode of action in Wistar rats. Teratology 38(2):17A, 1988. [A]

Rodriguez Gonzalez MD, Lima Perez MT, Sanabria Negrin JG: The effect of cyproheptadine chlorhydrate on rat embryonic development. Teratogenesis Carcinog Mutagen 3:439-446, 1983. [A]

Weinstein D, Ornoy A, Ben-Zur Z, Pfeifer Y, et al.: Teratogenicity of cyproheptadine in pregnant rats. Arch Int Pharmacodyn 215:345-349, 1975. [A]

CYTARABINE

Synonyms

Alexan, Ara-C, Arabinocytidine, Arabinofuranosylcytosine, Arabinosyl Cytosine, Arabinosylcytosine, Arabitin, Cyclocide, Cytosar, Cytosine Arabinoside

Summary

Cytarabine, a nucleoside analogue that inhibits DNA synthesis, is used parenterally in the treatment of leukemia.

Magnitude of Teratogenic Risk

Small To Moderate

Quality and Quantity of Data

Fair

Comment

Maternal use of cytarabine late in pregnancy may be associated with neonatal bone marrow suppression (see below).

No controlled epidemiological studies of congenital anomalies among infants born to women treated with cytarabine during pregnancy have been reported. Anecdotal descriptions of more than 50 pregnancies in which the mother was treated with cytarabine, usually in combination with other antineoplastic agents, have been reported (Gililland & Weinstein, 1983; Caligiuri & Mayer, 1989; Aviles et al., 1991). In the pregnancies that were continued to term, most of the infants appeared normal. Treatment in these cases was usually in the second and/or third trimester, but at least 11 normal infants have been reported whose mothers were treated with cytarabine during the first trimester of pregnancy.

Major limb malformations, including ectrodactyly and longitudinal hemimelia, have been reported in two infants whose mothers had been treated with cytarabine alone or with one other antineoplastic agent early in pregnancy (Wagner et al., 1980; Schafer, 1981). Although a causal relationship cannot be established on the basis of these anecdotal observations, the occurrence of similar defects in experimental animal studies supports a causal interpretation. Unexplained fetal death has been observed several times in pregnancies of women who were being treated with cytarabine and other antineoplastic agents (O'Donnell et al., 1979; Plows, 1982; Volkenandt et al., 1987; Caligiuri & Mayer, 1989).

Increased frequencies of limb defects, particularly ectrodactyly and other digital anomalies, were observed among the offspring of pregnant mice or rats treated with 2-3 or 8-67 times the human dose of cytarabine (Ritter et al., 1971; Rooze, 1983; Ortega et al., 1991). The effect showed typical responsiveness to dose and time of exposure. Abnormal brain and kidney development occurred in mice and rats born to animals that had been treated with 10-16 or 8-93 times the human dose of cytarabine late in pregnancy (Percy, 1975; Shimada et al., 1982; Matsutani et al., 1983; Ohno, 1984).

Pancytopenia, neutropenia, and thrombocytopenia have been reported in newborn infants of women treated with cytarabine in late pregnancy (Colbert et al., 1980; Pizzuto et al., 1980; Taylor & Blom, 1980). Bone marrow suppression is a recognized complication of cytarabine therapy in adults.

Key References

Aviles A, Diaz-Maqueo JC, Talavera A, et al.: Growth and development of children of mothers treated with chemotherapy during pregnancy: Current status of 43 children. Am J Hematol 36:243-248, 1991. [S]

Caligiuri MA, Mayer RJ: Pregnancy and leukemia. Semin Oncol 16(5):388-396, 1989. [R]

Colbert N, Najman A, Gorin NC, et al.: Acute leukaemia during pregnancy: Favourable course of pregnancy in two patients treated with cytosine arabinoside and anthracyclines. Nouv Press Med 12:175-178, 1980. [C]

Gililland J, Weinstein L: The effects of cancer chemotherapeutic agents on the developing fetus. Obstet Gynecol Surv 38(1):6-12, 1983. [C]

Matsutani T, Tamaru M, Hayakawa Y, et al.: A neurochemical study of developmental impairment of the brain caused by the administration of cytosine arabinoside during the fetal or neonatal period of rats. Neurochem Res 8(10):1295-1306, 1983. [A]

O'Donnell R, Costigan C, O'Connell LG: Two cases of acute leukaemia in pregnancy. Acta Haemat 61:298-300, 1979. [C]

Ohno M: Neuroanatomical study of somatomotor cortex in microcephalic mice induced by cytosine arabinoside. Brain Dev 6(6):528-538, 1984. [A]

Ortega A, Puig M, Domingo JL: Maternal and developmental toxicity of low doses of cytosine arabinoside in mice. Teratology 44:379-384, 1991. [A]

Percy DH: Teratogenic effects of the pyrimidine analogues 5-iododeoxyuridine and cytosine arabinoside in late fetal mice and rats. Teratology 11:103-118, 1975. [A]

Pizzuto J, Aviles A, Noriega L, et al.: Treatment of acute leukemia during pregnancy: Presentation of nine cases. Cancer Treat Rep 64(4-5):679-683, 1980. [S]

Plows CW: Acute myelomonocytic leukemia in pregnancy: Report of a case. Am J Obstet Gynecol 143(1):41-43, 1982. [C]

Ritter EJ, Scott WJ, Wilson JG: Teratogenesis and inhibition of DNA synthesis induced in rat embryos by cytosine arabinoside. Teratology 4:7-14, 1971. [A]

Rooze M: Correlations between necrotic patterns and limb skeletal defects induced by antimitotic drugs in the mouse. Prog Clin Biol Res 110(Pt. A):365-375, 1983. [A]

Schafer AI: Teratogenic effects of antileukemic chemotherapy. Arch Intern Med 141:514-515, 1981. [C]

Shimada M, Abe Y, Yamano T, et al.: The pathogenesis of abnormal cytoarchitecture in the cerebral cortex and hippocampus of the mouse treated transplacentally with cytosine arabinoside. Acta Neuropathol 58:159-167, 1982. [A]

Taylor G, Blom J: Acute leukemia during pregnancy. South Med J 73(10):1314-1315, 1980. [C]

Volkenandt M, Buchner T, Hiddemann W, van de Loo J: Acute leukaemia during pregnancy. Lancet 2:1521-1522, 1987. [C]

Wagner VM, Hill JS, Weaver D, Baehner RL: Congenital abnormalities in baby born to cytarabine treated mother. Lancet 2:98-99, 1980. [C]

CYTOMEGALOVIRUS

Synonyms

CMV

Summary

Cytomegalovirus (CMV), a member of the herpes group, is a DNA virus that usually produces asymptomatic infection in children and adults. Clinical disease may occur, however, and typically manifests as fever, malaise, and arthralgia or myalgia (Betts, 1980). Infection with CMV is almost universal in human populations by age 60 years; infection occurs at substantially younger ages in lower socioeconomic groups. Good professional hygiene among susceptible women with frequent exposure to CMV-infected individuals appears to be sufficient to prevent transmission (Balfour & Balfour, 1986; Nelson & Sullivan-Bolyai, 1987; Stagno, 1990; Tookey & Peckham, 1991).

Magnitude of Teratogenic Risk

Small

Quality and Quantity of Data

Good To Excellent

Comment

This risk is for primary maternal infection during pregnancy. The risk associated with secondary maternal infection is much lower.

The frequency of congenital CMV infection varies from 0.2-2.2% of newborns in various populations, with higher prevalence in lower socioeconomic groups (Stagno & Whitley, 1985; Yow et al., 1988; Stagno, 1990; Fowler & Pass, 1991; Griffiths et al., 1991). The presence of maternal antibody to CMV does not prevent fetal infection, but symptomatic manifestations are much less common among the infants of women with recurrent infection during pregnancy (Stagno et al., 1984; Stagno, 1990; Fowler et al., 1992).

About 10% of infants with congenital CMV infections exhibit serious clinical manifestations at birth (Stagno et al., 1984; Griffiths et al., 1991). Frequent features of symptomatic congenital CMV infection include intrauterine growth retardation, microcephaly, petechiae, hepatosplenomegaly, jaundice, and chorioretinitis (Pass et al., 1980; Weller & Hanshaw 1962; Stagno, 1990). Major cerebral migrational defects may be demonstrable on CT or MRI scan (Hayward et al., 1991). Of children with symptomatic congenital CMV infection who survive beyond infancy, 30% have microcephaly, 40-50% have mental retardation, 50% have neurological dysfunction, 60% have hearing loss, and 20% have ocular abnormalities (Williamson et al., 1982; Conboy et al., 1987). Symptomatic congenital CMV infection can occur after primary maternal infection at any stage of pregnancy, although adverse outcomes appear to be somewhat more likely with infection in the first half of gestation (Stagno et al., 1984; Griffiths & Baboonian, 1984; Stagno et al., 1986).

Ten to 25% of children with congenital CMV infection who are initially asymptomatic develop related abnormalities within the first few years of life (Saigal et al., 1982; Kumar et al., 1984; Stagno et al., 1984; Yow et al., 1988; Fowler et al., 1992). Manifestations may include sensorineural hearing loss, chorioretinitis, neurological deficits, and dental defects.

Fetal anomalies such as ventricular dilatation, ascites, cerebral calcification, and growth retardation resulting from intrauterine CMV infection can be diagnosed prenatally in the second and third trimester by ultrasound (Grose & Weiner, 1990; Lynch et al., 1991; Tassin et al., 1991). Amniocentesis and percutaneous umbilical blood sampling have been used to obtain fetal specimens for prenatal diagnosis of CMV infection, but interpretation of the results of these tests may be difficult (Grose & Weiner, 1990; Hohlfeld et al., 1991; Lynch et al., 1991; Lamy et al., 1992; Trofatter, 1992).

Perinatal CMV infection may occur due to passage of the infant through a contaminated birth canal, but this rarely seems to cause clinical illness (Stagno et al., 1984).

Experimental fetal infection has been demonstrated after maternal inoculation with CMV in guinea pigs, mice, and pigs (Edington et al., 1977, 1988; Griffith et al., 1982, 1986, 1990; Huang et al., 1986; Baskar et al., 1987; Fitzgerald & Shellam, 1991). Ventricular dilatation and leptomeningitis have been induced in fetal rhesus monkeys after intracerebral or intraamniotic injection of CMV (London et al., 1986).

Key References

Balfour CL, Balfour HH: Cytomegalovirus is not an occupational risk for nurses in renal transplant and neonatal units. Results of a prospective surveillance study. J Am Med Assoc 256:1909-1914, 1986. [E]

Baskar JF, Peacock J, Sulik KK, Huang E-S: Early-stage developmental abnormalities induced by murine cytomegalovirus. J Infect Dis 155:661-666, 1987. [A]

Betts RF: Syndromes of cytomegalovirus infection. Adv Intern Med 26:447-466, 1980. [R]

Conboy TJ, Pass RF, Stagno S, et al.: Early clinical manifestations and intellectual outcome in children with symptomatic congenital cytomegalovirus infection. J Pediatr 111:343-348, 1987. [S]

Edington N, Watt RG, Plowright WW, Wrathall AE, et al.: Experimental transplacental transmission of porcine cytomegalovirus. J Hyg (Camb) 78:243-251, 1977. [A]

Edington N, Wrathall AE, Done JT: Porcine cytomegalovirus (PCMV) in early gestation. Vet Microbiol 17:117-128, 1988. [A]

Fitzgerald NA, Shellam GR: Host genetic influences on fetal susceptibility to murine cytomegalovirus after maternal or fetal infection. J Infect Dis 163:276-281, 1991. [A]

Fowler KB, Pass RF: Sexually transmitted diseases in mothers of neonates with congenital cytomegalovirus infection. J Infect Dis 164:259-264, 1991. [E]

Fowler KB, Stagno S, Pass RF, et al.: The outcome of congenital cytomegalovirus infection in relation to maternal antibody status. N Engl J Med 326(10):663-667, 1992. [E]

Griffith BP, Chen M, Isom HC: Role of primary and secondary maternal viremia in transplacental guinea pig cytomegalovirus transfer. J Virol 64(5):1991-1997, 1990. [A]

Griffith BP, Lucia HL, Hsiung GD: Brain and visceral involvement during congenital cytomegalovirus infection of guinea pigs. Pediatr Res 16:455-459, 1982. [A]

Griffith BP, McCormick SR, Booss J, et al.: Inbred guinea pig model of intrauterine infection with cytomegalovirus. Am J Pathol 122:112-119, 1986. [A]

Griffiths PD, Baboonian C: A prospective study of primary cytomegalovirus infection during pregnancy: Final report. Br J Obstet Gynaecol 91:307-315, 1984. [E]

Griffiths PD, Baboonian C, Rutter D, Peckham C: Congenital and maternal cytomegalovirus infections in a London population. Br J Obstet Gynaecol 98:135-140, 1991. [E]

Grose C, Weiner CP: Prenatal diagnosis of congenital cytomegalovirus infection: Two decades later. Am J Obstet Gynecol 163(2):447-450, 1990. [R]

Hayward JC, Titelbaum DS, Clancy RR, Zimmerman RA: Lissencephaly-pachygyria associated with congenital cytomegalovirus infection. J Child Neurol 6:109-114, 1991. [S]

Hohlfeld P, Vial Y, Maillard-Brignon C, et al.: Cytomegalovirus fetal infection: Prenatal diagnosis. Obstet Gynecol 78:615-618, 1991. [S]

Huang Y-S, Chernoff N, Kavlock RJ, Kawanishi CY: The effects of maternal murine cytomegalovirus infection on the mouse conceptus at different gestational stages. Teratogenesis Carcinog Mutagen 6:331-338, 1986. [A]

Kumar ML, Nankervis GA, Jacobs IB, Ernhart CB, et al.: Congenital and postnatally acquired cytomegalovirus infections: Long-term follow-up. J Pediatr 104:674-679, 1984. [E]

Lamy ME, Mulongo KN, Gadisseux J-F, et al.: Prenatal diagnosis of fetal cytomegalovirus infection. Am J Obstet Gynecol 166:91-94, 1992. [S]

London WT, Martinez AJ, Houff SA, Wallen WC, et al.: Experimental congenital disease with Simian cytomegalovirus in rhesus monkeys. Teratology 33:323-331, 1986. [A]

Lynch L, Daffos F, Emanuel D, et al.: Prenatal diagnosis of fetal cytomegalovirus infection. Am J Obstet Gynecol 165:714-718, 1991. [S]

Nelson KE, Sullivan-Bolyai JZ: Preventing teratogenic viral infections in hospital employees: The cases of rubella, cytomegalovirus and varicella-zoster virus. Occupational Medicine: State of the Art Reviews 2(3):471-498, 1987. [R]

Pass RF, Stagno S, Myers GJ, Alford CA: Outcome of symptomatic congenital cytomegalovirus infection: Results of long-term longitudinal follow-up. Pediatrics 66:758-762, 1980. [S]

Saigal S, Lunyk O, Larke RB, Chernesky MA: The outcome in children with congenital cytomega-

lovirus infection. Am J Dis Child 136:896-901, 1982. [E]

Stagno S: Cytomegalovirus. In: Remington JS, Klein JO (eds). Infectious Diseases of the Fetus and Newborn Infant. Philadelphia: W.B. Saunders Co., 1990, pp 241-281. [O]

Stagno S, Pass RF, Cloud G, Britt WJ, et al.: Primary cytomegalovirus infection in pregnancy. Incidence, transmission to fetus, and clinical outcome. J Am Med Assoc 256:1904-1908, 1986. [E]

Stagno S, Pass RF, Dworsky ME, Britt WJ, et al.: Congenital and perinatal cytomegalovirus infections: Clinical characteristics and pathogenic factors. Birth Defects 20:65-85, 1984. [R]

Stagno S, Whitley RJ: Herpes virus infections of pregnancy. Part I: Cytomegalovirus and Epstein-Barr virus infections. N Engl J Med 313:1270-1274, 1985. [R]

Tassin GB, Maklad NF, Stewart RR, Bell ME: Cytomegalic inclusion disease: Intrauterine sonographic diagnosis using findings involving the brain. Am J Neuroradiol 12:117-122, 1991. [C]

Tookey P, Peckham CS: Does cytomegalovirus present an occupational risk? Arch Dis Child 66:1009-1010, 1991. [R]

Trofatter KF, Jr.: Cytomegalovirus. In: Gleicher N (ed). Principles and Practice of Medical Therapy in Pregnancy, 2nd ed. Norwalk, Conn: Appleton & Lange, 1992, pp 633-637. [R]

Weller TH, Hanshaw JB: Virologic and clinical observations on cytomegalic inclusion disease. N Engl J Med 266:1233-1244, 1962. [S]

Williamson WD, Desmond MM, LaFevers N, et al.: Symptomatic congenital cytomegalovirus. Disorders of language, learning, and hearing. Am J Dis Child 136:902-905, 1982. [S]

Yow MD, Williamson DW, Leeds LJ, Thompson P, et al.: Epidemiologic characteristics of cytomegalovirus infection in mothers and their infants. Am J Obstet Gynecol 158:1189-1195, 1988. [E]

DACARBAZINE

Synonyms

Biocarbazine R, Deticene, DTIC, DTIC-Dome, Imidazole Carboxamide

Summary

Dacarbazine is an antineoplastic drug that is administered intravenously in the treatment of malignant melanoma, Hodgkin's disease, and other malignancies.

Magnitude of Teratogenic Risk

Undetermined

Quality and Quantity of Data

Poor

Comment

Although the teratogenic risk of dacarbazine in humans is undetermined, the fact that this drug is cytotoxic raises concern that the risk could be substantial.

No epidemiological studies of congenital anomalies in infants born to women treated with dacarbazine during pregnancy have been reported. No congenital anomalies were seen among the children of 10 women treated with dacarbazine and other antineoplastic agents during pregnancy in one series (Aviles et al., 1991). Four of these women were treated during the first trimester.

Increased frequencies of central nervous system, limb, and craniofacial anomalies have been observed among the offspring of rats treated with 22-220 times the usual human dose of dacarbazine during pregnancy (Chaube, 1973). The teratogenic effect exhibited typical time of gestation and dose dependence. Increased frequencies of cleft palate and skeletal anomalies were seen among the offspring of rabbits treated with only about twice the human therapeutic dose of dacarbazine; maternal toxicity was also observed at this dose (Thompson et al., 1975).

Key References

Aviles A, Diaz-Maqueo JC, Talavera A, et al.: Growth and development of children of mothers treated with chemotherapy during pregnancy: Current status of 43 children. Am J Hematol 36:243-248, 1991. [S]

Chaube S: Protective effects of thymidine, 5-aminoimidazolecarboxamide and riboflavin against fetal abnormalities produced in rats by 5-(3,3-dimethyl-1-triazeno)imidazole-4-carboxamide. Cancer Res 33:2231-2240, 1973. [A]

Thompson DJ, Mollelo JA, Strebing RJ, Dyke IL: Reproduction and teratology studies with oncolytic agents in the rat and rabbit: II. 5-(3,3-dimethyl-1-triazeno)imidazole-4-carboxamide (DTIC). Toxicol Appl Pharmacol 33:281-290, 1975. [A]

DANAZOL

Synonyms

Chronogyn, Cyclomen, Danatrol, Danocrine, Danokrin, Danol, Ladogar, Winobanin

Summary

Danazol is an anabolic steroid that is given orally in the treatment of endometriosis, fibrocystic breast disease and hereditary angioedema. Danazol has androgenic and antiestrogenic activity.

Magnitude of Teratogenic Risk

Virilization Of Female Fetus: Moderate

Nongenital Congenital Anomalies: Undetermined

Quality and Quantity of Data

Virilization Of Female Fetus: Fair

Nongenital Congenital Anomalies: Poor

Comment

1) Virilization of the female fetus is likely to occur only with doses of greater than 200 mg/day.

2) A small risk cannot be excluded, but a high risk of nongenital congenital anomalies in the children of women treated with danazol during pregnancy is unlikely.

There were 23 virilized female infants born of 94 completed pregnancies known to the manufacturer in which the mother was treated with danazol (Brunskill, 1992). The series includes all previously published cases (Duck & Katayama, 1981; Castro-Magana et al., 1981; Wentz, 1982; Schwartz, 1982; Peress et al., 1982; Shaw, 1984; Rosa, 1984; Quagliarello & Greco, 1985; Kingsbury, 1985) and those reported voluntarily to regulatory agencies in the United States and Australia. The abnormality in the affected girls usually consisted of cliteromegaly, fused labia, and a urogenital sinus opening at the base of the clitoris. Exposure generally occurred from conception; the minimum duration of therapy in a virilized case was nine weeks. The minimum dose in a virilized case was 200 mg/day, but most virilized cases were associated with treatment at 800 mg/day. The frequency of virilization in female fetuses of women who have taken danazol during pregnancy cannot be determined from these data. Several other congenital anomalies were also observed among these danazol-exposed pregnancies, but there was no specificity or consistency among the anomalies to suggest a causal relationship (Brunskill, 1992).

No animal teratology studies of danazol have been published.

Key References

Brunskill PJ: The effects of fetal exposure to danazol. Br J Obstet Gynaecol 99:212-215, 1992. [S]

Castro-Magana M, Cheruvanky T, Collipp PJ, et al.: Transient adrenogenital syndrome due to exposure to danazol in utero. Am J Dis Child 135:1032-1034, 1981. [C]

Duck SC, Katayama KP: Danazol may cause female pseudohermaphroditism. Fertil Steril 35:230-231, 1981. [C]

Kingsbury AC: Danazol and fetal masculinization: A warning. Med J Aust 143:410-411, 1985. [C]

Peress MR, Kreutner AK, Mathur RS, Williamson HO: Female pseudohermaphroditism with somatic chromosomal anomaly in association with

in utero exposure to danazol. Am J Obstet Gynecol 142:708-709, 1982. [C]

Quagliarello J, Greco MA: Danazol and urogenital sinus formation in pregnancy. Fertil Steril 43(6):939-942, 1985. [C]

Rosa FW: Virilization of the female fetus with maternal danazol exposure. Am J Obstet Gynecol 149:99-100, 1984. [S]

Schwartz RP: Ambiguous genitalia in a term female infant due to exposure to danazol in utero. Am J Dis Child 136:474, 1982. [C]

Shaw RW, Farquhar JW: Female pseudohermaphroditism associated with danazol exposure in utero. Case report. Br J Obstet Gynaecol 91:386-389, 1984. [C]

Wentz AC: Adverse effects of danazol in pregnancy. Ann Intern Med 96:672-673, 1982. [R]

DANTHRON

Synonyms

Antrapurol, Chrysazin, Dantron, Dianthon, Dioxyanthrachinonum, Dorbane, Duolax, Roydan, Solven

Summary

Danthron is an anthraquinone laxative that is administered orally. It is often formulated in combination with docusate. Danthron is absorbed from the gastrointestinal tract.

Magnitude of Teratogenic Risk

Undetermined

Quality and Quantity of Data

None To Poor

Comment

A small risk cannot be excluded, but a high risk of congenital anomalies in the children of women treated with danthron during pregnancy is unlikely.

No epidemiological studies of congenital anomalies among infants born to women treated with danthron during pregnancy have been reported.

No teratogenic effect was observed among the offspring of pregnant rats treated with a danthron and docusate combination in doses 8-120 times those used in humans (Ichikawa & Yamamoto, 1980).

Key References

Ichikawa Y, Yamamoto Y: [Teratology study of solvents in rats]. Gendai Iryo 12:819-831, 1980. [A]

DAPSONE

Synonyms

Avlosulfon, Dermosone, Diaminodiphenylsulfone, Diaphenylsulfone, Disulone, Dubronax, Servidapson, Sulfona, Sulphadione, Sulphonyldianiline

Summary

Dapsone is a sulfone used in the treatment of dermatitis herpetiformis, malaria, and leprosy.

Magnitude of Teratogenic Risk

Undetermined

Quality and Quantity of Data

None

Comment

None

No epidemiological studies of congenital anomalies in infants born to women treated with dapsone during pregnancy have been reported.

No animal teratology studies of dapsone have been published.

Key References

None available.

DAUNORUBICIN

Synonyms

Acetyladriamycin, Cerubidine, Daunoblastin, Daunomycin, Leukaemomycin C, Ondena, Rubidomycin, Rubidomycine, Rubomycin C

Summary

Daunorubicin is an anthracycline glycoside antibiotic that is administered intravenously in the treatment of leukemia and other neoplasms. Daunorubicin appears to act by interfering with nucleic acid synthesis.

Magnitude of Teratogenic Risk

Small To Moderate

Quality and Quantity of Data

Poor To Fair

Comment

Because this is a cytotoxic agent, adverse effects may occur at any time during pregnancy.

No epidemiological studies of congenital anomalies among the infants of women treated with daunorubicin during pregnancy have been reported. Only two congenital defects (adherence of the iris to the lens in one child and polydactyly, which was familial, in another) were noted among 35 fetuses or infants of women treated with daunorubicin and other cancer chemotherapeutic agents during pregnancy (Sears & Reid, 1976; Gokal et al., 1976; Lillyman et al., 1977; Lowenthal et al., 1978; Gstottner et al., 1978; Kurshid & Saleen, 1978; Okun et al., 1979; Coser et al., 1979; Doney et al., 1979; Hamer et al., 1979; O'Donnell et al.,

1979; Schaison et al., 1979; Colbert et al., 1980; Tobias & Bloom, 1980; Alegre et al., 1982; Cantini & Yanes, 1984; Catanzarite & Ferguson, 1984; Reynoso et al., 1987; Volkenandt et al., 1987; Feliu et al., 1988; Turchi & Villasis, 1988). Only four patients have been reported who received chemotherapy during the first trimester of pregnancy; two of these women had apparently normal babies and two suffered spontaneous abortions within three weeks of treatment (Alegre et al., 1982; Zuazu et al., 1991). Many of the infants were born prematurely, and transient neonatal anemia, neutropenia, or pancytopenia was often observed in them (Okun et al., 1979; Doney et al., 1979; Colbert et al., 1980; Catanzarite & Ferguson, 1984; Reynoso et al., 1987). One infant born to a woman who received daunorubicin therapy during the third trimester of pregnancy was stillborn and exhibited diffuse myocardial necrosis (Schaison et al., 1979); this finding is of particular concern because daunorubicin is known to cause cardiac damage in children and adults.

Increased frequencies of fetal death and of malformations of the heart, eye, and genitourinary tract were observed among the offspring of rats treated during pregnancy with 1-4 times the human therapeutic dose of daunorubicin (Roux & Taillemite, 1969; Thompson et al., 1978). This treatment was also toxic to the mothers. No teratogenic effect was observed among the offspring of rabbits treated with less than the usual human dose of daunorubicin during pregnancy (Thompson et al., 1978).

Acquired structural chromosome abnormalities were observed in the cord blood of a clinically normal infant whose mother was treated with daunorubicin and other antineoplastic agents throughout the last half of pregnancy (Schleuning & Clemm, 1987). Genotoxic damage (an increased frequency of micronuclei) was induced in blastocysts of pregnant rats treated with 10 times the human dose of daunorubicin (Ornaghi & Giavini, 1989). The clinical significance of these observations is unknown.

Key References

Alegre A, Chunchurreta R, Rodriguez-Alarcon J, Cruz E, et al.: Successful pregnancy in acute promyelocytic leukemia. Cancer 49:152-153, 1982. [C]

Cantini E, Yanes B: Acute myelogenous leukemia in pregnancy. South Med J 77:1050-1052, 1984. [C]

Catanzarite VA, Ferguson JE II: Acute leukemia and pregnancy: A review of management and outcome, 1972-1982. Obstet Gynecol Surv 39:663-678, 1984. [C]

Colbert N, Najman A, Gorin NC, Blum F, et al.: Acute leukaemia during pregnancy: Favourable course of pregnancy in two patients treated with cytosine arabinoside and anthracyclines. Nouv Presse Med 9:175-178, 1980. [C]

Coser P, Prinroth O, Fabris P, et al.: Normales neugerborenes nach zytostatischer therapie bei akuter promyelozytenleukamie in der schwangerschaft. Blut 38:483, 1979. [C]

Doney KC, Kraemer KG, Shepard TH: Combination chemotherapy for acute myelocytic leukemia during pregnancy: Three case reports. Cancer Treat Rep 63:369-371, 1979. [C]

Feliu J, Juarez S, Ordonez A, et al.: Acute leukemia and pregnancy. Cancer 61:580-584, 1988. [C]

Gokal R, Durrant J, Baum JD, Bennett MJ: Successful pregnancy in acute monocytic leukaemia. Br J Cancer 34:299-302, 1976. [C]

Gstottner M, Frisch H, Dienstl FP: Delivery of a normal child after chemotherapy of acute promyelocytic leukaemia during pregnancy. Blut 36:171-174, 1978. [C]

Hamer JW, Beard MEJ, Duff GB: Pregnancy complicated by acute myeloid leukaemia. NZ Med J 89:212-213, 1979. [C]

Kurshid M, Saleen M: Acute leukemia in pregnancy. Lancet 2:534, 1978. [C]

Lillyman JS, Hill AS, Anderton KJ: Consequences of acute myelogenous leukemia in early pregnancy. Cancer 40:1300-1307, 1977. [C] & [R]

Lowenthal RM, Marsden KA, Newman NM, MJ Baikie, et al.: Normal infant after treatment of acute myeloid leukaemia in pregnancy with daunorubicin. Aust NZ J Med 8:431-432, 1978. [C]

O'Donnell R, Costigan C, O'Connell LG: Two cases of acute leukaemia in pregnancy. Acta Haemat 61:298-300, 1979. [C]

Okun DB, Groncy PK, Sieger L, Tanaka K: Acute leukemia in pregnancy: Transient neonatal myelosuppression after combination chemotherapy in the mother. Med Pediatr Oncol 7:315-319, 1979. [C]

Ornaghi F, Giavini E: Induction of micronuclei in pre-implantation rat embryos in vivo. Mutat Res 225:71-74, 1989. [A]

Reynoso EE, Shepherd FA, Messner HA, et al.: Acute leukemia during pregnancy: The Toronto leukemia study group experience with long-term follow-up of children exposed in utero to chemotherapeutic agents. J Clin Oncol 5:1098-1106, 1987. [C] & [R]

Roux C, Taillemite JL: Teratogenic action by rubidomycin in the rat. C R Soc Biol 163:1299-1302, 1969. [A]

Schaison G, Jacquillat C, Auclerc G, Weil M: Les risques foeto-embryonnaires des chimiotherapies. Bull Cancer 66:165, 1979. [C]

Schleuning M, Clemm C: Chromosomal aberrations in a newborn whose mother received cytotoxic treatment during pregnancy. N Engl J Med 317:1666-1667, 1987. [C]

Sears HF, Reid J: Granulocytic sarcoma. Cancer 37:1808-1813, 1976. [C]

Thompson DJ, Molello JA, Strebing RJ, Dyke IL: Teratogenicity of adriamycin and daunomycin in the rat and rabbit. Teratology 17:151-157, 1978. [A]

Tobias JS, Bloom HJG: Doxorubicin in pregnancy. Lancet 1:776, 1980. [C]

Turchi JJ, Villasis C: Anthracyclines in the treatment of malignancy in pregnancy. Cancer 61:435-440, 1988. [C] & [R]

Volkenandt M, Buchner T, Hiddemann W, van de Loo J: Acute leukaemia during pregnancy. Lancet 2:1521-1522, 1987. [C]

Zuazu J, Julia A, Sierra J, et al.: Pregnancy outcome in hematologic malignancies. Cancer 67:703-709, 1991. [S]

DEFEROXAMINE

Synonyms

Deferoxamide B, Deferoxamine Mesylate, Deferrioxamine B, Desferal, Desferal Mesylate, Desferan, Desferex, Desferin, Desferrioxamine B, Desferrioxamine Mesylate

Summary

Deferoxamine is an iron chelating agent. It is used in the treatment of acute iron intoxication and chronic iron overload. Oral preparations are poorly absorbed from the gastrointestinal tract.

Magnitude of Teratogenic Risk

None To Minimal

Quality and Quantity of Data

Poor

Comment

None

No epidemiological studies of congenital anomalies in infants born to women treated with deferoxamine during pregnancy have been reported. A few women who attempted suicide with iron tablets at various times during pregnancy and were treated with deferoxamine have been reported (Rayburn et al., 1983; Blanc et al., 1984; Olenmark et al., 1987; van Ameyde & Tenenbein, 1989; Tenenbein et al., 1989). None of their infants had congenital anomalies. Similarly, a normal infant was born to a woman treated with deferoxamine chronically during the first trimester of pregnancy for thalassemia (Thomas & Skalicka, 1980).

The frequency of fetal resorptions was not increased among the offspring of mice treated during pregnancy with 4-7 times the human dose of deferoxamine (Gower et al., 1990; Wells et al., 1991).

Key References

Blanc P, Hryhorczuk D, Danel I: Deferoxamine treatment of acute iron intoxication in pregnancy. Obstet Gynecol 64:12S-14S, 1984. [C]

Gower JD, Baldock RJ, O'Sullivan AM, et al.: Protection against endotoxin-induced foetal resorption in mice by desferrioxamine and ebselen. Int J Exp Pathol 71:433-440, 1990. [A]

Olenmark M, Biber B, Dottori O, Rybo G: Fatal iron intoxication in late pregnancy. J Toxicol Clin Toxicol 25:347-359, 1987. [C]

Rayburn WF, Donn SM, Wulf ME: Iron overdose during pregnancy: Successful therapy with deferoxamine. Am J Obstet Gynecol 147:717-718, 1983. [C]

Tenenbein M: Iron overdose during pregnancy. Vet Hum Toxicol 31(4):346, 1989. [S]

Thomas RM, Skalicka AE: Successful pregnancy in transfusion-dependent thalassaemia. Arch Dis Child 55:572-574, 1980. [C]

van Ameyde KJ, Tenenbein M: Whole bowel irrigation during pregnancy. Am J Obstet Gynecol 160:646-647, 1989. [C]

Wells PG, Davidovich O, Mark TM: Inhibition of murine phenytoin teratogenicity by the iron chelator deferoxamine. Toxicologist 11(1):293, 1991. [A]

DEHYDROCHOLIC ACID

Synonyms

Atrocholin, Cholan-DH, Chologon, Decholin, Hepahydrin, Idrocrine, Ketocholanic Acid, Medichol, Neocholan, Oxycholin, Triketocholanic Acid

Summary

Dehydrocholic acid is a semisynthetic bile acid. It is used to stimulate bile flow after gallbladder surgery and as a laxative.

Magnitude of Teratogenic Risk

Undetermined

Quality and Quantity of Data

None To Poor

Comment

A small risk cannot be excluded, but a high risk of congenital anomalies in the children of women treated with dehydrocholic acid during pregnancy is unlikely.

No epidemiological studies of congenital anomalies among the infants of women treated with dehydrocholic acid during pregnancy have been reported.

No teratogenic effect was observed among the offspring of rats or mice treated during pregnancy with dehydrocholic acid in doses 2-50 or 50 times those used in human (Skamoto & Ichihara, 1976).

Key References

Skamoto I, Ichihara K: Effects of dehychol on pregnant maternal bodies and embryos. Yonago Igaku Zasshi 27:111-121, 1976. [A]

DEMECARIUM

Synonyms

Bromure de Demecarium, Frumtosnil, Humorsol, Tonilen, Tosmicil, Tosmilen, Tosmilene, Visumatic, Visumiotic

Summary

Demecarium is a cholinesterase inhibitor used in topical ophthalmic preparations for treatment of glaucoma and strabismus.

Magnitude of Teratogenic Risk

Undetermined

Quality and Quantity of Data

None

Comment

A small risk cannot be excluded, but a high risk of congenital anomalies in the children of women treated with demecarium during pregnancy is unlikely.

No epidemiological studies of congenital anomalies among infants born to women treated with demecarium during pregnancy have been reported.

No mammalian teratology studies of demecarium have been published.

Please see agent summary on atropine for information on a related agent that has been more thoroughly studied.

Key References

None available.

DEMECLOCYCLINE

Synonyms

Actaciclina, Declomycin, Deme-Proter, Demethylchlortetracycline, Ledermicina, Ledermycin, Magis-Ciclina, Methylchlortetracycline, Mirciclina, Rynabron, Veraciclina

Summary

Demeclocycline, an antibiotic related to tetracycline, is administered orally in the treatment of bacterial and protozoal infections. It also inhibits antidiuretic hormone-induced water reabsorption and is used in the treatment of inappropriate ADH secretion.

Magnitude of Teratogenic Risk

Dental Staining: Small To Moderate

Malformations: None To Minimal

Quality and Quantity of Data

Dental Staining: Fair To Good

Malformations: Poor To Fair

Comment

None

The frequency of congenital anomalies was no greater than expected among the children of 90 women who were treated with demeclocycline during the first four lunar months of pregnancy or among the children of 280 women who were treated with this medication anytime in pregnancy in the Collaborative Perinatal Project (Heinonen et al., 1977).

Staining of the deciduous teeth has been observed in five children born to mothers who were treated with demeclocycline during the third trimester of pregnancy (Macaulay & Leistyna, 1964). This is similar to the dental staining observed with other antibiotics of the tetracycline class (Toaff & Ravid, 1966; Cohlan, 1977).

An increased frequency of congenital anomalies was observed among the offspring of pregnant mice treated with 6-12 times the human therapeutic dose of demeclocycline (Mangi et al., 1969).

Please see agent summary on tetracycline for information on a related drug that has been more thoroughly studied.

Key References

Cohlan SQ: Tetracycline staining of teeth. Teratology 15:27-130, 1977. [R]

Heinonen OP, Slone D, Shapiro S: Birth Defects and Drugs in Pregnancy. Littleton, Mass.: John Wright-PSG, 1977, pp 297-298, 301, 313, 435, 472, 485. [E]

Mangi Y, Mizutani M, Kaziwara R: Effects of demethylchortetracycline hydrochloride on the fetuses of experimental animals. I. Observation by cesarean section of CF1 mice at term (Personal communication), 1969. In: Nishimura H, Tanimura T (eds). Clinical Aspects of the Teratogenicity of Drugs. New York: American Elsevier Publishing Co, 1976, p 125. [A]

Macaulay JC, Leistyna JA: Preliminary observations on the prenatal administration of demethylchlortetracycline HCl. Pediatrics 34:423-424, 1964. [C]

Toaff R, Ravid R: Tetracyclines and the teeth. Lancet 2:281-282, 1966. [S]

DENOFUNGIN

Summary

Denofungin is an antibacterial and antifungal agent.

Magnitude of Teratogenic Risk

Undetermined

Quality and Quantity of Data

None

Comment

None

No epidemiological studies of congenital anomalies in infants born to women who used denofungin during pregnancy have been reported.

No animal teratology studies of denofungin have been published.

Key References

None available.

DESLANOSIDE

Synonyms

Cedilanid D, Deacetyllanatoside C, Desacetyl-Lanatoside C, Deslanatoside C

Summary

Deslanoside is a cardiac glycoside used to treat cardiac failure and dysrhythmias.

Magnitude of Teratogenic Risk

Undetermined

Quality and Quantity of Data

None

Comment

None

No epidemiological studies of congenital anomalies in infants born to women treated with deslanoside during pregnancy have been reported.

No animal teratology studies of deslanoside have been published.

Please see agent summary on digoxin for information on a related drug that has been studied.

Key References

None available.

DESMOPRESSIN

Synonyms

Adiuretin SD, Dav Ritter, DDAVP, Demopressin Acetate, Desmospray, Minirin, Minirin/DDAVP, Minurin, Stimate

Summary

Desmopressin is a synthetic antidiuretic hormone. It is administered intranasally or parenterally in the diagnosis and treatment of diabetes insipidus. Desmopressin is also used in the management of mild hemophilia and von Willebrand's disease.

Magnitude of Teratogenic Risk

Undetermined

None To Poor

Comment

None

No epidemiological studies of congenital anomalies in infants born to women treated with desmopressin during pregnancy have been reported. Three infants with congenital anomalies have been reported who were born to women treated throughout pregnancy with desmopressin for diabetes insipidus (Linder et al., 1986). One of these infants had Down's syndrome, another had complex congenital heart disease, and the third had growth retardation and developmental delay. A causal relationship has not been established.

No animal teratology studies of desmopressin have been published. Decreased renal concentrating ability was observed among the offspring of rats made hypotonic during pregnancy by administration of desmopressin in doses more than 100 times those used in humans (Lichardus et al., 1983).

Key References

Linder N, Matoth I, Ohel G, Yourish D, et al.: L-deamino-8-d-arginine vasopressin treatment in pregnancy and neonatal outcome: A report of three cases. Am J Perinatol 3:165-167, 1986. [C]

Lichardus B, Szaboova A, Foldes O, Ponec J, et al.: The impairment of osmoregulation in the rat offsprings of hyperadiuretic mothers is probably of renal nature. Exp Clin Endocrinol 82:107-110, 1983. [A]

DESONIDE

Synonyms

Apolar, Desfluorotriamcinolone, Desowen, Locapred, Prednacinolone, Sine-Fluor, Sterax, Steroderm, Topifug, Tridesilon

Summary

Desonide is a topical corticosteriod used to treat inflammatory and pruritic dermatoses.

Magnitude of Teratogenic Risk

Undetermined

Quality and Quantity of Data

None

Comment

A small risk cannot be excluded, but a high risk of congenital anomalies in the children of women treated with desonide during pregnancy is unlikely.

No epidemiological studies of congenital anomalies in infants born to women treated with desonide during pregnancy have been reported.

No animal teratology studies of desonide have been published.

Please see agent summary on triamcinolone for information on a related agent that has been studied.

Key References

None available.

DESOXIMETASONE

Synonyms

Actiderm, Desoxymethasone, Flubason, Ibaril, Stiedex, Topicort, Topiderm, Topisolon

Summary

Desoximetasone is a synthetic corticosteroid used topically to treat dermatologic disorders.

Magnitude of Teratogenic Risk

Undetermined

Quality and Quantity of Data

None To Poor

Comment

None

No epidemiological studies of congenital anomalies in infants born after maternal exposure to desoximetasone during pregnancy have been published.

The frequency of malformations was not increased among the offspring of rats and mice born of mothers subcutaneously injected with about 1-2 times the usual human topical dose of desoximetasone during pregnancy. At doses about 8 times that used topically in humans, cleft palate was induced in mice, but such doses were toxic to the mothers (Miyamoto et al., 1975).

Please see agent summary on cortisone for information on a related drug that has been more thoroughly studied.

Key References

Miyamoto M, Ohtsu M, Sugisaki T, Sakaguchi T: [Teratogenic effect of 9-fluoro-11-beta, 21-dihydroxy-16-alpha-methylpregna-1, 4-diene-3, 20-dione (A 41 304), a new anti-inflammatory agent, and of dexamethasone in rats and mice]. Nippon Yakurigaku Zasshi (Folia Pharmacol Japon) 71:367-378, 1975. [A]

DEXAMETHASONE

Synonyms

Aeroseb-Dex, Ak-Dex, Dalalone, Decaderm, Decadron, Decasone, Deronil, Deseronil, Dexasone, Dexone, Hexadrol, Maxidex, Oradexon, Respihaler Decadron

Summary

Dexamethasone is a synthetic adrenocortical steroid that is used to treat a variety of inflammatory and allergic disorders. Intravenous doses of dexamethasone up to 10 times those conventionally used orally are sometimes employed to treat shock. Substantial systemic absorption of dexamethasone from topical preparations may occur.

Magnitude of Teratogenic Risk

None To Minimal

Quality and Quantity of Data

Poor To Fair

Comment

Chronic use of dexamethasone at high doses may be associated with fetal growth retardation.

No epidemiological studies of congenital anomalies among infants born to women treated with dexamethasone early in pregnancy have been reported.

Dexamethasone treatment of pregnant women has been used to provide fetal therapy for congenital virilizing adrenal hyperplasia due to a genetic defect of 21-hydroxylase. Such therapy appears to prevent virilization of some female fetuses affected with this disease (David & Forest, 1984; Forest et al., 1989; Pang et al., 1990). No teratogenic effect of the therapy has been noted among these infants, a few of whom have been treated in the first trimester of gestation.

Maternal dexamethasone therapy in the late second or third trimester of pregnancy has been used to accelerate fetal lung maturation and prevent respiratory distress syndrome in prematurely born infants (Cosmi & DiRenzo, 1989; Roberts & Morrison, 1991). No growth, physical, motor, or developmental deficiencies attributable to such prenatal therapy were observed in a three-year follow-up study of 200 children delivered to treated women (Collaborative Group on Antenatal Steroid Therapy, 1984).

Scalp aplasia was observed among the offspring of rhesus monkeys treated in early pregnancy with dexamethasone in doses similar to or several times greater than those used in humans (Jerome & Hendrickx, 1988). Cranium bifidum occurred in one of the monkeys with scalp defects. Fetal weight and head circumference were reduced and dose-dependent alterations of brain histology were observed among the offspring of rhesus monkeys treated late in pregnancy with dexamethasone in doses within the human therapeutic range (Novy & Walsh, 1983; Uno et al., 1990).

Increased frequency of cleft palate occurs among the offspring of mice treated during pregnancy with 4-10 times the maximal human dose of dexamethasone (Pinsky & DiGeorge, 1965; Natsume et al., 1986). Fetal growth retardation and neonatal immune deficiency have been reported among the offspring of mice treated during pregnancy with dexamethasone in doses similar to those conventionally used in the treatment of asthma and inflammatory diseases in humans (Eishi et al., 1983). Increased frequencies of palatal, cardiac, and abdominal wall defects were observed among the offspring of rats treated during pregnancy with dexamethasone in doses within the human therapeutic range or several times greater (Vannier & Bremaud, 1985). Fetal and neonatal growth retardation were observed in other studies of the offspring of pregnant rats treated with dexamethasone in doses within the human therapeutic range (Garvey & Scott, 1981; Steiss et al., 1989). Congenital myopathy and fetal growth retardation were found among the offspring of minipigs treated during pregnancy with dexamethasone in doses similar to those conventionally used in the treatment of asthma and inflammatory diseases in humans (Jirmanova & Lojda, 1985).

Please see agent summary on prednisone/prednisolone for information on a related agent that has been more thoroughly studied.

Key References

Collaborative Group on Antenatal Steroid Therapy: Effects of antenatal dexamethasone administration in the infant: Long-term follow-up. J Pediatr 104(2):259-267, 1984. [E]

Cosmi EV, Di Renzo GC: Prevention and treatment of fetal lung immaturity. Fetal Ther 4(Suppl 1):52-62, 1989. [R]

David M, Forest MG: Prenatal treatment of congenital adrenal hyperplasia resulting from 21-hydroxylase deficiency. J Pediatr 105(5):799-803, 1984. [C]

Eishi Y, Hirokawa K, Hatakeyama S: Long-lasting impairment of immune and endocrine systems of offspring induced by injection of dexamethasone into pregnant mice. Clin Immunol Immunopathol 26:335-349, 1983. [A]

Forest MG, Betuel H, David M: Prenatal treatment in congenital adrenal hyperplasia due to 21-hydroxylase deficiency: Up-date 88 of the French Multicentric Study. Endocr Res 15(1&2):277-301, 1989. [S]

Garvey D, Scott J: Placental and fetal contra-indications of dexamethasone administration to pregnant rats. Experientia 37:6-8, 1981. [A]

Jerome CP, Hendrickx AG: Comparative teratogenicity of triamcinolone acetonide and dexamethasone in the rhesus monkey (Macaca mulatta). J Med Primatol 17:195-203, 1988. [A]

Jirmanova I, Lojda L: Dexamethasone applied to pregnant minisows induces splayleg in minipiglets. Zentralbl Veterinaermed Reihe A 32:445-458, 1985. [A]

Natsume N, Narukawa T, Kawai T: Teratogenesis of dexamethasone and preventive effect of vitamin B12. Int J Oral Maxillofac Surg 15:752-755, 1986. [A]

Novy MJ, Walsh SW: Dexamethasone and estradiol treatment in pregnant rhesus macaques: Effects on gestational length, maternal plasma hormones, and fetal growth. Am J Obstet Gynecol 145(8):920-931, 1983. [A]

Pang S, Pollack MS, Marshall RN, Immken L: Prenatal treatment of congenital adrenal hyperplasia due to 21-hydroxylase deficiency. N Engl J Med 322(2):111-115, 1990. [C] & [R]

Pinsky L, DiGeorge AM: Cleft palate in the mouse: A teratogenic index of glucocorticoid potency. Science 147:402-403, 1965. [A]

Roberts WE, Morrison JC: Pharmacologic induction of fetal lung maturity. Clin Obstet Gynecol 34(2):319-327, 1991. [R]

Steiss JE, Wright JC, Cox NR: Effects of perinatal high dose dexamethasone on skeletal muscle development in rats. Can J Vet Res 53:17-22, 1989. [A]

Uno H, Lohmiller L, Thieme C, et al.: Brain damage induced by prenatal exposure to dexamethasone in fetal rhesus macaques. I. Hippocampus. Dev Brain Res 53:157-167, 1990. [A]

Vannier B, Bremaud R: Induction of heart defects in the rat foetus with dexamethasone. Teratology 32(2):35A, 1985. [A]

DEXIVACAINE

Synonyms

Dexivacaina, Dexivacainum

Summary

Dexivacaine is a local anesthetic agent.

Magnitude of Teratogenic Risk

Undetermined

Quality and Quantity of Data

None

Comment

None

No epidemiological studies of congenital anomalies in children born to women exposed to dexivacaine during pregnancy have been reported.

No investigations of teratologic effects of dexivacaine in experimental animals have been published.

Key References

None available.

DEXPANTHENOL

Synonyms

Bepanten, D-Panthenol, Dexol, Ilopan, Panthoderm, Pantothenyl Alcohol

Summary

Dexpanthenol is the alcohol of pantothenic acid, a B vitamin, to which it is readily converted in the body. Dexpanthenol is given parenterally in large doses (100-200 times the U.S. recommended daily allowance) to prevent paralytic ileus and related disorders of gastrointestinal motility. Dexpanthenol is used in much smaller doses in vitamin supplements, topical dermatologic preparations, and cosmetics.

Magnitude of Teratogenic Risk

Undetermined

Quality and Quantity of Data

None

Comment

A small risk cannot be excluded, but a high risk of congenital anomalies in the children of women treated with dexpanthenol during pregnancy is unlikely.

No epidemiological studies of congenital anomalies in infants born to women treated with dexpanthenol during pregnancy have been reported.

No animal teratology studies of dexpanthenol have been published.

Key References

None available.

DEXTRANOMER

Synonyms

Debrisan, Debrisorb, Wound Cleaning Beads, Wound Cleaning Paste

Summary

Dextranomer is a polymer of dextran that is used to absorb fluids and thus promote healing in wounds.

Magnitude of Teratogenic Risk

Undetermined

Quality and Quantity of Data

None

Comment

A small risk cannot be excluded, but a high risk of congenital anomalies in the children of women treated with dextranomer during pregnancy is unlikely.

No epidemiological studies of congenital anomalies among infants born to women treated with dextranomer during pregnancy have been reported.

No animal teratology studies of dextranomer have been published.

Key References

None available.

DEXTROAMPHETAMINE

Synonyms

Amphetamine, Dexampex, Dexamphetamine, Dexedrine, Ferndex, Maxiton, Speed, Synatan, Uppers

Summary

Dextroamphetamine is a sympathomimetic agent and central nervous system stimulant. It is used as a stimulant, an anorectic, and in the treatment of narcolepsy.

Magnitude of Teratogenic Risk

Minimal

Quality and Quantity of Data

Fair To Good

Comment

None

The frequencies of congenital anomalies, of major malformations, and of minor anomalies were no greater than expected among the children of 367 women who took dextroamphetamine during the first four lunar months of pregnancy in the Collaborative Perinatal Project (Heinonen et al., 1977). Similarly, no association was observed with congenital anomalies in other cohort studies involving 52 children born to mothers who took dextroamphetamine or 347 children born to mothers who took some drug in the amphetamine group early in pregnancy (Nora et al., 1967; Milkovich & van den Berg, 1977). The frequency of congenital anomalies was not increased among the children of 1069 women who took dextroamphetamine anytime during pregnancy or 1694 children of women who took a drug of the amphetamine class anytime during pregnancy (Heinonen et al., 1983; Milkovich & van den Berg, 1977).

The results of case-control studies have been less consistent. Use of dextroamphetamine during early pregnancy was found more frequently than expected among the mothers of 458 infants with a variety of congenital anomalies (Nelson & Forfar, 1971) and among the mothers of 184 children with cardiovascular malformations (Nora et al., 1970). A history of maternal dextroamphetamine use during the period of fetal bile duct formation was observed with unusually high frequency among 11 infants with primary biliary atresia (Levin, 1971). The clinical importance of these observations is brought into question by their inconsistency with cohort studies.

Increased frequencies of fetal death and cardiac, skeletal, eye and other malformations have been reported among the offspring of mice treated with 80-160 times the dose of dextroamphetamine used in humans (Nora et al., 1965; Fein et al., 1987), but such doses are also toxic to the mothers. Persistent behavioral alterations occur among the offspring of mice and rats treated with dextroamphetamine during pregnancy in doses equivalent to and greater than those used in humans (Middaugh et al., 1974; Hitzemann et al., 1976; Adams et al., 1982; Holson et al., 1985). The relevance of these findings to the clinical use of dextroamphetamine in human pregnancy is uncertain.

Key References

Adams J, Buelke-Sam J, Kimmel CA, LaBorde JB: Behavioral alterations in rats prenatally exposed to low doses of d-amphetamine. Neurobehav Toxicol Teratol 4:63-70, 1982. [A]

Fein A, Shviro Y, Manoach M, Nebel L: Teratogenic effects of d-amphetamine sulphate: Histodifferentiation and electrocardiogram pattern of mouse embryonic heart. Teratology 35:27-34, 1987. [A]

Heinonen OP, Slone D, Shapiro S: Birth Defects and Drugs in Pregnancy. Littleton, Mass.: John Wright-PSG, 1977, pp. 346, 347, 350, 353, 355, 459, 491. [E]

Hitzemann BA, Hitzemann RJ, Brase DA, Loh HH: Influence of prenatal d-amphetamine administration on development and behavior of rats. Life Sci 18:605-612, 1976. [A]

Holson R, Adams J, Buelkje-Sam J, Gough B, et al.: d-amphetamine as a behavioral teratogen: Effects depend on dose, sex, age and task. Neurobehav Toxicol Teratol 7:753-758, 1985. [A]

Levin JN: Amphetamine ingestion with biliary atresia. J Pediatr 79(1):130-131, 1971. [S]

Middaugh LD, Blackwell LA, Santos III CA, Zemp JW: Effects of d-amphetamine sulfate given to pregnant mice on activity and on catecholamines in the brains of offspring. Dev Psychobiol 7(5):429-438, 1974. [A]

Milkovich L, van den Berg BJ: Effects of antenatal exposure to anorectic drugs. Am J Obstet Gynecol 129:637-642, 1977. [E]

Nelson MM, Forfar JO: Associations between drugs administered during pregnancy and congenital abnormalities of the fetus. Brit Med J 1:523-527, 1971. [E]

Nora JJ, McNamara DG, Fraser FC. Dexamphetamine sulfate and human malformations. Lancet 1:570-571, 1967. [E]

Nora JJ, Trasler DG, Fraser FC: Malformations in mice induced by dexamphetamine sulphate. Lancet 2:1021-1022, 1965. [A]

DEXTROMETHORPHAN

Synonyms

Balminil D.M., Benylin DM, Broncho-Grippol-DM, Brontyl, Cosylan, Delsym, Dextrorphan, DM Syrup, Hold, Pediacare-1, Robidex, Sedatuss

Summary

Dextromethorphan is an antitussive that is a component of many widely used cough medicines.

Magnitude of Teratogenic Risk

None

Quality and Quantity of Data

Poor To Fair

Comment

None

The frequencies of malformations in general, of major malformations, and of minor malformations were no greater than expected among the offspring of 300 women who used dextromethorphan during the first four lunar months of pregnancy in the Collaborative Perinatal Project (Heinonen et al., 1977). Similarly, in another cohort study that included 59 women who used dextromethorphan during the first trimester of pregnancy, the frequency of malformations in the infants was no greater than expected (Aselton et al., 1985). No association with congenital anomalies in the infants was observed among 580 women who took dextromethorphan anytime during pregnancy in the Collaborative Perinatal Project (Heinonen et al., 1977). The observation that of five women who gave birth to infants with agenesis of the cloacal membrane, all four who had respiratory symptoms during the first trimester of pregancy may have taken a cough medicine containing dextromethorphan is unlikely to be of causal significance, given the frequency of such illness and treatment in normal pregnancies (Robinson & Tross, 1984).

No teratology studies of dextromethorphan in experimental animals have been published.

Key References

Aselton P, Jick H, Milunsky A, Hunter JR, et al.: First-trimester drug use and congenital disorders. Obstet Gynecol 65:451-455, 1985. [S]

Heinonen OP, Slone D, Shapiro S: Birth Defects and Drugs in Pregnancy. Littleton, Mass.: John Wright-PSG, 1977, pp 379, 496. [E]

Robinson HB, Tross K: Agenesis of the cloacal membrane. A probable teratogenic anomaly. Perspect Pediatr Pathol 8:79-96, 1984. [S]

DEXTROTHYROXINE

Synonyms

Biotirmone, D-Thyroxine Sodium, Dethyrona, Dynothel, Lisolipin, Nadrothyron D, Travenon

Summary

Dextrothyroxine is the dextrorotatory stereoisomer of thyroxine. It is administered orally as an antilipidemic agent.

Magnitude of Teratogenic Risk

Undetermined

Quality and Quantity of Data

None

Comment

None

No epidemiological studies of congenital anomalies in infants whose mothers were treated with dextrothyroxine during pregnancy have been reported.

No animal teratology studies of dextrothyroxine have been published.

Please see agent summary on thyroxine for information on a related agent that has been more thoroughly studied.

Key References

None available.

DIAMOCAINE

Synonyms

Diamocaine Cyclamate

Summary

Diamocaine is a local anesthetic of the ester class.

Magnitude of Teratogenic Risk

Undetermined

Quality and Quantity of Data

None

Comment

None

No epidemiological studies of congenital anomalies in children born to women exposed to diamocaine during pregnancy have been reported.

No investigations of teratologic effects of diamocaine in experimental animals have been published.

Please see agent summary on procaine for information on a related drug that has been more thoroughly studied.

Key References

None available.

DIAZEPAM

Synonyms

Apozepam, E-Pam, Meval, Neo-Calme, Novodipam, Rival, Valium, Valrelease, Vivol

Summary

Diazepam is a widely used benzodiazepine. It is employed as a tranquilizer, skeletal muscle relaxant, preoperative medication, and adjunct to anticonvulsants in the treatment of seizures.

Magnitude of Teratogenic Risk

Minimal

Quality and Quantity of Data

Good

Comment

Neonatal behavioral alterations have been observed in infants born to women treated with diazepam during pregnancy, but it is not known what, if any, implications this has for long-term development of these children (see below).

Available epidemiological data regarding the risk of malformations among children born to women who took diazepam during pregnancy are inconsistent. The frequency of congenital anomalies was not increased among the infants of more than 150 women who took diazepam during the first trimester of pregnancy in two cohorts of the Boston Collaborative Drug Surveillance Program or among the infants of 60 women so treated in a French study (Jick et al., 1981; Crombie et al., 1975; Aselton et al., 1985). No association with maternal use of diazepam during pregnancy was seen in a case-control study involving 417 children with multiple congenital anomalies (Czeizel, 1988). In contrast, maternal use of diazepam during the first trimester of pregnancy was reported almost three times more frequently than expected in a case-control study involving 1427 children with various congenital anomalies (Bracken & Holford, 1981) and almost eight times more frequently than expected in another case-control study involving 222 affected children (Restrepo et al., 1990).

No association with maternal use of diazepam during the first trimester of pregnancy was found among the mothers of 611 children with oral clefts in a case-control study that was designed specifically to test the hypothesis that first-trimester exposure to diazepam increases the risk of cleft lip with or without cleft palate or of cleft palate alone (Rosenberg, 1983). This finding is supported by three other case-control studies involving 194, 522, and 1201 children with oral clefts, respectively (Saxen, 1975b; Czeizel, 1988), and by a cohort study in which the frequency of oral clefts was not increased among the children of 854 women who took diazepam during the first trimester of pregnancy (Shiono & Mills, 1984). The negative results in these studies cast doubt on a causal basis for previously reported associations with maternal use of diazepam or other benzodiazepines during the first trimester of pregnancy in 599, 111, and 49 children with oral clefts (Saxen, 1975a; Safra & Oakley, 1975; Aarskog, 1975).

Two case-control studies involving 383 and 390 children with cardiovascular malformations have suggested an association with maternal use of diazepam or related drugs during the first trimester of pregnancy (Rothman et al., 1979; Bracken & Holford, 1981). However, Bracken (1986) reanalyzed the data from his study and failed to find a significant association, and Rothman reported that no association was found in a follow-up study of another 298 children with congenital heart disease (Zierler & Rothman, 1985). No association with maternal use of diazepam during the first trimester of pregnancy was seen in case-control studies involving 150 children with ventricular septal defect or 90 chidren with conotruncal malformations (Tikkanen & Heinonen, 1991, 1992).

Decreased birth weight and head circumference were observed in a series of 17 infants born to women who took diazepam or other benzodiazepines during pregnancy (Laegreid et al., 1992a). The weights of these children had become normal by 10 months of age, but the head circumferences were still smaller than expected at 18 months (Laegreid et al., 1992b).

The suggestion that there exists a "benzodiazepine embryofetopathy" comprised of typical facial features, neurological dysfunction, and other anomalies (Laegreid et al., 1987, 1989, 1990, 1992b) is not generally accepted. Benzodiazepines (mostly diazepam) were identified much more frequently than expected in stored blood samples taken at the end of the first trimester of pregnancy from mothers of 18 children with congenital anomalies suspected of being manifestations of benzodiazepine teratogenesis in one investigation (Laegreid et al., 1990). Interpretation of this study is difficult because of possible biased ascertainment of cases.

An increased frequency of malformations has been demonstrated among the offspring of mice and hamsters treated with diazepam during pregnancy, but only at doses hundreds of times larger than those used in humans (Weber, 1985). Cleft palate is the abnormality most commonly seen in affected mice; neural tube defects are most common in hamsters. A typical dose-response relationship has been demonstrated (Barlow et al., 1980; Gill et al., 1981). Studies in rats and rabbits have generally not shown an increased frequency of malformations after maternal treatment with diazepam during pregnancy in doses as much as 150 times those usually employed in humans (Weber, 1985; Esaki et al., 1981).

Diazepam treatment of rats, mice and cats late in gestation causes persistent abnormalities of central nervous system biochemistry and function in the offspring (Weber, 1985; Kellogg, 1988; De Salvia et al., 1990; Barbier et al., 1991). Alterations of behavior and the ability to respond to stress are frequently observed. *In humans, treatment of the mother with diazepam during the third trimester of pregnancy or during delivery has resulted in apnea, hypotonia, and hypothermia in the newborn* (Owen et al., 1972; Cree et al., 1973; Gillberg, 1977; Speight, 1977; Laegreid et al., 1992a). Tremors, irritability, and hypertonia reminiscent of neonatal narcotic withdrawal occur in some babies born to mothers treated with diazepam chronically in the third trimester (Rementeria & Bhatt, 1977). Exposure of a pregnant woman to diazepam causes loss of beat-to-beat variability of fetal heart rate (Scher et al., 1972) and decreased fetal movement (Birger et al., 1980). In one study of 17 children born to mothers who took diazepam or other benzodiazepines during pregnancy, delayed gross motor development was observed at six and ten months, but at 18 months few differences from controls were apparent (Laegreid et al., 1992b).

A few apparently normal infants have been reported whose mothers took toxic doses of diazepam during pregnancy (Cerqueira et al, 1988; Czeizel, 1988). In most of these cases, the toxic ingestion occurred after the first trimester.

Key References

Aarskog D: Association between maternal intake of diazepam and oral clefts. Lancet 2:921, 1975. [E]

Aselton P, Jick H, Milunsky A, Hunter JR, et al.: First-trimester drug use and congenital disorders. Obstet Gynecol 65:451-455, 1985. [S]

Barbier P, Breteaudeau J, Autret E, Bertrand P, et al.: Effects of prenatal exposure to diazepam on exploration behavior and learning retention in mice. Dev Pharmacol Ther 17:35-43, 1991. [A]

Barlow SM, Knight AF, Sullivan FM: Diazepam-induced cleft palate in the mouse: The role of endogenous maternal corticosterone. Teratology 21:149-155, 1980. [A]

Birger M, Homburg R, Insler V: Clinical evaluation of fetal movements. Int J Gynaecol Obstet 18:377-382, 1980. [S]

Bracken MB, Holford TR: Exposure to prescribed drugs in pregnancy and association with congenital malformations. Obstet Gynecol 58:336-344, 1981. [E]

Cerqueira MJ, Olle C, Bellart J, Baro F, et al.: Intoxication by benzodiazepines during pregnancy. Lancet 1:1341, 1988. [S]

Cree JE, Meyer J, Hailey DM: Diazepam in labour: Its metabolism and effect on the clinical condition and thermogenesis of the newborn. Br Med J 4:251-255, 1973. [S]

Crombie DL, Pinsent RF, Fleming DM, Rumeau-Rouquette C, Goujard J, Huel G: Fetal effects of tranquilizers in pregnancy. [Letter to the Editor.] N Engl J Med 293:198-199, 1975. [E]

Czeizel A: Lack of evidence of teratogenicity of benzodiazepine drugs in Hungary. Reprod Toxicol 1:183-188, 1988. [E]

De Salvia MA, Cagiano R, Lacomba C, Cuomo V: Neurobehavioral changes produced by developmental exposure to benzodiazepines. Dev Pharmacol Ther 15:173-177, 1990. [R]

Esaki K, Sakai Y, Yanagita T: Effects of oral administration of alprazolam (TUS-1) on rabbit fetus. Jitchuken Zenrinsho Kenkyuho 7:79-90, 1981. [A]

Gill TS, Guram MS, Geber WF: Comparative study of the teratogenic effects of chlordiazepoxide and diazepam in the fetal hamster. Life Sci 29:2141-2147, 1981. [A]

Gillberg C: "Floppy infant syndrome" and maternal diazepam. Lancet 2:244, 1977. [C]

Jick H, Holmes LB, Hunter JR, Madsen S, et al.: First-trimester drug use and congenital disorders. JAMA 246:343-346, 1981. [S]

Kellogg CK: Benzodiazepines: Influence on the developing brain. Prog Brain Res 73:207-228, 1988. [R]

Laegreid L, Hagberg G, Lundberg A: The effect of benzodiazepines on the fetus and the newborn. Neuropediatrics 23:18-23, 1992a. [E]

Laegreid L, Hagberg G, Lundberg A: Neurodevelopment in late infancy after prenatal exposure to benzodiazepines - A prospective study. Neuropediatrics 23:60-67, 1992b. [E]

Laegreid L, Olegard R, Conradi N, et al.: Congenital malformations and maternal consumption of benzodiazepines: A case-control study. Dev Med Child Neurol 32:432-441, 1990. [E]

Laegreid L, Olegard R, Wahlstrom J, Conradi N: Abnormalities in children exposed to benzodiazepines in utero. Lancet 1:108-109, 1987. [S]

Laegreid L, Olegard R, Walstrom J, Conradi N: Teratogenic effects of benzodiazepine use during pregnancy. J Pediatr 114:126-131, 1989. [S]

Owen JR, Irani SF, Blair AW: Effect of diazepam administered to mothers during labour on temperature regulation of neonate. Arch Dis Child 47:107-110, 1972. [S]

Rementeria JL, Bhatt K: Withdrawal symptoms in neonates from intrauterine exposure to diazepam. J Pediatr 90:123-126, 1977. [C]

Restrepo M, Munoz N, Day N, et al.: Birth defects among children born to a population occupationally exposed to pesticides in Colombia. Scand J Work Environ Health 16:239-246, 1990. [E]

Rosenberg L, Mitchell AA, Parsells JL, Pashayan H, et al.: Lack of relation of oral clefts to diazepam use during pregnancy. N Engl J Med 309:1282-1285, 1983. [E]

Rothman KJ, Fyler DC, Goldblatt A, Kreidberg MB: Exogenous hormones and other drug exposures of children with congenital heart disease. Am J Epidemiol 109:433-439, 1979. [E]

Safra MJ, Oakley GP: Association between cleft lip with or without cleft palate and prenatal exposure to diazepam. Lancet 2:478-479, 1975. [E]

Saxen I: Associations between oral clefts and drugs taken during pregnancy. Int J Epidemiol 4:37-44, 1975a. [E]

Saxen I: Epidemiology of cleft lip and palate. Int J Prev Soc Med 29:103-110, 1975b. [E]

Scher J, Hailey DM, Beard RW: The effects of diazepam on the fetus. J Obstet Gynaecol Br Commonw 79:635-638, 1972. [S]

Shiono PH, Mills JL: Oral clefts and diazepam use during pregnancy. [Letter to the editor.] N Engl J Med 311:919-920, 1984. [E]

Speight ANP: Floppy-infant syndrome and maternal diazepam and/or nitrazepam. Lancet 1:878, 1977. [C]

Tikkanen J, Heinonen OP: Risk factors for conal malformations of the heart. Eur J Epidemiol 8(1):48-57, 1992. [E]

Tikkanen J, Heinonen OP: Risk factors for ventricular septal defect in Finland. Public Health 105:99-112, 1991. [E]

Weber LWD: Benzodiazepines in pregnancy -- academical debate or teratogenic risk? Biol Res Pregnancy 6:151-167, 1985. [R]

Zierler S, Rothman KJ: Congenital heart disease in relation to maternal use of Bendectin and other drugs in early pregnancy. N Engl J Med 313:347-352, 1985. [E]

DIAZOXIDE

Synonyms

Diazossido, Eudemine, Hyperstat, Hypertonalum, Mutabase, Proglicem, Proglycem

Summary

Diazoxide is a thiazide used intravenously in the acute treatment of hypertension and orally, in smaller doses, in the treatment of hypoglycemia.

Magnitude of Teratogenic Risk

Undetermined

Quality and Quantity of Data

Poor

Comment

None

No epidemiological studies of congenital anomalies among the infants of women treated with diazoxide during pregnancy have been reported.

No teratogenic effect is said to have occurred among the offspring of rats or dogs treated with diazoxide during pregnancy in one study (Anonymous, 1971), but insufficient data are provided to assess this report.

Alterations of neonatal glucose homeostasis, other abnormalities of perinatal adaptation, fetal bradycardia, and cessation of labor have been observed in women treated intravenously with diazoxide late in pregnancy (Morris et al., 1977; Neuman et al., 1979; Smith et al., 1982; Michael, 1986). Histological evidence of pancreatic islet cell damage has been observed among the offspring of sheep and goats treated late in pregnancy with intravenous diazoxide in doses similar to those used in humans (Boulos et al., 1971). Abnormalities of body and scalp hair growth have been noted in four infants born to women treated with oral diazoxide during the last trimester of pregnancy (Milner & Chouksey, 1972).

Please see agent summary on chlorothiazide for information on a related agent that has been more thoroughly studied.

Key References

Anonymous: Diazoxide: A review of its pharmacological properties and therapeutic use in hypertensive crises. Drugs 2:114-115, 1971. [A] & [R]

Boulos BM, Davis LE, Almond CH, Jackson RL: Placental transfer of diazoxide and its hazardous effect on the newborn. J Clin Pharmacol 11:206-210, 1971. [A]

Michael CA: Intravenous labetalol and intravenous diazoxide in severe hypertension complicating pregnancy. Aust NZ J Obstet Gynaec 26:26-29, 1986. [S]

Milner RDG, Chouksey SK: Effects of fetal exposure to diazoxide in man. Arch Dis Child 47:537-543, 1972. [C]

Morris JA, Arce JJ, Hamilton CJ, Davidson EC, et al.: The management of severe preeclampsia and eclampsia with intravenous diazoxide. Obstet Gynecol 49(6):675-680, 1977. [S]

Neuman J, Weiss B, Rabello Y, Cabal L, et al.: Diazoxide for the acute control of severe hypertension complicating pregnancy. A pilot study. Obstet Gynecol 53(3)(Suppl.):50S-55S, 1979. [C]

Smith MJ, Aynsley-Green A, Redman CWG: Neonatal hyperglycaemia after prolonged maternal treatment with diazoxide. Br Med J 284:1234, 1982. [C]

DIBROMOCHLOROPRO-PANE

Synonyms

DBCP, Fumagon, Fumazone, Nemabrom, Nemafume, Nemagon, Nemanax, Nemapaz, Nematox

Summary

Dibromochloropropane is a brominated organochlorine compound that is used in agriculture as a nematodocidal soil fumigant. The U.S. OSHA standard for occupational exposure to dibromochloropropane is 1 ppb as an 8-hour time-weighted average (Babich & Davis, 1981).

Magnitude of Teratogenic Risk

Undetermined

Quality and Quantity of Data

Poor

Comment

The toxic effects of high doses of this agent on the male reproductive system (see below) raise concern about possible mutagenic effects on cells in the developing embryo.

No significant correlation was observed between the level of dibromochloropropane contamination in the parents' drinking water and the birth weight, sex ratio, or presence of congenital anomalies among 46,328 infants in Fresno County, California (Whorton et al., 1989).

Occupational exposure of men to high levels of dibromochloropropane has been associated with the development of infertility and oligospermia or azoospermia (Whorton, 1983; Whorton & Foliart, 1983). The frequency of congenital anomalies does not appear to be unusually high among the children of men with heavy exposure to dibromochloropropane (Postashnik & Phillip, 1988), but a reduced

male/female sex ratio has been reported among such children (Potashnik et al., 1984).

The frequency of malformations was not increased among the offspring of rats treated orally with 12.5-50.0 mg/kg/d of dibromochloropropane in one study (Ruddick & Newsome, 1979). Fetal growth retardation and increased frequencies of fetal and perinatal death were observed among the offspring of rats treated during pregnancy with dibromochoropropane in doses of 10-40 mg/kg/d (Shaked et al., 1988).

At adulthood, male rat offspring prenatally exposed to 25 mg/kg/d of dibromochloropropane for two, four, or six days during the critical period of sexual differentiation exhibited significant impairment in development of both the interstitial and tubular components of the testis. Adult males treated for four or six days of fetal life also displayed aberrant sexual behavior (Warren et al., 1988).

Key References

Babich H, Davis DL: Dibromochloropropane (DBCP): A review. Sci Total Environ 17:207-221, 1981. [R]

Potashnik G, Goldsmith J, Insler V: Dibromochloropropane-induced reduction of the sex-ratio in man. Andrologia 16:213-218, 1984. [E]

Potashnik G, Phillip M: Lack of birth defects among offspring conceived during or after paternal exposure to dibromochloropropane (DBCP). Andrologia 20:90-94, 1988. [S]

Ruddick JA, Newsome WH: A teratogenicity and tissue distribution study on dibromochloropropane in the rat. Bull Environ Contam Toxicol 21:483-487, 1979. [A]

Shaked I, Sod-Moriah UA, Kaplanski J, et al.: Reproductive performance of dibromochloropropane-treated female rats. Int J Fertil 33(2):129-133, 1988. [A]

Warren DW, Ahmad N, Rudeen PK: The effects of fetal exposure to 1,2-dibromochloropropane on adult male reproductive function. Biol Reprod 39:707-716, 1988. [A]

Whorton MD: Dibromochloropropane health effects. Environ Occup Med 11:573-577, 1983. [R]

Whorton MD, Foliart DE: Mutagenicity, carcinogenicity and reproductive effects of dibromochloropropane (DBCP). Mutat Res 123:13-30, 1983. [R]

Whorton MD, Wong O, Morgan RW, Gordon N: An epidemiologic investigation of birth outcomes in relation to dibromochloropropane contamination in drinking water in Fresno County, California, USA. Int Arch Occup Environ Health 61:403-407, 1989. [E]

DIBUCAINE

Synonyms

Benzolin, Cincaine Chloride, Cinchocaine, Cincocaina, Cinkain, Dermacaine, Nupercainal, Percaine, Sovcaine

Summary

Dibucaine is a local anesthetic of the amide class.

Magnitude of Teratogenic Risk

Undetermined

Quality and Quantity of Data

None

Comment

A small risk cannot be excluded, but there is no indication that the risk of congenital anomalies in the children of women treated with dibucaine during pregnancy is likely to be great.

No epidemiological studies of congenital anomalies in children born to women exposed to dibucaine during pregnancy have been reported.

No investigations of teratologic effects of dibucaine in experimental animals have been published.

Please see agent summary on lidocaine for information on a related agent that has been studied.

Key References

None available.

DICLOXACILLIN

Synonyms

Dichlor-Stapenor, Dicloxin, Dycill, Dynapen, Maclicine, Pathocil, Totocillin

Summary

Dicloxacillin is an antibiotic related to penicillin. Dicloxacillin is usually administered orally in the treatment of infections by penicillinase-producing bacteria.

Magnitude of Teratogenic Risk

None To Minimal

Quality and Quantity of Data

Poor To Fair

Comment

None

The frequency of congenital anomalies was no greater than expected among the children of 86 women treated with dicloxacillin during the first trimester of pregnancy in the Boston Collaborative Drug Surveillance Program (Aselton et al., 1985).

In two studies reported only as abstracts, no evidence of teratogenic effect was noted among the offspring of rabbits treated with dicloxacillin in doses that were in the human therapeutic range but were maternally toxic in rabbits (Madissoo et al., 1967; Brown et al., 1968).

Please see agent summary on penicillin for information on a related agent that has been more thoroughly studied.

Key References

Aselton P, Jick H, Milunsky JR, et al.: First-trimester drug use and congenital disorders. Obstet Gynecol 65:451-455, 1985. [S]

Brown DM, Harper KH, Palmer AK, Tesh SA: Effect of antibiotics upon pregnancy in the rabbit. Toxicol Appl Pharmacol 12:295, 1968. [A]

Madissoo H, Johnston CD, Scott WJ, et al.: Toxicologic and teratologic studies on antibiotics in rabbits. Toxicol Appl Pharmacol 10:379, 1967. [A]

DICUMAROL

Synonyms

Acadyl, Apekumarol, Baracoumin, Bishy-droxycoumarin, Cumid, Dicoumarin, Dicumol, Dufalone, Melitoxin

Summary

Dicumarol is a coumarin anticoagulant that is administered orally.

Magnitude of Teratogenic Risk

Moderate

Quality and Quantity of Data

Fair To Good

Comment

It seems likely that maternal use of dicumarol during pregnancy is associated with teratogenic and perinatal risks similar to those of warfarin. Please see warfarin summary for information on this closely related drug that has been studied more thoroughly.

In a series of 78 pregnancies in women who were treated with dicumarol for cardiac valve prostheses, there were 35 (45%) abortions and 43 liveborn infants (Quaini et al.,

1986). Among the latter, four infants had petechiae or cutaneous hematomas, one child had cleft lip and palate, and another had abnormal occipital calcification, hypoplasia of the nasal cartilage, choanal stenosis, and fatal respiratory insufficiency. The features in this last infant are typical of those that may be caused by maternal use during pregnancy of warfarin, a closely related drug (Hall et al., 1980). Among 29 infants born to women treated with dicumarol during pregnancy whose cases were reported prior to 1965, there were six fetal deaths, three of which were demonstrably associated with hemorrhage, and two liveborn infants who had intracranial hemorrhage (Villasanta, 1965). In addition, one child had optic atrophy, microcephaly, and cerebral agenesis, but it is uncertain which anticoagulant this mother took during pregnancy (Quenneville et al., 1959). In another series of 20 pregnancies among women treated with dicumarol, four of the infants were stillborn (Fillmore & McDevitt, 1970).

Fatal neonatal hemorrhage was often observed among the offspring of dogs and rabbits treated during pregnancy with dicumarol in doses similar to those used in humans (Quick, 1946; Kraus et al., 1949). Fetal death occurred frequently among the offspring of rabbits and mink treated during pregnancy with dicumarol in doses within or below the human therapeutic range (Kraus et al., 1949; Kangas & Makela, 1974).

It seems likely that dicumarol is associated with teratogenic risks similar to those of warfarin. Please see agent summary on warfarin for information on this related drug that has been more thoroughly studied.

Key References

Fillmore SJ, McDevitt E: Effects of coumarin compounds on the fetus. Ann Intern Med 73:731-735, 1970. [S]

Hall JG, Pauli RM, Wilson KM: Maternal and fetal sequelae of anticoagulation during pregnancy. Am J Med 68:122-40, 1980. [R]

Kangas J, Makela J: Dikumarols abortframkallande effekt hos mink. Nord Veterinaermed 26:444-447, 1974. [A]

Kraus AP, Perlow S, Singer K: Danger of dicumarol treatment in pregnancy. JAMA 139:758-762, 1949. [A]

Quaini E, Vitali E, Colombo T, et al.: Complicanze materne e fetali in 105 gravidanze di portatrici di protesi valvolari cardiache. Minerva Ginecol 38:217-224, 1986. [S]

Quenneville G, Barton B, McDevitt E, et al.: The use of anticoagulants for thrombophlebitis during pregnancy. Am J Obstet Gynecol 77:1135-1149, 1959. [E]

Quick AJ: Experimentally induced changes in the prothrombin level of the blood. III. Prothrombin concentration of new-born pups of a mother given dicumarol before parturition. J Biol Chem 164:371-376, 1946. [A]

Villasanta U: Thromboembolic disease in pregnancy. Am J Obstet Gynecol 93:142-160, 1965. [R]

DICYCLOMINE

Synonyms

Bentyl, Bentylol, Formulex, Menospasm, Merbentyl, Or-Tyl, Spasmoban, Viscerol

Summary

Dicyclomine is an anticholinergic agent with peripheral effects similar to, but considerably weaker than, those of atropine. Dicyclomine is one of three components originally included in Bendectin, an antinauseant that was widely used in pregnancy before its withdrawal from the market. Dicyclomine was removed from Bendectin when the product was reformulated (in 1976 in the United States).

Magnitude of Teratogenic Risk

None

Quality and Quantity of Data

Good

Comment

Many studies of dicyclomine as a component of bendectin are available. Please see bendectin agent summary for more information.

The frequency of congenital anomalies was no greater than expected among the infants of 97 women who took dicyclomine alone during the first trimester of pregnancy (Aselton et al., 1985).

The frequency of malformations was not increased among the offspring of rats or rabbits treated during pregnancy with 10 to 100 times the usual human dose of dicyclomine (Gibson et al., 1968).

Key References

Aselton P, Jick H, Milunsky A, Hunter JR, et al.: First-trimester drug use and congenital disorders. Obstet Gynecol 65:451-455, 1985. [S]

Gibson JP, Staples RE, Larson EJ, Kuhn WL, et al.: Teratology and reproduction studies with an antinauseant. Toxicol Appl Pharmacol 13:439-447, 1968. [A]

DIETHYLPROPION

Synonyms

Adiposan, Amfepramone Hydrochloride, Apistate, Dietil Retard, Nobensine-75, Regenon Retard, Regibon, Sinapet, Tenuate

Summary

Diethylpropion is a sympathomimetic agent used as an anorectic.

Magnitude of Teratogenic Risk

None

Quality and Quantity of Data

Fair

189

Comment

None

The frequency of congenital anomalies was not significantly increased among the children of 40 women who took diethylpropion during the first four lunar months of pregnancy or of 225 women who took this drug anytime during pregnancy in the Collaborative Perinatal Project (Heinonen et al., 1977). Similarly, no association between maternal use of diethylpropion during pregnancy and congenital anomalies in the infants was observed in a cohort study performed among the patients of more than one hundred North American obstetrical practices (Bunde & Leyland, 1965). This investigation included 1232 infants born to women who used this drug during pregnancy; in 271 of these pregnancies treatment began in the first 100 days of gestation.

The frequency of malformations was no greater than expected among the offspring of rats or mice treated during pregnancy with diethylpropion in doses, respectively, 4-10 and 10-33 times those used in humans (Cahen et al., 1964).

Key References

Bunde CA, Leyland HM: A controlled retrospective survey in evaluation of teratogenicity. J New Drugs 5:193-198, 1965. [S]

Cahen R, Sautai M, Montagne J, Pessonnier J: Experiments on the teratogenic effect of 2-diethylaminopro-piophenone. Med Exp Int J Exp Med 10:201-224, 1964. [A]

Heinonen OP, Slone D, Shapiro S: Birth Defects and Drugs in Pregnancy. Littleton, Mass.: John Wright-PSG, 1977, pp 346-347, 439. [E]

DIETHYLSTILBESTROL

Synonyms

APS Stilboestrol, DES, Desma, Dicorvin, Pabestrol, Stilbestrol Dipropionate, Stilbocream, Stilboestrol, Stilphostrol

Summary

Diethylstilbestrol (DES) is a nonsteroidal synthetic estrogen that is used in treatment of ovarian insufficiency and as a postcoital contraceptive. DES has also been employed to inhibit lactation and in palliative treatment of breast carcinoma.

Magnitude of Teratogenic Risk

For Clear Cell Carcinoma Of The Cervix: Minimal To Small

For Genital Tract Anomalies In Females: Small To Moderate

For Genital Tract Anomalies In Males: Minimal

For Nongenital Congenital Anomalies: None To Minimal

Quality and Quantity of Data

For Clear Cell Carcinoma Of The Cervix: Good

For Genital Tract Anomalies In Females: Fair To Good

For Genital Tract Anomalies In Males: Poor To Fair

For Nongenital Congenital Anomalies: Fair To Good

Comment

None

Adenosis and other abnormalities of the vagina are very common among the daughters of women who were treated with diethystilbestrol in pregnancy. Gross structural abnormalities of the cervix or vagina occur in about one-fourth and histological abnormalities of the vaginal epithelium in at least one-third to one-half of women whose mothers took DES during gestation (Herbst et al., 1975; Bibbo, 1979; Robboy et al., 1981; Stillman, 1982; Robboy et al., 1984; Kaufman et al., 1984; Vessey, 1989).

Malformations, such as T-shaped uterus, constricting bands of the uterine cavity, uterine hypoplasia, or para-ovarian cysts, also occur with increased frequency.

Several studies suggest that development of clear cell adenocarcinoma, a rare tumor of the vagina or cervix, is associated with in utero exposure to DES (Herbst et al., 1971; Stillman, 1982; Walker, 1984; Melnick et al., 1987; Vessey, 1989; Herbst & Anderson, 1990; Sharp & Cole, 1990). In a registry that includes more than 500 cases of clear cell adenocarcinoma of the vagina diagnosed in the United States since 1971, prenatal exposure to DES was reported in 60% of patients in whom maternal history was available (Melnick et al., 1987; Herbst & Anderson, 1990). The median age at which malignancy was diagnosed was 19 years. The risk that a woman whose mother took DES during pregnancy will develop clear cell adenocarcinoma of the vagina or cervix by age 34 is estimated to be about 1/1000 (Melnick et al., 1987; Vassey, 1989; Herbst & Anderson, 1990). The risk of vaginal or cervical squamous cell intraepithelial neoplasia has been estimated to be about twice as great as expected among women who were exposed in utero to DES (Robboy et al., 1984; Bornstein et al., 1988). Available data on genital tract neoplasms among women exposed to DES in utero are subject to several potential biases, and some authors question whether the observed associations between prenatal DES exposure and malignancy are causal (McFarlane et al., 1986; Bornstein et al., 1988; Edelman, 1989).

Ectopic implantation, miscarriage, and premature delivery are more common than expected among the pregnancies of women whose mothers took DES during gestation (Barnes et al., 1980; Herbst et al., 1980, 1981; Sandberg, 1981; Linn et al., 1988; de Hass et al., 1991). Some studies have also shown an increased frequency of infertility among these women (Herbst et al., 1980; Senekjian, et al., 1988). This may be a result of the uterine abnormalities associated with prenatal DES exposure (Berger & Alper, 1986; Kaufman et al., 1986).

Some studies suggest that epididymal cysts, hypoplastic testes, cryptorchidism, and abnormalities on semen analysis are more fre-
quent than expected among the sons of mothers treated with DES during pregnancy (Bibbo et al., 1977; Gill et al., 1979; Shy et al., 1984). Such abnormalities have not been found to be associated with prenatal DES exposure in other investigations (Vessey et al., 1983; Leary et al., 1984). An association between maternal treatment with DES during pregnancy and subsequent development of testicular cancer in their sons has been suggested, but the data are inconsistent (Gershman & Stolley, 1988; Vessey, 1989).

In the Collaborative Perinatal Project, a large cohort study in which genital abnormalities of the type discussed above would not be detected, the frequencies of congenital anomalies in general, of major malformations, and of minor anomalies were no greater than expected among the children of 164 women treated with DES during the first four lunar months of pregnancy (Heinonen et al., 1977). Similarly, the frequency of congenital anomalies was not increased among the children of 233 women treated with this drug anytime during pregnancy.

Depression, anxiety, eating disorders, altered psychosexual behavior, and variations in cognitive function have been reported with increased frequency among adult children of women treated with DES during pregnancy (Vessey et al., 1983; Meyer-Bahlburg & Ehrhardt, 1986; Ehrhardt et al., 1989; Lish et al., 1991; Gustavson et al., 1991; Reinisch & Sanders, 1992). The effects observed have varied in different studies and may be related, at least in part, to the perceived burden of being a "DES daughter or son" rather than to prenatal exposure to DES per se (Fried-Cassorla et al., 1987).

Gross and microscopic genital tract abnormalities similar to those found in humans have been observed among the offspring of monkeys treated during pregnancy with DES in doses within the human therapeutic range (Hendrickx et al., 1979, 1988; Johnson et al., 1981; Thompson et al., 1981; Walker, 1989). Similar findings have been reported in mice, rats, hamsters, guinea pigs, and ferrets (McLachlan et al., 1980; Walker 1980; Gilloteaux et al., 1982; Miller et al., 1982; Baggs & Miller, 1983; Newbold et al., 1983, 1987a, b; Walker, 1983a, b; Newbold & McLachlan, 1985; Davies & Lefkowitz, 1987; Bullock et al., 1988; Rothschild et al., 1988; Walker, 1989). Histological alterations have also been observed in human fetal genital tract tissue grown in nude mice treated with DES in doses similar to those used in humans (Cunha et al., 1987; Sugimura et al., 1988). Neoplasms of the uterus, vagina, breast, rete testis, and testis were seen among the offspring of DES-treated rodents in some studies (Miller et al., 1982; Newbold & McLachlan, 1982; Walker, 1983a, 1989; Newbold et al., 1986, 1987b; Lopez et al., 1988; Bullock et al., 1988). Increased rates of uterine and ovarian neoplasms were observed in the second generation after intrauterine exposure in one investigation (Turusov et al., 1992). It is difficult to envision a pathogenic mechanism that could account for this effect.

Key References

Baggs RB, Miller RK: Induction of urogenital malformation by diethylstilbestrol in the ferret. Teratology 27:28A, 1983. [A]

Barnes AB, Colton T, Gundersen J, Noller KL, et al.: Fertility and outcome of pregnancy in women exposed in utero to diethylstilbestrol. N Engl J Med 302:609-613, 1980. [E]

Berger MJ, Alper MM: Intractable primary infertility in women exposed to diethylstilbestrol in utero. J Reprod Med 31(4):231-235, 1986. [E]

Bibbo M: Transplacental effects of diethylstilbestrol. In: Grundmann E (ed). Perinatal Pathology. New York: Springer-Verlag, 1979, pp 191-211. [R]

Bibbo M, Gill WB, Azizi F, et al.: Follow-up study of male and female offspring of DES-exposed mothers. Obstet Gynecol 49(1):1-8, 1977. [E]

Bornstein J, Adam E, Adler-Storthz K, et al.: Development of cervical and vaginal squamous cell neoplasia as a late consequence of in utero exposure to diethylstilbestrol. Obstet Gynecol Surv 43(1):15-21, 1988. [R]

Bullock BC, Newbold RR, McLachlan JA: Lesions of testis and epididymis associated with prenatal diethylstilbestrol exposure. Environ Health Perspect 77:29-31, 1988. [A]

Cunha GR, Taguchi O, Namikawa R, et al.: Teratogenic effects of clomiphene, tamoxifen, and

diethylstilbestrol on the developing human female genital tract. Hum Pathol 18(11):1132-1143, 1987. [A]

Davies J, Lefkowitz J: Delayed effects of prenatal or postnatal exposure to diethylstilbestrol in the adult female guinea pig. Acta Anat 130:351-358, 1987. [A]

de Haas I, Harlow BL, Cramer DW, Frigoletto FD: Spontaneous preterm birth: A case-control study. Am J Obstet Gynecol 165:1290-1296, 1991. [E]

Edelman DA: Diethylstilbestrol exposure and the risk of clear cell cervical and vaginal adenocarcinoma. Int J Fertl 34(4):251-255, 1989. [R]

Ehrhardt AA, Meyer-Bahlburg HFL, Rosen LR, et al.: The development of gender-related behavior in females following prenatal exposure to diethylstilbestrol (DES). Horm Behav 23(4):526-541, 1989. [E]

Fried-Cassorla M, Scholl TO, Borow LD, et al.: Depression and diethylstilbestrol exposure in women. J Reprod Med 32(11):847-850, 1987. [E]

Gershman ST, Stolley PD: A case-control study of testicular cancer using Connecticut tumour registry data. Int J Epidemiol 17(4):738-742, 1988. [E]

Gill WB, Schumacher GFB, Bibbo M, et al.: Association of diethylstilbestrol exposure in utero with cryptorchidism, testicular hypoplasia and semen abnormalities. J Urol 122:36-39, 1979. [E]

Gilloteaux J, Paul RJ, Steggles AW: Upper genital tract abnormalities in the Syrian hamster as a result of in utero exposure to diethylstilbestrol. Virchows Arch [Pathol Anat] 398:163-183, 1982. [A]

Gustavson CR, Gustavson JC, Noller KL, et al.: Increased risk of profound weight loss among women exposed to diethylstilbestrol in utero. Behav Neural Biol 55:307-312, 1991. [E]

Heinonen OP, Slone D, Shapiro S: Birth Defects and Drugs in Pregnancy. Littleton, Mass.: John Wright-PSG, 1977, pp 389-391, 433. [E]

Hendrickx AG, Benirschke K, Thompson RS, Ahern JK, et al.: The effects of prenatal diethylstilbestrol (DES) exposure on the genitalia of pubertal Macaca mulatta. I. Female offspring. J Reprod Med 22:233-240, 1979. [A]

Hendrickx AG, Prahalada S, Binkerd PE: Long-term evaluation of the diethylstilbestrol (DES) syndrome in adult female rhesus monkeys (Macaca mulatta). Reproductive Toxicol 1:253-261, 1988. [A]

Herbst AL, Anderson D: Clear cell adenocarcinoma of the vagina and cervix secondary to intrauterine exposure to diethylstilbestrol. Semin Surg Oncol 6(6):343-346, 1990. [S]

Herbst AL, Hubby MM, Azizi F, Makii MM: Reproductive and gynecologic surgical experience in diethylstilbestrol-exposed daughters. Am J Obstet Gynecol 141:1019-1028, 1981. [E]

Herbst AL, Hubby MM, Blough RR, Azizi F: A comparison of pregnancy experience in DES-exposed and DES-unexposed daughters. J Reprod Med 24:62-69, 1980. [E]

Herbst AL, Poskanzer DC, Robboy SJ, Friedlander L, et al.: Prenatal exposure to stilbestrol. A prospective comparison of exposed female offspring with unexposed controls. N Engl J Med 292:334-339, 1975. [E]

Herbst AL, Ulfelder H, Poskanzer DC: Adenocarcinoma of the vagina. Association of maternal stilbestrol therapy with tumor appearance in young women. N Engl J Med 284(16):878-881, 1971. [E]

Johnson LD, Palmer AE, King NW, Hertig AT: Vaginal adenosis in Cebus apella monkeys exposed to DES in utero. Obstet Gynecol 57:629-635, 1981. [A]

Kaufman RH, Adam E, Noller K, et al.: Upper genital tract changes and infertility in diethylstilbestrol-exposed women. Am J Obstet Gynecol 154(6):1312-1318, 1986. [S]

Kaufman RH, Noller K, Adam E, Irwin J, et al.: Upper genital tract abnormalities and pregnancy outcome in diethylstilbestrol-exposed progeny. Am J Obstet Gynecol 148:973-984, 1984. [S]

Leary FJ, Resseguie LJ, Kurland LT, et al.: Males exposed in utero to diethylstilbestrol. JAMA 252(21):2984-2989, 1984. [E]

Linn S, Lieberman E, Schoenbaum SC, et al.: Adverse outcomes of pregnancy in women exposed to diethylstilbestrol in utero. J Reprod Med 33(1):3-7, 1988. [E]

Lish JD, Ehrhardt AA, Meyer-Bahlburg HFL, et al.: Gender-related behavior development in females exposed to diethylstilbestrol (DES) in utero: An attempted replication. J Am Acad Child Adolesc Psychiatry 30(1):29-37, 1991. [E]

Lopez J, Ogren L, Verjan R, et al.: Effects of perinatal exposure to a synthetic estrogen and progestin on mammary tumorigenesis in mice. Teratology 38:129-134, 1988. [A]

McFarlane MJ, Feinstein AR, Horwitz RI: Diethylstilbestrol and clear cell vaginal carcinoma. Reappraisal of the epidemiologic evidence. Am J Med 81:855-863, 1986. [R]

McLachlan JA, Newbold RR, Bullock BC: Long-term effects on the female mouse genital tract associated with prenatal exposure to diethylstilbestrol. Cancer Res 40:3988-3999, 1980. [A]

Melnick S, Cole P, Anderson D, et al.: Rates and risks of diethylstilbestrol-related clear-cell adenocarcinoma of the vagina and cervix. N Engl J Med 316(9):514-516, 1987. [S]

Meyer-Bahlburg HFL, Ehrhardt AA: Prenatal diethylstilbestrol exposure: Behavioral consequences in humans. Monogr Neural Sci 12:90-95, 1986. [E]

Miller RK, Baggs RB, Odoroff CL, McKenzie RC: Transplacental carcinogenicity of diethyltilbestrol (DES): A Wistar rat model. Teratology 25:62A, 1982. [A]

Newbold RR, Bullock BC, McLachlan JA: Adenocarcinoma of the rete testis. Diethylstilbestrol-induced lesions of the mouse rete testis. AJP 125(3):625-628, 1986. [A]

Newbold RR, Bullock BC, McLachlan JA: Mullerian remnants of male mice exposed prenatally to diethylstilbestrol. Teratogenesis Carcinog Mutagen 7:377-389, 1987a. [A]

Newbold RR, Bullock BC, McLachlan JA: Testicular tumors in mice exposed in utero to diethylstilbestrol. J Urol 138:1446-1450, 1987b. [A]

Newbold RR, McLachlan JA: Diethylstilbestrol associated defects in murine genital tract development. Estrogens Environ (Proc Symp) 2nd:288-318, 1985. [A]

Newbold RR, McLachlan JA: Vaginal adenosis and adenocarcinoma in mice exposed prenatally or neonatally to diethylstilbestrol. Cancer Res 42:2003-2011, 1982. [A]

Newbold RR, Tyrey S, Haney AF, McLachlan JA: Developmentally arrested oviduct: A structural and functional defect in mice following prenatal exposure to diethylstilbestrol. Teratology 27:417-426, 1983. [A]

Reinisch JM, Sanders SA: Effects of prenatal exposure to diethylstilbestrol (DES) on hemispheric laterality and spatial ability in human males. Horm Behav 25:62-75, 1992. [E]

Robboy SJ, Noller KL, O'Brien P, Kaufman RH, et al.: Increased incidence of cervical and vaginal dysplasia in 3,980 diethylstilbestrol-exposed young women. Experience of the National Collaborative Diethylstilbestrol Adenosis Project. JAMA 252:2979-2983, 1984. [E]

Robboy SJ, Szyfelbein WM, Goellner JR, Kaufman RH, et al.: Dysplasia and cytologic findings in 4,589 young women enrolled in Diethylstilbestrol-Adenosis (DESAD) project. Am J Obstet Gynecol 140:579-586, 1981. [E]

Rothschild TC, Calhoon RE, Boylan ES: Genital tract abnormalities in female rats exposed to diethylstilbestrol in utero. Reprod Toxicol 1(3):193-202, 1988. [A]

Sandberg EC, Riffle NL, Higdon JV, Getman CE: Pregnancy outcome in women exposed to diethylstilbestrol in utero. Am J Obstet Gynecol 140:194-205, 1981. [E]

Senekjian EK, Potkul RK, Frey K, et al.: Infertility among daughters either exposed or not exposed to diethylstilbestrol. Am J Obstet Gynecol 158:493-498, 1988. [E]

Sharp GB, Cole P: Vaginal bleeding and diethylstilbestrol exposure during pregnancy: Relationship to genital tract clear cell adenocarcinoma and vaginal adenosis in daughters. Am J Obstet Gynecol 164(4):994-1001, 1990. [E]

Shy KK, Stenchever MA, Karp LE, et al.: Genital tract examinations and zona-free hamster egg penetration tests from men exposed in utero to diethylstilbestrol. Fertil Steril 42(5):772-778, 1984. [E]

Stillman RJ: In utero exposure to diethylstilbestrol: Adverse effects on the reproductive tract and reproductive performance in male and female offspring. Am J Obstet Gynecol 142:905-921, 1982. [R]

Sugimura Y, Cunha GR, Yonemura CU, et al.: Temporal and spatial factors in diethylstilbestrol-induced squamous metaplasia of the developing human prostate. Hum Pathol 19(2):133-139, 1988. [A]

Thompson RS, Hess DL, Binkerd PE, Hendrickx AG: The effects of prenatal diethylstilbestrol exposure on the genitalia of pubertal Macaca mulatta. II. Male offspring. J Reprod Med 26:309-316, 1981. [A]

Turusov VS, Trukhanova LS, Parfenov YD, Tomatis L: Occurrence of tumours in the descendants of CBA male mice prenatally treated with diethylstilbestrol. Int J Cancer 50:131-135, 1992. [A]

Vessey MP: Epidemiological studies of the effects of diethystilboestrol. IARC Sci Publ (96):335-348, 1989. [R]

Vessey MP, Fairweather DVI, Norman-Smith B: A randomized double-blind controlled trial of the value of stilboestrol therapy in pregnancy: Long-term follow-up of mothers and their offspring. Br J Obstet Gynaecol 90:1007-1017, 1983. [E]

Walker BE: Animal models of prenatal exposure to diethylstilboestrol. IARC Sci Publ (96):349-364, 1989. [R]

Walker BE: Reproductive tract anomalies in mice after prenatal exposure to DES. Teratology 21:313-321, 1980. [A]

Walker BE: Transplacental exposure to diethylstilbestrol. Issues Rev Teratol 2:157-187, 1984. [R]

Walker BE: Uterine tumors in old female mice exposed prenatally to diethylstilbestrol. J Nat Canc Inst 70:477-484, 1983a. [A]

Walker BE: Complications of pregnancy in mice exposed prenatally to DES. Teratology 27:73-80, 1983b. [A]

DIFENOXIN

Synonyms

Difenossina, Difenoxilic Acid, Difenoxina, Difenoxinum, Difenoxylic Acid, Diphenoxin, Diphenoxylic Acid

Summary

Difenoxin, an active metabolite of diphenoxylate, is chemically related to narcotics. Difenoxin is administered orally in the treatment of diarrhea.

Magnitude of Teratogenic Risk

Undetermined

Quality and Quantity of Data

None

Comment

None

No epidemiological studies of congenital anomalies in infants born to women who were treated with difenoxin during pregnancy have been reported.

No animal teratology studies of difenoxin have been published.

Please see agent summary on meperidine for information on a related agent that has been studied.

Key References

None available.

DIFLORASONE

Synonyms

Bexilona, Dermonilo, Diflorasona, Florone, Flutone, Fulixan, Maxiflor, Murode, Psorcon, Sterodelta

Summary

Diflorasone is a fluorinated corticosteroid that is used topically in the treatment of various dermatoses. Diflorasone may be systemically absorbed after topical application.

Magnitude of Teratogenic Risk

Undetermined

Quality and Quantity of Data

None To Poor

Comment

A small risk cannot be excluded, but a high risk of congenital anomalies in the children of women treated with diflorasone during pregnancy is unlikely.

No epidemiological studies of congenital anomalies among infants born to women treated with diflorasone during pregnancy have been reported.

Increased frequencies of palatal, cardiac, and other congenital anomalies were observed among the offspring of rabbits treated during pregnancy with topical diflorasone in a dose that was sufficient to produce maternal toxicity (0.016 mg/kg/d) (Narama, 1984). No effect was seen with lower doses. No increase in the frequency of malformations was observed among the offspring of pregnant rats treated subcutaneously with doses of diflorasone that caused maternal toxicity (0.045 mg/kg/d or greater), but fetal growth and developmental retardation and increased perinatal mortality were seen (Suzuki & Narama, 1984; Satoh et al., 1984).

Key References

Narama I: Reproduction studies of diflorasone diacetate (DDA). (4) Teratogenicity study in rabbits by percutaneous administration. Oyo Yakuri 28(2):241-250, 1984. [A]

Satoh T, Narama I, Odani Y: Reproduction studies of diflorasone diacetate (DDA). (2) Teratogenicity study in rats by subcutaneous administration. Oyo Yakuri 28(2):207-224, 1984. [A]

Suzuki T, Narama I: Reproduction studies of diflorasone diacetate (DDA). (1) Fertility study in rats by subcutaneous administration. Oyo Yakuri 28(2):195-205, 1984. [A]

DIFLUNISAL

Synonyms

Adomal, Algobid, Difludol, Dolobid, Fluniget, Renflos, Unisal

Summary

Diflunisal is a salicylate analgesic used orally in the treatment of arthritis.

Magnitude of Teratogenic Risk

Undetermined

Quality and Quantity of Data

Poor

Comment

A small risk cannot be excluded, but there is no indication that the risk of congenital anomalies in the children of women treated with diflunisal during pregnancy is likely to be great.

No epidemiological studies of congenital anomalies in children born to women who used diflunisal during pregnancy have been reported.

No teratogenic effect was observed among the offspring of cynomolgus monkeys treated with 1-3 times the human therapeutic dose of diflunisal during pregnancy (Rowland et al., 1977). The frequency of malformations was not increased among the offspring of rats or rabbits treated during pregnancy with diflunisal in doses, respectively, 1-4 and 1-2 times those used in humans (Nakatsuka & Fujii, 1979; Clark et al., 1984). In rabbits, increases in fetal death and vertebral anomalies were observed with higher doses, but these were toxic to the mothers.

Please see agent summary on aspirin for information on a related agent that has been more thoroughly studied.

Key References

Clark RL, Robertson RT, Minsker DH, Cohen SM, et al.: Diflunisal-induced maternal anemia as a cause of teratogenicity in rabbits. Teratology 30:319-332, 1984. [A]

Nakatsuka T, Fujii T: Comparative teratogenicity study of diflunisal (MK-647) and aspirin in the rat. Oyo Yakuri 17:551-557, 1979. [A]

Rowland JM, Robertson RT, Cukierski M, et al.: Evaluation of the teratogenicity and pharmacokinetics of diflunisal in cynomolgus monkeys. Fundam Appl Toxicol 8:51-58, 1987. [A]

DIGOXIN

Synonyms

Digitalis Lanata, Digomal, Dixina, Lanoxicaps, Lanoxin, Novodigal, Prodigox

Summary

Digoxin is the prototype of a widely used class of drugs, the cardiac glycosides. These agents are employed in the treatment of heart failure and cardiac arrhythmias.

Magnitude of Teratogenic Risk

None To Minimal

Quality and Quantity of Data

Fair

Comment

None

The frequency of congenital anomalies was no greater than expected among the infants of 142 women who were treated with digoxin in the first trimester of pregnancy in a large cohort study (Aselton et al., 1985). Similarly, the frequency of congenital anomalies was not increased among the children of 52 women treated with cardiac glycosides in the first four lunar months of pregnancy or of 129 women treated with these agents anytime in pregnancy in the Collaborative Perinatal Project (Heinonen et al., 1977).

No teratogenic effect has been observed among the offspring of either rats or rabbits treated during pregnancy with cardiac glycosides in doses hundreds of times greater than those used in humans (Hatano, 1976; Nagaoka et al., 1976).

A significantly shortened gestation and labor were observed among 22 women who took cardiac glycosides during pregnancy in one study (Weaver & Pearson, 1973) but not in another study of similar size (Ho et al., 1980).

Fetal cardiac arrhythmia and hydrops have been treated successfully during the second half of pregnancy by administration of digoxin to the mother or directly to the fetus (Wladimiroff et al., 1985; Weiner et al., 1988; Maeda et al., 1988).

Maternal digitalis toxicity may cause serious or even fatal arrhythmias in the fetus or neonate (Sherman & Locke, 1960; Potondi, 1966).

Key References

Aselton P, Jick H, Milunsky A, Hunter JR, et al.: First-trimester drug use and congenital disorders. Obstet Gynecol 65:451-455, 1985. [S]

Hatano M, Nagaoka T, Osuka F, Shigemura T: Reproduction studies of beta-methyldigoxin. 1. Teratogenicity study in rats. Kiso To Rinsho (Clin Rep) 10:579-593, 1976. [E]

Heinonen OP, Slone D, Shapiro S: Birth Defects and Drugs in Pregnancy. Littleton, Mass.: John Wright-PSG, 1977, pp 441, 496. [E]

Ho PC, Chen TY, Wong V: The effect of maternal cardiac disease and digoxin administration on labour, fetal weight and maturity at birth. Aust NZ J Obstet Gynaecol 20:24-27, 1980. [E]

Maeda H, Shimokawa H, Nakano H: Effects of intrauterine treatment on nonimmunologic hydrops fetalis. Fetal Ther 3(4):198-209, 1988. [S]

Nagaoka T, Osuka F, Shigemura T, Hatano M: Teratogenicity test of beta-methyldigoxin (beta-MD). Kiso To Rinsho (Clin Rep) 10:405-411, 1976. [A]

Potondi A: Congenital rhabdomyoma of the heart and intrauterine digitalis poisoning. J Forensic Sci 11:81-88, 1966. [C]

Sherman JL, Locke RV: Transplacental neonatal digitalis intoxication. Am J Cardiol 6:834-837, 1960. [C]

Weaver JB, Pearson JF: Influence of digitalis on time of onset and duration of labour in women with cardiac disease. Br Med J 3:519-520, 1973. [E]

Weiner CP, Thompson MIB: Direct treatment of fetal supraventricular tachycardia after failed transplacental therapy. Am J Obstet Gynecol 158:570-573, 1988. [C]

Wladimiroff JW, Stewart PA: Treatment of fetal cardiac arrhythmias. Br J Hosp Med 34:134-140, 1985. [R]

DIHYDROERGOTAMINE

Synonyms

D.H.E. 45, Dihydroergotamine Mesylate, Dihydroergotamine Tartrate

Summary

Dihydroergotamine is an ergot derivative used in treatment of migraine and vascular headache. It also has mild vasoconstrictive and oxytocic effects.

Magnitude of Teratogenic Risk

Undetermined

Quality and Quantity of Data

None To Poor

Comment

1) A small risk cannot be excluded, but there is no indication that the risk of congenital anomalies in the children of women treated with dihydroergotamine during pregnancy is likely to be great.

2) Use of dihydroergotamine late in pregnancy may be associated with premature onset of labor.

No epidemiological studies of congenital anomalies in infants whose mothers took dihydroergotamine during pregnancy have been reported.

No animal teratology studies of dihydroergotamine have been published.

Premature labor has been observed after administration of dihydroergotamine to a woman at the thirty-sixth week of pregnancy (Lippert & Bohm, 1982). In view of the known oxytocic activity of dihydroergotamine, this association may be causal (Lippert & Bohm, 1984).

Key References

Lippert TH, Bohm HR: [Risk of treatment with dihydroergotamine in pregnancy]. Geburtsh u Frauenheilk 42:866-867, 1982. [C]

Lippert TH, Bohm HR: [Risk of treatment with dihydroergotamine in pregnancy]. Geburtsh u Frauenheilk 44:403-405, 1984. [C]

DIHYDROXYACETONE

Synonyms

Chromelin, Dihyxal, Otan, Oxantin, Oxatone, Soleal, Triulose, Vitadye, Viticolor

Summary

Dihydroxyacetone is applied topically to enhance pigmentation through activation of melanocytes.

Magnitude of Teratogenic Risk

Undetermined

Quality and Quantity of Data

None

Comment

None

No epidemiological studies of congenital anomalies among infants born to women who used dihydroxyacetone during pregnancy have been reported.

No animal teratology studies of dihydroxyacetone have been published.

Please see the agent summary on methoxsalen for information on an agent with similar activity.

Key References

None available.

DILOXANIDE

Synonyms

Entamide, Furamide

Summary

Diloxanide is an oral antiparasitic agent used to treat amebiasis.

Magnitude of Teratogenic Risk

Undetermined

Quality and Quantity of Data

None

Comment

None

No epidemiological studies of congenital anomalies among the children of women treated with diloxanide during pregnancy have been reported.

No animal teratology studies of diloxanide have been published.

Key References

None available.

DILTIAZEM

Synonyms

Cardizem, CRD-401, Herbesser, Latiazem Hydrochloride, Masdil, Tildiem

Summary

Diltiazem is a calcium channel-blocking agent used in the management of angina pectoris.

Magnitude of Teratogenic Risk

Undetermined

Quality and Quantity of Data

None To Poor

Comment

None

No epidemiological studies of congenital anomalies among infants born to women treated with diltiazem during pregnancy have been reported.

A dose-dependent increase in the frequency of embryonic loss was observed among pregnant rabbits, mice, and rats treated with diltiazem in doses respectively 2, 2, and 6 or more times those used in humans (Ariyuki, 1975). Malformations of the limbs and tail were observed in the offspring of rabbits and rats, but not mice, treated with similar doses. No significant teratogenic effect was observed among the offspring of animals of these three species treated with smaller doses of diltiazem during pregnancy. The relevance, if any, of these findings to the therapeutic use of diltiazem in human pregnancy is unknown.

Diltiazem, in doses 7 times those used clinically, inhibits labor in rats at term (Hahn et al., 1984). This effect has not been studied in humans.

Key References

Ariyuki F: Effects of diltiazem hydrochloride on embryonic development: Species differences in the susceptibility and stage specificity in mice, rats, and rabbits. Okajimas Folia Anat Jpn 52:103-117, 1975. [A]

Hahn DW, McGuire JL, Vanderhoof M, Ericson E, et al.: Evaluation of drugs for arrest of premature labor in a new animal model. Am J Obstet Gynecol 148:775-778, 1984. [A]

DIMERCAPROL

Synonyms

BAL, BAL in Oil, British Anti-Lewisite, Sulfactin

Summary

Dimercaprol is a chelating agent that is administered intramuscularly in the treatment of lead, gold, mercury, and arsenic poisoning.

Magnitude of Teratogenic Risk

Undetermined

Quality and Quantity of Data

None To Poor

Comment

None

No epidemiological studies of congenital anomalies among infants born to women treated with dimercaprol during pregnancy have been reported.

The frequency of malformations was not increased among the offspring of mice treated with dimercaprol in a daily dose 2-3 times that used in humans (Hood & Pike, 1972; Hood & Vedel-Macrander, 1984). Skeletal malformations were found more often than expected in the offspring of pregnant mice treated with 60 times the human therapeutic dose of dimercaprol in another study (Nishimura & Takagaki, 1959).

Key References

Hood RD, Pike CT: BAL alleviation of arsenate-induced teratogenesis in mice. Teratology 6:235-238, 1972. [A]

Hood RD, Vedel-Macrander GC: Evaluation of the effect of BAL (2,3-dimercaptopropanol) on arsenite-induced teratogenesis in mice. Toxicol Appl Pharmacol 73:1-7, 1984. [A]

Nishimura H, Takagaki S: Developmental anomalies in mice induced by 2,3-dimercaptopropanol (BAL). Anat Rec 135:261-267, 1959. [A]

DIMETHISOQUIN

Synonyms

Chinisocaine Hydrochloride, Haenal, Isochinol, Pruralgan, Pruralgin, Quinisocaine Hydrochloride, Quotane

Summary

Dimethisoquin is a surface anesthetic.

Magnitude of Teratogenic Risk

Undetermined

Quality and Quantity of Data

None

Comment

None

No epidemiological studies of congenital anomalies in children born to women exposed to dimethisoquin during pregnancy have been reported.

No investigations of teratologic effects of dimethisoquin in experimental animals have been published.

Key References

None available.

DIMETHYL SULFOXIDE (DMSO)

Synonyms

Deltan, Demasorb, Demavet, Demeso, DMSO, Dolicur, Dromisol, Gamasol 90, Hyadur, Infiltrina, Somipront, Syntexan

Summary

Dimethyl sulfoxide (DMSO) is an organic solvent that is widely used in industry. It is employed medically as a bladder irrigant in symptomatic treatment of cystitis and as a topical therapy for scleroderma. Dimethyl sulfoxide is absorbed after topical application.

Magnitude of Teratogenic Risk

Undetermined

Quality and Quantity of Data

None To Poor

Comment

None

No epidemiological studies of congenital anomalies among infants born to women treated with dimethyl sulfoxide during pregnancy have been reported.

Increased frequencies of central nervous system, facial, skeletal, and other malformations were observed among the offspring of hamsters and mice treated with very large doses (>5 g/kg/d) of dimethyl sulfoxide during pregnancy (Ferm, 1966; Robens, 1969; Staples & Pecharo, 1973), but no consistent teratogenic effect was seen among the offspring of pregnant mice given DMSO in smaller doses (0.1-2.8 g/kg/d) (Anonymous, 1968; Nomura et al., 1984). In rats and rabbits, increased frequencies of fetal death were observed with doses of 5-10 or 1-3 g/kg/d, respectively (Caujolle et al., 1967; Schumacher et al., 1968; Staples & Pecharo, 1973). The relevance of these findings to usual human exposures to dimethyl sulfoxide is unknown.

Key References

Anonymous: Evaluation of carcinogenic, teratogenic, and mutagenic activities of selected pesticides and industrial chemicals. 2. Teratogenic study in mice and rats. NTIS (National Technical Information Service) Report/PB223 160, 1968. [A]

Caujolle FME, Caujolle DH, Cros SB, Calvet MMJ: Limits of toxic and teratogenic tolerance of dimethyl sulfoxide. NY Acad Sci 141:110-125, 1967. [A]

Ferm VH: Congenital malformations induced by dimethyl sulphoxide in the golden hamster. J Empryol Exp Morphol 16:49-54, 1966. [A]

Nomura T, Kurokawa N, Isa Y, et al.: Induction of lymphorecticular neoplasia and malformations by prenatal treatment with 1,3-di(4-sulfamoyl-phenyl)-triazene in mice. Carcinogenesis 5(5):571-575, 1984. [A]

Robens JF: Teratologic studies of carbaryl, diazinon, norea, disulfiram, and thiram in small laboratory animals. Toxicol Appl Pharmacol 15:152-163, 1969. [A]

Schumacher H, Blake DA, Gurian JM, Gillette JR: A comparison of the teratogenic activity of thalidomide in rabbits and rats. J Pharmacol Exp Ther 160:189-200, 1968. [A]

Staples RE, Pecharo MM: Species differences in DMSO-induced teratology. Acta Univ Carol Med Monogr 61:131-133, 1973. [A]

DINITROPHENOL

Synonyms

Aldifen, Dinofan, Maroxol-50, Nitro Kleenup, Nitrophene, Solfo Black B

Summary

Dinitrophenol is used as an insecticide, as a wood preservative, and in the manufacture of dyes. Dinitrophenol markedly increases metabolism and is highly toxic to humans. It has been administered systemically to induce weight loss. Dinitrophenol is readily absorbed through intact skin or, as a vapor, through the lungs.

Magnitude of Teratogenic Risk

Undetermined

Quality and Quantity of Data

None To Poor

Comment

Dinitrophenol may pose a teratogenic risk under conditions of exposure in which maternal toxicity occurs, such as when it is taken to induce weight loss.

No epidemiological studies of congenital anomalies among infants born to women exposed to dinitrophenol during pregnancy have been reported.

The frequency of malformations was not increased among the offspring of rats treated with 30-40 mg/kg/d of dinitrophenol although increased rates of maternal and fetal death were observed (Goldman & Yakovac, 1964). In another study employing similar doses and published as a letter to the editor, a slightly increased frequency of anophthalmia and microphthalmia is said to have occurred (Klein Obbink & Dalderup, 1964).

Please see agent summary on dinoseb for information on a related agent that has been more thoroughly studied.

Key References

Goldman AS, Yakovac WC: Salicylate intoxication and congenital anomalies. Arch Environ Health 8:648-656, 1964. [A]

Klein Obbink HJ, Dalderup LM: Effect of acetylsalicylic acid on fetal mice and rats. Lancet 2:152, 1964. [A]

DINOSEB

Synonyms

Basanite, Butaphene, Caldon, Dinitrobutyl-phenol, DNBP, Premerge, Subitex

Summary

Dinoseb is a dinitrophenol derivative that is widely used as an herbicide. Dinoseb acts as a cumulative toxin and may be absorbed into the body after ingestion, inhalation, or through the skin.

Magnitude of Teratogenic Risk

Undetermined

Quality and Quantity of Data

Poor

Comment

The risk of congenital anomalies may be substantial in the children of women who are exposed to maternally toxic doses of dinoseb during pregnancy.

No epidemiological studies of congenital anomalies among infants born to women exposed to dinoseb during pregnancy have been reported.

Increased frequencies of fetal death and of malformations including imperforate anus and skeletal defects have been observed among the offspring of mice treated with dinoseb in doses that were maternally toxic (17.7 mg/kg/d or greater) but not in lower doses (10.0-15.8 mg/kg/d) (Gibson, 1973). Increased frequencies of malformations, especially of the eye, were seen among the offspring of pregnant rats fed a diet containing 200 ppm of dinoseb, a dose that causes substantial maternal toxicity (Giavini et al., 1986, 1989). Increased frequencies of CNS and skeletal anomalies were reportedly seen among the offspring of rabbits treated with 10 mg/kg/d of dinoseb, a dose that did not produce apparent maternal toxicity (Anonymous, 1986).

Supplemental Information for Environmental and Occupational Exposures

Occupational Exposure: Human exposure to dinoseb occurs primarily during its application as a herbicide, fungicide, or dessicant. Agricultural workers and their families are also at risk to exposure, indirectly, via contaminated clothing (Anonymous, 1986).

    Aerial and Spray Applicators
        Dermal: 0.32-146 mg/hr. Wind shifts can produce exposures as high as 1700 mg/hr in flaggers (Anonymous, 1986).
        Respiratory (Spray applicators): 0.12 mg/hr. (HSDB(R), 1990).

Occupational Re-EntryValues: Unavailable.

Odor Threshold: Unavailable.

Permissible Exposure Limit In Air: Unavailable.

No Effects Level: 3 mg/kg/day (Anonymous, 1986).

Maximum Residue Allowed In Clothing: Unavailable.

Immediately Dangerous To Life Or Health Value: Unavailable. Symptoms of acute toxicity occur with ingestion of 3-5 mg/kg or equivalent exposure by other routes.

Toxic Signs And Symptoms (HSDB(R), 1990; POISINDEX(R), 1990):
    Acute (onset within a few hours of exposure):
        Yellow staining of skin and hair; staining of sclerae and urine with potentially toxic amounts
        Profuse sweating, high fever, tachypnea, cyanosis, tachycardia, cardiac arrythmias, hypertension
        Headache, thirst, confusion, anxiety, restlessness, mania, lassitude, coma, or inappropriate sense of well-being
    Muscle weakness
    Jaundice
    Albuminuria, hematuria, pyuria, azotemia

Chronic (Kurt et al., 1986; Finkel, 1983):

Cataracts
Weight loss
Skin rash
Liver damage
Renal damage
Neutropenia

LD50 (Dermal):

Guinea Pig: 200-300 mg/kg
Humans: 75 mg/kg (Spencer et al., 1948)

LD50 (Oral):

Guinea Pig: 20-40 mg/kg (Bough et al., 1965)
Mouse: 20-40 mg/kg (Bough et al., 1965)
Rat: 60 mg/kg (Spencer, 1982)

Tests For Exposure: Dinoseb can be detected in the plasma and urine by gas chromatography.

Key References

Anonymous: Decision and emergency order suspending the registrations of all pesticide products containing dinoseb. Federal Register 51(198):36634-36649, 1986. [O]

Bough RG, Cliffe EE, Lessel B: Comparative toxicity and blood level studies on binapacryl and DNBP. Toxicol Appl Pharmacol 7:353-360, 1965. [A]

Finkel AJ: Herbicides: Dinitrophenols. In: Hamilton and Hardy's Industrial Toxicology, 4th ed. Boston: John Wright-PSG, 1983, pp 301-302. [R]

Giavini E, Broccia ML, Prati M, Cova D, Rossini L: Teratogenicity of dinoseb: Role of the diet. Bull Environ Contam Toxicol 43:215-219, 1989. [A]

Giavini E, Broccia ML, Prati M, Vismara C: Effect of method of administration on the teratogenicity of dinoseb in the rat. Arch Environ Contam Toxicol 15:377-384, 1986. [A]

Gibson JE: Teratology studies in mice with 2-sec-butyl-4,6-dinitrophenol (dinoseb). Fd Cosmet Toxicol 11:31-43, 1973. [A]

HSDB [database online]. Bethesda, Md.: National Library of Medicine, 1985- [updated 1990]. Available from: National Library of Medicine; BRS Information Technologies, McLean, Va. [O]

Kurt TL, Anderson R, Petty C, et al.: Dinitrophenol in weight loss. The poison center and public safety. Vet Human Toxicol 28:574-575, 1986. [S]

POISINDEX(R): POISINDEX Substance Indentification (CD-ROM version). Denver, CO: Micromedex, 1990. [O]

Spencer F, Tat S-L: Reproductive toxicity in pseudopregnant and pregnant rats following post-implantational exposure: Effects of the herbicide dinoseb. Pestic Biochem Physiol 18:150-157, 1982. [A]

Spencer HC, Rowe VK, Adams EM, et al.: Toxicological studies on laboratory animals of certain alkyldinitrophenols used in agriculture. J Ind Toxicol 30:73-87, 1948. [A]

DIOXYBENZONE

Synonyms

Advastab 47, Benzophenone 8, Spectra-Sorb UV 24

Summary

Dioxybenzone is used topically as a sunscreen.

Magnitude of Teratogenic Risk

Undetermined

Quality and Quantity of Data

None

Comment

None

No epidemiological studies of congenital anomalies in infants whose mothers used dioxybenzone during pregnancy have been reported.

No animal teratology studies of dioxybenzone have been published.

Key References

None available.

DIPERODON

Synonyms

Diothane Ointment, Diperocaine

Summary

Diperodon is a surface anesthetic.

Magnitude of Teratogenic Risk

Undetermined

Quality and Quantity of Data

None

Comment

A small risk cannot be excluded, but there is no indication that risk of congenital anomalies in the children of women treated with diperodon during pregnancy is likely to be great.

No epidemiological studies of congenital anomalies in children born to women exposed to diperodon during pregnancy have been reported.

No investigations of teratologic effects of diperodon in experimental animals have been published.

Key References

None available.

DIPHENHYDRAMINE

Synonyms

Benadryl, Benylin, Dimedrolum, Ephedramine, Histergan, Insomnal, Nytol, Pheramin, Sleep-eze 3, Sominex 2

Summary

Diphenhydramine is an antihistamine that is commonly used to treat allergic reactions, coughs and colds, nausea and vomiting, and Parkinson's disease.

Magnitude of Teratogenic Risk

None To Minimal

Quality and Quantity of Data

Fair To Good

Comment

None

The frequencies of congenital anomalies in general, of major malformations, minor anomalies, and major categories of congenital anomalies were no greater than expected among the children of 595 women who took diphenhydramine during the first four lunar months of pregnancy in the Collaborative Perinatal Project (Heinonen et al., 1977). The frequency of congenital anomalies among the children of 2948 women who took this drug anytime during pregnancy was also no greater than expected. Similarly, the frequency of malformations was no greater than expected among the infants of a total of 631 women who used diphenhydramine during the first trimester of pregnancy in two cohorts of the Boston Collaborative Drug Surveillance Program (Jick et al., 1981; Aselton et al., 1985).

First-trimester maternal exposure to diphenhydramine was more frequent than expected in one case-control study of 590 children with oral clefts (Saxen, 1974), but this association was not apparent in the

Collaborative Perinatal Project (Heinonen et al., 1977). If there is an increased risk of cleft palate in infants born to women who use diphenhydramine early in pregnancy, the magnitude of this risk is probably less than 1%.

No definite increase in the frequency of malformations was observed among the offspring of mice treated with diphenhydramine in doses 8-33 times those used clinically (Iuliucci & Gautieri, 1971; Jones-Price et al., 1982a, b). No teratogenic effect was observed among the offspring of rats or rabbits treated during pregnancy with diphenhydramine in doses <1-17 or <1-3 times those used in humans (Schardein et al., 1971; Jones-Price et al., 1983). Alterations of behavior have been observed among the offspring of rats treated with three times the human dose of diphenhydramine during pregnancy (Chiavegatto et al., 1989).

Uterine hyperstimulation and associated fetal compromise have been reported in women given diphenhydramine during labor (Hay & Wood, 1967; Hara et al., 1980).

Key References

Aselton P, Jick H, Milunsky A, Hunter JR, et al.: First-trimester drug use and congenital disorders. Obstet Gynecol 65:451-455, 1985. [S]

Chiavegatto S, Bernardi MM, de-Souza-Spinosa H: Effects of prenatal diphenydramine administration on sexual behavior in rats. Braz J Med Biol Res 22:729-732, 1989. [A]

Hara GS, Carter RP, Krantz KE: Dramamine in labor: Potential boon or a possible bomb? J Kans Med Soc 81:134-136, 155, 1980. [S]

Heinonen OP, Slone D, Shapiro S: Birth Defects and Drugs in Pregnancy. Littleton, Mass.: John Wright-PSG, 1977, pp 437, 475. [E]

Iuliucci JD, Gautieri RF: Morphine-induced fetal malformation. II: Influence of histamine and diphenhydramine. J Pharmaceut Sci 60:420-424, 1971. [A]

Jick H, Holmes LB, Hunter JR, Madsen S, et al.: First-trimester drug use and congenital disorders. JAMA 246:343-346, 1981. [S]

Jones-Price C, Ledoux TA, Reel JR, Langhoff-Paschke L: Teratologic evaluation of diphenhydramine hydrochloride (CAS No. 147-24-0) in CD-1 mice. NTIS (National Technical Information Service) Report/PB83-163055, 1982b. [E]

Jones-Price C, Ledoux TA, Reel JR, Langhoff-Paschke L: Teratologic evaluation of diphenhydramine hydrochloride (CAS No. 147-24-0) in CD rats. NTIS (National Technical Information Service) Report/PB83-180612, 1983. [A]

Jones-Price C, Ledoux TA, Reel JR, Langhoff-Paschke L, et al.: Teratologic evaluation of diphenhydramine hydrochloride (CAS No. 147-24-0) administered to CD-1 mice on gestational days 11 through 14. NTIS (National Technical Information Service) Report/ PB83-148684, 1982a. [A]

Saxen I: Cleft palate and maternal diphenhydramine intake. Lancet 1:407-408, 1974. [E]

Schardein JL, Hentz DL, Petrere JA, Kurtz SM: Teratogenesis studies with diphenhydramine HCL. Toxicol Appl Pharmacol 18:971-976, 1971. [A]

DIPHENIDOL

Synonyms

Ansmin, Avomol, Difenidol Hydrochloride, Vontril, Vontrol

Summary

Diphenidol is used for the treatment of vertigo and the control of nausea and vomiting. It is chemically unrelated to other commonly used antiemetics.

Magnitude of Teratogenic Risk

Undetermined

Quality and Quantity of Data

None

Comment

None

No epidemiological studies of congenital anomalies in infants born to women who were treated with diphenidol during pregnancy have been reported.

No animal teratology studies of diphenidol have been published.

Key References

None available.

DIPHENOXYLATE

Summary

Diphenoxylate is chemically related to narcotics but has no analgesic action. It decreases intestinal motility and is used to treat acute and chronic diarrhea. It is formulated in combination with atropine to prevent abuse.

Magnitude of Teratogenic Risk

Undetermined

Quality and Quantity of Data

None To Poor

Comment

None

No adequate epidemiological study of malformations in infants born to women who used diphenoxylate during pregnancy has been reported.

Fetal death was substantially increased among pregnant rats that were treated with 75-125 times the maxiumum human dose of diphenoxylate (Wang et al., 1987). The relevance of this observation to the therapeutic use of diphenoxylate in human pregnancy is uncertain.

Key References

Wang NG, Guan MZ, Lei HP: [Studies on the effect of the combined use of dl-15methyl-prostaglandin F2 alpha methyl ester with diphenoxylate hydrochloride in early pregnancy in rats]. Chung

Kuo I Hsueh Ko Hsueh Yuan Hsueh Pao 9:414-417, 1987. [A]

DIPHENYLPYRALINE

Synonyms

Allerzine, Anti-Hist, Diafen, Hispril, Histalert, Histryl, Kolton, Lergoban

Summary

Diphenylpyraline is an oral antihistaminic agent. It is used in the treatment of allergic conditions.

Magnitude of Teratogenic Risk

Undetermined

Quality and Quantity of Data

None To Poor

Comment

A small risk cannot be excluded, but a high risk of congenital anomalies in the children of women treated with diphenylpyraline during pregnancy is unlikely.

No epidemiological studies of congenital anomalies among infants born to women treated with diphenylpyraline during pregnancy have been reported.

The frequency of malformations was no greater than expected among the offspring of rats or mice treated during pregnancy with diphenylpyraline in doses respectively 6-94 and 8-24 times those used in humans (Knoche & Konig, 1964; King et al., 1965).

Key References

King CTG, Weaver SA, Narrod SA: Antihistamines and teratogenicity in the rat. J Pharmacol Exp Therapeut 147:391-398, 1965. [A]

Knoche VC, Konig J: Zur pranatalen Toxizitat von Diphenylpyralin-8-chlor-theophyllinat unter Berucksichtigung von Erfahrungen mit Thalidomid und Coffein. Arzneimittelforsch 14:415-424, 1964. [A]

DIPHTHERIA ANTITOXIN

Synonyms

Equine Diphtheria Antitoxin

Summary

Diphtheria antitoxin is a purified antiserum containing equine antibodies against the toxin of Corynebacterium diphtheriae. Diphtheria antitoxin is administered intramuscularly or intravenously in the treatment of diphtheria.

Magnitude of Teratogenic Risk

Undetermined

Quality and Quantity of Data

None

Comment

None

No epidemiological studies of congenital anomalies in infants whose mothers were treated with diphtheria antitoxin during pregnancy have been reported.

No animal teratology studies of diphtheria antitoxin have been published.

Key References

None available.

DIPOTASSIUM PHOSPHATE

Synonyms

Dipotassium Monophosphate, Potassium Biphosphate, Potassium Monophosphate

Summary

Dipotassium phosphate has been used orally as a saline cathartic and parenterally in the treatment of electrolyte disturbances.

Magnitude of Teratogenic Risk

Undetermined

Quality and Quantity of Data

None

Comment

A small risk cannot be excluded, but a high risk of congenital anomalies in the children of women treated with dipotassium phosphate during pregnancy is unlikely.

No epidemiological studies of congenital anomalies in infants whose mothers were treated with dipotassium phosphate during pregnancy have been reported.

No animal teratology studies of dipotassium phosphate have been published.

Key References

None available.

DIPYRIDAMOLE

Synonyms

Dipramol, Peridamol, Persantin

Summary

Dipyridamole is an antithrombotic agent. It has been used in pregnancy in an attempt to prevent fetal growth retardation and fetal death. It is also employed as a vasodilator in the long-term management of angina pectoris.

Magnitude of Teratogenic Risk

None To Minimal

Quality and Quantity of Data

Poor To Fair

Comment

None

Maternal therapy with dipyridamole and aspirin may prevent recurrence of fetal growth retardation and fetal death in women who have had previously affected pregnancies (Beaufils et al., 1985; Wallenburg & Rotmans, 1987; Uzan et al., 1991). No increase in congenital anomalies or other adverse effects among the infants was observed in controlled trials of 119, 48, and 30 high-risk pregnancies in women who were treated with dipyridamole and aspirin in the second and third trimesters of pregnancy (Beaufils et al., 1985, 1986; Wallenburg & Rotmans, 1987; Uzan et al., 1991). Although a variety of congenital anomalies have been observed in children whose mothers were treated with dipyridamole during pregnancy, no consistent pattern of malformations is apparent and the frequency of anomalies in these series does not seem unusually high (Tejani, 1973; Ibarra-Perez et al., 1976; Chen et al., 1982). A causal relationship cannot be inferred from these observations.

Fetal loss is frequent among women with artifical heart valves who are treated during pregnancy with warfarin and may be even higher in those treated with both warfarin and dipyridamole (Ibarra-Perez et al., 1976; Sareli et al., 1989). The clinical significance of this is unclear.

No animal teratology studies of dipyridamole have been published.

Key References

Beaufils M, Uzan S, Donsimoni R, Colau JC: Prevention of pre-eclampsia by early antiplatelet therapy. Lancet 1:840-842, 1985. [S]

Beaufils M, Uzan S, Donsimoni R, Colau JC: Prospective controlled study of early antiplatelet therapy in prevention of preeclampsia. Adv Nephrol 15:87-94, 1986. [E]

Chen WWC, Chan CS, Lee PK, Wang RYC, et al.: Pregnancy in patients with prosthetic heart valves: An experience with 45 pregnancies. Q J Med 51:358-365, 1982. [S]

Ibarra-Perez C, Arevalo-Toledo N, Alvarez-De La Cadena O, Noriega-Guerra L: The course of pregnancy in patients with artificial heart valves. Am J Med 61:504-512, 1976. [S]

Sareli P, England MJ, Berk MR, et al.: Maternal and fetal sequelae of anticoagulation during pregnancy in patients with mechanical heart valve prostheses. Am J Cardiol 63:1462-1465, 1989. [E]

Tejani N: Anticoagulant therapy with cardiac valve prosthesis during pregnancy. Obstet Gynecol 42:785-793, 1973. [R] & [C]

Wallenburg HCS, Rotmans N: Prevention of recurrent idiopathic fetal growth retardation by low-dose aspirin and dipyridamole. Am J Obstet Gynecol 157(5):1230-1235, 1987. [E]

Uzan S, Beaufils M, Breart G, et al.: Prevention of fetal growth retardation with low-dose aspirin: Findings of the EPREDA trial. Lancet 337(8755):1427-1431, 1991. [E]

DIPYRITHIONE

Synonyms

Omadine MDS

Summary

Dipyrithione is a topical antifungal and antibacterial agent used in antidandruff shampoos and as a preservative in cosmetics.

Quality and Quantity of Data

None To Poor

Comment

None

No epidemiological studies of congenital anomalies in infants born to women who used dipyrithione during pregnancy have been reported.

No significant increase in the frequency of malformations was observed among the offspring of pigs or rats treated cutaneously with large amounts of dipyrithione during pregnancy (Wedig et al., 1977; Johnson et al., 1984). Similarly, the frequency of malformations was not consistently increased among the offspring of rats or mice given large doses of this agent systemically during pregnancy (Wedig et al., 1977; Inoue, 1978).

Key References

Inoue K: [Reproduction studies of 2,2'-dithiodipyridine-1, 1'-dioxide (DS) in mice. (2) Teratogenicity study.] Oyo Yakuri (Pharmacometrics) 15:1169-1184, 1978. [A]

Johnson DE, Schardein JL, Mitoma C, Wedig JH: Reproductive toxicological evaluation of omadine MDS. Fund Appl Toxicol 4:81-90, 1984. [A]

Wedig JH, Kennedy GL, Jenkins DH, Keplinger ML: Teratologic evaluation of the magnesium sulfate adduct of [2,2'-dithio-bis-(pyridine-1-oxide)] in swine and rats. Toxicol Appl Pharmacol 42:561-570, 1977. [A]

DISODIUM PHOSPHATE

Synonyms

Dibasic Sodium Phosphate, Disodium Hydrophosphate, Disodium Orthophosphate, Disodium Phosphoric Acid, DSP, Joulie's Solution, Natrium Phosphoricum, Soda Phosphate, Sodium Hydrogen Phosphate, Sodium Phosphate, Dibasic

Summary

Disodium phosphate is used to treat electrolyte disorders.

Magnitude of Teratogenic Risk

Undetermined

Quality and Quantity of Data

None

Comment

A small risk cannot be excluded, but a high risk of congenital anomalies in children of women treated with disodium phosphate during pregnancy is unlikely.

No epidemiological studies of congenital malformations in infants whose mothers were treated with disodium phosphate during pregnancy have been reported.

No animal teratology studies of disodium phosphate have been published.

Key References

None available.

DISOPYRAMIDE

Synonyms

Dirythmin, Durbis, Norpace, Ritmodan, Rythmodan

Summary

Disopyramide is an oral cardiac antiarrhythmic agent with anticholinergic and local anesthetic properties.

Magnitude of Teratogenic Risk

Undetermined

Quality and Quantity of Data

None To Poor

Comment

None

No epidemiological studies of congenital anomalies in children born to women treated with disopyramide during pregnancy have been reported.

No increase in the frequency of malformations was observed in the offspring of pregnant rats, mice, or rabbits treated with disopyramide in doses, respectively, 2-9, <1-9, and 1-4 times those used in humans (Jequier et al., 1970; Esaki et al., 1981, 1983; Umemura et al., 1981; 1984).

Disopyramide induces uterine contractions and delivery when administered to pregnant women at term (Tadmor et al., 1990). Administration of disopyramide at 32 weeks gestation to a woman with cardiac arrhythmia was associated with premature onset of labor (Leonard et al., 1978).

Key References

Esaki K, Umemura T, Yanagita T: Teratogenicity of intragastric administration of disopyramide phosphate in rabbits. Jitchuken Zenrinsho Kenkyuho 9(1):83-92, 1983. [A]

Esaki K, Yanagita T: Effects of intravenous administration of disopyramide phosphate on the rabbit fetus. Jitchuken Zenrinsho Kenkyuho (Preclin Rep Cent Inst Exp Animal) 7:189-198, 1981. [A]

Jequier R, Deraedt R, Plongeron R, Vannier B: [Pharmacology and toxicology of disopiramide.] Minerva Med 61 (Suppl):3689-3693, 1970. [R]

Leonard RF, Braun TE, Levy AM: Initiation of uterine contractions by disopyramide during pregnancy. N Engl J Med 299:84-85, 1978. [C]

Tadmor OP, Keren A, Rosenak D, et al.: The effect of disopyramide on uterine contractions during pregnancy. Am J Obstet Gynecol 162:482-486, 1990. [E]

Umemura T, Esaki K, Ando K, et al.: Effects of intragastric administration of disopyramide phosphate on reproduction in rats. III. Experiment on drug administration during the organogenesis period. CIEA (Cent Inst Exp Anim) Preclin Rep 10:87-110, 1984. [A]

Umemura T, Sasa H, Esaki K, Takada K, et al.: Effects of disopyramide phosphate on reproduction in the rats. II. Experiments on drug administration during the organogenesis periods. Jitchuken Zenrinsho Kenkyuho (Preclin Rep Cent Inst Exp Animal) 7:157-173, 1981. [A]

DISULFIRAM

Synonyms

Antabuse, Antietanol, Ethyldithiourame, Refusal, Ro-Sulfiram-500, Tetraethylthiuram

Summary

Disulfiram, an inhibitor of acetaldehyde dehydrogenase, is used in the treatment of alcoholism.

Magnitude of Teratogenic Risk

None To Minimal

Quality and Quantity of Data

Poor

Comment

The risk of fetal alcohol syndrome may be unusually high in women who drink heavily despite taking disulfiram during pregnancy.

In a prospectively-ascertained series of infants, all of whose mothers took disulfiram during pregnancy, no malformations were noted among the seven infants whose mothers did not drink, but three of six infants whose mothers did drink had fetal alcohol syndrome (Jones et al., 1991). A variety of limb and other anomalies have been noted anecdotally among a few children whose mothers took disulfiram during the first trimester of pregnancy, but no consistent pattern of malformations was observed (Favre-Tissot et al., 1965; Nora et al., 1977; Gardner and Clarkson, 1981; Dehaene et al., 1984). These findings do not permit any conclusion regarding the possible teratogenicity of disulfiram.

The frequency of malformations was no greater than expected among the offspring of hamsters, rats, or mice treated with disulfiram during pregnancy in doses, respectively, 25-50, 5-10, and 3-30 times those used in humans (Robens, 1969; Salgo and Oster, 1974; Lambert et al., 1980; Thompson & Folb, 1985). Increased rates of fetal death occurred in some experiments, usually in association with maternal toxicity.

Key References

Dehaene P, Titran M, Dubois D: [Pierre Robin Syndrome and heart malformations in a newborn infant. The role of disulfiram during pregnancy]. Nouv Presse Med 13:1394-1395, 1984. [C]

Favre-Tissot M, Delatour P: Psychopharmacologie et teratogenese a propos du disulfirame: Essai experimental. Annales Medico-psychologiques 1:735-740, 1965. [C] & [A]

Gardner RJM, Clarkson JE: A malformed child whose previously alcoholic mother had taken disulfiram. N Z Med J 93:184-186, 1981. [C]

Jones KL, Chambers CC, Johnson KA: The effect of disulfiram on the unborn baby. Teratology 43(5):438, 1991. [S]

Lambert GH, Papp LA, Nishiura B: Disulfiram (D) and the fetal alcohol syndrome (FAS). Pediatri Res 14:586, 1980. [A]

Nora AH, Nora JJ, Blu J: Limb-reduction anomalies in infants born to disulfiram treated alcoholic mothers. Lancet 2:664, 1977. [O]

Robens JF: Teratologic studies of carbaryl, diazinon, norea, disulfiram, and thiram in small laboratory animals. Toxicol Appl Pharmacol 15:152-163, 1969. [A]

Salgo MP, Oster G: Fetal resorption induced by disulfiram in rats. J Reprod Fert 39:375-377, 1974. [A]

Thompson PAC, Folb PI: The effects of disulfiram on the experimental C3H mouse embryo. J Appl Toxicol 5(1):1-10, 1985. [A]

DIVALPROEX

Synonyms

Semisodium Valproate, Valproate Semisodium, Valproate Semisodico, Valproate Semisodique

Summary

Divalproex is an oral antiepileptic agent. It is supplied in the form of enteric-coated tablets, and therefore is uniformly and reliably absorbed.

Magnitude of Teratogenic Risk

Undetermined

Quality and Quantity of Data

None

Comment

The risk of divalproex is probably similar to valproic acid because this agent is metabolized to valproic acid.

No epidemiological studies of congenital anomalies in infants born to women treated with divalproex during pregnancy have been reported.

No animal teratology studies of divalproex have been published.

Please see agent summary on valproic acid for information on a related agent that has been more thoroughly studied.

Key References

None available.

DOBUTAMINE

Synonyms

Compound 81929, Dobutrex, Inotrex

Summary

Dobutamine is a sympathomimetic agent with primarily beta-adrenergic action. It is administered intravenously to improve cardiac function in congestive heart failure and after cardiac surgery.

Magnitude of Teratogenic Risk

None

Quality and Quantity of Data

None To Poor

Comment

None

No epidemiological studies of congenital anomalies in infants born to women treated with dobutamine during pregnancy have been published.

The frequency of malformations was no greater than expected among the offspring of rats or rabbits treated respectively with up to 5 or up to 2 times the usual human daily dose of dobutamine during pregnancy (Nagaoka et al., 1979).

Key References

Nagaoka T, Fuchigami K, Shigemura T, Takatouka K, et al.: Reproductive studies on S-1000 (dobutamine hydrochloride). Yakuri to Chiryo 7:1691-1763, 1979. [A]

DOCONAZOLE

Synonyms

R 34000

Summary

Doconazole is an antifungal agent.

Magnitude of Teratogenic Risk

Undetermined

Quality and Quantity of Data

None

Comment

None

No epidemiological studies of congenital anomalies in infants born to women who used doconazole during pregnancy have been reported.

No animal teratology studies of doconazole have been published.

Key References

None available.

DOCUSATE

Synonyms

Afko-Lube, Colace, Dialose, Diocto, Dioeze, Diosuccin, Molatoc, Pro-Sof, Regutol, Stulex

Summary

Docusate is an anionic surfactant that is taken orally as a stool softener. Docusate is also used as a dispersing and emulsifying agent.

Magnitude of Teratogenic Risk

None To Minimal

Quality and Quantity of Data

Fair

Comment

None

The frequency of congenital anomalies was no higher than expected among the infants of 792 women who took docusate during the first trimester of pregnancy in two cohorts of the Boston Collaborative Drug Surveillance Program (Jick et al., 1981; Aselton et al., 1985). Similarly, there was no increase in the frequency of congenital anomalies observed among the children of 30 women who took docusate during the first four lunar months of pregnancy or of 116 women who took this medication anytime during pregnancy in the Collaborative Perinatal Project (Heinonen et al., 1977).

No consistent teratogenic effect was observed among the offspring of rats given 4.5-70 times the usual human dose of docusate in combination with danthron (a purgative) in one study (Ichikawa & Yamamoto, 1980).

Key References

Aselton P, Jick H, Milunsky A, Hunter JR, et al.: First-trimester drug use and congenital disorders. Obstet Gynecol 65(4):451-455, 1985. [S]

Heinonen OP, Slone D, Shapiro S: Birth Defects and Drugs in Pregnancy. Littleton, Mass.: John Wright-PSG, 1977, pp 385, 442. [E]

Ichikawa Y, Yamamoto Y: Teratology study of solven in rats. Gendai Ivyo (JPN) 12:819, 1980. [A]

Jick H, Holmes LB, Hunter JR, Madsen S, et al.: First-trimester drug use and congenital disorders. JAMA 246(4):343-346, 1981. [S]

DOXEPIN

Synonyms

Adapin, Co-Dox, Novoxapin, Quitaxon, Sinequan, Sinquan, Spectra

Summary

Doxepin is a tricyclic antidepressant with strong sedative action.

Magnitude of Teratogenic Risk

Undetermined

Quality and Quantity of Data

Poor

Comment

None

No epidemiological studies of congenital anomalies among the children of women treated with doxepin during pregnancy have been reported.

An increased frequency of fetal loss and neonatal death was reported among the offspring of rats and rabbits treated with doxepin during pregnancy in doses 40-100 times those used clinically (Owaki et al., 1971a, b). These doses were toxic to the mothers in the rat experiments. No increase in the frequency of malformations was observed in the offspring of animals treated during pregnancy with doxepin in doses 2-40 times (rabbit) or 4-100 times (rat) those used in humans.

Key References

Owaki Y, Momiyama H, Onodera N: Effects of doxepin hydrochloride administered to pregnant rabbits upon the fetuses. Oyo Yakuri 5:905-912, 1971a. [A]

Owaki Y, Momiyama H, Onodera N: Effects of doxepin hydrochloride administered to pregnant rats upon the fetuses and their postnatal development. Oyo Yakuri 5:913-924, 1971b. [A]

DOXORUBICIN

Synonyms

Adriamycin, Adriblastin, Adriblastina, Adriblastine, Farmiblastina

Summary

Doxorubicin is an anthracycline glycoside antibiotic. It is used intravenously in the treatment of leukemia, lymphomas, and a variety of solid tumors.

Magnitude of Teratogenic Risk

Undetermined

Quality and Quantity of Data

Poor To Fair

Comment

Although the risk of doxorubicin is unknown, it may be substantial because it is an antineoplastic agent.

Of 18 reported cases of women treated with doxorubicin and other antineoplastic agents during pregnancy, 17 infants were born alive and one fetus died in utero in temporal association with the therapy (Karp et al., 1983). The mothers of 15 infants were treated after the period of organogenesis or at unspecified times in pregnancy; no malformations were apparent in any of these babies (Lowenthal et al., 1982; Dara et al., 1981; Pizzuto et al., 1980; Webb, 1980; Karp et al., 1983; Newcomb et al., 1978; Metz et al., 1989; Hassenstein & Riedel, 1978; Garg & Kochupillai, 1985; Khurshid & Saleem, 1978; Tobias & Bloom, 1980;

Gililland & Weinstein, 1983; Brusamolino et al., 1989; Garcia et al., 1981). Two pregnant women were treated with doxorubicin and other antineoplastic agents during the period of embryogenesis. One woman had a therapeutic abortion; the abortus could not be examined fully but had a missing digit on one foot (Thomas & Andes, 1982). The other woman had a child with imperforate anus, small size, and microcephaly (Murray et al., 1984). It is uncertain whether the doxorubicin, the other antineoplastic agents, or some other factor caused these fetal anomalies.

A significantly higher than expected frequency of first trimester occupational exposure to doxorubicin and other antineoplastic drugs was observed in a case-control study of 124 nurses who had had a fetal loss (Selevan et al, 1985). No causal inference is possible on the basis of this investigation alone.

Increased frequencies of gastrointestinal anomalies, cardiovascular malformations, bladder hypoplasia, dilatation of the renal pelvis and ureter, and other abnormalities were observed among the offspring of rats treated during pregnancy with doxorubicin in doses similar to, but more frequent, than those used in humans (Thompson et al., 1978; Kavlock et al., 1986). Malformations were not increased among the offspring of pregnant rabbits treated with somewhat smaller doses of doxorubicin, but fetal loss was common (Thompson et al., 1978).

Key References

Brusamolino E, Lazzarino M, Morra E, et al.: Combination chemotherapy with alternating MOPP-ABVD in advanced Hodgkin's disease. Haematologica (Pavia) 74(2):173-179, 1989. [C]

Dara P, Slater LM, Armentrout SA: Successful pregnancy during chemotherapy for acute leukemia. Cancer 47:845-846, 1981. [C]

Garcia V, San Miguel J, Borrasca AL: Doxorubicin in the first trimester of pregnancy. Ann Intern Med 94:547, 1981. [C]

Garg A, Kochupillai V: Non-Hodgkin's lymphoma in pregnancy. South Med J 78(10):1263-1264, 1985. [C]

Gililland J, Weinstein L: The effects of cancer chemotherapeutic agents on the developing fetus. Obstet Gynecol Surv 38(1):6-13, 1983. [C] & [R]

Hassenstein E, Riedel H. Zur teratogenitat von adriamycin. Ein Fallbericht. Geburtshilfe Fraunheilkd 38:131-133, 1978. [C]

Karp GI, von Oeyen P, Valone F, et al.: Doxorubicin in pregnancy: Possible transplacental passage. Cancer Treat Rep 67(9):773-777, 1983. [C]

Kavlock RJ, Rogers EH, Rehnberg BF: Renal functional teratogenesis resulting from adriamycin exposure. Teratology 33:213-220, 1986. [A]

Khurshid M, Saleem M: Acute leukaemia in pregnancy. Lancet 2:534-535, 1978. [C]

Lowenthal R, Funnell CF, Hope DM, et al.: Normal infant after combination chemotherapy including teniposide for Burkitt's lymphoma in pregnancy. Med Pediatr Oncol 10:165-169, 1982. [C]

Metz SA, Day TG, Pursell SH: Adjuvant chemotherapy in a pregnant patient with endodermal sinus tumor of the ovary. Gynecol Oncol 32:371-374, 1989. [C]

Murray CL, Reichert JA, Anderson J, et al.: Multimodal cancer therapy for breast cancer in the first trimester of pregnancy. JAMA 252(18):2607-2608, 1984. [C]

Newcomb M, Balducci L, Thigpen JT, et al.: Acute leukemia in pregnancy. Successful delivery after cytarabine and doxorubicin. JAMA 239(25):2691-2692, 1978. [C]

Pizzuto J, Aviles A, Noriega L, Niz J, et al.: Treatment of acute leukemia during pregnancy: Presentation of nine cases. Cancer Treat Rep 64(4-5):679-683, 1980. [S]

Selevan SG, Lindbohm M-L, Hornung RW, et al.: A study of occupational exposure to antineoplastic drugs and fetal loss in nurses. N Engl J Med 313(19):1173-1178, 1985. [E]

Thomas L, Andes WA: Fetal anomaly associated with successful chemotherapy for Hodgkin's disease during the first trimester of pregnancy. Clin Res 30(2):424A, 1982. [C]

Thompson DJ, Molello JA, Strebing RJ, et al.: Teratogenicity of adriamycin and daunomycin in the rat and rabbit. Teratology 17:151-158, 1978. [A]

Tobias JS, Bloom HJG: Doxorubicin in pregnancy. Lancet 1:776, 1980. [C]

Webb GA: The use of hyperalimentation and chemotherapy in pregnancy: A case report. Am J Obstet Gynecol 137(2):263-266, 1980. [C]

DOXYCYCLINE

Synonyms

Doryx, Doxy-100, Doxy-Caps, Doxy-Lemmon, Doxy-Tabs, Vibra-Tabs, Vibracina, Vibramycin, Vivox

Summary

Doxycycline is a potent tetracycline antibiotic used in the treatment of a wide variety of infections.

Magnitude of Teratogenic Risk

Malformations: Undetermined

Dental Staining: High

Quality and Quantity of Data

Malformations: None To Poor

Dental Staining: Excellent

Comment

1) A small risk cannot be excluded, but there is no indication that the risk of malformations in the children of women treated with doxycycline during pregnancy is likely to be great.

2) Tetracyclines cause staining of the primary dentition in fetuses exposed during the second or third trimester of pregnancy (Toaff & Ravid, 1966; Cohlan, 1977).

No epidemiological studies of congenital anomalies in infants born to women who took doxycycline during pregnancy have been reported.

No teratogenic effect was noted in the offspring of pregnant mice, rats, or rabbits given about 100 times the usual human dose of doxycycline (Cahen & Fave, 1972).

Please see agent summary on tetracycline for information on a related drug that has been more thoroughly studied.

Key References

Cahen RL, Fave A: Absence of teratogenic effect of 6-alpha-deoxy-5 oxytetracycline. Fed Proc Fed Am Soc Exp Biol 31:238, 1972. [A]

Cohlan SQ: Tetracycline staining of teeth. Teratology 15:127-130, 1977. [R]

Toaff R, Ravid R: Tetracyclines and the teeth. Lancet 2:281-282, 1966. [S]

DOXYLAMINE

Synonyms

Alsadorm, Decapryn, Doxised, Gittalun, Histadoxylamine Succinate, Hoggar, Mereprime, Sanalepsi-N, Sedaplus, Somnil

Summary

Doxylamine is an oral antihistaminic agent. Its major uses have been as a hypnotic and as a component of Bendectin, an antinauseant. In these preparations, the dose of doxylamine administered daily is about 1/8 the maximum employed when the drug is used as an antihistaminic.

Magnitude of Teratogenic Risk

None

Quality and Quantity of Data

Good To Excellent

Comment

In most of the available studies, doxylamine has been used as a component of the antinauseant, Bendectin. Please see Bendectin summary for more information.

The Collaborative Perinatal Project included 1169 infants exposed to doxylamine as an antinauseant during the first trimester and 1700 infants exposed at anytime during gestation. The frequency of congenital anomalies was no different in these children than in unexposed controls (Heinonen et al., 1977). No association with maternal use of doxylamine during the first trimester of pregnancy was observed in a case-control study of 298 children with congenital heart disease (Zierler & Rothman, 1985).

The frequency of malformations was not increased among the offspring of rats or rabbits treated with 3-33 times the maximum human dose of doxylamine during pregnancy in one study (Gibson et al., 1968). In contrast, McBride reported increased frequencies of eye, limb, and other malformations were observed in another laboratory among the offspring of rabbits treated with doxylamine in doses 7-111 times the maximum used in humans (McBride, 1984; McBride & Hicks, 1987); maternal death was frequent with such doses. Limb and tail malformations were reported among the offspring of a marmoset monkey treated during pregnancy with 38 times the maximum human dose of doxylamine; abortion was consistently induced by higher doses (McBride, 1985). The validity of these studies by McBride has been cast into doubt by allegations of scientific fraud.

Key References

Gibson JP, Staples RE, Larson EJ, Kuhn WL, et al.: Teratology and reproduction studies with an antinauseant. Toxicol Appl Pharmacol 13:439-447, 1968. [A]

Heinonen OP, Slone D, Shapiro S: Birth Defects and Drugs in Pregnancy. Littleton, Mass.: John Wright-PSG, 1977, pp 323, 437. [E]

McBride WG: Doxylamine succinate induced dysmorphogenesis in the marmoset (Callithrix jacchus). IRCS Med Sci 13:225-226, 1985. [A]

McBride WG: Teratogenic effect of doxylamine succinate in New Zealand white rabbits. IRCS Med Sci 12:536-537, 1984. [A]

McBride WG, Hicks LJ: Acetylcholine and choline levels in rabbit fetuses exposed to anti-

cholinergics. Int J Dev Neurosci 5:117-125, 1987.
[A]

Zierler S, Rothman KJ: Congenital heart disease in relation to maternal use of Bendectin and other drugs in early pregnancy. N Engl J Med 313:347-352, 1985. [E]

DROCODE

Synonyms

Bicodein, DF 118, DHC Continus, Dihydrocodeine Tartrate, Fortuss, Hydrocodeine, Paracodin, Remedacen, Rikodeine, Tiamon

Summary

Drocode is a narcotic analgesic used for relief of mild-to-moderate pain.

Magnitude of Teratogenic Risk

Undetermined

Quality and Quantity of Data

None

Comment

None

No epidemiological studies of congenital anomalies in infants born to women who used drocode during pregnancy have been reported.

No animal teratology studies of drocode have been published.

Please see agent summary on codeine for information on a related drug that has been more thoroughly studied.

Key References

None available.

DROPERIDOL

Synonyms

Dehydrobenzperidol, Dridol, Droleptan, Halkan, Inapsin, Inoval, Properidol, Sintodril

Summary

Droperidol is a butyrophenone major tranquilizer. It is used as a preoperative medication and in the treatment of acute psychiatric illness.

Magnitude of Teratogenic Risk

Undetermined

Quality and Quantity of Data

None

Comment

None

No epidemiological studies of congenital anomalies in infants born to women treated with droperidol during pregnancy have been reported.

No teratologic studies of droperidol in mammals have been published.

Please see agent summary on haloperidol for information on a related agent that has been studied.

Key References

None available.

DYCLONINE

Synonyms

Dyclone, Dyclocaini Chloridum, Sucrets

Summary

Dyclonine is a local anesthetic that is used topically.

Magnitude of Teratogenic Risk

Undetermined

Quality and Quantity of Data

None

Comment

None

No epidemiological studies of congenital anomalies in children born to women exposed to dyclonine during pregnancy have been reported.

No investigations of teratologic effects of dyclonine in experimental animals have been published.

Key References

None available.

ECHOTHIOPHATE

Synonyms

Echodide, Ecofilina, Ecostigmine Iodide, Ecothiopate, Iodeto de Fosfolina, Phospholine, Phospholinjodid

Summary

Echothiophate is a very long-lasting cholinesterase inhibitor. It is used as an ophthalmic preparation in the treatment of glaucoma and strabismus.

Magnitude of Teratogenic Risk

Undetermined

Quality and Quantity of Data

None

Comment

None

No epidemiological studies of congenital anomalies in infants born to women treated with echothiophate during pregnancy have been reported.

No animal teratology studies of echothiophate have been published.

Please see agent summary on neostigmine for information on a related agent that has been studied.

Key References

None available.

ECONAZOLE

Synonyms

Econacort

Summary

Econazole is an imidazole antifungal agent. Systemic and topical preparations are available; the latter are poorly absorbed from the skin or vagina.

Magnitude of Teratogenic Risk

Undetermined

Quality and Quantity of Data

Poor

Comment

A small risk cannot be excluded, but a high risk of congenital anomalies in the children of women treated with econazole during pregnancy is unlikely.

No malformations were observed among 107 infants born to one series of women treated with topical econazole for vaginal candidiasis during pregnancy; treatment occurred at an average gestational age of 30 weeks (Goormans et al., 1985). No epidemiological studies of congenital anomalies among children born to women treated with systemic econazole during pregnancy have been reported.

The frequency of malformations was not increased among the offspring of pregnant rats or rabbits treated with 3-11 or 2-5 times the human systemic dose of econazole (Thienpont et al., 1975; Maruoka et al., 1978).

Please see agent summary on miconazole for information on a related agent that has been studied.

Key References

Goormans E, Beek JM, Declercq JA, Loendersloot EW, et al.: Efficacy of econazole (gynopevaryl 150) in vaginal candidosis during pregnancy. Curr Med Res Opin 9:371-377, 1985. [E]

Maruoka H, Kadota Y, Ueshima M, Uesako T, et al.: Toxicological studies on econazole nitrate: 6. Teratological studies in mice and rabbits. Iyakuhin Kenkyu 9:955-970, 1978. [A]

Thienpont D, Van Cutsem J, Van Nueten JM, Niemegeers CJE, et al.: Biological and toxicological properties of econazole, a broad-spectrum antimycotic. Arzneimittelforsch 25:224-230, 1975. [A]

EDROPHONIUM

Synonyms

Antirex, Edrofonio Cloruro, Enlon, Oedrophanium, Tensilon

Summary

Edrophonium is a rapid-acting cholinesterase inhibitor that is administered intravenously. It is used to test for myasthenia gravis and in treatment of cardiac arrhythmias.

Magnitude of Teratogenic Risk

Undetermined

Quality and Quantity of Data

None

Comment

A small risk cannot be excluded, but a high risk of congenital anomalies in the children of women treated with edrophonium during pregnancy is unlikely because of its short duration of action.

No epidemiological studies of congenital anomalies among infants born to women treated with edrophonium during pregnancy have been reported.

No teratology studies of edrophonium in mammals have been published.

Please see agent summary on atropine for information on a related agent that has been more thoroughly studied.

Key References

None available.

ELECTROCONVULSIVE THERAPY

Synonyms

ECT, Electrical Shock Therapy

Summary

High-voltage electrical shock is used in the treatment of some psychiatric illnesses.

Magnitude of Teratogenic Risk

None To Minimal

Quality and Quantity of Data

Poor To Fair

Comment

None

219

The frequency of congenital anomalies did not appear to be unusual among children born to 318 women who received electroconvulsive therapy during pregnancy (Impastato et al., 1964).

No animal teratology studies of high voltage electrical shock have been published.

Key References

Impastato DJ, Gabriel AR, Lardaro HH: Electric and insulin shock therapy during pregnancy. Dis Nerv Syst 25:542-546, 1964. [S]

EMETINE

Synonyms

Hemometina

Summary

Emetine is an ipecacuanha alkaloid that inhibits protein synthesis. Emetine is administered parenterally in the treatment of intestinal and hepatic amebiasis. Elimination of emetine from the body occurs very slowly; the drug has been detected in the urine two months after the cessation of treatment.

Magnitude of Teratogenic Risk

Undetermined

Quality and Quantity of Data

None To Poor

Comment

Although the risk of congenital anomalies among infants born to women treated with emetine during pregnancy is unknown, the fact that it inhibits protein synthesis raises concern that the risk could be substantial.

No epidemiological studies of congenital anomalies among infants born to women treated with emetine during pregnancy have been reported.

Increased frequencies of cardiac malformations and of fetal death were observed among the offspring of rats treated during pregnancy with 5 times the usual human dose of emetine (Ritter et al., 1982).

Key References

Ritter EJ, Scott WJ, Wilson JG, Mathinos PR, et al.: Potentiative interactions between caffeine and various teratogenic agents. Teratology 25:95-100, 1982. [A]

EMOTIONAL STRESS

Synonyms

Maternal Stress, Stress

Summary

The belief that maternal emotional stress or "impressions" can cause congenital anomalies exists in many cultures (Warkany, 1971), but scientific study of this effect is very difficult (Scialli, 1988). The experience of emotional stress is perceived differently by various individuals, and the ability to recall and determine the magnitude of stressful events during pregnancy is likely to be different after the birth of an abnormal baby than after a normal delivery. Animal experiments are especially hard to interpret because it is impossible to compare the quality and severity of experimentally induced stress in animals with naturally occurring emotional stress in humans.

Magnitude of Teratogenic Risk

Undetermined

Quality and Quantity of Data

Poor

Comment

A small risk cannot be excluded, but there is no indication that the risk of congenital anomalies in the children of women under emotional stress during pregnancy is likely to be great.

The frequency of congenital anomalies among 1263 infants born to women who had requested but were refused induced abortion early in pregnancy was greater than among control infants in one study (Blomberg, 1980), but the data are insufficient to conclude that this association is due to differences in maternal stress between the two groups. An increased frequency of "emotional shock" during pregnancy was observed in a retrospective case-control study of 1419 infants with various congenital anomalies, but the author felt that the association was unlikely to be causal (Record, 1958). An increased frequency of "emotional stress" during the first trimester of pregnancy was observed in one case-control study involving 599 children with facial clefts but not in two others involving 194 and 246 affected children (Saxen, 1975; Fraser & Warburton, 1964). Premature delivery and low birth weight have been associated with increased maternal stress late in pregnancy (Newton et al., 1979; Newton & Hunt, 1984).

An increased frequency of congenital anomalies including cleft palate, limb defects, and neural tube defects has been reported among rodents subjected during pregnancy to stress induced by factors such as shipping, crowding, restraint, light, and electrical shock (Arvay et al., 1961; Rosenzweig, 1966; Brown et al., 1972; Hamburgh et al., 1974). Fetal and embryonic loss has also been induced by such factors as well as by loud noise, although noise-induced maternal stress has not generally altered the frequency of malformations in the offspring (Warkany & Kalter, 1962; Kimmel et al., 1976; Nawrot et al., 1980). Long-lasting alterations of behavior have been observed in mice and rats born to mothers subjected to a variety of kinds of stress during pregnancy (Masterpasqua et al., 1976; Deitchman et al., 1977; Barlow et al., 1978; Meisel et al., 1979; Politch & Herrenkohl, 1979). Fetal bradycardia has been induced by maternal stress in late pregnancy in monkeys (Myers, 1975; Morishima et al., 1978, 1979).

Key References

Arvay A, Nagy T, Bazso J: The importance of neurotropic overload stimuli in the genesis of congenital malformations. Biol Neonat 3:1-23, 1961. [A]

Barlow SM, Knight AF, Sullivan FM: Delay in postnatal growth and development of offspring produced by maternal restraint stress during pregnancy in the rat. Teratology 18:211-218, 1978. [A]

Blomberg S: Influence of maternal distress during pregnancy on fetal malformations. Acta Psychiatr Scand 62:315-330, 1980. [E]

Brown KS, Johnston MC, Niswander JD: Isolated cleft palate in mice after transportation during gestation. Teratology 5:119-124, 1972. [A]

Deitchman R, Sanders RE, Burkholder J, Newman I: Effects of prenatal crowding on behavior of rodent mothers and offspring. Psychol Rep 40:327-338, 1977. [A]

Fraser FC, Warburton D: No association of emotional stress or vitamin supplement during pregnancy to cleft lip or palate in man. Plast Reconstr Surg 33:395-399, 1964. [E]

Hamburgh M, Mendoza LA, Rader M, Lang A, et al.: Malformations induced in offspring of crowded and parabiotically stressed mice. Teratology 10:31-38, 1974. [A]

Kimmel CA, Cook RO, Staples RE: Teratogenic potential of noise in mice and rats. Toxicol Appl Pharmacol 36:239-245, 1976. [A]

Masterpasqua F, Chapman RH, Lore RK: The effects of prenatal psychological stress on the sexual behavior and reactivity of male rats. Dev Psychobiol 9:403-411, 1976. [A]

Meisel RL, Dohanich GP, Wark IL: Effects of prenatal stress on avoidance acquisition, open-field performance and lordotic behavior in male rats. Physiol Behav 22:527-530, 1979. [A]

Morishima HO, Pedersen H, Finster M: The influence of maternal psychological stress on the fetus. Am J Obstet Gynecol 131:286-290, 1978. [A]

Morishima HO, Ych MN, James LS: Reduced uterine blood flow and fetal hypoxemia with acute maternal stress: Experimental observation in the pregnant baboon. Am J Obstet Gynecol 134:270-275, 1979. [A]

Myers RE: Maternal psychological stress and fetal asphyxia: A study in the monkey. Am J Obstet Gynecol 122:47-59, 1975. [A]

Nawrot PS, Cook RO, Staples RE: Embryotoxicity of various noise stimuli in the mouse. Teratology 22:279-289, 1980. [A]

Newton RW, Hunt LP: Psychosocial stress in pregnancy and its relation to low birth weight. Br Med J 288:1191-1194, 1984. [E]

Newton RW, Webster PAC, Binu PS, Maskrey N, et al: Psychosocial stress in pregnancy and its relation to the onset of premature labour. Br Med J 2:411-413, 1979. [E]

Politch JA, Herrenkohl LR: Prenatal stress reduces maternal aggression by mice offspring. Physiol Behav 23:415-418, 1979. [A]

Record RG: Environmental influences in the etiology of congenital malformations. Proc R Soc Med 51:147-148, 1958. [E]

Rosenzweig A: Psychological stress in cleft palate etiology. J Dent Res 45:1585-1593, 1966. [A]

Saxen I: Epidemiology of cleft lip and palate: A chance to rule out chance correlations. Brit J Prev Soc Med 29:103-110, 1975. [E]

Scialli AR: Is stress a developmental toxin? Reproductive Toxicology 1(3):163-171, 1988. [R]

Warkany J: Maternal Impressions. In: Congenital Malformations: Notes and Comments, Chicago: Year Book Medical Publishers, 1971, pp 12-15. [R]

Warkany J, Kalter H: Maternal impressions and congenital malformations. Plast Reconstr Surg 30:628-637, 1962. [A]

ENALAPRIL

Synonyms

Converten, Enapren, Innovace, Naprilene, Pres, Renitec, Reniten, Xanef

Summary

Enalapril is an angiotensin-converting enzyme (ACE) inhibitor that is administered orally in the treatment of hypertension.

Magnitude of Teratogenic Risk

First-Trimester Use: Undetermined

Use Later In Pregnancy: Moderate

Quality and Quantity of Data

First-Trimester Use: Poor

Use Later In Pregnancy: Fair To Good

Comment

1) A small risk cannot be excluded, but a high risk of congenital anomalies in the children of women treated with enalapril during pregnancy is unlikely.

2) There is a substantial risk of oligohydramnios and fetal distress or death in hypertensive women treated with enalapril in the latter part of pregnancy. The effect may be related to the pharmacological action of this drug on the fetus (see below).

No epidemiological studies of congenital anomalies among the infants of women treated with enalapril during pregnancy have been reported.

Oligohydramnios and fetal anuria and neonatal pulmonary hypoplasia, renal failure, joint contractures, and death have been repeatedly observed after maternal treatment with enalapril or related drugs during pregnancy (Rothberg & Lorenz, 1984; Schubiger et al., 1988; Broughton-Pipkin et al., 1989; Mehta & Modi, 1989; Scott & Purohit, 1989; Anonymous, 1989; Rosa et al., 1989; Boutroy, 1989; Cunniff et al., 1990; Hulton et al., 1990; Brent & Beckman, 1991; Hanssens et al., 1991). Women who require such treatment have hypertension which may be severe, and hypertension per se is known to be associated with similar fetal and neonatal complications. Although no epidemiological studies are available to permit apportionment of risk, it appears that these complications are unusually common in the pregnancies of hypertensive women who are treated with ACE inhibitors

(Anonymous, 1989; Rosa et al., 1989; Boutroy, 1989; Hulton et al., 1990; Brent & Beckman, 1991; Hanssens et al., 1991). It is important to note that these effects do not appear to reflect abnormal embryogenesis but rather a pharmacologic response of the fetus to enalapril during the second half of gestation (Brent & Beckman, 1991; Martin et al., 1992).

Two cases have been reported in which hypocalvaria, an unusual underdevelopment of the skull bones, and other skeletal anomalies occurred in the infants of women treated with enalapril throughout pregnancy (Mehta & Modi, 1989; Cunniff et al., 1990). Four infants with similar unusual skull defects have been observed after maternal treatment throughout pregnancy with other ACE inhibitors (Duminy & Berger, 1981; Rothberg & Lorenz, 1984; Barr & Cohen, 1991).

The frequency of congenital anomalies was no greater than expected among the offspring of rats treated with 15-1500 times the usual human dose of enalapril during pregnancy in one study (Fujii et al., 1985), but in another study fetal growth retardation and incomplete skull ossification were observed after treatment of pregnant rats with 19 times the human dose of enalapril (Valdes et al., 1992). Increased frequencies of fetal death but not of malformations were observed among the offspring of rabbits treated during pregnancy with 4-40 times the human dose of enalapril (Minsker et al., 1990). Fetal death occurred only when the drug was administered during the last portion of pregnancy. Fetal hypotension has been demonstrated when pregnant sheep were given 2.5 times the human dose of enalapril (Broughton Pipkin & Wallace, 1986).

Please see agent summary on captopril for information on a related agent that has been studied.

Key References

Anonymous: Are ACE inhibitors safe in pregnancy? Lancet 2:482-483, 1989. [O]

Barr M Jr, Cohen MM: ACE inhibitor fetopathy and hypocalvaria: The kidney-skull connection. Teratology 44:485-495, 1991. [C]

Boutroy MJ: Fetal effects of maternally administered clonidine and angiotensin-converting enzyme inhibitors. Dev Pharmacol Ther 13:199-204, 1989. [R]

Brent RL, Beckman DA: Angiotensin-converting enzyme inhibitors, and embryopathic class of drugs with unique properties: Information for clinical teratology counselors. Teratology 43:543-546, 1991. [O]

Broughton Pipkin F, Baker PN, Symonds EM: ACE inhibitors in pregnancy. Lancet 2:96-97, 1989. [C]

Broughton Pipkin F, Wallace CP: The effect of enalapril (MK421), an angiotensin converting enzyme inhibitor, on the conscious pregnant ewe and her foetus. Br J Pharmacol 87:533-542, 1986. [A]

Cunniff C, Jones KL, Phillipson J, Benirschke K, et al.: Oligohydramnios sequence and renal tubular malformation associated with maternal enalapril use. Am J Obstet Gynecol 162:187-189, 1990. [C]

Duminy PC, Burger PT: Fetal abnormality associated with the use of captopril during pregnancy. S Afr Med J 60:805, 1981. [C]

Fujii T, Nakatsuka T, Hanada S, Komatsu T, et al.: MK-421: Oral teratogenicity study in the rat. Yakuri to Chiryo 13:519-528, 1985. [A]

Hanssens M, Keirse MJNC, Vankelecom F, Van Assche FA: Fetal and neonatal effects of treatment with angiotensin-converting enzyme inhibitors in pregnancy. Obstet Gynecol 78:128-135, 1991. [R]

Hulton SA, Thomson PD, Cooper PA, Rothberg AD: Angiotensin-converting enzyme inhibitors in pregnancy may result in neonatal renal failure. S Afr Med J 78:673-676. 1990. [C]

Martin RA, Jones KL, Mendoza A, et al.: Effect of ACE inhibition on the fetal kidney: Decreased renal blood flow. Teratology 46:317-321, 1992. [E]

Mehta N, Modi N: Ace inhibitors in pregnancy. Lancet 2:96, 1989. [C]

Minsker DH, Bagdon WJ, MacDonald JS, et al.: Maternotoxicity and fetotoxicity of an angiotensin-converting enzyme inhibitor, enalapril, in rabbits. Fundam Appl Toxicol 14:461-470, 1990. [A]

Rosa FW, Bosco LA, Graham CF, et al.: Neonatal anuria with maternal angiotensin-converting enzyme inhibition. Obstet Gynecol 74:371-374, 1989. [S]

Rothberg AD, Lorenz R: Can captopril cause fetal and neonatal renal failure? Pediatr Pharmacol 4:189-192, 1984. [C]

Schubiger G, Flury G, Nussberger J: Enalapril for pregnancy-induced hypertension: Acute renal failure in a neonate. Ann Intern Med 108(2):215-216, 1988. [C]

Scott AA, Purohit DM: Neonatal renal failure: A complication of maternal antihypertensive therapy. Am J Obstet Gynecol 160, 1223-1224, 1989. [C]

Valdes G, Marinovic D, Falcon C, et al.: Placental alterations, intrauterine growth retardation and teratogenicity associated with enalapril use in pregnant rats. Biol Neonate 61:124-130, 1992. [A]

ENCAINIDE

Synonyms
Enkaid, MJ-9067

Summary
Encainide is used for the treatment of cardiac arrhythmias.

Magnitude of Teratogenic Risk
Undetermined

Quality and Quantity of Data
None

Comment
None

No epidemiological studies of congenital anomalies in infants born to women treated with encainide during pregnancy have been reported.

No animal teratology studies of encainide have been published.

Key References
None available.

ENFLURANE

Synonyms
Alyrane, Efrane, Ethrane, Inhelthran, Methylflurether

Summary
Enflurane is a general anesthetic that is administered by inhalation.

Magnitude of Teratogenic Risk
Undetermined

Quality and Quantity of Data
None To Poor

Comment
None

No epidemiological studies of congenital anomalies in children born to women exposed to enflurane during pregnancy have been reported.

Limb and abdominal wall defects were observed more often than expected in the offspring of rabbits treated with anesthetic doses of enflurane during pregnancy (Ramazzatto & Carlin, 1978). Similarly, increased frequencies of cleft palate, skeletal variations, and fetal growth retardation were found among the offspring of mice exposed repeatedly during pregnancy to anesthetic doses of enflurane (Wharton et al., 1981). In contrast, no teratogenic effect was observed among the offspring of rats or mice treated repeatedly during pregnancy with enflurane in similar anesthetic doses in another study (Saito et al., 1974). Long-lasting deficits in learning function were observed among the offspring of mice treated repeatedly with anesthetic doses of enflurane during pregnancy (Chalon et al., 1981). The relevance of these observations to the teratogenic risk associated with enflurane anesthesia in a pregnant woman is uncertain.

Malformation frequencies were no greater than expected among the offspring of mice or rats treated repeatedly during pregnancy with enflurane in subanesthetic doses similar to or greater than those encountered occupationally in humans (Pope & Persaud, 1978; Wharton et al., 1981; Green et al., 1982).

Key References

Chalon J, Tang C-K, Ramanathan S, et al.: Exposure to halothane and enflurane affects learning function of murine progeny. Anesth Analg 60(11):794-797, 1981. [A]

Green CJ, Monk SJ, Knight JF, Dore C, et al.: Chronic exposure of rats to enflurane 200 P.P.M.: No evidence of toxicity or teratogenicity. Br J Anaesth 54:1097-1104, 1982. [A]

Pope WDB, Persaud TVN: Foetal growth retardation in the rat following chronic exposure to the inhalation anaesthetic enflurane. Experientia 34:1332-1333, 1978. [A]

Ramazzotto LJ, Carlin RD: Ethrane-teratogenicity. A preliminary report. J Dent Res 57 (Spec Iss A):289, 1978. [A]

Saito N, Urakawa M, Ito R: [Influence of enflurane on fetus and growth after birth in mice and rats]. Oyo Yakuri 8:1269-1276, 1974. [A]

Wharton RS, Mazze RI, Wilson AI: Reproduction and fetal development in mice chronically exposed to enflurane. Anesthesiology 54:505-510, 1981. [A]

ENILCONAZOLE

Synonyms

Deccozil, Florasan, Fungaflor, Fungazil, Imazalil

Summary

Enilconazole is an antifungal agent used in agriculture.

Magnitude of Teratogenic Risk

Undetermined

Quality and Quantity of Data

Poor

Comment

None

No epidemiological studies of congenital anomalies in infants whose mothers were exposed to enilconazole during pregnancy have been reported.

No malformations were found among the offspring of rats or rabbits treated orally with 5-80 or 0.6-2.5 mg/kg/d of enilconazole during pregnancy (Thienpont et al., 1981).

Key References

Thienpont D, Van Cutsem J, Van Cauteren H, Marsboom R: The biological and toxicological properties of imazalil. Arzneimittelforsch 31:309-315, 1981. [A]

ENOXIMONE

Synonyms

Fenoximone, Perfan

Summary

Enoximone is a cardiotonic drug.

Magnitude of Teratogenic Risk

Undetermined

Quality and Quantity of Data

None

Comment

None

No epidemiological studies of congenital anomalies in infants born to women treated with enoximone during pregnancy have been reported.

No animal teratology studies of enoximone have been published.

Key References

None available.

EPHEDRINE

Synonyms

Eciphin, Fedrin, Sanedrine

Summary

Ephedrine is a sympathomimetic drug used to treat nasal congestion, bronchospasm, urinary incontinence, and congestive heart failure. Topical preparations are used to relieve blood-shot eyes.

Magnitude of Teratogenic Risk

None To Minimal

Quality and Quantity of Data

Poor To Fair

Comment

None

The frequencies of congenital anomalies in general, of major malformations, and of minor anomalies were no greater than expected among the children of 373 women who used ephedrine during the first four lunar months of pregnancy in the Collaborative Perinatal Project (Heinonen et al., 1977). Similarly, the frequency of congenital anomalies was not increased among the children of 873 women who used ephedrine anytime during pregnancy in this study. No association with maternal ephedrine use during the first trimester of pregnancy was seen in case-control studies of 76 children with gastroschisis and 416 children with various congenital anomalies thought to have a vascular pathogenesis (Werler et al., 1992).

Increased fetal heart rate and beat-to-beat variability have been observed in association with maternal ephedrine treatment during labor (Wright et al., 1981).

A dose-dependent increase in the frequency of cardiac anomalies, primarily ventricular septal defects, was observed among the offspring of rats treated during pregnancy with ephedrine in doses 3-1700 times the single dose used in humans (or 1-420 times the human daily dose) in a study that has only been published in abstract form (Kanai et al., 1986).

Key References

Heinonen OP, Slone D, Shapiro S: Birth Defects and Drugs in Pregnancy. Littleton, Mass.: John Wright-PSG, 1977, pp 346, 347, 439, 491. [E]

Kanai T, Nishikawa T, Satoh A, et al.: Cardiovascular teratogenicity of ephedrine in rats. Teratology 34:469, 1986. [A]

Werler MM, Mitchell AA, Shapiro S: First trimester maternal medication use in relation to gastroschisis. Teratology 45:361- 367, 1992. [E]

Wright RG, Shnider SM, Levinson G, et al.: The effect of maternal administration of ephedrine on fetal heart rate and variability. Obstet Gynecol 57:734-738, 1981. [S]

EPINEPHRINE

Synonyms

Adrenaline, Bronkaid Mist, Dysne-Inhal, Epifrin, Epipen, Epitrate, Glaucon, Medi-haler-Epi, Primatene, Sus-Phrine, Vaponefrin

Summary

Epinephrine is a direct-acting sympatho-mimetic hormone released from the adrenal medulla in response to stress. Epinephrine is administered therapeutically to alleviate bronchospasm and other allergic conditions.

Magnitude of Teratogenic Risk

None To Minimal

Quality and Quantity of Data

Fair

Comment

None

The frequency of congenital anomalies was increased among the children of 189 women treated with epinephrine during the first four lunar months of pregnancy in the Collaborative Perinatal Project, but this increase was due entirely to mild defects that had highly variable rates of occurrence at participating institutions (Heinonen et al., 1977). The frequency of congenital anomalies was not increased among the children of 508 women who were treated with epinephrine anytime during pregnancy in this study.

Disruptions of limb development can be produced by injection of epinephrine directly into rat or rabbit fetuses in doses thousands of times greater than those used clinically (Jost et al., 1964; Jost et al., 1969). Cataracts can be induced in rat fetuses under similar conditions (Pitel & Lerman, 1962). No teratogenic effect was observed among the offspring of pregnant rats given continuous infusions of epinephrine at a dose about 8 times that used in humans (Trend & Bruce, 1989). An increased frequency of cleft palate was observed in the offspring of one strain of mice, but not another, treated during pregnancy with epinephrine in doses 40-80 times those used in humans (Loevy & Roth, 1968; Blaustein et al., 1971). An increased frequency of fetal loss was reported in pregnant mice and rabbits given, respectively, 200 and 85 times the human therapeutic dose of epinephrine (Loevy & Roth, 1968; Auletta, 1971). The frequency of malformations was not increased among the offspring of hamsters treated during pregnancy with 25 times the human subcutaneous dose of epinephrine (Hirsch & Fritz, 1981). Behavioral alterations have been noted in the offspring of rats treated with epinephrine during pregnancy in doses 140-430 times those used in humans (Thompson et al., 1963). The clinical relevance of these observations is unknown.

Fetal asphyxia can be produced in term rhesus monkey fetuses by administration of epinephrine to their mothers in doses similar to those used in human therapy (Adamsons et al., 1971).

Key References

Adamsons K, Mueller-Heubach E, Myers RE: Production of fetal asphyxia in the rhesus monkey by administration of catecholamines to the mother. Am J Obstet Gynecol 109:248-262, 1971. [A]

Auletta FJ: Effect of epinephrine on implantation and foetal survival in the rabbit. J Reprod Fertil 27:281-282, 1971. [A]

Blaustein FM, Feller R, Rosenzweig S: Effect of ACTH and adrenal hormones on cleft palate frequency in CD-1 mice. J Dent Res 50:609-612, 1971. [A]

Heinonen OP, Slone D, Shapiro S: Birth Defects and Drugs in Pregnancy. Littleton, Mass.: John Wright-PSG, 1977, pp 346-347, 439. [E]

Hirsch KS, Fritz HI: Teratogenic effects of mescaline, epinephrine, and norepinephrine in the hamster. Teratology 23:287-291, 1981. [A]

Jost A, Petter C, Duval G, Maltier JP, et al.: [Effect of adrenalin on the division of blood between the fetus and placenta: Hemodynamic factors of certain congenital lesions of the limbs]. C R Acad Sc Paris 259:3086-3088, 1964. [A]

Jost A, Roffi J, Courtat M: Congenital amputations determined by the BR gene and those induced by adrenalin infection in the rabbit fetus. In: Swinyard CA (ed). Limb Development and Deformity: Problems of Evaluation and Rehabilitation. Springfield, Ill.: Charles C Thomas Publisher, 1969, pp 187-199. [A]

Loevy H, Roth BF: Induced cleft palate development in mice: Comparison between the effect of epinephrine and cortisone. Anat Rec 160:386, 1968. [A]

Pitel M, Lerman S: Studies on the fetal rat lens. Effects of intrauterine adrenalin and noradrenalin. Invest Ophthalmol 1:406-412, 1962. [A]

Thompson WR, Goldenberg L, Watson J, Watson M: Behavioral effects of maternal adrenalin infection during pregnancy in rat offspring. Psychol Rep 12:279-284, 1963. [A]

Trend SC, Bruce NW: Resistance of the rat embryo to elevated maternal epinephrine concentrations. Am J Obstet Gynecol 160:498-501, 1989. [A]

EPSTEIN-BARR VIRUS

Synonyms

Infectious Mononucleosis, Kissing Disease, Mononucleosis

Summary

Epstein-Barr virus (EBV) is a member of the herpes virus group. It is the usual causative agent of infectious mononucleosis, but many EBV infections are asymptomatic. Serological evidence of previous EBV infection is almost universal among adults; infection occurs earlier in life in individuals of lower socioeconomic groups.

Magnitude of Teratogenic Risk

None To Minimal

Quality and Quantity of Data

Poor To Fair

Comment

None

No association was observed between serological evidence of active EBV infection in the mother and major or minor malformations, prematurity, or growth retardation among the infants born to 500 pregnant women tested for EBV in the first trimester (Fleisher & Bolognese, 1983). No abnormalities were observed among the infants of three women who had symptomatic infectious mononucleosis during the first trimester of pregnancy (Fleisher & Bologonese, 1984). Another cohort study of 719 pregnancies showed a statistically significant correlation between maternal serological evidence of primary or reactivated EBV infection and prematurity, fetal malformations, growth retardation, or fetal death (Icart et al., 1981). The meaning of this association is uncertain, however, because possible confounding factors were not considered, the malformations were not described and the overall frequency of malformations was only 1.7%, suggesting considerable underascertainment.

Placental inflammation was consistently observed in one study of five pregnancies terminated because of maternal mononucleosis in the first trimester (Ornoy et al., 1982). Several infants with malformations and serological or clinical evidence of prenatal EBV infection have been reported; cataracts have been observed in three such infants, congenital heart disease in two, and diffuse myocarditis in two (Goldberg et al., 1981; Ornoy et al., 1982). However, given the fact that more than half of pregnant women in some populations can be shown to have evidence of active EBV infection (Fleisher & . Bolognese, 1983), no causal inference can be made from such observations (Arvin & Yeager, 1990). If maternal EBV infection produces damage in the embryo or fetus, it appears to do so only rarely.

No animal teratology studies of EBV have been published.

Key References

Arvin AM, Yeager AS: Other viral infections of the fetus and newborn. In: Remington JS, Klein JO (eds). Infectious Diseases of the Fetus and Newborn Infant. Philadelphia: W.B. Saunders Co., 1990, pp 516-527. [O]

Fleisher G, Bologonese R: Infectious mononucleosis during gestation: Report of three women and their infants studied prospectively. Pediatr Infect Dis 3:308-311, 1984. [C]

Fleisher G, Bolognese R: Persistent Epstein-Barr virus infection and pregnancy. J Infect Dis 147:982-986, 1983. [E]

Goldberg GN, Fulginiti VA, Ray CG, Ferry P, et al.: In utero Epstein-Barr virus (infectious mononucleosis) infection. JAMA 246:1579-1581, 1981. [C]

Icart J, Didier J, Dalens M, Chabanon G, et al.: Prospective study of Epstein Barr virus (EBV) infection during pregnancy. Biomedicine 34:160-163, 1981. [S]

Ornoy A, Dudai M, Sadovsky E: Placental and fetal pathology in infectious mononucleosis. A possible indicator for Epstein-Barr virus teratogenicity. Diagn Gynecol Obstet 4:11-16, 1982. [S]

ERGOLOID MESYLATES

Synonyms

Circanol, Co-Dergocrine Mesylate, Dacoren, Deapril-ST, DH-Erogotoxin-Forte, Hydergin, Nehydrin, Niloric Tablets, Progeril

Summary

Ergoloid mesylates are mixtures of hydrogenated ergot alkaloids used to treat symptoms of mild to moderate mental impairment in elderly patients.

Magnitude of Teratogenic Risk

Undetermined

Quality and Quantity of Data

None To Poor

Comment

None

No epidemiological studies of congenital anomalies in infants whose mothers took ergoloid mesylates during pregnancy have been reported.

No studies of malformations in the offspring of experimental animals treated with ergoloid mesylates during pregnancy have been published. Birth weight was decreased among rats born to mothers that had been administered ergoloid mesylates during pregnancy in doses 50 times that used in humans (Sommer & Buchanan, 1955).

Key References

Sommer AF, Buchanan AR: Effects of ergot alkaloids on pregnancy and lactation in the albino rat. Am J Physiol 180:296-300, 1955. [A]

ERGOTAMINE

Synonyms

Ergostat, Ergotamin Medihaler, Gynergeen, Megral, Wigrettes

Summary

Ergotamine is an ergot alkaloid that acts as a vasoconstrictor. Ergotamine is used in the treatment of migraine headaches and premenstrual tension.

Magnitude of Teratogenic Risk

Minimal

Quality and Quantity of Data

Fair To Good

Comment

Risk assessment is for therapeutic use of ergotamine; a substantial risk of congenital anomalies may be possible at maternally toxic doses.

In a case-control study of 9460 children with various congenital anomalies, the frequency of maternal use of ergotamine during the first three months or anytime in pregnancy was no greater than expected (Czeizel, 1989). In this preliminary study, an eight-fold difference in the rate of neural tube defects was observed, but this observation was based on only four affected and exposed pregnancies and therefore needs further confirmation. The frequency of congenital anomalies was not increased among the children of 25 women who were treated with ergotamine during the first four lunar months of pregnancy in the Collaborative Perinatal Project (Heinonen et al., 1977). The frequency of congenital anomalies was no higher than expected among 924 children of women who had migraine headaches (Wainscott et al., 1978). Seventy-one percent of these women are said to have taken ergotamine at some time, but it is not known whether or not the drug was taken during their pregnancies. Various congenital anomalies attributed to vascular disruption have been reported in individual infants whose mothers took ergotamine during pregnancy; no causal inference can be made on the basis of these anecdotal observations (Peeden et al., 1979; Graham et al., 1983; Hughes & Goldstein, 1988; Verloes et al., 1990). Intrauterine death has been observed in a pregnant woman who took a toxic overdose of ergotamine in a suicide attempt (Au et al., 1985).

Increased frequencies of embryonic and fetal death were found among pregnant mice, rats, and rabbits treated during pregnancy with 830-2500, 83-830, and 8-250 times the usual human dose of ergotamine, respectively (Grauwiler & Schon, 1973). Delayed osseous maturation and fetal growth retardation were seen at some of the higher doses that were also toxic to the mothers but not at lower doses that were not. An increased frequency of malformations was found only among the offspring of rabbits treated with the highest dose of ergotamine during gestation. No teratogenic effect was noted among the offspring of pregnant pigs treated with about five times the human therapeutic dose of ergotamine (Bailey et al., 1973).

Key References

Au KL, Woo JSK, Wong VCW: Intrauterine death from ergotamine overdosage. Eur J Obstet Gynecol Reprod Biol 19:313-315, 1985. [C]

Bailey J, Wrathall AE, Mantle PG: The effect of feeding ergot to gilts during early pregnancy. Br Vet J 129:127-133, 1973. [A]

Czeizel A: Teratogenicity of ergotamine. J Med Genet 26:69-71, 1989. [E]

David TJ: Nature and etiology of the Poland anomaly. N Eng J Med 287:487-489, 1972. [S]

Graham JM, Marin-Padilla M, Hoefnagel D: Jejunal atresia associated with Cafergot ingestion during pregnancy. Clin Pediatr (Phila) 22(3):226-228, 1983. [C]

Grauwiler J, Schon H: Teratological experiments with ergotamine in mice, rats, and rabbits. Teratology 7:227-235, 1973. [A]

Heinonen OP, Slone D, Shapiro S: Birth Defects and Drugs in Pregnancy. Littleton, Mass.: John Wright-PSG, 1977, pp 358-360. [E]

Hughes HE, Goldstein DA: Birth defects following maternal exposure to ergotamine, beta blockers, and caffeine. J Med Genet 25:396-399, 1988. [C]

Peeden JN, Wilroy RS, Soper RG: Prune perineum. Teratology 20:233-236, 1979. [C]

Verloes A, Emonts P, Dubois M, et al.: Paraplegia and arthrogryposis multiplex of the lower extremities after intrauterine exposure to ergotamine. J Med Genet 27:213-216, 1990. [C]

Wainscott G, Volans GN, Sullivan FM, et al.: The outcome of pregnancy in women suffering from migraine. Postgrad Med J 54:98-102, 1978. [E]

ERYTHRITYL TETRANITRATE

Synonyms

Cardilate, Eritritile Tetranitrate, Erythritol Tetranitrate, Tetranitrol

Summary

Erythrityl tetranitrate is a vasodilator used for treatment of angina pectoris.

Magnitude of Teratogenic Risk

Undetermined

Quality and Quantity of Data

None

Comment

None

No epidemiological studies of congenital anomalies in infants born to women treated with erythrityl tetranitrate during pregnancy have been reported.

No animal teratology studies of erythrityl tetranitrate have been published.

Please see agent summary on nitroglycerine for information on a related agent that has been studied.

Key References

None available.

ERYTHROMYCIN

Synonyms

E-Mycin E Liquid, EryDerm, EryPed Granules, Ery-Tab, Ilotycin Gluceptate, Pediamycin, Wyamycin

Summary

Erythromycin is a macrolide antibiotic. It is widely used to treat a variety of infections, especially in patients allergic to penicillins.

Magnitude of Teratogenic Risk

None

Quality and Quantity of Data

Fair To Good

Comment

None

The frequency of congenital anomalies was no greater than expected among the children of 79 women treated with erythromycin during the first four lunar months of pregnancy or the children of 230 women treated anytime in pregnancy in the Collaborative Perinatal Project (Heinonen et al., 1977). Similarly, no increase in the frequency of congenital anomalies was observed in either of two cohorts of the Boston Collaborative Drug Surveillance Program that included children of 100-200 and 260 women who were treated with erythromycin during the first trimester of pregnancy (Jick et al., 1981; Aselton et al., 1985). The frequency of congenital anomalies was no greater than expected among the infants of 398 women treated with erythromycin during the second or third trimester of pregnancy in a controlled trial of antibiotic therapy for vaginal infections (McCormack et al., 1987). No medication-related adverse effects have been noted among the infants of women treated for vaginal infections with erythromycin during the second of third trimester of pregnancy in other therapeutic trials (Ryan et al., 1990; McGregor et al., 1990; Cohen et al., 1990; Eschenbach et al., 1991).

No increase in the frequency of malformations was observed among the offspring of rats treated with <1-20 times the usual human dose of erythromycin or among the offspring of mice treated with 40 times the usual human dose of erythromycin during pregnancy (Takaya, 1965; Moriguchi et al., 1972a, b).

Key References

Aselton P, Jick H, Milunsky A, Hunter JR, et al.: First-trimester drug use and congenital disorders. Obstet Gynecol 65:451-455, 1985. [S]

Cohen I, Veille J-C, Calkins BM: Improved pregnancy outcome following successful treatment of chlamydial infection. JAMA 263:3160-3163, 1990. [E]

Eschenbach DA, Nugent RP, Rao AV, et al.: A randomized placebo-controlled trial of erythromycin for the treatment of Ureaplasma urealyticum to prevent premature delivery. Am J Obstet Gynecol 164:734-742, 1991. [E]

Heinonen OP, Slone D, Shapiro S: Birth Defects and Drugs in Pregnancy. Littleton, Mass.: John Wright-PSG, 1977, pp 297, 301. [E]

Jick H, Holmes LB, Hunter JR, Madsen S, et al.: First-trimester drug use and congenital disorders. JAMA 246:343-346, 1981. [R]

McCormack WM, Rosner B, Lee Y-H, Munoz A, et al.: Effect of birth weight of erythromycin treatment of pregnant women. Obstet Gynecol 69:202-207, 1987. [E]

McGregor JA, French JI, Richter R, et al.: Cervicovaginal microflora and pregnancy outcome: Results of a double-blind, placebo-controlled trial of erythromycin treatment. Am J Obstet Gynecol 163:1580-1591, 1990. [E]

Moriguchi M, Fujita M, Koeda T: Teratological studies on SF-837 in mice. Jpn J Antibiot 25:193-198, 1972b. [A]

Moriguchi M, Fujita M, Koeda T: Teratological studies on SF-837 in rats. Jpn J Antibiot 25:187-192, 1972a. [A]

Ryan GM Jr, Abdella TN, McNeeley SG, et al.: Chlamydia trachomatis infection in pregnancy and effect of treatment on outcome. Am J Obstet Gynecol 162:34-39, 1990. [E]

Takaya M: Teratogenic effects of antibodies. J Osaka City Med Cen 14:107-115, 1965. [A]

ETHACRYNIC ACID

Synonyms

Edecril, Edecrin, Edecrina, Hydromedin, Reomax, Taladren

Summary

Ethacrynic acid is a loop diuretic used to treat edema.

Magnitude of Teratogenic Risk

Undetermined

Quality and Quantity of Data

None To Poor

Comment

None

No epidemiological studies of congenital anomalies among infants born to women treated with ethacrynic acid during pregnancy have been reported. Nephrolithiasis has been observed in an infant born to a woman with severe diabetes mellitus and hypertension who was treated during pregnancy with ethacrynic acid, captopril, and other medications (Fischer et al., 1988). No causal inference can be made from this single anecdotal report.

No animal teratology studies of ethacrynic acid have been published.

Key References

Fischer AF, Parker BR, Stevenson DK: Nephrolithiasis following in utero diuretic exposure: An unusual case. Pediatrics 81(5):712-714, 1988. [C]

ETHAMBUTOL

Synonyms

Aethambutolum, Diambutol, Etambutol, Etambutolo, Myambutol, Tibutol

Summary

Ethambutol is used orally in the treatment of tuberculosis.

Magnitude of Teratogenic Risk

None To Minimal

Quality and Quantity of Data

Poor To Fair

Comment

None

The frequency of congenital anomalies was not increased among 303 children born to women treated with ethambutol during pregnancy (Jentgens, 1973). Congenital anomalies were noted in 2.2% of 638 infants born to women treated with ethambutol during pregnancy in a series compiled from published cases, including those of Jentgens (Snider et al., 1980). Of these women, 320 were treated during the first four months of pregnancy. No recurrent pattern of anomalies was observed among the infants.

No animal teratology studies of ethambutol have been published.

Key References

Jentgens H: Antituberkulose chemotherapie und schwangerschaftsabbruch. Prax Pneumol 27:479-488, 1973. [E]

Snider DE, Layde PM, Johnson MW, et al.: Treatment of tuberculosis during pregnancy. Am Rev Respir Dis 122:65-79, 1980. [R]

ETHAVERINE

Synonyms

Cardiostron, Circubid, Ethaquin, Ethatab, Ethavex, Ethylpapaverine, Isovex, Papetherine Hydrochloride, Pavaspan, Perperine

Summary

Ethaverine is a phosphodiesterase inhibitor that is administered orally as an anti-spasmodic and anti-arrhythmic agent.

Magnitude of Teratogenic Risk

Undetermined

Quality and Quantity of Data

None

Comment

None

No epidemiological studies of congenital anomalies among the infants of women who were treated with ethaverine during pregnancy have been reported.

No animal teratology studies of ethaverine have been published.

Please see agent summary on papaverine for information on a related agent that has been studied.

Key References

None available.

ETHCHLORVYNOL

Synonyms

Alvinol, Arvynol, Etclorvinol, Normosan, Placidyl, Serenesil

Summary

Ethchlorvynol is used as an oral hypnotic and sedative agent.

Magnitude of Teratogenic Risk

Undetermined

Quality and Quantity of Data

None To Poor

Comment

None

No epidemiological studies of congenital anomalies among infants born to women treated with ethchlorvynol during pregnancy have been reported.

No studies of congenital anomalies in the offspring of experimental animals treated with ethchlorvynol during pregnancy have been published. Behavioral alterations have been observed among the offspring of rats treated during pregnancy with 1-4 times the human therapeutic dose of ethchlorvynol (Peters & Hudson, 1981). The clinical importance of this finding is unknown.

Symptoms of neonatal withdrawal, including jitteriness, irritability, and hypotonia, have been observed in the infant of a woman who took ethchlorvynol as a hypnotic throughout the last three months of pregnancy (Rumak & Walravens, 1973).

Key References

Peters MA, Hudson PM: The effects of totigestational exposure to ethchlorvynol on development and behavior. Ecotoxicol Environ Safety 5:494-502, 1981. [A]

Rumack BH, Walravens PA: Neonatal withdrawal following maternal ingestion of ethchlorvynol (placidyl). Pediatr 52:714-715, 1973. [C]

ETHER

Synonyms

Acetic Ether, Diethyl Ether, Diethyl Oxide, Ethyl Ether, Ethyl Oxide

Summary

Ether (diethyl ether) is a general anesthetic administered by inhalation. It is rarely used now.

Magnitude of Teratogenic Risk

Undetermined

Quality and Quantity of Data

Poor

Comment

None

No epidemiological studies of congenital anomalies in children born to women exposed to ether anesthesia during pregnancy have been reported.

The frequency of malformations was no greater than expected among the offspring of mice and rats subjected repeatedly to ether anesthesia during pregnancy, but decreased head growth and an increased frequency of skeletal variations and fetal resorptions were noted in the offspring of exposed mice (Lindskog, 1958; Schwetz & Becker, 1970). The relevance of these observations to the risks associated with ether exposure in human pregnancy is unknown.

Key References

Lindskog BI: On the influence of ether narcosis on embryo development in mice with special reference to repeated cesarean sections. Acta Anat 33:208-214, 1958. [A]

Schwetz BA, Becker BA: Embryotoxicity and fetal malformations of rats and mice due to maternally administered ether. Toxicol Appl Pharmacol 17:275, 1970. [A]

ETHINAMATE

Synonyms

Etinamate, Etinamato, Valamin, Valaminetten, Valmid, Valmidate, Volamin

Summary

Ethinamate is a non-barbiturate sedative and hypnotic that is administered orally to induce sleep.

Magnitude of Teratogenic Risk

Undetermined

Quality and Quantity of Data

None To Poor

Comment

None

No epidemiological studies of congenital anomalies among infants born to women treated with ethinamate during pregnancy have been reported.

The frequency of congenital anomalies was said to have been slightly increased among the offspring of mice treated with 20 times the human dose of ethinamate in one study published only as an abstract (Harris & Morgan, 1969). Insufficient information is available to assess this study.

Key References

Harris JWS, Morgan PR: Aetiology of cleft palate induced by meclozine, buclizine and hydroxyzine. In: Fraser FC (ed). 3rd International Conference Congenital Malformations: 47 (Abstract). Amsterdam: Excerpta Med, 1969. [A]

ETHINYL ESTRADIOL

Synonyms

Estinyl, Feminone, Linoral, Norlestrin, Novestrol, Primogyn, Progynon C

Summary

Ethinyl estradiol is a synthetic estrogen that is widely used to treat menopausal symptoms and menstrual disorders, and, in combination with a progestin, for oral contraception. Ethinyl estradiol is also employed in doses 2-40 times greater for palliative treatment of breast cancer.

Magnitude of Teratogenic Risk

None

Quality and Quantity of Data

Good

Comment

None

The frequency of congenital anomalies was not significantly increased among the infants of 89 women who took ethinyl estradiol during the first four lunar months of pregnancy or of 98 women who took this drug anytime during pregnancy in the Collaborative Perinatal Project (Heinonen et al., 1977). In a case-control study, use during pregnancy of ethinyl estradiol alone or in combination with a progestin was no more frequent than expected among the mothers of 171 infants with congenital anomalies (Spira et al., 1972). Similarly, the frequency of hormonal pregnancy tests using ethinyl estradiol and norethindrone (a progestin) during the second month of pregnancy was not increased among the mothers of 194 infants with major malformations or 551 infants with minor anomalies (Kullander & Kallen, 1976).

No alteration in the frequency of congenital anomalies was apparent among the offspring of three species of nonhuman primates treated during pregnancy with ethinyl estradiol in combination with norethindrone (a progestin) in doses 10-100 times those used for human contraception (Hendrickx et al., 1987). Embryonic loss and genital alterations were observed at higher doses in cynomolgus monkeys, but such doses were also toxic to the mothers. Pregnancy loss occurred in rhesus monkeys treated with this drug combination at 100 times the human contraceptive dose (Prahlada & Hendrickx, 1983). The frequency of extragenital malformations was not increased among the offspring of pregnant mice, rats or rabbits treated with 20-2000, 10-500, or 1-75 times the human contraceptive dose of ethinyl estradiol (Morris, 1970; Chemnitius et al., 1979; Yasuda et al., 1981; Joshi et al., 1983), although pregnancy loss was frequent at the higher doses in rodents.

Alterations of gonadal and internal genital tract morphology were observed among the offspring of mice treated during pregnancy with 20-2000 times the human contraceptive dose of ethinyl estradiol (Yasuda et al., 1981, 1986, 1987, 1988). Increases in uterine weight were noted among the offspring of pregnant rats treated with 4-400 times the human contraceptive dose of ethinyl estradiol (Harmon et al., 1989). Cryptorchidism was found with increased frequency among the offspring of a genetically-predisposed strain of mice treated during pregnancy with 200 times the human contraceptive dose of ethinyl estradiol (Walker et al., 1990). The clinical significance of these observations is uncertain.

Key References

Chemnitius KH, Oettel M, Lemke H: Teratogenic effects of ethinyloestradiol sulfonate) in Wistar rats. In: Benesova A, Rychter Z, Jelinek R (eds). Evaluation of Embryotoxicity, Mutagenicity and Carcinogenicity Risks in New Drugs. Proc 3rd Symp Toxicol Test for Safety of New Drugs. Prague, USSR: Univ Karlova-Praha, 1979, pp 75-81. [A]

Harmon JR, Branham WS, Sheehan DM: Transplacental estrogen responses in the fetal rat: Increased uterine weight and ornithine decarboxylase activity. Teratology 39:253-260, 1989. [A]

Heinonen OP, Slone D, Shapiro S: Birth Defects and Drugs in Pregnancy. Littleton, Mass.: John Wright-PSG, 1977, pp 389-391, 443. [E]

Hendrickx AG, Korte R, Leuschner F, Neumann BW, et al.: Embryotoxicity of sex steroidal hormone combinations in nonhuman primates: I. Norethisterone acetate + ethinylestradiol and progesterone + estradiol benzoate (Macaca mulatta, Macaca fascicularis, and Papio cynocephalus). Teratology 35:119-127, 1987. [A]

Joshi NJ, Ambani LM, Munshi SR: Evaluation of teratogenic potential of a combination of norethisterone and ethinyl estradiol in rats. Indian J Exp Biol 21:591-596, 1983. [A]

Kullander S, Kallen B: A prospective study of drugs and pregnancy. 3. Hormones. Acta Obstet Gynecol Scand 55:221-224, 1976. [S]

Morris JM: Postcoital antifertility agents and their teratogenic effect. Contraception 2:85-97, 1970. [A]

Prahalada S, Hendrickx AG: Embryotoxicity of norlestrin, a combined synthetic oral contraceptive, in rhesus macaques (Macaca mulatta). Teratology 27:215-222, 1983. [A]

Spira N, Goujard J, Huel G, Rumeau-Rouquette C: [Investigation into the teratogenic action of sex hormones first results of an epidemiologic survey involving 20,000 women.] Rev Med 41:2683-2694, 1972. [S]

Walker AH, Bernstein L, Warren DW, et al.: The effect of in utero ethinyl oestradiol exposure on the risk of cryptorchid testis and testicular teratoma in mice. Br J Cancer 62(4):599-602, 1990. [A]

Yasuda Y, Kihara T, Nishimura H: Effect of ethinyl estradiol on development of mouse fetuses. Teratology 23:233-239, 1981. [A]

Yasuda Y, Konishi H, Tanimura T: Leydig cell hyperplasia in fetal mice treated transplacentally with ethinyl estradiol. Teratology 33:281-288, 1986. [A]

Yasuda Y, Konishi H, Tanimura T: Ovarian follicular cell hyperplasia in fetal mice treated transplacentally with ethinyl estradiol. Teratology 36:35-43, 1987. [A]

Yasuda Y, Ohara I, Konishi H, Tanimura T: Long-term effects on male reproductive organs of prenatal exposure to ethinyl estradiol. Am J Obstet Gynecol 159(5):1246-1250, 1988. [A]

ETHIONAMIDE

Synonyms

Etimid, Etionid, Thiodine, Trecator, Trescatyl

Summary

Ethionamide is a thioamide derivative used in the treatment of tuberculosis and leprosy.

Magnitude of Teratogenic Risk

Undetermined

Quality and Quantity of Data

Poor

Comment

A small risk cannot be excluded, but a high risk of congenital anomalies in the children of women treated with ethionamide during pregnancy is unlikely.

No congenital anomalies were noted among the children of 40 women treated with ethionamide beginning early in pregnancy in one series (Zierski, 1966).

Slightly increased frequencies of malformations were observed among the offspring of mice and rats treated during pregnancy with ethionamide in doses respectively 2.5-12 and 10 times those used in humans (Takekoshi, 1965; Fujimori et al., 1965; Khan & Azam, 1969). Typical dose-dependence of the teratogenic effect was demonstrated in mice. In another study in rats, only skeletal variations were observed with increased frequency at these doses and no increase in defects was observed after maternal treatment with doses similar to those used clinically (Dluzniewski & Gastol- Lewinska, 1971). No increase in fetal malformations but an increased fetal loss rate was noted after treatment of pregnant rabbits with ethionamide in doses similar to those used in humans (Dluzniewski & Gastol-Lewinska, 1971). Increased frequencies of malformations and fetal growth retardation were seen among the offspring of rabbits treated during pregnancy with 5-10 times the human dose of ethionamide (Khan & Azam, 1969).

Key References

Dluzniewski A, Gastol-Lewinska L: The search for teratogenic activity of some tuberculostatic drugs. Diss Pharm Pharmacol 23:383-392, 1971. [A]

Fujimori H, Yamada F, Shibukawa N, et al.: The effect of tuberculostatics on the fetus: An experimental production of congenital anomaly in rats by ethionamide. Proc Congen Anom Res Assoc Japan 5:34-35, 1965. [A]

Khan I, Azam A: Study of teratogenic activity of trifluoperazine, amitriptyline, ethionamide and thalidomide in pregnant rabbits and mice. Proc Eur Soc Study Drug Toxic 10:235-242, 1969. [A]

Takekoshi S: Effects of hydroxymethylpyrimidine on isoniazid- and ethionamide-induced teratosis. Gunma J Med Sci 14:233-244, 1965. [A]

Zierski M: Effects of ethionamide on the development of the human fetus. Gruzlica 34:349-352, 1966. [S]

ETHOHEPTAZINE

Synonyms

Aethoheptazin, Ethyl Heptazine, Panalgin, Zactane, Zactipar

Summary

Ethoheptazine is an opioid analgesic administered orally for pain.

Magnitude of Teratogenic Risk

None To Minimal

Quality and Quantity of Data

Poor To Fair

None

The frequency of congenital anomalies was no higher than expected among the children of 60 mothers who were treated with ethoheptazine during the first four lunar months of pregnancy, or of 300 mothers who were treated with the drug anytime during pregnancy in the Collaborative Perinatal Project (Heinonen et al., 1977).

No animal teratology studies of ethoheptazine have been published.

Please see agent summary on meperidine for information on a related agent that has been more thoroughly studied.

Key References

Heinonen OP, Slone D, Shapiro S: Birth Defects and Drugs in Pregnancy. Littleton, Mass.: John Wright-PSG, 1977, pp 287-288, 434, 485. [E]

ETHOSUXIMIDE

Synonyms

Emeside, Ethosuccimide, Ethymal, Petinimid, Petnidan, Pyknolepsinum, Suxinutin, Zarondan, Zarontin

Summary

Ethosuximide is a succinimide anticonvulsant used to treat petit mal epilepsy.

Magnitude of Teratogenic Risk

Undetermined

Quality and Quantity of Data

Poor

Comment

Although a risk of teratogenicity has not been demonstrated for this agent, animal studies and *analogy to other anticonvulsants raise concern that such a risk may exist.*

No adequate epidemiological studies of congenital anomalies among the infants of women who were treated with ethosuximide during pregnancy have been reported.

Increased frequencies of skeletal, central nervous system, and other anomalies were observed among the offspring of rats, mice, hamsters, and rabbits treated during pregnancy with ethosuximide in doses respectively <1-25, 6-36, <1-18, and <1-7 times those used in humans (Dluzniewski et al., 1979; Sullivan & McElhatton, 1977; El-Sayed et al., 1983). The clinical relevance of these observations is unclear.

Key References

Dluzniewski A, Gastol-Lewinska L, Kulej-Grodecka A, Kwiatek H, et al.: Teratogenic activity of ethosuximide in rats, hamsters, and rabbits. In: Benasova, O, Rychter A and Jelinek R (eds). Evaluation of Embryotoxicity, Mutagenicity, and Carcinogenicity Risks in New Drugs. Proc 3rd Symp on Toxicol Test for Safety of New Drugs. Prague: Univ Karlova-Praha, 1979, pp 59-68. [A]

El-Sayed MGA, Aly AE, Kadri M, Moustafa AM: Comparative study on the teratogenicity of some antiepileptics in the rat. East Afr Med J 60:407-415, 1983. [A]

Sullivan FM, McElhatton PR: Comparison of the teratogenic activity of the antiepileptic drugs carbamazepine, clonazepam, ethosuximide, phenobarbital, phenytoin and primidone in mice. Toxicol Appl Pharmacol 40:365-378, 1977. [A]

ETHOTOIN

Synonyms

Etotoina, Peganone

Summary

Ethotoin is a hydantoin anticonvulsant.

Magnitude of Teratogenic Risk

Small To Moderate

Quality and Quantity of Data

Poor To Fair

Comment

None

No adequate epidemiological studies of congenital anomalies in infants born to women treated with ethotoin during pregnancy have been published. Three children with features characteristic of fetal hydantoin syndrome whose mothers took ethotoin but no other phenytoin anticonvulsant during pregnancy have been reported (Finnell & DiLiberti, 1983; Waller et al., 1978). These observations suggest that maternal use of ethotoin during pregnancy may be associated with the occurrence of this pattern of anomalies *(See phenytoin agent summary for more information on the fetal hydantoin syndrome).*

An increased frequency of skeletal and other malformations similar to those found with other hydantoin anticonvulsants was seen among the offspring of mice treated with 5-11 times the human therapeutic dose of ethotoin during pregnancy (Brown et al., 1982). The relevance of this observation to the clinical use of ethotoin in human pregnancy is unknown.

Key References

Brown NA, Shull G, Kao J, Goulding EH, et al.: Teratogenicity and lethality of hydantoin de-rivatives in the mouse: Structure--toxicity relation-ships. Toxicol Appl Pharmacol 64:271-288, 1982. [A]

Finnell RH, DiLiberti JH: Hydantoin-induced teratogenesis: Are arene oxide intermediates really responsible? Helv Paediat Acta 38:171-177, 1983. [C]

Wallar PH, Genstler DE, George CC: Multiple systemic and periocular malformations associated with the fetal hydantoin syndrome. Ann Opthalmol 10:1568-1572, 1978. [C]

ETHYL CHLORIDE

Synonyms

Aethylium Chloratum, Anodynon, Chelen, Chlorethyl, Chloroethane, Hydrochloric Ether, Monochloroethane, Narcotile

Summary

Ethyl chloride has been used as an inhalational anesthetic. It is sometimes employed as a topi-cal anesthetic because it has a low boiling point and produces intense cold on evaporation.

Magnitude of Teratogenic Risk

Undetermined

Quality and Quantity of Data

None

Comment

None

No epidemiological studies of congenital anomalies in children born to women exposed to ethyl chloride during pregnancy have been reported.

No studies of teratologic effects of ethyl chloride in experimental animals have been published.

Key References

None available.

ETHYLENE

Synonyms

Acetene, Athylen, Elayl, Ethene

Summary

Ethylene is a general anesthetic that is administered by inhalation. It is rarely used for this purpose now.

Magnitude of Teratogenic Risk

Undetermined

Quality and Quantity of Data

None

Comment

None

No epidemiological studies of congenital anomalies in children born to women exposed to ethylene during pregnancy have been reported.

No studies of teratologic effects of ethylene in experimental animals have been published.

Key References

None available.

ETHYLENE OXIDE

Synonyms

ETO, Oxirane

Summary

Ethylene oxide is a colorless gas that is widely used in the chemical and plastics industries, as an agricultural fungicide, and to sterilize surgical instruments. Ethylene oxide is readily absorbed after inhalation or dermal exposure.

Magnitude of Teratogenic Risk

Spontaneous Abortions: Minimal To Small

Congenital Anomalies: Minimal

Quality and Quantity of Data

Spontaneous Abortions: Fair

Congenital Anomalies: Poor

Comment

None

A higher incidence of spontaneous abortions was found in a cohort of 146 pregnancies of Finnish hospital staff exposed to ethylene oxide (8-hour weighted mean concentrations in the range of 0.1-0.5 ppm) when compared to apparently unexposed hospital staff (Hemminki et al., 1982, 1983). The study found a lower than expected adjusted rate of miscarriage among controls (7.7%) rather than a higher than expected frequency among the exposed group (12.7%). The investigation has been criticized on methodological grounds (Gordon & Meinhardt, 1983; Austin, 1983) and was not confirmed in a more recent case control study of 164 spontaneous abortions and 34 infants with congenital anomalies reported by the same authors (Hemminki et al., 1985). A higher incidence of spontaneous abortions has also been reported in 95 pregnancies of women exposed to atmospheric concentrations of ethylene oxide of 0.55 ppm or less in an organic chemical factory when compared to unexposed plant administrators (Yakubova, 1976). The rate of miscarriage in the exposed women was about what would be expected in the general population (16%) while the rate among the controls was again inexplicably low (8%).

Increased frequencies of fetal death and craniofacial and skeletal anomalies were observed among the offspring of pregnant mice treated intravenously with ethylene oxide in a dose of 150 mg/kg/d but not 75 mg/kg/d

(LaBorde & Kimmel, 1980); maternal toxicity was also evident at the higher dose. The incidence of congenital anomalies was not increased among the offspring of pregnant rats exposed by inhalation to 10-150 ppm of ethylene oxide for 6-7 hrs/day, but maternal toxicity and a reduction in fetal weight, length, and skeletal ossification were observed at the highest doses (Snellings et al., 1982; Hardin et al., 1983). No increase in the frequency of congenital anomalies was found among the offspring of rabbits treated during pregnancy with intravenous ethylene oxide at doses of 9-36 mg/kg/d or with inhalational exposure at 150 ppm for 7 hours per day, although fetal death and maternal toxicity were often seen at the higher doses (Hardin et al., 1983; Jones-Price et al., 1983). The relevance of these observations to human occupational exposure to ethylene oxide during pregnancy is unknown.

Increased frequencies of fetal death, growth retardation, hydrops, and malformations of the skeleton, palate, eye, heart, and abdominal wall were found among the offspring of female mice exposed by inhalation to 900-1200 ppm of ethylene oxide shortly after fertilization (Generoso et al., 1987; Rutledge & Generoso, 1989; Polifka et al., 1992). This early period of development is generally thought to be resistant to the induction of malformations, and the mechanism underlying the striking effect that occurs in mice with high doses of ethylene oxide is unknown (Katoh et al., 1989).

Supplemental Information For Environmental And Occupational Exposures

Occupational Exposure: Human exposure to ethylene oxide occurs primarily in sterilization facilities and in chemical production plants (WHO, 1985; Hine et al, 1981).
Production Plants:
Typical time-weighted exposures: 0.01-2.20 ppm. Occasionally exposures up to 82 ppm can be measured (WHO, 1985).
Worst-case peak exposures: Up to 9400 ppm (Flores, 1983).
Sterilization Facilities:

Typical exposures of 5-10 ppm for 20 minutes occur when the door to the sterilization chamber is opened. Peak concentrations up to 1000 ppm have been measured (HSDB (R), 1992).
Occupational Re-Entry Values: Unavailable.
Odor Threshold: 50-700 ppm (Clayton & Clayton, 1981; CHRIS, 1990). The odor of ethylene oxide resembles that of ether. Ethylene oxide causes rapid olfactory fatigue (Hine et al, 1981).
Permissible Exposure Limit In Air (8 Hour, Time-Weighted Average For Occupational Exposure): 1 ppm (ACGIH, 1991).
No Effects Level: 5-10 ppm (HSDB (R), 1992).
Maxiumum Residue Allowed In Clothing: 200 ppm (Poisindex (R), 1989).
Immediately Dangerous To Life Or Health Value: 800 ppm (NIOSH, 1990).
Toxic Signs And Symptoms (POISINDEX (R), 1992; HSDB (R), 1992; Hathaway et al., 1991):
Acute (occur with brief single exposures of more than 200 ppm):
Cough, dyspnea, pulmonary edema
Conjunctivitis, corneal injury (with splash contact)
Headache, lethargy, malaise, dizziness, stupor, coma
Muscle twitching
Vomiting
Skin irritation at 100 ppm or more in clothing burns
Peripheral neuropathy, memory impairment
Cataracts
Chronic (occur with continuous 8 hour exposures above 200 ppm):
Peripheral neuropathy, memory impairment Cataracts
LC50 (Inhalation):
Dog: 973 ppm/4 hr (HSDB (R), 1992)
Mouse: 836 ppm/4 hr (HSDB (R), 1992).

241

Rat: 1462 ppm/4 hr (HSDB (R), 1992).

LD50 (Oral):

Guinea Pig: 270 mg/kg (HSDB (R), 1992).

Rat: 330 mg/kg (HSDB (R), 1992).

Tests For Exposure: Blood or urine concentrations of ethylene oxide can be measured by flame-ionization gas chromatography (Brugnone et al., 1986). Blood levels in workers exposed to the threshold limit value (1 ppm) should not exceed 10 mcg/L. Alveolar breath concentrations should not exceed 0.5 mg/cu m.

The measurement of hemoglobin adducts (Calleman et al., 1978; Ehrenberg et al., 1974), urinary 2-hydroxyethylmercapturic acid (Gerin & Tardif, 1986), or lymphocyte sister chromatid exchange (Yager et al., 1983; Hogstedt et al., 1983) to monitor ethylene oxide exposure is considered experimental.

Key References

ACGIH: 1991-1992 Threshold Limit Values For Chemical Substances and Physical Agents and Biological Exposure Indices. Cincinnati, Ohio: Am Conference Govt Ind Hyg, 1991, p. 21. [O]

Austin SG: Spontaneous abortions in hospital sterilising staff. (Letter to the editor). Br Med J 286:1976, 1983. [O]

Brugnone F, Perbellini L, Faccini GB, Pasini F, et al.: Ethylene oxide exposure. Biological monitoring by analysis of alveolar air and blood. Int Arch Occup Environ Health 58:105-112, 1986. [S]

Calleman CJ, Ehrenberg L, Jansson B, et al.: Monitoring and risk assessment by means of alkyl groups in hemoglobin in persons occupationally exposed to ethylene oxide. J Environ Pathol Tox 2:427-442. [E]

CHRIS: CHRIS Hazardous Chemical Data. Washington, D.C: U.S. Department of Transportation, U.S. Coast Guard, 1990. [R]

Clayton GD, Clayton FE: Patty's Industrial Hygiene and Toxicology, 3rd ed.: Vol 2A Toxicology. New York: Wiley-Interscience, 1981. [R]

Ehrenberg L, Hiesche K, Osterman-Goger S, et al.: Evaluation of genetic risks of alkylating agents: Tissue doses in the mouse from air contaminated with ethylene oxide. Mut Res 24:83-103, 1974. [A]

Flores GH: Controlling exposure to alkene oxides. Chem Eng Preg 79:39-43, 1983. [E]

Generoso WM, Rutledge JC, Cain KT, Hughes LA, et al.: Exposure of female mice to ethylene oxide within hours after mating leads to fetal malformation and death. Mutat Res 176:269-274, 1987. [A]

Gerin M and Tardif R: Urinary N-acetyl-S-2-hydroxyethyl-L-cysteine in rats as biological indicator of ethylene oxide exposure. Fund Appl Toxicol 7:419-423, 1986. [A]

Gordon J, Meinhardt TJ: Ethylene oxide-- spontaneous abortions. (Letter to the editor) Br Med J 286:1976-1977, 1983. [O]

Hardin BD, Niemeier RW, Sikov MR, Hackett PL: Reproductive-toxicologic assessment of the epoxides ethylene oxide, propylene oxide, butylene oxide, and styrene oxide. Scand J Work Environ Health 9:94-102, 1983. [A]

Hathaway GJ, Proctor NH, Hughes JP, Fischman ML (eds): Proctor and Hughes' Chemical Hazards of the Workplace. New York: Van Nostrand Reinhold, 1991, pp 292-294. [R]

HSDB [database online]. Bethesda, Md: National Library of Medicine, 1985- [updated 1992]. Available from: National Library of Medicine; BRS Information Technologies, McLean, Va. [O]

Hemminki K, Mutanen P, Niemi M-L: Spontaneous abortions in hospital staff engaged in sterilizing instruments with chemical agents. Br Med J 285:1461-1463, 1982. [E]

Hemminki K, Mutanen P, Saloniemi I, Niemi M-L, et al.: Spontaneous abortions in hospital staff engaged in sterilizing instruments with chemical agents. Br Med J 285:1461-1463, 1982. [E]

Hemminki K, Kyyronen P, Lindbohm M-L: Spontaneous abortions and malformations in the offspring of nurses exposed to anaesthetic gases, cytostatic drugs, and other potential hazards in hospitals. Based on registered information outcome. J Epidemiol Comm Health 39:141-147, 1985. [E]

Hine C, Rowe VK, White ER, Darmer KI, et al.: Epoxy Compounds. In: Clayton GD and Clayton FE (eds). Patty's Industrial Hygiene and Toxicology, Vol 2A. Toxicology. New York: John Wiley & Sons, 1981, pp 2141-2186. [R]

Hogstedt B, Gullberg B, Hedner K, Kolnig AM, et al.: Chromosome aberrations and micronuclei in bone marrow cells and peripheral blood lymphocytes in humans exposed to ethylene oxide. Hereditas 98:105-113, 1983. [E]

Jones-Price C, Marks TA, Ledoux TA, Reel JR, et al.: Teratologic evaluation of ethylene oxide (CAS No. 75-21-8) in New Zealand white rabbits. NTIS Report PB83-242016, 1983. [A]

Katoh M, Cacheiro NL, Cornett CV, et al.: Fetal anomalies produced subsequent to treatment of zygotes with ethylene oxide or ethyl methanesulfonate are not likely due to the usual genetic causes. Mutat Res 210(2):337-344, 1989. [A]

LaBorde JB, Kimmel CA: The teratogenicity of ethylene oxide administered intravenously to mice. Toxicol Appl Pharmacol 56:16-22, 1980. [A]

NIOSH: Pocket Guide to Chemical Hazards. Cincinnati, Ohio: National Institute for Occupational Safety and Health, 1990. [O]

Poisindex (R) Information System. Denver, Colo.: Micromedex, 1989. [O]

Polifka JE, Rutledge JC, Kimmel GL, et al.: Skeletal deviations in mice offspring following zygotic exposure to ethylene oxide. Teratology 43(5):444, 1991. [A]

Rutledge JC, Generoso WM: Fetal pathology produced by ethylene oxide treatment of the murine zygote. Teratology 39:563-572, 1989. [A]

Snellings WM, et al: Teratology study in Fischer 344 rats exposed to ethylene oxide by inhalation. Toxicol Appl Pharmacol 64:476-481, 1982. [A]

WHO (World Health Organization): Ethylene Oxide. In: Environmental Health Criteria 55. Geneva, Switzerland: United Nations Environment Program, International Labor Organization, 1985. [R]

Yakubova ZN, Shamova HA, Muftaknova FA, Shilova LF: Gynaecological disorders in workers engaged in ethylene oxide production. Kazan Med Zh 57:558-560, 1976. [E]

Yager JW, Hines CJ, Spear RC: Exposure to ethylene oxide at work increases sister-chromatid exchanges in human peripheral lymphocytes. Science 219:1221-1223, 1983. [E]

ETHYLNOREPIN-EPHRINE

Synonyms

Bronkephrine, Butanefrine, Butanephrine

Summary

Ethylnorepinephrine is a sympathomimetic agent that is administered parenterally in the treatment of bronchial asthma.

Magnitude of Teratogenic Risk

Undetermined

Quality and Quantity of Data

None

Comment

None

No epidemiological studies of congenital anomalies in infants born to women treated with ethylnorepinephrine during pregnancy have been reported.

No animal teratology studies of ethylnorepinephrine have been published.

Key References

None available.

ETHYNODIOL DIACETATE

Synonyms

Femulen, Metrulen, Mutrulen, Ovulen

Summary

Ethynodiol diacetate is a synthetic progestin that is used alone or in combination with an estrogenic compound as an oral contraceptive and in treatment of menstrual disorders.

Magnitude of Teratogenic Risk

None To Minimal

Quality and Quantity of Data

Poor To Fair

Comment

This risk estimate is for virilization of the genitalia in a female fetus. The estimate is based on studies involving use of progestational hormones at doses that are often much greater than those currently employed.

Maternal use of ethynodiol diacetate was no more frequent than expected among 171 infants with congenital anomalies in one case-control study (Spira et al., 1972).

The frequency of malformations was no greater than expected among the offspring of rats treated during pregnancy with ethynodiol diacetate in combination with an estrogenic agent in doses 10-100 times those used in human contraception, although increased fetal loss was observed among pregnant animals treated with 24 or more times the usual human dose of ethynodiol diacetate alone (Saunders & Elton, 1967). Similarly, malformations were no more frequent than expected among the offspring of rabbits treated during pregnancy with ethynodiol diacetate alone or in combination with an estrogenic agent in doses 1-25 or more times greater than those used in huamn contraception (Saunders & Elton, 1967).

Key References

Saunders FJ, Elton RL: Effects of ethynodiol diacetate and mestranol in rats and rabbits, on conception, on the outcome of pregnancy and on the offspring. Toxicol Appl Pharmacol 11:229-244, 1967. [A]

Spira N, Goujard J, Huel G, et al.: Investigation into the teratogenic action of sex hormones: First results of an epidemiologic survey involving 20,000 women. Rev Med 41:2683-2694, 1972. [E]

ETIDOCAINE

Synonyms

Duranest

Summary

Etidocaine is a local anesthetic of the amide class.

Magnitude of Teratogenic Risk

Undetermined

Quality and Quantity of Data

None

Comment

A small risk cannot be excluded, but there is no indication that the risk of congenital anomalies in the children of women treated with etidocaine during pregnancy is likely to be great.

No epidemiological studies of congenital anomalies in children born to women given etidocaine during pregnancy have been reported.

No animal teratology studies of etidocaine have been published.

Please see agent summary on lidocaine for information on a related agent that has been studied.

Key References

None available.

ETIDRONATE

Synonyms

Calcimux, Didronel, Disodium Ethydronate, Etidron, Sodium Ethydronate, Tetrasodium Etidronate

Summary

Etidronate is a diphosphonate administered orally in the treatment of abnormal ossification.

Magnitude of Teratogenic Risk

Undetermined

Quality and Quantity of Data

Poor

Comment

None

No epidemiological studies of congenital anomalies among the infants of women treated with etidronate during pregnancy have been published.

An increased frequency of central nervous system, craniofacial, and other anomalies was observed among the offspring of pregnant mice treated with about 10 times the human therapeutic dose of etidronate (Sakiyama et al., 1986). Alterations of ossification were observed among the offspring of rats treated with 1.5-5 times the human dose of etidronate during pregnancy in one study (Rohnelt, 1975). In another study, the frequency of malformations was not increased among the offspring of rats or rabbits treated during pregnancy with etidronate in doses 7-22 or 1-5 times those used therapeutically in humans (Nolen & Buehler, 1971).

Key References

Nolen GA, Buehler EV: The effects of disodium etidronate on the reproductive functions and embryogeny of albino rats and New Zealand rabbits. Toxicol Appl Pharmacol 18:548-561, 1971. [A]

Rohnelt M: Teratogenicity of diphosphonates in rats. In: Neubert D, Merker HJ, (eds). New Approaches to the Evaluation of Abnormal Embryonic Development. Stuttgart: Thieme, 1975, pp 728-745. [A]

Sakiyama Y, Yamamoto H, Soeda Y, et al.: The effect of ethane-1-hydroxy-1, 1-diphosphonate (EHDP) on fetal mice during pregnancy. Part 2. External anomalies. J Osaka Dent Univ 20(2):91-100, 1986. [A]

ETOMIDATE

Synonyms

Amidate, Hypnodil, Hypnomidate, Metomidate Hydrochloride, Sibul

Summary

Etomidate is a short-acting non-barbiturate intravenous anesthetic.

Magnitude of Teratogenic Risk

Undetermined

Quality and Quantity of Data

None To Poor

Comment

None

No epidemiological studies have been reported of congenital anomalies in children born to women who had been treated during pregnancy with etomidate.

The frequency of malformations was no greater than expected among the offspring of rats treated during pregnancy with etomidate in doses 40 times those used to induce anesthesia in humans (Doenicke & Haehl, 1977).

Key References

Doenicke A, Haehl M: Teratogenicity of etomidate. Anaesthesiol Resuscitation 106:23-24, 1977. [A]

ETOPOSIDE

Synonyms

Epipodophyllotoxin, Etopol, Vepesid

Summary

Etoposide is a semisynthetic podophyllin derivative that inhibits DNA synthesis. Etoposide is used as an antineoplastic agent.

Magnitude of Teratogenic Risk

Undetermined

Quality and Quantity of Data

Poor To Fair

Comment

Although the teratogenic risk of etoposide in humans is undetermined, the fact that this drug is cytotoxic raises concern that the risk could be substantial.

No epidemiological studies of congenital anomalies among infants born to women treated with etoposide during pregnancy have been reported. Anecdotal observations of at least nine infants whose mothers were treated with etoposide during gestation have been reported (Choo et al., 1985; Raffles et al., 1989; Aviles et al., 1991). None of these babies, including at least two born to mothers treated in the first trimester of pregnancy, had malformations. Leukopenia and hearing loss were observed in one child who was born at 27 weeks gestation (Raffles et al., 1989).

Increased frequencies of congenital anomalies, fetal death, and fetal growth retardation were observed among the offspring of rats and mice treated with 3-4 and <1 times the human therapeutic dose of etoposide during pregnancy (Sieber et al., 1978; Hiramatsu, 1985; Takahashi et al., 1986a). The most frequent structural anomalies observed involved the brain, eyes, and skeleton. Doses that caused fetal damage often produced evidence of maternal toxicity as well. No teratogenic effect was observed among the offspring of pregnant rabbits treated with etoposide in doses similar to those used in humans (Takahashi et al., 1986b).

Key References

Aviles A, Diaz-Maqueo JC, Talavera A, et al.: Growth and development of children of mothers treated with chemotherapy during pregnancy: Current status of 43 children. Am J Hematol 36:243-248, 1991. [S]

Choo YC, Chan SY, Wong LC, Ma HK: Ovarian dysfunction in patients with gestational trophoblastic neoplasia treated with short intensive courses of etoposide (VP-16-213). Cancer 55(10):2348-2352, 1985. [S]

Hiramatsu Y, Suzuki T, Okada K, et al.: Safety study of etoposide (NK 171). 8. Oral administration in pre and post implantation period in rats. Kiso to Rinsho (Clin Rep)19:3885-3896, 1985. [A]

Raffles A, Williams J, Costeloe K, Clark P: Transplacental effects of maternal cancer chemotherapy. Case Report. Br J Obstet Gynaecol 96:1099-1100, 1989. [C]

Sieber SM, Whang-Peng J, Botkin C, Knutsen T: Teratogenic and cytogenetic effects of some plant-derived antitumor agents (vincristine, colchicine, maytansine, VP-16-213 and VM-26) in mice. Teratology 18:31-48, 1978. [A]

Takahashi N, Kai S, Kohmura H, et al.: Reproduction studies of VP16-213. II. Oral administration to rats during the period of fetal organogenesis. J Toxicol Sci 11(Suppl 1):195-225, 1986a. [A]

Takahashi N, Kai S, Kohmura H, et al.: Reproduction studies of VP16-213. III. Oral administration to rabbits during the period of fetal organogenesis. J Toxicol Sci 11(Suppl 1):227-239, 1986b. [A]

ETOXADROL

Summary

Etoxadrol is an anesthetic.

Magnitude of Teratogenic Risk

Undetermined

Quality and Quantity of Data

None

Comment

None

No epidemiological studies of congenital anomalies in children born to women exposed to etoxadrol during pregnancy have been reported.

No investigations of teratologic effects of etoxadrol in experimental animals have been published.

Key References

None available.

ETRETINATE

Synonyms

Ethyl Etrinoate, Tegison, Tigason

Summary

Etretinate is a retinoid that is administered orally in the treatment of psoriasis.

Magnitude of Teratogenic Risk

High

Quality and Quantity of Data

Fair

Comment

Etretinate persists in the body for an extremely long time after administration; the drug has been detected in the serum one to two years or more after cessation of therapy (Digiovanna et al., 1984; Rinck et al., 1989). The length of time that teratogenic effects of etretinate may occur after discontinuation of therapy is unknown (Mitchell, 1992).

No epidemiological studies of congenital anomalies among the infants of women treated with etretinate during pregnancy have been reported. At least four cases of neural tube and other central nervous system (CNS) defects and three cases of craniofacial and skeletal abnormalities have been observed among the infants of women treated with etretinate during pregnancy (Happle et al., 1984; Rosa et al., 1986). The anomalies in these infants have not been fully described, but appear generally similar to those seen among the offspring of experimental animals treated with etretinate during pregnancy. No malformations were observed among nine infants born to women treated with etretinate during pregnancy who were identified prior to knowledge of the outcome (Mitchell, 1992). This series consists of cases reported to the manufacturer; no information is provided regarding the time, duration, or dose of treatment.

A woman who conceived four months after cessation of etretinate therapy had a fetus with hypoplasia of one leg (Grote et al., 1985), another woman who conceived seven months after stopping etretinate therapy had a fetus with cardiovascular and renal malformations (Verloes et al., 1990), and another woman whose etretinate therapy ended 51 weeks prior to conception gave birth to a baby with CNS and craniofacial features consistent with retinoic acid embryopathy (Lammer, 1988). Although a causal relationship between maternal etretinate therapy and the fetal anomalies in these cases cannot be established with certainty, they do raise concern that the teratogenic potential of etretinate may be manifested long after maternal therapy is stopped. Among 32 births identified prospectively in women who became pregnant within two years of stopping therapy with etretinate, there was only one infant with a congenital anomaly, and this appeared to be unrelated to etretinate (Mitchell, 1992).

Etretinate is teratogenic in experimental animals at doses similar to or just above those used in humans. Increased frequencies of CNS, craniofacial, and limb malformations as well as of fetal death have been observed among the offspring of pregnant mice, rats, rabbits, and hamsters treated respectively with <1-133, 4-50, 2, and 3-250 times the human therapeutic dose of etretinate (Hummler & Schupbach, 1981; Aikawa et al., 1982; Williams et al., 1984; Kochhar et al., 1989; Willhite et al., 1989; Agnish et al., 1990; Lofberg et al., 1990; Turton et al., 1992). Typical dose and time of exposure dependence of this teratogenic effect has been demonstrated (Aikawa et al., 1982; Williams et al., 1984; Kochhar et al., 1989; Agnish et al., 1990).

Please see agent summary on isotretinoin for information on a related agent that has been more thoroughly studied.

Key References

Agnish ND, Vane FM, Rusin G, et al.: Teratogenicity of etretinate during early pregnancy in the rat and its correlation with maternal plasma concentrations of the drug. Teratology 42:25-33, 1990. [A]

Aikawa M, Sato M, Noda A, Ukada K: Toxicity study of etretinate. 3. Reproduction segment II study in rats. Yakuri to Chiryo 10:5095-5115, 1982. [A]

DiGiovanna JJ, Zech LA, Ruddel ME, Gantt G, et al.: Etretinate: Persistent serum levels of a potent teratogen. Clin Res 32:579A, 1984. [O]

Grote W, Harms D, Janig U, Kietzmann H, et al.: Malformation of fetus conceived 4 months after termination of maternal etretinate treatment. Lancet 1:1276, 1985. [C]

Happle R, Traupe H, Bounameaux Y, Fisch T: Teratogenic effects of etretinate in humans. Dtsch Med Wochenschr 109:1476-1480, 1984. [S]

Hummler H, Schupbach ME: Studies in reproductive toxicology and and mutagenicity with Ro 10-9359. In: C.E. Orfanos et al. (eds). Retinoids. New York: Springer-Verlag, 1981, pp 49-59. [A]

Kochhar DM, Penner JD, Minutella LM: Biotransformation of etretinate and developmental toxicity of etretin and other aromatic retinoids in teratogenesis bioassays. Drug Metab Dispos 17(6):618-624, 1989. [A]

Lammer EJ: Embryopathy in infant conceived one year after termination of maternal etretinate. Lancet 2:1080-1081, 1988. [C]

Lofberg B, Reiners J, Spielmann H, Nau H: Teratogenicity of steady-state concentrations of etretinate and metabolite acitretin maintained in maternal plasma and embryo by intragastric infusion during organogenesis in the mouse: A possible model for the extended elimination phase in human therapy. Dev Pharmacol Ther 15:45-51, 1990. [A]

Mitchell AA: Oral retinoids. What should the prescriber know about their teratogenic hazards among women of child-bearing potential? Drug Safety 7(2):79-85, 1992. [R]

Rinck G, Gollnick H, Organos CE: Duration of contraception after etretinate. Lancet 1(8642):845-846, 1989. [S]

Rosa FW, Wilk AL, Kelsey FO: Teratogen update: Vitamin A congeners. Teratology 33:355-364, 1986. [E]

Turton JA, Willars GB, Haselden JN, et al.: Comparative teratogenicity of nine retinoids in the rat. Int J Exp Pathol 73:551-563, 1992. [A]

Verloes A, Dodinval P, Koulischer L, et al.: Etretinate embryotoxicity 7 months after discontinuation of treatment. [Letter] Am J Med Genet 37:437-438, 1990. [C]

Willhite CC, Wier PJ, Berry DL: Dose response and structure-activity considerations in retinoid-induced dysmorphogenesis. Crit Rev Toxicol 20(2):113-135, 1989. [R]

Williams KJ, Ferm VH, Willhite CC: Teratogenic dose-response relationships of etretinate in the golden hamster. Fundam Appl Toxicol 4:977-982, 1984. [A]

EUPROCIN

Synonyms

Isopentylhydrocupreine Dihydrochloride

Summary

Euprocin is a local anesthetic that has been used topically.

Magnitude of Teratogenic Risk

Undetermined

Quality and Quantity of Data

None

Comment

None

No epidemiological studies of congenital anomalies in children born to women exposed to euprocin during pregnancy have been reported.

No investigations of teratologic effects of euprocin in experimental animals have been published.

Key References

None available.

FACTOR IX COMPLEX

Synonyms

Konyne-HT, Profilnine Heat-Treated, Proplex SX-T, Proplex T

Summary

Factor IX complex is a preparation of partially purified Factor IX and other blood clotting factors obtained from human plasma. Factor IX complex is used in the treatment of hemophilia B (Christmas disease) and certain other clotting factor deficiencies.

Magnitude of Teratogenic Risk

Undetermined

Quality and Quantity of Data

None

Comment

A small risk cannot be excluded, but a high risk of congenital anomalies in the children of women treated with factor IX complex during pregnancy is unlikely.

No epidemiological studies of congenital anomalies among infants born to women treated with factor IX complex during pregnancy have been reported.

No animal teratology studies of factor IX complex have been published.

Key References

None available.

FAMOTIDINE

Synonyms

Famodil, Fanox, Gaster, Gastridin, Gastrion, Motiax, Pepcid, Pepdul, Tamin

Summary

Famotidine is a histamine H2-receptor antagonist used in the treatment of peptic ulcer and gastric hypersecretory states.

Magnitude of Teratogenic Risk

Undetermined

Quality and Quantity of Data

None To Poor

Comment

None

No epidemiological studies of congenital anomalies among infants born to women treated with famotidine during pregnancy have been reported.

The frequency of malformations was not increased among the offspring of rats or rabbits treated during pregnancy with famotidine in doses 38-2500 or 38-625 times that used in humans (Shibata et al., 1983; Burek et al., 1985).

Please see agent summary on cimetidine for information on a related drug that has been studied.

Key References

Burek JD, Majka JA, Bokelman DL: Famotidine: Summary of preclinical safety assessment. Digestion 32(Suppl 1):7-14, 1985. [A]

Shibata M, Kawano K, Shiobara Y: Teratological study of famotidine (YM-11170) administered orally to rats. Oyo Yakuri 26:489-497, 1983. [A]

FENOPROFEN

Synonyms

Fenopron, Fepron, Feprona, Nalfon, Nalgesic, Progesic

Summary

Fenoprofen is a non-steroidal anti-inflammatory agent with analgesic and antipyretic actions. It is used to treat pain and rheumatic disorders.

Magnitude of Teratogenic Risk

Undetermined

Quality and Quantity of Data

None To Poor

Comment

None

No epidemiological studies of congenital anomalies in the children of women who took fenoprofen during pregnancy have been reported.

In one study published only as an abstract, no teratogenic effects were noted in the offspring of rats or rabbits treated during pregnancy with fenoprofen in doses 1.5-2.5 times those used clinically (Emmerson et al., 1973).

Premature closure of the ductus arteriosus was observed among the offspring of rats treated near term with fenoprofen in doses equivalent to or slightly larger than those used in humans (Powell & Cochrane, 1978; Momma et al., 1984). Similar abnormalities of perinatal cardiovascular adaptation were reported in human neonates whose mothers took drugs that are pharmacologically similar to fenoprofen late in pregnancy [*see agent summary on indomethacin for further discussion*]. Such problems have not been reported in the infants of women who took fenoprofen near term, but clinical experience with this drug in human pregnancy is limited.

Several prostaglandin inhibitors including fenoprofen have been shown to block or delay labor in rats (Powell & Cochrane, 1978). Similar effects have been observed in humans with other drugs of this class (Zuckerman et al., 1974; Grella & Zanor, 1978), but such studies have not been reported for fenoprofen.

Key References

Emmerson JL, Gibson WR, Pierce EC, Todd GC: Preclinical toxicology of fenoprofen. Toxicol Appl Pharmacol 25:444, 1973. [A]

Grella P, Zanor P: Premature labor and indomethacin. Prostaglandins 16:1007-1017, 1978. [S]

Momma K, Hagiwara H, Konishi T: Constriction of fetal ductus arteriosus by non-steroidal anti-inflammatory drugs: Study of additional 34 drugs. Prostaglandins 28:527-536, 1984. [A]

Powell JG, Cochrane RL: The effects of the administration of fenoprofen or indomethacin to rat dams during late pregnancy, with special reference to the ductus arteriosus of the fetuses and neonates. Toxicol Appl Pharmacol 45:783-796, 1978. [A]

Zuckerman H, Reiss U, Rubinstein I: Inhibition of human premature labor by indomethacin. Obstet Gynecol 44:787-792, 1974. [S]

FENTICONAZOLE

Synonyms

REC 15/1476

Summary

Fenticonazole is an antifungal agent.

Magnitude of Teratogenic Risk

Undetermined

Quality and Quantity of Data

None

Comment

None

No epidemiological studies of congenital anomalies in infants born to women who used fenticonazole during pregnancy have been reported.

No animal teratology studies of fenticonazole have been published.

Key References

None available.

FILGRASTIM

Synonyms

G-CSF, Granulocyte Colony Stimulating Factor, Neupogen, rhG-CSF

Summary

Filgrastim is recombinant human granulocyte colony stimulating factor. It is administered parenterally in the treatment of neutropenia and non-myeloid malignancies.

Magnitude of Teratogenic Risk

Undetermined

Quality and Quantity of Data

None

Comment

None

No epidemiological studies of congenital anomalies in infants whose mothers were treated with filgrastim during pregnancy have been reported.

No animal teratology studies of filgrastim have been published.

Key References

None available.

FILIPIN

Summary

Filipin is an antifungal agent.

Magnitude of Teratogenic Risk

Undetermined

Quality and Quantity of Data

None

Comment

None

No epidemiological studies of congenital anomalies in infants born to women who used filipin during pregnancy have been reported.

No animal teratology studies of filipin have been published.

Key References

None available.

FLAVOXATE

Synonyms

Bladderon, Flavossato, Flavoxato, Relaxant, Urispas

Summary

Flavoxate is an oral antispasmodic agent that is used to treat disorders of the lower urinary tract.

Magnitude of Teratogenic Risk

Undetermined

Quality and Quantity of Data

None

Comment

None

No epidemiological studies of congenital anomalies in infants whose mothers were treated with flavoxate during pregnancy have been reported.

No animal teratology studies of flavoxate have been published.

Key References

None available.

FLECAINIDE

Synonyms

R 818, Tambocor

Summary

Flecainide is an antiarrhythmic agent that is administered orally to treat cardiac arrhythmias.

Magnitude of Teratogenic Risk

Undetermined

Quality and Quantity of Data

None To Poor

Comment

None

No epidemiological studies of congenital anomalies in infants born to women treated with flecainide during pregnancy have been reported. An infant without congenital anomalies was born to a woman treated with flecainide throughout pregnancy (Wagner et al., 1990).

An increased frequency of congenital anomalies was observed among the offspring of pregnant rats treated with 2.5 times the human therapeutic dose of flecainide (Nishimura et al., 1989); an increased rate of fetal death was seen with 7 times the human dose.

Maternal or direct fetal administration of flecainide has been used to treat fetal cardiac arrhythmias in the third trimester of pregnancy (Gembruch et al., 1988; MacPhail & Walkinshaw, 1988; Wren & Hunter, 1988; Perry et al., 1991).

Key References

Gembruch U, Hansmann M, Bald R: Direct intrauterine fetal treatment of fetal tachyarrhythmia with severe hydrops fetalis by antiarrhythmic drugs. Fetal Ther 3:210-215, 1988. [S]

MacPhail S, Walkinshaw SA: Fetal supraventricular tachycardia: Detection by routine auscultation and successful in-utero management. Case Report. Br J Obstet Gynaecol 95:1073-1076, 1988. [C]

Nishimura O, Okada B, Ohsumi I, et al.: Reproduction study of flecainide teratological study in rats with oral administration. Kiso To Rinsho 23(5):331-348, 1989. [A]

Perry JC, Ayres NA, Carpenter RJ Jr: Fetal supraventricular tachycardia treated with flecainide acetate. J Pediatr 118:303-305, 1991. [C]

Wagner X, Jouglard J, Moulin M, et al.: Co-administration of flecainide acetate and sotalol during pregnancy: Lack of teratogenic effects, passage across the placenta, and excretion in human breast milk. Am Heart J 119:700-702, 1990. [C]

Wren C, Hunter S: Maternal administration of flecainide to terminate and suppress fetal tachycardia. Br Med J 296:249, 1988. [C]

FLOXURIDINE

Synonyms

Deoxyfluorouridine, Floxiridina, Fluorodeoxyuridine, FUDR

Summary

Floxuridine is an inhibitor of DNA synthesis used to treat malignant neoplasms. It is usually administered by arterial infusion but intravenous infusion, which requires doses 50 times as great, has also been used.

Magnitude of Teratogenic Risk

Undetermined

Quality and Quantity of Data

None To Poor

Comment

Although the risk of floxuridine is undetermined, it may be substantial because it is an antineoplastic agent.

No epidemiological studies of congenital anomalies among the infants of women treated with floxuridine during pregnancy have been reported.

Increased frequencies of skeletal, central nervous system, and other anomalies occurred among the offspring of rats treated with floxuridine during pregnancy in doses 2000-12,500 times that used for arterial infusion in humans (Murphy, 1960; Ritter, 1984). The relevance of these observations to the therapeutic use of floxuridine is unknown.

Key References

Murphy ML: Teratogenic effects of tumour-inhibiting chemicals in the foetal rat. In: Wolstenholme GEW, O'Connor CM (eds). Congenital Malformations (Ciba Foundation Symposium). Boston: Little, Brown and Co., 1960, pp 78-114. [A]

Ritter EJ: Potentiation of teratogenesis. Fundam Appl Toxicol 4(3):352-359, 1984. [A]

FLUCYTOSINE

Synonyms

Alcobon, Ancobon, Ancotil, Flucitosina

Summary

Flucytosine is an antifungal agent used to treat severe systemic mycotic infections.

Magnitude of Teratogenic Risk

Undetermined

Quality and Quantity of Data

None To Poor

Comment

None

No epidemiological studies of congenital anomalies in infants born to women treated with flucytosine during pregnancy have been reported.

Increased frequencies of fetal death and of facial clefts and skeletal malformations occurred in the offspring of rats treated during pregnancy with flucytosine in doses 4.5-27 times that used in humans (Chaube & Murphy, 1969). Typical effects of dose and time of gestation were demonstrated in these experiments; no teratogenic effect was observed after maternal treatment with 3.5 times the human therapeutic dose of flucytosine. The relevance of these observations to the clinical use of flucytosine in human pregnancy is unknown.

Key References

Chaube S, Murphy ML: The teratogenic effects of 5-fluorocytosine in the rat. Canc Res 29:554-557, 1969. [A]

FLUNISOLIDE

Synonyms

AeroBid, Nasalide

Summary

Flunisolide is a synthetic glucocorticoid used by inhalation to treat asthma and, at a much lower dose, by nasal instillation to treat allergic rhinitis.

Magnitude of Teratogenic Risk

Undetermined

Quality and Quantity of Data

Poor

Comment

A small risk cannot be excluded, but a high risk of congenital anomalies in the children of women treated with flunisolide during pregnancy is unlikely.

No epidemiological studies of congenital anomalies among the infants of women treated with flunisolide during pregnancy have been reported.

Increased frequencies of cleft palate and other anomalies have been observed among the offspring of mice and rats treated during pregnancy with flunisolide in doses 5 and 2.5 times those used in the therapy of asthma in humans (Itabashi et al., 1982; Tamagawa et al., 1982). Teratogenic effects were not seen with lower doses in either strain. The relevance of these findings to the clinical use of flunisolide in human pregnancy is unknown.

Please see agent summary on beclomethasone for information on a related drug that has been more thoroughly studied.

Key References

Itabashi M, Inoue T, Yokota M, Takehara K, et al.: Reproduction studies on flunisolide in rats. 2. Oral administration during the period of organogenesis. Oyo Yakuri (Pharmacometrics) 24(5):643-659, 1982. [A]

Tamagawa M, Hatori M, Ooi A, Nishioeda R, et al.: Comparative teratological study of flunisolide in mice. Oyo Yakuri (Pharmacometrics) 24(6):741-750, 1982. [A]

FLUOCINONIDE

Synonyms

FAPG Cream, Lidemol, Lidex, Lyderm, Metosyn

Summary

Fluocinonide is a synthetic glucocorticoid used topically in treatment of dermatologic disorders.

Magnitude of Teratogenic Risk

Undetermined

Quality and Quantity of Data

None

Comment

None

No epidemiological studies of malformations in infants born to women who used fluocinonide during pregnancy have been reported.

No animal teratology studies of fluocinonide have been published.

Key References

None available.

FLUORIDE

Synonyms

Fluorigard, Fluorineed, Fluoritab, Flura Drops, Karidium, Pediaflor, Phos-Flur, Thera Flur

Summary

Fluoride salts are given orally, added to public water supplies, and included in toothpastes to prevent dental decay. They are also used in a 25-50 fold greater dose to treat osteoporosis.

Magnitude of Teratogenic Risk

When Used For Dental Prophylaxis: None To Minimal

When Used To Treat Osteoporosis: Undetermined

Quality and Quantity of Data

When Used For Dental Prophylaxis: Poor To Fair

When Used To Treat Osteoporosis: None To Poor

Comment

None

The frequency of congenital anomalies was not significantly increased among the children of 122 women who took fluoride during the first four lunar months of pregnancy or among the children of 1422 women who took fluoride anytime during pregnancy in the Collaborative Perinatal Project (Heinonen et al., 1977). The dose of fluoride taken by these women is not stated in the report.

The suggestion that an association may exist between fluoridation of drinking water and the frequency of Down's syndrome in a community (Rapaport, 1956) appears to be incorrect (Needleman et al., 1974; Erickson et al., 1980).

Administration of supplemental fluoride to women during the second and third trimesters of pregnancy has been advocated to reduce the frequency of dental caries in their children, but the value of such treatment is controversial (Driscoll, 1981; Glenn et al., 1982, 1984; Musselman, 1983; Speirs et al., 1983; Glenn & Glenn, 1987).

Increased frequencies of fetal resorption, fetal growth retardation, and skeletal alterations have been observed among the offspring of pregnant mice given water fluoridated at 20-30 times the level recommended for humans (Fleming & Greenfield, 1954; Larez et al., 1980). Increased frequencies of fetal death have been reported after injection of pregnant rats with 1-20 times the dose of fluorine used in humans to treat osteoporosis (Devoto et al., 1972). Retarded ossification but no external malformations were noted among the offspring of pregnant rats given fluoride during pregnancy in 2-10 times the dose used to treat osteoporosis in women (Goto, 1968; Horvath, 1989). No teratogenic effect was observed among the offspring of pregnant rats or dogs fed diets containing 460 ppm of fluorine (Marks et al., 1984; Shellenberg et al., 1990). The clinical significance of these observations is unknown.

Key References

Devoto FCH, Perrotto BM, Bordoni NE, Arias NH: Effect of sodium fluoride on the placenta in the rat. Arch Biol 17:371-374, 1972. [A]

Driscoll WS: A review of clinical research on the use of prenatal fluoride administration for prevention of dental caries. J Dent Child 48:109-117, 1981. [R]

Erickson JD: Down syndrome, water fluoridation, and maternal age. Teratology 21:177-180, 1980. [E]

Fleming HS, Greenfield VS: Changes in the teeth and jaws of neonatal Webster mice after administration of NaF and CaF2 to the female parent during gestation. J Dent Res 33:780-788, 1954. [A]

Glenn FB, Glenn WD III: Optimum dosage for prenatal fluoride supplementation (PNF): Part IX. J Dent Child 54:445-450, 1987. [R]

Glenn FB, Glenn WD III, Duncan RC: Fluoride tablet supplementation during pregnancy for caries immunity: A study of the offspring produced. Am J Obstet Gynecol 143:560-564, 1982. [E]

Glenn FB, Glenn WD, Duncan RC: Prenatal fluoride tablet supplementation and improved molar occlusal morphology: Part V. J Dent Child 51:19-23, 1984. [E]

Goto K: Effects of sodium fluoride on the fetuses and sucklings in Wistar strain albino rats. Congen Anom 8:46, 1968. [A]

Heinonen OP, Slone D, Shapiro S: Birth Defects and Drugs in Pregnancy. Littleton, Mass.: John Wright-PSG, 1977, pp 401-404, 444, 479, 497. [E]

Horvath C: Does fluoride interfere with normal gestation of the rat? Teratology 40:285, 1989. [A]

Larez A, Ochoa Y, Aponte N, Montenegro M, et al.: Sodium fluoride, fetotoxicity and oral experimental teratogeny in rats. Toxicol Aspects (Int Congr Eur Assoc Poison Control Cent 9th 1980) 0:528-540, 1980. [A]

Marks TA, Schellenberg D, Metzler CM, et al.: Effect of dog food containing 460 ppm fluoride on rat reproduction. J Toxicol Environ Health 14(5-6):707-714, 1984. [A]

Musselman RJ: Prenatal fluoride supplements to inhibit dental caries. Am J Obstet Gynecol 147:225, 1983. [O]

Needleman HL, Pueschel SM, Rothman KJ: Fluoridation and the occurrence of Down's syndrome. N Engl J Med 291:821-823, 1974. [E]

Rapaport I: Contribution a l'etude du mongolism: Role pathogenique du fluor. Bull Acad Natl Med (Paris) 140:529-531, 1956. [E]

Shellenberg D, Marks TA, Metzler CM, et al.: Lack of effect of fluoride on reproductive performance and development in Shetland sheepdogs. Vet Hum Toxicol 32(4):309-314, 1990. [A]

Speirs RL: The value of prenatally administered fluoride. Dent Update 10:43-46, 49-51, 1983. [R]

FLUOROURACIL

Synonyms

Adrucil, Efudex, Efudix, Fluoroplex, Fluracil, Fluril, 5-FU

Summary

Fluorouracil, a pyrimidine analog, is an inhibitor of DNA and RNA synthesis that is used as an antineoplastic agent. It is administered intravenously or topically. Variable absorption of topical preparations occurs.

Magnitude of Teratogenic Risk

Undetermined

Quality and Quantity of Data

Poor To Fair

Comment

The risk related to this agent, although undetermined, may be substantial because it interferes with dna synthesis.

No epidemiological studies of congenital anomalies among infants born to women treated with fluorouracil during pregnancy have been reported. Multiple congenital anomlies were observed in the fetus of a woman treated with fluorouracil during pregnancy (Stephens et al., 1980), but a causal relationship seems unlikely in this case because treatment did not occur until organogenesis was complete. Several anecdotal cases have been reported in which infants without malformations have been born to women treated with intravenous or vaginal fluorouracil during pregnancy (Stadler & Knowles, 1971; Geggie, 1982; Turchi & Villasis, 1988; Kopelman & Miyazawa, 1990; Odom et al., 1990). Only two cases involved exposure during the period of organogenesis; one was with with intravenous administration and the other a vaginal preparation (Turchi & Villasis, 1988; Kopelman & Miyazawa, 1990). In another case in which large doses of fluorouracil were administered intravenously late in pregnancy, the infant manifested apparent drug toxicity briefly in the newborn period (Stadler & Knowles, 1971).

Increased frequencies of skeletal and other malformations have been observed among the offspring of pregnant mice, rats, and hamsters treated with fluorouracil in doses respectively 1-4, 1.5-3, and 2-8 times those used therapeutically in humans (Dagg, 1960; Chaube & Murphy, 1968; Wilson et al., 1969; Shah & MacKay, 1977; Naya et al., 1990). The teratogenic effect was shown to exhibit typical response to dose and time of gestation (Dagg, 1960; Wilson et al., 1969). Limited teratological studies of fluorouracil in rhesus monkeys have been inconclusive (Wilson, 1971a, b).

Key References

Chaube S, Murphy ML: The teratogenic effects of the recent drugs active in cancer chemotherapy. Adv Teratol 30:181-237, 1968. [A]

Dagg CP: Sensitive stages for the production of developmental abnormalities in mice with 5-Fluorouracil. Am J Anat 106:89-96, 1960. [A]

Geggie PHS: Breast cancer in pregnant women. Can Med Ass J 127:358-359, 1982. [C]

Kopelman JN, Miyazawa K: Inadvertent 5-fluorouracil treatment in early pregnancy: A report of three cases. Reprod Toxicol 4:233-235, 1990. [C]

Naya M, Noguchi M, Mataki Y, et al.: Effects of L-2-oxothiazolidine-4-carboxylate, a cysteine pro-drug, on teratogenicity of 5-fluorouracil in mice. Hiroshima J Med Sci 39(3):79-82, 1990. [A]

Odom LD, Plouffe Jr L, Butler WJ: 5-fluorouracil exposure during the period of conception: Report on two cases. Am J Obstet Gynecol 163(1):76-77, 1990. [C]

Shah RM, MacKay RA: Comparative teratogenicity of two anticancer drugs in hamster. Anat Rec 187:710, 1977. [A]

Stadler HE, Knowles J: Fluorouracil in pregnancy: Effect on the neonate. JAMA 217(2):214-215, 1971. [C]

Stephens JD, Golbus MS, Miller TR, Wilber RR, et al.: Multiple congenital anomalies in a fetus exposed to 5-fluorouracil during the first trimester. Am J Obstet Gynecol 137(6):747-749, 1980. [C]

Turchi JJ, Villasis C: Anthracyclines in the treatment of malignancy in pregnancy. Cancer 61:435-440, 1988. [C] & [R]

Wilson JG: Abnormalities of intrauterine development in non-human primates. Acta Endocrinol 166 (Suppl):261-292, 1971b. [A]

Wilson JG: Use of rhesus monkeys in teratological studies. Fed Proc 30(1):104-109, 1971a. [A]

Wilson JG, Jordan RL, Schumacher H: Potentiation of the teratogenic effects of 5-Fluorouracil by natural pyrimidines. I. Biological aspects. Teratology 2:91-98, 1969. [A]

FLUOXETINE

Synonyms

Prozac

Summary

Fluoxetine is an oral antidepressant which selectively inhibits the re-uptake of serotonin.

Magnitude of Teratogenic Risk

None

Quality and Quantity of Data

Poor To Fair

Comment

None

The frequency of congenital anomalies was no greater than expected among the infants of 98 women who took fluoxetine during the first trimester of pregnancy in a cohort study performed at four teratogen information services (Pastuszak et al., 1993). The frequency of congenital anomalies did not appear unusual among the infants born of 44 pregnancies that occurred in women who were taking part in clinical trials of fluoxetine or among the children of 219 women voluntarily reported to the manufacturer because they took this medication during pregnancy (Goldstein, 1990; Shader, 1992).

The frequency of malformations was not increased among the offspring of rats or rabbits treated during pregnancy with fluoxetine in doses respectively 1-8 or 2-9 times those used in humans (Byrd et al., 1989; Hoyt et al., 1989).

Key References

Byrd RA, Brophy GT, Markham JK: Developmental toxicology studies of fluoxetine hydrochloride (I) administered orally to rats and rabbits. Teratology 39(5):444, 1989. [A]

Goldstein DJ: Outcome of fluoxetine-exposed pregnancies. Am J Hum Genetics 47:A136, 1990. [S]

Hoyt JA, Byrd RA, Brophy GT, et al.: A reproduction study of fluoxetine hydrochloride (I) administered in the diet to rats. Teratology 39(5):459, 1989. [A]

Pastuszak A, Schick-Boschetto B, Zuber C, Feldkamp M, et al.: Pregnancy outcome following first trimester exposure to fluoxetine (Prozac). JAMA 269:2246-2248, 1993. [E]

Shader RI: Does continuous use of fluoxetine during the first trimester of pregnancy present a high risk for malformation or abnormal development to the exposed fetus? J Clin Psychopharmacol 12:441, 1992. [R]

FLUOXYMESTERONE

Synonyms

Androfluorene, Fluotestin, Halotestin, Ora-Testryl, Oralsterone, Oratestin, Testoral, Ultandren, Ultandrene

Summary

Fluoxymesterone is an androgenic hormone that is administered orally.

Magnitude of Teratogenic Risk

Undetermined

Quality and Quantity of Data

Poor

Comment

Because of the pharmacological action of this agent, maternal use of fluoxymesterone during pregnancy would be expected to produce virilization of the external genitalia of a female fetus.

No epidemiological studies of congenital anomalies among infants born to women who took fluoxymesterone during pregnancy have been reported.

Virilization of the external genitalia was observed among female offspring of rats treated with about twice the human dose of fluoxymesterone in one study (Jost, 1960); similar treatment caused pregnancy loss in another investigation (Tache & Tache, 1974).

Key References

Jost A: The action of various sex steriods and related compounds on the growth and sexual differentiation of the fetus. Acta Endocrinol 34 (Suppl 50):119-123, 1960. [A]

Tache Y, Tache J: Interruption of pregnancy in rats by various fluoroandrostane derivatives. J Reprod Fert 39:319-327, 1974. [A]

FLURANDRENOLIDE

Synonyms

Cordran, Drenison

Summary

Flurandrenolide is a synthetic glucocorticoid that is used as a topical anti-inflammatory agent.

Magnitude of Teratogenic Risk

Undetermined

Quality and Quantity of Data

Poor

Comment

A small risk cannot be excluded, but a high risk of congenital anomalies in the children of women treated with flurandrenolide during pregnancy is unlikely.

No epidemiological studies of congenital anomalies in infants whose mothers used flurandrenolide during pregnancy have been reported.

No animal teratology studies of flurandrenolide have been published.

Please see agent summary on hydrocortisone for information on a related agent that has been studied.

Key References

None available.

FLURAZEPAM

Synonyms

Benozil, Dalmane, Somlan, Valdorm

Summary

Flurazepam is a benzodiazepine derivative with hypnotic action.

Magnitude of Teratogenic Risk

None To Minimal

Quality and Quantity of Data

Poor

Comment

None

No epidemiological studies of congenital anomalies among infants born to women treated with flurazepam during pregnancy have been reported.

Rats and mice orally administered flurazepam during embryogenesis at levels 8, 25, and 50 times the usual human dose and rabbits orally administered flurazepam in doses 8, 25, and 75 times the usual human dose during embryogenesis did not have an increased frequency of malformations (Irikura et al., 1977; Noda et al., 1977).

Please see the agent summary on diazepam for information on a related drug which has been more thoroughly studied.

Key References

Irikura T, Hosomi J, Suzuki H, et al.: Teratological study on flurazepam free base in mice and rats. Oyo Yakuri 14:659-667, 1977. [A]

Noda K, Hirabayashi M, Irikura T, et al.: Teratological study on flurazepam free base in rabbits. Oyo Yakuri 14:801-804, 1977. [A]

FLUROXENE

Synonyms

2,2,2-Trifluoroethyl Vinyl Ether

Summary

Fluroxene is a general anesthetic administered by inhalation.

Magnitude of Teratogenic Risk

Undetermined

Quality and Quantity of Data

Poor

Comment

None

No epidemiological studies of congenital anomalies in children born to women exposed to fluroxene during pregnancy have been reported.

No investigations of teratologic effects of fluroxene in experimental animals have been published.

Key References

None available.

FOMOCAINE

Synonyms

Erbocain

Summary

Fomocaine is a local anesthetic that has been used topically.

Magnitude of Teratogenic Risk

Undetermined

Quality and Quantity of Data

None

Comment

None

No epidemiological studies of congenital anomalies in children born to women exposed to fomocaine during pregnancy have been reported.

No investigations of teratologic effects of fomocaine in experimental animals have been published.

Please see agent summary on procaine for information on a related agent that has been studied.

Key References

None available.

FORMALDEHYDE

Synonyms

Formalin, Formol, Ivalon, Karsan

Summary

Formaldehyde is a simple hydrocarbon that is used as a disinfectant, a tissue preservative, and in cosmetics. Formaldehyde is a common component of resins used in the paint, clothing, paper, plastics, and construction industries. Formaldehyde is absorbed through the lungs and gastrointestinal tract. The maximum permissible level for occupational exposure to formaldehyde in air is 1 ppm as an 8-hour time-weighted average (Hathaway, 1991). Formalin is an aqueous solution of formaldehyde.

Magnitude of Teratogenic Risk

None To Minimal

Quality and Quantity of Data

Poor To Fair

Comment

None

A weak association with occupational exposure to formaldehyde during the first trimester of pregnancy was observed in a case-control study of 188 cosmetologists who had had miscarriages (OR= 1.8, 95% CI 1.0-2.4) (John, 1991). In contrast, no significant association was observed with maternal occupational exposure to formaldehyde during the first three months of pregnancy in a case-control study of 164 nurses who had had spontaneous abortions and 34 nurses whose infants had congenital anomalies (Hemminki et al., 1985).

The frequency of malformations was no greater than expected among the offspring of mice, rats, hamsters, or dogs treated during pregnancy with formaldehyde by various routes in doses far above the human permissible exposure level (Marks et al., 1980; Hurni & Ohder, 1973; Overman, 1985; Feinman, 1988; Saillenfait et al., 1989; Martin, 1990). Evidence of maternal toxicity was observed in many of these studies.

Key References

Feinman SE: Formaldehyde genotoxicity and teratogenicity. In: Feinman SE (ed): Formaldehyde Sensitivity and Toxicity. Boca Raton: CRC Press, 1988, pp 167-178. [R]

Hathaway GJ, Proctor NH, Hughes JP, Fischman ML (eds): Proctor and Hughes' Chemical Hazards of the Workplace, 3rd ed. New York: Van Nostrand Reinhold, 1991, p 305. [R]

Hemminki K, Kyyronen P, Lindbohm M-L: Spontaneous abortions and malformations in the offspring of nurses exposed to anaesthetic gases, cytostatic drugs, and other potential hazards in hospitals, based on registered information of outcome. J Epidemiol Community Health 39:141-147, 1985. [E]

Hurni H, Ohder H: Reproduction study with formaldehyde and hexamethylenetetramine in beagle dogs. FD Cosmet Toxicol 11:459-462, 1973. [A]

John EM: Spontaneous abortions among cosmetologists. NTIS (National Technical Information Service) Report/PB91-222703, 1991. [E]

Marks TA, Worthy WC, Staples RE: Influence of formaldehyde and SonacideR (potentiated acid glutaraldehyde) on embryo and fetal development in mice. Teratology 22:51-58, 1980. [A]

Martin WJ: A teratology study of inhaled formaldehyde in the rat. Reprod Toxicol 4:237-239, 1990. [A]

Overman DO: Absence of embryotoxic effects of formaldehyde after percutaneous exposure in hamsters. Toxicol Lett 24:107-110, 1985. [A]

Saillenfait AM, Bonnet P, De Ceaurriz J: The effects of maternally inhaled formaldehyde on embryonal and foetal development in rats. Food Chem Toxicol 27(8):545-548, 1989. [A]

FRAMYCETIN

Synonyms

Framygen, Isofra, Isoframicol, Perframyl, Sofra, Soframycin, Tuttomycin

Summary

Framycetin is an aminoglycoside antibiotic that is administered topically in the treatment of skin, eye, and ear infections and orally in enteric infections. It is poorly absorbed after these exposures.

Magnitude of Teratogenic Risk

Undetermined

Quality and Quantity of Data

None

Comment

A small risk cannot be excluded, but a high risk of congenital anomalies in the children of women treated with framycetin during pregnancy is unlikely.

No epidemiological studies of congenital anomalies in infants whose mothers were

261

treated with framycetin during pregnancy have been reported.

No animal teratology studies of framycetin have been published.

Please see agent summary on neomycin for information on a related agent that has been studied.

Key References

None available.

FUNGIMYCIN

Summary

Fungimycin is an antifungal agent.

Magnitude of Teratogenic Risk

Undetermined

Quality and Quantity of Data

None

Comment

None

No epidemiological studies of congenital anomalies in infants born to women who used fungimycin during pregnancy have been reported.

No animal teratology studies of fungimycin have been published.

Key References

None available.

FURAZOLIDONE

Synonyms

Dialidene, Enterar, Furaxone, Giardil, Medaron, Nifurazolidone

Summary

Furazolidone is an antimicrobial nitrofuran. It is given orally in the treatment of diarrhea and used locally to treat vaginal infections. Systemic absorption is poor.

Magnitude of Teratogenic Risk

None To Minimal

Quality and Quantity of Data

Poor To Fair

Comment

None

The frequency of congenital anomalies was no greater than expected among the children of 132 women treated with oral furazolidone during the first four lunar months of pregnancy in the Collaborative Perinatal Project (Heinonen et al., 1977).

Increased frequencies of fetal death were observed among pregnant mice treated with 90-250 times the human dose of furazolidone during pregnancy, but maternal toxicity was also frequent at the higher doses (Jackson and Robson, 1957). No congenital anomalies were observed among the offspring in this study, but too few fetuses were studied to draw meaningful conclusions.

Key References

Heinonen OP, Slone D, Shapiro S: Birth Defects and Drugs in Pregnancy. Littleton, Mass.: John Wright-PSG, 1977, pp 299, 302. [E]

Jackson D, Robson JM: The action of furazolidone on pregnancy. J Endocrin 15:355-359, 1957. [A]

FUROSEMIDE

Synonyms

Frusemide, Lasix, Neo-Renal, Novosemide, SK-Furosemide, Uritol

Summary

Furosemide is a diuretic used in the treatment of hypertension.

Magnitude of Teratogenic Risk

Undetermined

Quality and Quantity of Data

Poor

Comment

1) A small risk cannot be excluded, but there is no indication that the risk of congenital anomalies in the children of women treated with furosemide is likely to be great.

2) Possible effects on perinatal electrolyte balance are discussed below.

No adequate epidemiological studies of congenital anomalies among children of women treated with furosemide during pregnancy have been reported.

An increased frequency of fetal loss has been observed in rabbits treated early in pregnancy with furosemide at a dose about 10 times the maximum used in humans (Godde & Grote, 1975). The frequency of malformations was no greater than expected among the offspring of mice treated with 17-100 times or of rats treated with 25-50 times the maximum human dose of furosemide during pregnancy (Robertson et al., 1981; Hayasaka et al., 1984). Skeletal anomalies occurred at 40-100 times or at 4-50 times the human therapeutic dose in mice and rats, respectively (Robertson et al., 1981; Hayasaka et al., 1984; Sterz et al., 1985). Decreased renal maturation has been reported among the offspring of rats treated with 6 times

the human dose of furosemide during pregnancy (Mallie et al., 1985). The relevance, if any, of these observations to the clinical use of furosemide in pregnant women is unclear.

Pharmacologic effects of furosemide have been demonstrated in the fetus after maternal administration of the drug (Wladimiroff, 1975), and some workers have suggested that this effect may be useful in assessing fetal urinary obstruction (Barrett et al., 1983). Furosemide is cleared from the circulation considerably more slowly in the neonate, especially if born prematurely, than in adults. *Thus, babies born to mothers who have recently taken furosemide may be at risk of developing electrolyte disturbances as a result of the pharmacological actions of the drug* (Vert et al., 1982). Furosemide can displace bilirubin from albumin and may pose a risk to prenatally exposed newborns who become jaundiced (Turmen et al., 1982).

Key References

Barrett RJ, Rayburn WF, Barr M: Furosemide (Lasix) challenge test in assessing bilateral fetal hydronephrosis. Am J Obstet Gynecol 147:846-847, 1983. [C]

Godde VE, Grote W: Animal experimental investigations on the dysionic genesis of intrauterine malformations. Arzneimittelforsch 25:809-813, 1975. [A]

Hayasaka I, Uchiyama K, Murakami K, et al.: Teratogenicity of azosemide, a loop diuretic, in rats, mice and rabbits. Cong Anom 24:111-121, 1984. [A]

Mallie JP, Gerard A, Gerard H: Does the in-utero exposure to furosemide delay the renal maturation? Pediatr Pharmacol 5:131-138, 1985. [A]

Robertson RT, Minsker DH, Bokelman DL, Durano G, et al.: Potassium loss as a causative factor for skeletal malformations in rats produced by indacrinone: A new investigational loop diuretic. Toxicol Appl Pharmacol 60:142-150, 1981. [A]

Sterz H, Sponer G, Neubert P, Hebold G: A postulated mechanism of beta-sympathomimetic induction of rib and limb anomalies in rat fetuses. Teratology 31:401-412, 1985. [A]

Turmen T, Thom P, Louridas AT, LeMorvan P, et al.: Protein binding and bilirubin displacing properties of bumetanide and furosemide. J Clin Pharmacol 22:551-556, 1982. [O]

Vert P, Broquaire M, Legagneur M, Morselli PL: Pharmacokinetics of furosemide in neonates. Eur J Clin Pharmacol 22:39-45, 1982. [S]

Wladimiroff JW: Effect of furosemide on fetal urine production. Br J Obstet Gynaecol 82:221-224, 1975. [S]

GASOLINE

Synonyms

Benzin, Petrol, Petroleum Benzin, Petroleum Ether, Petroleum Spirit, Solvent Hexane, Wundbenzin

Summary

Gasoline is a variable mixture of volatile hydrocarbons including paraffins, olefins, cycloparaffins, and aromatic compounds. Tetraethyl lead, methanol, and other agents may be added during manufacture. Gasoline is used as a fuel and solvent. Ingestion of gasoline causes pneumonitis, shock, cardiac arrhythmias, convulsions, coma, and death. Gasoline is sometimes "sniffed" by inhalent abusers. The Threshold Limit Value for occupational exposure to gasoline vapor as an 8-hour time-weighted average is 300 ppm (900 mg/cu m) (Anonymous, 1989).

Magnitude of Teratogenic Risk

Undetermined

Quality and Quantity of Data

None To Poor

Comment

None

No epidemiological studies of infants born to mothers exposed to large amounts of gasoline during pregnancy have been reported. Two children with profound mental retardation, neurological dysfunction, and minor dysmorphic features whose mothers had abused gasoline to "get high" during pregnancy have been reported (Hunter et al., 1979). No causal inference can be made on the basis of this anecdotal observation, but the resemblance of the abnormalities in these children to those reported in children born to women who abused toluene during pregnancy suggests a causal relationship (Hersh et al., 1985; Hersh, 1989).

No teratogenic effect was observed among the offspring of rats exposed to 400-1600 ppm of gasoline for six hours daily during pregnancy (Schreiner, 1983; Anonymous, 1989).

Key References

Anonymous: Gasoline. J Appl Toxicol 9(3):203-210, 1989. [O]

Hersh JH: Toluene embryopathy: Two new cases. J Med Genet 26(5):333-337, 1989. [C]

Hersh JH, Podruch PE, Rogers G, Weisskopf B: Toluene embryopathy. J Pediatr 106:922-927, 1985. [C]

Hunter AGW, Thompson D, Evans JA: Is there a fetal gasoline syndrome? Teratology 20:75-79, 1979. [C]

Schreiner CA: Petroleum and petroleum products: A brief review of studies to evaluate reproductive effects. Adv Mod Environ Toxicol 3:29-45, 1983. [R]

GEMEPROST

Synonyms

Cervegem, ONO 802, Preglandin

Summary

Gemeprost is a synthetic prostaglandin analogue that is used in vaginal suppositories to soften and dilate the uterine cervix prior to pregnancy termination.

Magnitude of Teratogenic Risk

Undetermined

Quality and Quantity of Data

None To Poor

Comment

Gemeprost is used to induce abortion, and therefore pregnancies are unlikely to continue after exposure.

No epidemiological studies of congenital anomalies among infants born to women treated with gemeprost during pregnancy have been reported.

No teratogenic effect was observed among the offspring of pregnant rats treated intravaginally with gemeprost in doses 1-10 times those used in humans (Petrere et al., 1984a). Maternal and embryonic death often occurred among pregnant rabbits treated intravaginally with <1-2.5 times the human therapeutic dose of gemeprost, but the frequency of malformations among surviving fetuses was not increased (Petrere et al., 1984b).

Key References

Petrere JA, Humphrey RR, Sakowski R, et al.: Teratology study with the synthetic prostaglandin ONO-802 given intravaginally to rabbits. Teratogenesis Carcinog Mutagen 4:225-231, 1984b. [A]

Petrere JA, Humphrey RR, Sakowski R, et al.: Two-phase teratology study with the synthetic prostaglandin ONO-802 given intravaginally to rats. Teratogenesis Carcinog Mutagen 4:233-243, 1984a. [A]

GEMFIBROZIL

Synonyms

CL-719, Lopid

Summary

Gemfibrozil is administered orally to treat hyperlipidemia.

Magnitude of Teratogenic Risk

Undetermined

Quality and Quantity of Data

None To Poor

Comment

None

No epidemiological studies of congenital anomalies in infants whose mothers were treated with gemfibrozil during pregnancy have been reported.

No teratogenic effect was observed among the offspring of rats or rabbits given 4-12 or 2.5-8 times the usual human dose of gemfibrozil during pregnancy (Fitzgerald et al., 1987).

Key References

Fitzgerald JE, Petrere JA, de la Iglesia FA: Experimental studies on reproduction with the lipid-regulating agent gemfibrozil. Fundam Appl Toxicol 8:454-464, 1987. [A]

GENTAMICIN

Synonyms

Cidomycin, Garamycin, Gentacidin

Summary

Gentamicin is an aminoglycoside antibiotic used topically and parenterally to treat infections.

Undetermined

Quality and Quantity of Data

Poor

Comment

1) A small risk cannot be excluded, but there is no indication that the risk of malformations in children of women treated with gentamicin during pregnancy is likely to be great.

2) Because it is an aminoglycoside, maternal gentamicin treatment during pregnancy may be associated with an increased risk for fetal auditory nerve or renal damage. This has not been demonstrated to date in humans, however.

No epidemiological studies of congenital anomalies among infants born to women treated with gentamicin during pregnancy have been reported.

Increased frequencies of fetal death were observed among the offspring of pregnant mice treated with 1-12 times the human dose of gentamicin during pregnancy (Nishio et al., 1987). A slightly increased rate of congenital anomalies was seen at the lower but not the higher dose. Typical aminoglycoside nephrotoxicity was observed among the offspring of rats treated with 10-25 times the maximum human dose of gentamicin during pregnancy (Mallie et al., 1984; Gilbert et al., 1987, 1991; Chahoud et al., 1988; Gossrau et al., 1990; Smaoui et al., 1991). Maternal nephrotoxicity regularly occurred under these conditions. Hearing loss was demonstrated among the offspring of pregnant rats fed a magnesium-deficient diet and treated with 12.5-37.5 times the maximum human dose of gentamicin; this effect was not seen in animals treated similarly but fed a normal diet (Gunther et al., 1989). Hearing loss also occurred in the mothers in these experiments. The relevance of these findings to the clinical use of gentamicin in human pregnancy is unknown.

Please see agent summary on streptomycin for information on a related agent that has been more thoroughly studied.

Key References

Chahoud I, Stahlmann R, Merker H-J, Neubert D: Hypertension and nephrotoxic lesions in rats 1 year after prenatal exposure to gentamicin. Arch Toxicol 62:274-284, 1988. [A]

Gilbert T, Lelievre-Pegorier M, Malienou R, Meulemans A, et al.: Effects of prenatal and postnatal exposure to gentamicin on renal differentiation in the rat. Toxicology 43:301-313, 1987. [A]

Gilbert T, Lelievre-Pegorier M, Merlet-Benichou C: Long-term effects of mild oligonephronia induced in utero by gentamicin in the rat. Pediatr Res 30(5):450-456, 1991. [A]

Gossrau R, Graf R, Chahoud J, et al.: Enzyme histochemical and histological changes in the adult rat kidney after prenatal gentamicin exposure. Z Mikrosk Anat Forsch 104(3):385-394, 1990. [A]

Gunther T, Rebentisch E, Ising H, Vormann J: Enhanced ototoxicity of gentamicin in maternal and fetal rats due to magnesium deficiency. Magnesium-Bull 11:19-21, 1989. [A]

Mallie JP, Gerard H, Gerard A: Gentamicin administration to pregnant rats: Effect on fetal renal development in utero. Dev Pharmacol Ther 7 (Suppl 1): 89-92, 1984. [A]

Nishio A, Ryo S, Miyao N: Effects of gentamicin, exotoxin and their combination on pregnant mice. The Bulletin of the Faculty of Agriculture, Kagoshima University 37:129-136, 1987. [A]

Smaoui H, Mallie J-P, Cheignon M, et al.: Glomerular alterations in rat neonates after transplacental exposure to gentamicin. Nephron 59:626-631, 1991. [A]

GENTIAN VIOLET

Synonyms

Basic Violet 3, Crystal Violet, Methylrosaniline Chloride, Methylviolett

Summary

Gentian violet is a basic dye used topically in the treatment of candidal and other infections.

Magnitude of Teratogenic Risk

None To Minimal

Quality and Quantity of Data

Poor To Fair

Comment

None

The frequency of congenital anomalies was not significantly increased among the children of 40 women treated topically with gentian violet in the Collaborative Perinatal Project (Heinonen et al., 1977).

No teratogenic effect was observed among the offspring of pregnant rats given 2.5-5.0 mg/kg/d of gentian violet by gavage (Wolkowski-Tyl et al., 1983a; Kimmel et al., 1986). Increased frequencies of renal and skeletal anomalies were observed among the offspring of rats treated with 10 mg/kg/d of gentian violet, but such doses produced substantial maternal toxicity. The frequency of congenital anomalies was not increased among the offspring of pregnant rabbits treated by gavage with gentian violet in maternally toxic doses (0.5-2.0 mg/kg/d) (Wolkowski-Tyl et al., 1983b; Kimmel et al., 1986). The doses used in these experiments are quite large; gentian violet tampons used by women contain 5 mg of the dye.

Key References

Heinonen OP, Slone D, Shapiro S: Birth Defects and Drugs in Pregnancy. Littleton, Mass.: John Wright-PSG, 1977, pp 298, 300, 302. [E]

Kimmel CA, Price CJ, Tyl RW, Ledoux TA, et al.: Developmental toxicity of gentian violet (GV) in rats and rabbits. Teratology 33:64C-65C, 1986. [A]

Wolkowski-Tyl R, Jones-Price C, Reel JR, Ledoux TA, et al.: Teratologic evaluation of gentian violet (CAS No. 548-62-9) in CD rats. NTIS(National Technical Information Service) Report/PB83-155754, 1983a. [A]

Wolkowski-Tyl R, Jones-Price C, Reel JR, Marr MC, et al.: Teratologic evaluation of gentian violet (CAS No. 548-62-9) in New Zealand white rabbits. NTIS (National Technical Information Service) Report/PB83-182519, 1983b. [A]

GLIPIZIDE

Synonyms

Glibenese, Glucotrol, Glydiazinamide, Mindiab, Minidiab, Minodiab

Summary

Glipizide is a sulphonylurea compound used to treat non-insulin-dependent diabetes.

Magnitude of Teratogenic Risk

Undetermined

Quality and Quantity of Data

None

Comment

None

No epidemiological studies of congenital anomalies in infants whose mothers were treated with glipizide during pregnancy have been reported.

No animal teratology studies of glipizide have been published.

Please see agent summary on chlorpropamide for information on a related agent that has been studied.

Key References

None available.

GLUTETHIMIDE

Synonyms

Alfimid, Doriden, Dorimide, Elrodorm, Glimid, Noxiron, Noxyron, Rigenox, Sarodormin

Summary

Glutethimide is a piperidinedione used as an oral hypnotic agent.

Magnitude of Teratogenic Risk

None To Minimal

Quality and Quantity of Data

Poor To Fair

Comment

1) These risks are for usual therapeutic doses. The risk with toxic doses such as those that may be encountered in suicide attempts may be substantially greater.

2) Glutethimide may produce perinatal effects (see below).

The frequency of congenital anomalies was increased among the children of 67 women who took glutethimide during the first four lunar months of pregnancy in the Collaborative Perinatal Project, but this increase was due entirely to inguinal hernias, an anomaly that was subject to considerable nonuniformity in reporting (Heinonen et al., 1977). The frequency of congenital anomalies was no greater than expected among the children of 640 women who took glutethimide anytime during pregnancy in this study.

Two fetal deaths and three children with mental retardation have been reported among the offspring of 17 pregnancies in which the mothers took toxic doses of glutethimide, usually in combination with other drugs in a suicide attempt (Kurtz et al., 1966; Bello et al., 1981; Czeizel et al., 1984, 1988). The fetal deaths were attributed to the toxic ingestions, but the mental retardation may have had other familial causes. There were no major malformations observed among any of these children, but only two were exposed during the first trimester of gestation (Czeizel et al., 1984, 1988).

The frequency of malformations was no greater than expected among the offspring of mice, rats, or rabbits treated with glutethimide during pregnancy in doses 5-50, 5-50, or 10-40 times those used in humans, although fetal death, skeletal variations, and growth retardation were often seen (Tuchmann-Duplessis & Mercier-Parot, 1963a, b; McColl et al., 1967; Kalter, 1972).

Transient respiratory depression and withdrawal symptoms have been observed in infants born to women who took glutethimide late in pregnancy (Asnes & Lamb, 1969; Reveri et al., 1977).

Key References

Asnes RS, Lamb JM: Neonatal respiratory depression secondary to maternal analgesics, treated by exchange transfusion. Pediatrics 43:94-96, 1969. [C]

Bello GV, Moshirpur J, Sklar GS: Coma caused by drug abuse in pregnancy. Mt Sinai J Med 48:66-78, 1981. [C] & [R]

Czeizel A, Szentesi I, Szekeres I, Glauber A, et al.: Pregnancy outcome and health conditions of offspring of self-poisoned pregnant women. Acta Paediatr Hung 25(3):209-236, 1984. [E]

Czeizel A, Szentesi I, Szekeres I, Molnar G: A study of adverse effects on the progeny after intoxication during pregnancy. Arch Toxicol 62:1-7, 1988. [E]

Heinonen OP, Slone D, Shapiro S: Birth Defects and Drugs in Pregnancy. Littleton, Mass.: John Wright-PSG, 1977, pp 280, 335-337, 341, 344, 438, 476, 491. [E]

Kalter H: Teratogenicity, embryolethality, and mutagenicity of drugs of dependence. In: Mule SJ, Brill H (eds). Chemical and Biological Aspects of Drug Dependence. Cleveland, Ohio: CRC Press, 1972, pp 413-445, 1972. [R] & [A]

Kurtz GG, Michael UF, Morosi HJ, Vaamonde CA: Hemodialysis during pregnancy. Arch Intern Med 118:30-32, 1966. [C]

McColl JD, Robinson S, Globus M: Effect of some therapeutic agents on the rabbit fetus. Toxicol Appl Pharmacol 10:244-252, 1967. [A]

Reveri M, Pyati SP, Pildes RS: Neonatal withdrawal symptoms associated with glutethimide (doriden) addiction in the mother during pregnancy. Clin Pediatr 16:424-425, 1977. [C]

Tuchmann-Duplessis H, Mercier-Parot L: Effect of glutethimide, a hypnotic, on gestation and fetal development of the rat, mouse and rabbit. C R Hebd Acad Sci 256:1841-1843, 1963a. [A]

Tuchmann-Duplessis H, Mercier-Parot L: Effect of increasing doses of glutethimide (Doriden) on gestation and fetal development in the rabbit. C R Soc Biol 157:5-8, 1963b. [A]

GLYBURIDE

Synonyms

Diabeta, Glibenclamide, Glucolon, Gluconorm, Glycbenzcyclamide, Glycolande, Micronase, Orabetic

Summary

Glyburide is an oral sulfonylurea used to treat non-insulin-dependent diabetes mellitus.

Magnitude of Teratogenic Risk

None To Minimal

Quality and Quantity of Data

Poor To Fair

Comment

None

No adequate epidemiological studies of congenital anomalies among infants born to women who took glyburide during pregnancy have been reported.

The frequency of congenital anomalies was not increased among the offspring of rats, mice, or rabbits treated during pregnancy with glyburide in doses, respectively, <1-6600 or more, <1-6600 or more, and <1-1100 or more times that used in humans (Miyamoto et al., 1970; Baeder & Sakaguchi, 1969). In another series of experiments from the same workers, an increased frequency of ocular anomalies was observed among the offspring of rats treated with glyburide in doses 1000 times those used in humans for a smaller portion of pregnancy (Miyamoto et al., 1977), but this finding was not reproduced in a similar study from a different laboratory (Nishi & Kaito, 1976).

Key References

Baeder VC, Sakaguchi T: Teratologic studies on HB 419. Arzneimittelforsch 19 (Suppl):1419-1420, 1969. [A]

Miyamoto M, Ohtsu M, Kumai M, Takayama K, et al.: Influence of N-[4-(2-(5-Chloro-2-methoxybenzamido)-ethyl)-phenylsulfonyl]-N'-cyclohexylurea (HB-419) on embryos. Oyo Yakuri (Pharmacometrics), 4:271-283, 1970. [A]

Miyamoto M, Sakaguchi T, Midorikawa O. Teratogenic effects of sulfonylureas and insulin in rats. Cong Anom 17:31-37, 1977. [A]

Nishi R, Kaito H: Effects of hypoglycemic agents on development of the eye of rat embryos. Acta Soc Ophthalmol Jap 80:1248-1254, 1976. [A]

GLYCERIN

Synonyms

Glycerol, Glyrol, Ophthalgan, Osmoglyn, Oxydermine

Summary

Glycerin is an organic alcohol that is used as a laxative, lubricant, and emollient and to reduce intraocular and intracranial pressure.

Magnitude of Teratogenic Risk

Undetermined

No epidemiological studies of congenital anomalies in the infants of women who used glycerin during pregnancy have been reported.

No teratogenic effect was observed among the offspring of mice, rats, or rabbits given large doses of glycerin (more than 1 g/kg/d) during pregnancy (Food and Drug Research Lab, 1974).

Key References

Food and Drug Research Lab: Teratologic evaluation of FDA 71-89 (glycerol: glycerine) in mice, rats, and rabbits. NTIS (National Technical Information Service) Report/PB-234 876, 1974. [A]

GOLD SODIUM THIOMALATE

Synonyms

Myochrysine

Summary

Gold sodium thiomalate is used by injection to treat rheumatoid arthritis.

Magnitude of Teratogenic Risk

None To Minimal

Quality and Quantity of Data

Poor To Fair

Comment

None

No epidemiological studies of congenital anomalies in infants born to women treated with gold sodium thiomalate during pregnancy have been reported. The frequency of malformations did not seem to be increased among 119 children born to women who had been treated with gold compounds during early pregnancy in one clinical series (Miyamoto et al., 1974).

Increased frequencies of skeletal, central nervous system, and other malformations were observed among the offspring of rats and rabbits treated during pregnancy with gold sodium thiomalate in doses 21-630 and 7-315 times those used in humans (Szabo et al., 1978a, b). Maternal toxicity occurred throughout much of this dose range in both species. No teratogenic effect was seen among the offspring of pregnant rats treated with 10 times the usual human dose of this drug. The relevance of these observations to the therapeutic use of gold sodium thiomalate in human pregnancy is unknown.

Key References

Miyamoto T, Miyaji S, Horiuchi Y, Hara M, et al.: [Gold therapy in bronchial asthma--Special emphasis upon blood level of gold and its teratogenicity.] Nippon Naika Gakkai Zasshi 63:1190-1197, 1974. [S]

Szabo KT, DiFebbo ME, Phelan DG: The effects of gold-containing compounds on pregnant rabbits and their fetuses. Vet Pathol 15 (Suppl 5):97-102, 1978a. [A]

Szabo KT, Guerriero FJ, Kang YJ: The effects of gold-containing compounds on pregnant rats and their fetuses. Vet Pathol 15 (Suppl 5):89-96, 1978b. [A]

GOLD-198

Synonyms

Colloidal Gold Au 198 Injection, Gold Au 198 Injection

Summary

Gold-198 is a short-lived radio-isotope of colloidal gold used by local injection to treat malignant effusions and rheumatoid arthritis. Gold-198 is also administered intravenously for imaging studies of the reticuloendothelial system. Gold-198 emits beta and gamma particles.

Magnitude of Teratogenic Risk

Undetermined

Quality and Quantity of Data

None

Comment

Administration of gold-198 during pregnancy may be associated with a risk of radiation damage to the embryo or fetus. Calculations of embryonic or fetal radiation exposure should be made to assess this risk.

No epidemiolgical studies have been reported of congenital anomalies in infants born to women who had been given gold-198 during pregnancy.

No animal teratology studies of gold-198 have been published.

Key References

None available.

GONADORELIN

Synonyms

Luforan, Lutal, Lutamin, Relefact LH-RH, Relisorm L, Stimu-LH

Summary

Gonadorelin is the decapeptide leutinizing hormone-releasing hormone. It is administered
parenterally in the assessment and treatment of pituitary dysfunction and infertility.

Magnitude of Teratogenic Risk

Undetermined

Quality and Quantity of Data

None To Poor

Comment

A small risk cannot be excluded, but a high risk of congenital anomalies in the children of women treated with gonadorelin during pregnancy is unlikely.

No epidemiological studies of congenital anomalies among infants born to women treated with gonadorelin during pregnancy have been reported. High rates of early spontaneous abortion and multifetal pregnancies have been observed after ovulation induction with gonadorelin in infertile women (Homburg et al., 1989). These are expected complications of ovulation induction in such patients. None of the infants delivered of 71 continuing pregnancy in this series was noted to have a congenital anomaly.

The frequency of malformations was not increased among the offspring of rats treated with 1-200 times the human dose of gonadorelin during pregnancy (Tanabe et al., 1974). No teratogenic effect was observed among the offspring of rats, mice, or rabbits treated during pregnancy with gonadorelin in doses 2-50 times those used in humans in one study that has only been published as an abstract (Hemm et al., 1974).

Key References

Hemm RD, Arslanoglou L, Pollock JJ: Comparative teratogenicity studies of a synthetic gonadotrophin releasing hormone. Teratology 9:19A, 1974. [A]

Homburg R, Eshel A, Armar NA, et al.: One hundred pregnancies after treatment with pulsatile luteinising hormone releasing hormone to induce ovulation. BMJ 298:809-812, 1989. [S]

GRAMICIDIN

Synonyms

Bafucin, Gramacidine S, Gramoderm, Mytrex F Cream, Ointment

Summary

Gramicidin is an antimicrobial polypeptide that is employed topically for dermatologic and ophthalmic infections, often in combination with other antimicrobials.

Magnitude of Teratogenic Risk

None

Quality and Quantity of Data

Poor

Comment

None

The frequency of anomalies was no greater than expected among infants born to 61 women exposed to gramicidin during the first trimester or 96 women exposed anytime during gestation in the Collaborative Perinatal Project (Heinonen et al., 1977).

No experimental animal studies of the teratogenicity of gramicidin have been reported.

Key References

Heinonen OP, Slone D, Shapiro S: Birth Defects and Drugs in Pregnancy. Littleton, Mass.: John Wright-PSG, 1977, pp 297, 301, 435. [E]

GRISEOFULVIN

Synonyms

Curling Factor, Fulvicin, Grifulvin, Gris-PEG, Grisactin, Spirofulvin

Summary

Griseofulvin is an antifungal agent that is given orally to treat infections of the skin, nails, and hair.

Magnitude of Teratogenic Risk

Undetermined

Quality and Quantity of Data

Poor

Comment

A small risk cannot be excluded, but a high risk of congenital anomalies in the children of women treated with griseofulvin during pregnancy is unlikely.

No epidemiological studies of congenital anomalies among the children of women treated with griseofulvin during pregnancy have been reported. Rosa et al. (1987) reported two cases in which the mother took griseofulvin early in pregnancy and gave birth to conjoined twins. In contrast, none of 86 cases of conjoined twins identified in eight birth defects registries were associated with maternal griseofulvin treatment during pregnancy (Metneki & Czeizel, 1987; Knudsen, 1987).

Fetal death was observed with increased frequency among the offspring of rats and mice treated with griseofulvin during pregnancy in doses 75-250 times those used in humans (Klein & Beall, 1972; Jindra et al., 1979). In rats, fetal growth retardation was observed with maternal treatment during pregnancy with griseofulvin in doses 6-75 times that used clinically (Klein & Beall, 1972). Increased frequencies of major skeletal anomalies were observed in the offspring of rats treated with 62-75 times the human dose and mice treated with 250 times the human dose of griseofulvin during pregnancy (Klein & Beall, 1972; Jindra et al., 1979). A variety of skeletal and central nervous system malformations were observed among the offspring of cats treated with several times the human dose of griseofulvin during pregnancy (Scott et al., 1975). The relevance of these observations to the clinical use of griseofulvin in human pregnancy is unknown.

Key References

Jindra J, Aujezdska A, Janousek V: Embryotoxic effect of high doses of griseofulvin on the skeleton of the albino mouse. In: Benesova O, Rychter Z, Jelinek R (eds). Evaluation of Embryotoxicity, Mutagenicity and Carcinogenicity Risks in New Drugs. Proc 3rd Symp Toxicol Test for Safety of New Drugs. Prague: Univ Karlova-Praha, 1979, pp 161-165. [A]

Klein MF, Beall JR: Griseofulvin: A teratogenic agent. Science 175:1483-1484, 1972. [A]

Knudsen LB: No association between griseofulvin and conjoined twinning [letter]. Lancet 2:1097, 1987. [S]

Metneki J, Czeizel A: Griseofulvin teratology. Lancet 1:1042, 1987. [S]

Rosa FW, Hernandez C, Carlo WA: Griseofulvin teratology, including two thoracopagus conjoined twins. Lancet 1:171, 1987. [O]

Scott FW, De LaHunta A, Schultz RD, et al.: Teratogenesis in cats associated with griseofulvin therapy. Teratology 11:79-86, 1975. [A]

GUAIFENESIN

Synonyms

Breonesin, Glyceryl Guaiacolate, Glycotuss, Glytuss, Humibid, Hytuss, Motussin, Robitussin, Tedral Expectorant

Summary

Guaifenesin, an expectorant, is a component of many proprietary cough mixtures.

Magnitude of Teratogenic Risk

None

Quality and Quantity of Data

Fair

Comment

None

The frequency of malformations was no greater than expected among the children of more than 925 women who took guaifenesin in the first trimester of pregnancy in the Boston Collaborative Drug Surveillance Program (Jick et al., 1981; Aselton et al., 1985). Similarly, the frequency of congenital anomalies was not increased among the infants of 197 women who used guaifenesin in the first four lunar months, or the infants of 1336 women who used the drug anytime in pregnancy in the Collaborative Perinatal Project (Heinonen et al., 1977).

No animal teratology studies of guaifenesin have been published.

Key References

Aselton P, Jick H, Milunsky A, Hunter JR, et al.: First-trimester drug use and congenital disorders. Obstet Gynecol 65:451-455, 1985. [S]

Heinonen OP, Slone D, Shapiro S: Birth Defects and Drugs in Pregnancy. Littleton, Mass.: John Wright-PSG, 1977, pp 378-379, 496. [E]

Jick H, Holmes LB, Hunter JR, Madsen S, et al.: First-trimester drug use and congenital disorders. JAMA 246:343-346, 1981. [S]

GUANABENZ

Synonyms

Guanabenzo, Rexitene, Wytensin

Summary

Guanabenz is an alpha-adrenergic agonist used as an oral anti-hypertensive agent.

Magnitude of Teratogenic Risk

Undetermined

Quality and Quantity of Data

None To Poor

Comment

A small risk cannot be excluded, but a high risk of congenital anomalies in the children of women treated with guanabenz during pregnancy is unlikely.

No epidemiological studies of congenital anomalies among the infants of women treated with guanabenz during pregnancy have been reported.

The frequency of malformations was no greater than expected among the offspring of rats and rabbits treated with guanabenz during pregnancy in doses 1-15 and 1-10 times those used clinically (Akatsuka et al., 1982a, b). An increased incidence of fetal death occurred in association with signs of maternal toxicity in rats treated with this drug in the higher doses studied.

Key References

Akatsuka K, Hashimoto T, Takeuchi K, Kogure M: Reproduction study of guanabenz, a new antihypertensive agent (4). Teratological test in rabbits. J Tox Sci 7(Suppl 2):141-150, 1982b. [A]

Akatsuka K, Hashimoto T, Takeuchi K, Yanagisawa Y: Reproduction study of guanabenz, a new antihypertensive agent (2). Teratological test in rats. J Tox Sci 7(Suppl 2):107-121, 1982a. [A]

GUANADREL

Synonyms

Hylorel

Summary

Guanadrel is an oral antihypertensive agent used in the treatment of hypertension.

Magnitude of Teratogenic Risk

Undetermined

Quality and Quantity of Data

None

Comment

None

No epidemiological studies of congenital anomalies in infants whose mothers were treated with guanadrel during pregnancy have been reported.

No animal teratology studies of guanadrel have been published.

Key References

None available.

GUANETHIDINE

Synonyms

Antipres, DOPOM, Ismelin, Normoten, Solo-Ethidine, Visutensil

Summary

Guanethidine is a sympathetic blocking agent used to treat hypertension.

Magnitude of Teratogenic Risk

Undetermined

Quality and Quantity of Data

None To Poor

Comment

None

No epidemiological studies of congenital anomalies among infants born to women treated with guanethidine during pregnancy have been reported.

No obvious increase in malformations was noted among the offspring of rats treated with 1-4 times the usual human dose of guanethidine in two studies (West, 1962; Evans & Burnstock, 1979), but careful teratological evaluation of the pups was not performed.

Key References

Evans BK, Burnstock G: Chronic guanethidine treatment of female rats including effects on the fetus. J Reprod Fert 56:715-724, 1979. [A]

West GB: Drugs and rat pregnancy. J Pharm Pharmacol 14:828-830, 1962. [A]

GUANFACINE

Synonyms

Entulic, Estulic, Sandoz, Tenex

Summary

Guanfacine is an oral antihypertensive agent.

Magnitude of Teratogenic Risk

Undetermined

Quality and Quantity of Data

Poor

Comment

None

No epidemiological studies of congenital anomalies among the infants of women treated with guanfacine during pregnancy have been reported.

The frequency of malformations was not consistently increased among the offspring of mice or rabbits treated during pregnancy with guanfacine in doses 8-33 times those used in humans (Esaki & Hirayama, 1979; Esaki & Nakayama, 1979).

Please see agent summary on clonidine agent for information on a related agent that has been studied.

Key References

Esaki K, Hirayama M: Effects of oral administration of BS100-141 on reproduction in the mouse. II. Experiments on drug administration during the period of fetal development. Jitchuken Zenrinsho Kenkyuho 5(2):117-123, 1979. [A]

Esaki K, Nakayama T: Effects of oral administration of BS100-141 on the rabbit fetus. Jitchuken Zenrinsho Kenkyuho 5(2):129-136, 1979. [A]

HALAZEPAM

Synonyms

Paxipam

Summary

Halazepam is a benzodiazepine used orally as an antianxiety agent.

Magnitude of Teratogenic Risk

Undetermined

Quality and Quantity of Data

None To Poor

Comment

None

No epidemiological studies of congenital anomalies in infants whose mothers were treated with halazepam during pregnancy have been reported.

No teratogenic effects were observed among the offspring of rats or rabbits treated during pregnancy with halazepam in doses equivalent to <1-60 or up to 40 times those used in humans (Beall, 1972).

Please see agent summary on diazepam for information on a related agent that has been more thoroughly studied.

Key References

Beall JR: Study of the teratogenic potential of diazepam and SCH 12041. Can Med Assoc J 106:1061, 1972. [A]

HALCINONIDE

Synonyms

Halcicomb, Halciderm, Halcimat, Halcort, Halog

Summary

Halcinonide is a synthetic glucocorticoid that is administered topically in the treatment of various steroid-responsive skin disorders. Absorption through the skin is possible if sufficiently large amounts are used.

Magnitude of Teratogenic Risk

Undetermined

Quality and Quantity of Data

None

Comment

A small risk cannot be excluded, but a high risk of congenital anomalies in the children of women treated with halcinonide during pregnancy is unlikely.

No epidemiological studies of congenital anomalies in infants whose mothers used halcinonide during pregnancy have been reported.

No animal teratology studies of halcinonide have been published.

Please see agent summary on hydrocortisone for information on a related agent that has been more thoroughly studied.

Key References

None available.

HALOPERIDOL

Synonyms

Dozic, Fortunan, Haldol, Halosten, Serenace, Sigaperidol

Summary

Haloperidol is a major tranquilizer used in the treatment of psychosis, Tourette syndrome, mania, and severe hyperactivity. It is occasionally employed as an antinauseant or anxiolytic.

Magnitude of Teratogenic Risk

None To Minimal

Quality and Quantity of Data

Fair

Comment

None

The frequency of malformations was not increased among a cohort of infants born to 98 women treated with haloperidol during pregnancy (90 in the first trimester) (van Waes & van de Velde, 1969). These women were treated for hyperemesis gravidarum; the dose of haloperidol used was substantially less than that generally employed for psychiatric illness. Two isolated cases of infants with limb reduction defects born to women who used haloperidol during the period of limb morphogenesis have been reported (Dieulangard et al., 1966; Kopelman et al., 1975). No cause-and-effect inference can be made from such anecdotal observations.

A slightly increased frequency of micromelia and a high rate of fetal death were observed among the offspring of rats treated during pregnancy with haloperidol in a dose about 70 times that used clinically (Druga et al., 1980). Cleft palate has been reported among the offspring of pregnant rats and mice treated repectively with haloperidol in doses greater than 80 times or 2 times those used in humans (Szabo & Brent, 1974), and increased frequencies of central nervous system and skeletal malformations were observed among the offspring of mice treated with 10-18 times the human dose of haloperidol (Jurand & Martin, 1990). No teratogenic effect was observed among the offspring of rats, mice, or rabbits treated during pregnancy with haloperidol in lower doses (Bertelli et al., 1968; Hamada & Hashiguchi, 1978). Increased rates of embryonic death and malformation have been observed among the offspring of hamsters treated with haloperidol during pregnancy in doses 70-130 times those used in humans (Gill et al., 1982). Malformations of the brain and skull were most common, and a typical dose-response relationship was seen. Treatment with doses 10-25 times those used clinically was not teratogenic.

Long-lasting alterations of behavior have been noted among the offspring of pregnant rats treated with haloperidol in doses similar to or greater than those used in humans (Hull et al., 1984; Cuomo et al., 1985; Scalzo et al., 1989). The relevance of these observations to the risks associated with therapeutic use of haloperidol in human pregnancy is unknown.

Transient neonatal tardive dyskinesia has been observed in an infant whose mother was treated with haloperidol during pregnancy (Sexson & Barak, 1989). Such neurological symptoms are a recognized complication of haloperidol therapy in children and adults.

Key References

Bertelli PA, Polani PE, Spector R, Seller MJ, et al.: The effect of Haloperidol on pregnancy and foetal growth in rodents. Arzneimittelforsch 18:1420-1424, 1968. [A]

Cuomo V, Cagiano R, Renna G, Serinelli A, et al.: Comparative evaluation of the behavioural consequences of prenatal and early postnatal exposure to haloperidol in rats. Neurobehav Toxicol Teratol 7:489-492, 1985. [A]

Dieulangard P, Coignet J, Vidal JC: On a case of phocomelia: Possibly caused by medication. Bull Fed Soc Gynecol Obstet Lang Fr 18:85-87, 1966. [C]

Druga A, Nyitray M, Szaszovszky E: Experimental teratogenicity of structurally similar compounds with or without piperazine-ring: A preliminary report. Pol J Pharmacol Pharm 32:199-204, 1980. [A]

Gill TS, Guram MS, Geber WF: Haloperidol teratogenicity in the fetal hamster. Dev Pharmacol Ther 4:1-5, 1982. [A]

Hamada Y, Hashiguchi M: Teratogenicity of butyrophenone derivatives in mice. Teratology 18:148, 1978. [A]

Hull EM, Nishita JK, Bitran D: Perinatal dopamine-related drugs demasculinize rats. Science 224:1011-1013, 1984. [A]

Jurand A, Martin LVH: Teratogenic potential of two neurotropic drugs, haloperidol and dextromoramide, tested on mouse embryos. Teratology 42:45-54, 1990. [A]

Kopelman AE, McCullar FW, Heggeness L: Limb malformations following maternal use of haloperidol. JAMA 231:62-64, 1975. [C]

Scalzo FM, Ali SF, Holson RR: Behavioral effects of prenatal haloperidol exposure. Pharmacol Biochem Behav 34:727-731, 1989. [A]

Sexson WR, Barak Y: Withdrawal emergent syndrome in an infant associated with maternal haloperidol therapy. J Perinatol 9:170-172, 1989. [C]

Szabo KT, Brent RL: Species differences in experimental teratogenesis by tranquillizing agents. Lancet 1:565, 1974. [A]

van Waes AV, van de Velde E: Safety evaluation of haloperidol in the treatment of hyperemesis gravidarum. J Clin Pharmacol 9:224-227, 1969. [E]

HALOPROGIN

Synonyms

Mycanden, Mycilan, Polik

Summary

Haloprogin is an antimicrobial agent used topically to treat fungal infections. A small proportion of the applied dose is absorbed.

Magnitude of Teratogenic Risk

Undetermined

Quality and Quantity of Data

Poor

Comment

None

No epidemiological studies of congenital anomalies in infants born to women treated with haloprogin during pregnancy have been reported.

No animal teratology studies of haloprogin have been published.

Key References

None available.

HALOTHANE

Synonyms

Alotano, Fluopan, Fluothane, Halovis, Somnothane

Summary

Halothane is a general anesthetic that is administered by inhalation. Occupational exposure to halothane may occur among operating room personnel, dentists, and veterinarians. The occupational exposure limit for halothane in air as an 8-hour time-weighted average is 50 ppm (404 mg/cu m) (Hathaway et al., 1991).

Magnitude of Teratogenic Risk

Undetermined

Quality and Quantity of Data

Poor

Comment

A small risk cannot be excluded, but there is no indication that the risk of congenital anomalies in the children of women treated with halothane during pregnancy is likely to be great.

The frequency of congenital anomalies was not significantly increased among the children of women who had received halothane anesthesia during the first four lunar months of pregnancy in the Collaborative Perinatal Project, but the study included only 25 exposed pregnancies (Heinonen et al., 1977).

Fetal death, growth retardation, and malformations were very frequent among the offspring of mice repeatedly anesthetized with halothane during pregnancy in one study, but such treatment usually produced maternal death (Wharton et al., 1978, 1979). In contrast, no teratogenic effect or maternal toxicity was observed in rats or rabbits after similar treatment (Kennedy et al., 1976; Mazze et al., 1986). Long-lasting behavioral abnormalities have been observed among the offspring of pregnant rats and mice treated with halothane in various doses, some of which are near the human occupational exposure limit (Dudley et al., 1977; Smith et al., 1978; Koeter & Rodier, 1986; Levin & Bowman, 1986; Rodier et al., 1986; Baeder & Albrecht, 1990; Levin et al., 1990).

The effects on the embryo or fetus of maternal treatment during pregnancy with halothane in doses in the range of human occupational exposure have been studied repeatedly in mice and rats, but the results are not entirely consistent. In most studies, such exposure does not cause fetal malformations or death, although an increased frequency of developmental delay and skeletal variants sometimes occurs at doses just below the anesthetic range (Pope et al., 1978; Wharton et al., 1978, 1979; Popova et al., 1979; Lansdown et al., 1982; Mazze et al., 1988).

An increased frequency of chromosomal aberrations was observed in bone marrow cells and spermatogonia of rats treated chronically with a mixture of halothane and nitrous oxide in doses similar to human occupational exposure (Coate et al., 1979a, b). No such changes were observed in somatic cells of Chinese hamsters or mice anesthetized with halothane or in the fetuses of female Chinese hamsters anesthetized with halothane just prior to conception (Basler & Rohrborn, 1981).

Key References

Baeder Ch, Albrecht M: Embryotoxic/teratogenic potential of halothane. Int Arch Occup Environ Health 62:263-271, 1990. [A]

Basler A, Rohrborn G: Lack of mutagenic effects of halothane in mammals in vivo. Anesthesiology 55:143-147, 1981. [A]

Coate WB, Kapp RW, Lewis TR: Chronic exposure to low concentrations of halothane--nitrous oxide: Reproductive and cytogenetic effects in the rat. Anesthesiology 50:310-318, 1979a. [A]

Coate WB, Kapp RW, Ulland BM, Lewis TR: Toxicity of low concentration long-term exposure to an airborne mixture of nitrous oxide and halothane. J Environ Pathol Toxicol 2:209-231, 1979b. [A]

Dudley AW, Chang LW, Dudley MA, Bowman RE, et al.: Review of effects of chronic exposure to low levels of halothane. Neurotoxicology 1:137-145, 1977. [R]

Hathaway GJ, Proctor NH, Hughes JP, Fischman ML (eds): Proctor and Hughes' Chemical Hazards of the Workplace, 3rd ed. New York: Van Nostrand Reinhold, 1991, pp 316-317. [O]

Heinonen OP, Slone D, Shapiro S: Birth Defects and Drugs in Pregnancy. Littleton, Mass.: John Wright-PSG, 1977, pp 358-360. [E]

Kennedy GL, Smith SH, Keplinger ML, Calandra JC: Reproductive and teratologic studies with halothane. Toxicol Appl Pharmacol 35:467-474, 1976. [A]

Koeter HBWM, Rodier PM: Behavioral effects in mice exposed to nitrous oxide or halothane: Prenatal vs. postnatal exposure. Neurobehav Toxicol Teratol 8:189-194, 1986. [A]

Lansdown ABG, Pope WDB, Halsey MJ, Bateman PE: Analysis of fetal development in rats following maternal exposure to subanesthetic concentrations of halothane. Teratology 26:11-16, 1982. [A]

Levin ED, Bowman RE: Behavioral effects of chronic exposure to low concentrations of halothane during development in rats. Anesth Analg 65:653-659, 1986. [A]

Levin ED, DeLuna R, Uemura E, Bowman RE: Long-term effects of developmental halothane exposure on radial arm maze performance in rats. Behav Brain Res 36:147-154, 1990. [A]

Mazze RI, Fujinaga M, Baden JM: Halothane prevents nitrous oxide teratogenicity in Sprague-Dawley rats; folinic acid does not. Teratology 38:121-127, 1988. [A]

Mazze RI, Fujinaga M, Rice SA, Harris SB, et al.: Reproductive and teratogenic effects of nitrous oxide, halothane, isoflurane, and enflurane in Sprague-Dawley rats. Anesthesiology 64:339-344, 1986. [A]

Pope WDB, Halsey MJ, Lansdown ABG, Simmonds A, et al.: Fetotoxicity in rats following chronic exposure to halothane, nitrous oxide, or methoxyflurane. Anesthesiology 48:11-16, 1978. [A]

Popova S, Virgieva T, Atanasova J, Atanasov A, et al.: Embryotoxicity and fertility study with halothane subanesthetic concentration in rats. Acta Anaesth Scand 23:505-512, 1979. [A]

Rodier PM, Koeter HBWM: General activity from weaning to maturity in mice exposed to halothane or nitrous oxide. Neurobehav Toxicol Teratol 8:195-199, 1986. [A]

Smith RF, Bowman RE, Katz J: Behavioral effects of exposure to halothane during early development in the rat: Sensitive period during pregnancy. Anesthesiology 49:319-323, 1978. [A]

Wharton RS, Mazze RI, Baden JM, Hitt BA, et al.: Fertility, reproduction and postnatal survival in mice chronically exposed to halothane. Anesthesiology 48:167-174, 1978. [A]

Wharton RS, Wilson AI, Mazze RI, Baden JM, et al.: Fetal morphology in mice exposed to halothane. Anesthesiology 51:532-537, 1979. [A]

HAMYCIN

Synonyms

Hamicina, Primamycin

Summary

Hamycin is a polyene antibiotic used to treat fungal and trichomonal infections.

Magnitude of Teratogenic Risk

Undetermined

Quality and Quantity of Data

None

Comment

None

No epidemiological studies of congenital anomalies in infants born to women treated with hamycin during pregnancy have been reported.

No animal teratology studies of hamycin have been published.

Key References

None available.

HEPARIN

Synonyms

Calciparine, Hep-Flush, Hep-Lock, Hepsal, Liquaemin, Minihep, Monoparin, Multiparin, Pump-Hep, Uniparin

Summary

Heparin is a sulfated glycosaminoglycan prepared from mammalian tissue. It is administered parenterally to prevent blood clotting. When given during pregnancy, standard heparin does not directly affect the thrombotic mechanism in the fetus, but certain low molecular weight heparin preparations may (Andrew et al., 1986), even though neither form appears to cross the placenta (Forestier et al., 1987; Omri et al., 1989).

Magnitude of Teratogenic Risk

None To Minimal

Quality and Quantity of Data

Fair

Comment

Because of its anticoagulant activity, there may be an increased risk of maternal hemorrhage associated with the use of heparin during pregnancy.

Three hundred fifty five cases in which the mother was treated with heparin during pregnancy were identified in the published literature prior to 1986 (Ginsberg et al., 1989a; Ginsberg & Hirsh, 1989). The overall rate of "adverse outcomes" was 21.7%, but most of these were associated with severe toxemia, glomerulonephritis, a history of recurrent miscarriage, or other maternal factors that are known to be associated with adverse pregnancy outcome. If these cases were excluded, the rates of prematurity (6.8%) and fetal or neonatal death (2.5%) were similar to those expected in the general population. Only three of the 317 liveborn infants in this series had congenital anomalies, which were different in each case (Ginsberg et al., 1989a). It seems likely that the presence of these comorbid conditions among the heparin-treated pregnancies accounts for the conclusion in an earlier review (Hall et al., 1980) that at least one-third of pregnancies in women treated with heparin have abnormal outcomes (Nageotte et al., 1981; Howie, 1986; Ginsberg et al., 1989a; Ginsberg & Hirsh, 1989). The frequencies of miscarriage, stillbirth, prematurity, and congenital anomalies did not appear to be unusual in a retrospective series of 100 consecutive pregnancies in women treated with heparin (Ginsberg et al., 1989b); 34 of these pregnancies were treated in the first trimester.

No teratogenic effect was observed among the offspring of rats or rabbits treated during pregnancy with heparin in doses <1-4 times those used clinically (Lehrer & Becker, 1974; Bertoli & Borelli, 1986). At doses 12 times those used clinically, increased rates of embryonic death were seen in both species (Lehrer & Becker, 1974).

Key References

Andrew M, Ofosu F, Fernandez A, et al.: A low molecular weight heparin alters the fetal coagulation system in the pregnant sheep. Thromb Haemost 55(3):342-346, 1986. [A]

Bertoli D, Borelli G: Peri- and postnatal, teratology and reproductive studies of a low molecular weight heparin in rats. Arzneimittelforsch 36:1260-1263, 1986. [A]

Forestier F, Daffos F, Rainaut M, Toulemonde F: Low molecular weight heparin (CY 216) does not cross the placenta during the third trimester of pregnancy. Thromb Haemost 57(2):234, 1987. [S]

Ginsberg JS, Hirsh J: Anticoagulants during pregnancy. Annu Rev Med 40:79-86, 1989. [R]

Ginsberg JS, Hirsh J, Turner C, et al.: Risks to the fetus of anticoagulant therapy during pregnancy. Thromb Haemost 61(2):197-203, 1989a. [R]

Ginsberg JS, Kowalchuk G, Hirsh J, et al.: Heparin therapy during pregnancy. Arch Intern Med 149:2233-2236, 1989b. [S]

Hall JG, Pauli RM, Wilson KM: Maternal and fetal sequelae of anticoagulation during pregnancy. Am J Med 68(1):122-140, 1980. [R]

Howie PW: Anticoagulants in pregnancy. Clin Obstet Gynaecol 13(2):349-363, 1986. [R]

Lehrer SB, Becker BA: Effects of heparin on fetuses of pregnant rats and rabbits. Teratology 9:A26-A27, 1974. [A]

Nageotte MP, Freeman RK, Garite TJ, Block RA: Anticoagulation in pregnancy. Am J Obstet Gynecol 141:472-473, 1981. [O]

Omri A, Delaloye JF, Andersen H, Bachmann F: Low molecular weight heparin novo (LHN-1) does not cross the placenta during the second trimester of pregnancy. Thromb Haemost 61(1):55-56, 1989. [E]

HEPATITIS B IMMUNE GLOBULIN

Synonyms

H-BIG, Hep-B-Gammagee, HyperHep

Summary

Hepatitis B immune globulin is an antibody preparation made from the plasma of human donors who are immune to hepatitis B virus. Hepatitis B immune globulin is administered parenterally to provide passive immunity to people who have been exposed to hepatitis B virus.

Magnitude of Teratogenic Risk

Undetermined

Quality and Quantity of Data

None

Comment

A small risk cannot be excluded, but a high risk of congenital anomalies in the children of women treated with hepatitis B immune globulin during pregnancy is unlikely.

No epidemiological studies of congenital anomalies among infants born to women treated with hepatitis B immune globulin during pregnancy have been reported.

No animal teratology studies of hepatitis B immune globulin have been published.

Please see agent summary on rho(d) immune globulin for information on a related agent that has been more thoroughly studied.

Key References

None available.

HEPATITIS B VACCINE

Synonyms

Engerix-B, Heptavax-B, Recombivax HB

Summary

Hepatitis B vaccines contain either hepatitis B surface antigen produced by recombinant DNA technology or inactivated and purified hepatitis B viral protein obtained from human plasma. Hepatitis B vaccine is administered parenterally to impart active immunity to hepatitis B virus.

Magnitude of Teratogenic Risk

Undetermined

Quality and Quantity of Data

None To Poor

Comment

A small risk cannot be excluded, but a high risk of congenital anomalies in the children of women who were treated with hepatitis B vaccine during pregnancy is unlikely.

No abnormalities were found among the infants of 10 women who were immunized with hepatitis B vaccine during the first trimester of pregnancy in one series (Levy & Koren, 1991). No "abnormal birth defects" were observed among the infants of 72 women vaccinated with hepatitis B vaccine in the third trimester of pregnancy in another study (Ayoola & Johnson, 1987).

No animal teratology studies of hepatitis B vaccine have been published.

Key References

Ayoola EA, Johnson AOK: Hepatitis B vaccine in pregnancy: Immunogenicity, safety and transfer of antibodies to infants. Int J Gynaecol Obstet 25:297-301, 1987. [S]

Levy M, Koren G: Hepatitis B vaccine in pregnancy: Maternal and fetal safety. Am J Perinatol 8(3):227-232, 1991. [S]

HEPTACHLOR

Synonyms

Heptox

Summary

Heptachlor is an organochloride insecticide that is used extensively for termite control. Heptachlor has also been used on corn, cereal crops, vegetables, and seeds. The 1989 U.S. OSHA Permissible Exposure Limit for heptachlor in air is 0.5 mg/cu m as a time-weighted average for an 8-hour exposure. Heptachlor can be absorbed through the lungs, skin, and gastrointestinal tract.

Magnitude of Teratogenic Risk

None To Minimal

Quality and Quantity of Data

Poor To Fair

Comment

None

Incidence rates of 23 major congenital anomalies or classes of congenital anomalies were not greater than expected among 20,614 infants born on the island of Oahu, Hawaii, during a period in which the entire milk supply was contaminated with heptachlor residues in excess of 0.1 ppm (Le Marchand et al., 1986).

The frequency of congenital anomalies was not increased among the offspring of rats fed diets containing 0.3-10 ppm of heptachlor during pregnancy (Eisler, 1968). Similarly, no teratogenic effect was observed among the offspring of rats fed 5-20 mg/kg/d of heptachlor during pregnancy despite the fact that maternal toxicity was evident at the highest dose (Yamaguchi et al., 1987). In another study, decreased litter size and an increased frequency of cataracts were observed among the offspring of rats fed 6 mg/kg/d of heptachlor during pregnancy (Mestitzova, 1967).

Key References

Eisler M: Heptachlor: Toxicology and safety evaluation. Ind Med Surg 37(11):840-844, 1968. [R] & [A]

Le Marchand L, Kolonel LN, Siegel BZ, et al: Trends in birth defects for a Hawaiian population exposed to heptachlor and for the United States. Arch Environ Health 41(3):145-148, 1986. [E]

Mestitzova M: On reproduction studies and the occurrence of cataracts in rats after long-term feeding of the insecticide heptachlor. Experientia 23(1):42-43, 1967. [A]

Yamaguchi M, Tanaka S, Kawashima K, et al.: Effects of heptachlor on fetal developments of rats. Bull Natl Inst Hyg Sci (Tokyo) 0:33-36, 1987. [A]

HEROIN

Synonyms

Black Tar, China White, Diacetylmorphine, Diamorphine Hydrochloride, Heroine, Junk, Smack

Summary

Heroin is an opiate narcotic that is widely abused. Outside of the U.S., heroin is used medically to relieve severe pain and cough.

Magnitude of Teratogenic Risk

None To Minimal

Quality and Quantity of Data

Fair

Comment

Neonatal withdrawal symptoms often occur among infants born to women who regularly use heroin during pregnancy (see below).

Epidemiological studies of malformations in the children of women who used heroin during pregnancy deal with addicted populations who use the drug illicitly. Such women often abuse other drugs, alcohol, and cigarettes and have poor nutritional and health status. Moreover, the dose of heroin used and the period of gestation during which it was used are usually unknown. Nevertheless, the frequency of malformations does not appear unusually high in most cohorts and clinical series of infants born to heroin-addicted mothers (Stone et al., 1971; Naeye et al., 1973; Stimmel & Adamsons, 1976; Kandall et al., 1977; Levy & Koren, 1990; Little et al., 1991). A statistically significant increase in the frequency of malformations was observed in one study of 830 infants born to narcotic-dependent mothers (Ostrea & Chavez, 1979), but the frequency of malformations in children born to addicts in this study was about what would be expected in general (2.4%), while the frequency in control infants was inexplicably low (0.5%). Although several anecdotal reports of children with congenital anomalies born to heroin-addicted mothers have been published, no consistent pattern of malformations has been observed (Rothstein & Gould, 1974), and no causal inference is possible.

Intrauterine growth retardation, perinatal death, and a variety of other perinatal complications have frequently been observed in the offspring of narcotic-addicted mothers (Zelson et al., 1971; Kandall et al., 1977; Oleske, 1977; Fricker & Segal, 1978; Lifschitz et al., 1983; Gregg et al., 1988; Little et al., 1990, 1991; Lam et al., 1992), but it is unclear whether these effects are due to fetal exposure to heroin or to the generally poor health of these mothers. Subsequent growth of these children appears to be normal in most cases although head circumference may continue to be somewhat smaller than expected (Lifschitz et al., 1985; Chasnoff et al., 1986; Lifschitz & Wilson, 1991; Little et al., 1991).

Neonatal withdrawal symptoms are observed in 40-80% of infants born to heroin-addicted women (Rothstein & Gould, 1974; Kandall et al., 1977; Fricker & Segal, 1978; Alroomi et al., 1988; Lam et al., 1992). Withdrawal symptoms include tremors, irritability, sneezing, vomiting, fever, diarrhea, and occasionally seizures. Although the duration of these symptoms is sometimes prolonged, it is usually less than three weeks. Sudden infant death syndrome and behavioral and intellectual deficits have been reported with increased frequency in older children whose mothers were addicted to heroin during pregnancy (Finnegan, 1979, 1985; Hutchings, 1982; Chasnoff et al., 1986; Wilson, 1989, 1992; van Baar, 1990; Kandall & Gaines, 1991), but the occurrence of other social and health problems in these families makes interpretation of such reports with respect to cause difficult.

Increased frequencies of central nervous system and other malformations have been observed among the offspring of mice treated during pregnancy with single doses of heroin 100-150 times those usually used in humans (Jurand, 1980, 1985). Significantly increased frequencies of central nervous system and other malformations were also observed in the offspring of hamsters injected with heroin during pregnancy in doses 200-1000 times those used by humans (Geber & Schramm, 1975). Typical dose-dependence of this teratogenic effect was observed. The relevance of these findings to human use of heroin during pregnancy is unknown.

Higher-than-expected frequencies of acquired chromosomal aberrations in peripheral blood lymphocytes have been reported in narcotic addicts (Kushnick et al., 1972; Amarose & Norusis, 1976). Similar findings were observed in the infants of narcotic-addicted women in one study (Amarose & Norusis, 1976) but not in another (Kushnick et al., 1972). Evidence from an investigation in rhesus monkeys supports the possibility that maternal heroin use may cause somatic cell chromosome breakage in infants (Fischman et al., 1983), but the clinical relevance of this observation is unknown.

Key References

Alroomi LG, Davidson J, Evans TJ, Galea P, et al.: Maternal narcotic abuse and the newborn. Arch Dis Child 63(1):81-83, 1988. [S]

Amarose AP, Norusis MJ: Cytogenetics of methadone-managed and heroin-addicted pregnant women and their newborn infants. Am J Obstet Gynecol 124:635-640, 1976. [S]

Chasnoff IJ, Burns KA, Burns WJ, Schnoll SH: Prenatal drug exposure: Effects on neonatal and infant growth development. Neurobehav Toxicol Teratol 8:357-362, 1986. [E]

Finnegan LP: Effects of maternal opiate abuse on the newborn. Fed Proc Fed Am Soc Exp Biol 44:2314-2317, 1985. [R]

Finnegan LP: In utero opiate dependence and sudden infant death syndrome. Clin Perinatol 6(1):163-180, 1979. [E] & [R]

Fischman HK, Roizin L, Moralishvili E, Albu P, et al.: Clastogenic effects of heroin in pregnant monkeys and their offspring. Mutat Res 118:77-89, 1983. [A]

Fricker HS, Segal S: Narcotic addiction, pregnancy, and the newborn. Am J Dis Child 132:360-366, 1978. [E]

Geber WF, Schramm LC: Congenital malformations of the central nervous system produced by narcotic analgesics in the hamster. Am J Obstet Gynecol 123:705-713, 1975. [A]

Gregg JEM, Davidson DC, Weindling AM: Inhaling heroin during pregnancy: Effects on the baby. Br Med J 296:754, 1988. [E]

Hutchings DE: Methadone and heroin during pregnancy: A review of behavioral effects in human and animal offspring. Neurobehav Toxicol Teratol 4:429-434, 1982. [R]

Jurand A: The interference of naloxone hydrochloride in the teratogenic activity of opiates. Teratology 31:235-240, 1985. [A]

Jurand A: Malformations of the central nervous system induced by neurotropic drugs in mouse embryos. Dev Growth Differ 22(1):61-78, 1980. [A]

Kandall SR, Albin S, Gartner LM, Lee K-S, et al.: The narcotic-dependent mother: Fetal and neonatal consequences. Early Hum Dev 1/2:159-169, 1977. [E]

Kandall SR, Gaines J: Maternal substance use and subsequent sudden infant death syndrome (SIDS) in offspring. Neurotoxicol Teratol 13(2):235-240, 1991. [R]

Kushnick T, Robinson M, Tsao C: Narcotic addicts and their newborns. J Med Soc N J 69:727-728, 1972. [O]

Lam SK, To WK, Duthie SJ, Ma HK: Narcotic addiction in pregnancy with adverse maternal and perinatal outcome. Aust NZ J Obstet Gynaecol 32(3):216-221, 1992. [E]

Levy M, Koren G: Obstetric and neonatal effects of drugs of abuse. Emerg Med Clin North Am 8(3):633-652, 1990. [R]

Lifschitz MH, Wilson GS: Patterns of growth and development in narcotic-exposed children. NIDA Res Monogr 114:323-339, 1991. [R]

Lifschitz MH, Wilson GS, Smith EO, Desmond MM: Factors affecting head growth and intellectual function in children of drug addicts. Pediatrics 75:269-274, 1985. [E]

Lifschitz MH, Wilson GS, Smith EO, Desmond MM: Fetal and postnatal growth of children born to narcotic-dependent women. J Pediatr 102:686-691, 1983. [E]

Little BB, Snell LM, Klein VR, Gilstrap LC III, et al.: Maternal and fetal effects of heroin addiction during pregnancy. J Reprod Med 35(2):159-162, 1990. [E]

Little BB, Snell LM, Knoll KA, Ghali FE, et al.: Heroin abuse during pregnancy: Effects on perinatal outcome and early childhood growth. Am J Hum Biol 3:463-468, 1991. [E]

Naeye RL, Blanc W, Leblanc W, Khatamee MA: Fetal complications of maternal heroin addiction: Abnormal growth, infections, and episodes of stress. J Pediatr 83:1055-1061, 1973. [E]

Oleske JM: Experiences with 118 infants born to narcotic-using mothers. Clin Pediatr 16:418-423, 1977. [E]

Ostrea EM, Chavez CJ: Perinatal problems (excluding neonatal withdrawal) in maternal drug addiction: A study of 830 cases. J Pediatr 94:292-295, 1979. [E]

Rothstein P, Gould JB: Born with habit. Infants of drug-addicted mothers. Pediatr Clin North Am 21:307-321, 1974. [R]

Stimmel B, Adamsons K: Narcotic dependency in pregnancy. Methadone maintenance compared to use of street drugs. JAMA 235:1121-1124, 1976. [E]

Stone ML, Salerno LJ, Green M, Zelson C: Narcotic addiction in pregnancy. Am J Obstet Gynecol 109:716-723, 1971. [S]

van Baar A: Development of infants of drug dependent mothers. J Child Psychol Psychiat 31(6):911-920, 1990. [E]

Wilson GS: Clinical studies of infants and children exposed prenatally to heroin. Ann NY Acad Sci 562:183-194, 1989. [E]

Wilson GS: Heroin use during pregnancy: Clinical studies of long-term effects. In: Sonderegger TB (ed). Perinatal Substance Abuse: Research Findings and Clinical Implications. Baltimore: Johns Hopkins Univ Press, 1992, 224-238. [R]

Zelson C, Rubio E, Wasserman E: Neonatal narcotic addiction: 10 years of observation. Pediatrics 48:178-189, 1971. [S]

HERPES SIMPLEX VIRUS

Synonyms

Herpes

Summary

Herpes simplex is a double-stranded DNA virus that occurs in two types. Type 1 infections usually involve the oral cavity; type 2 infections usually involve the genital region.

Most infections of either type are asymptomatic, but systemic illness occasionally occurs with primary infection. Once it occurs, infection is persistent, and periodic reactivation with recurrent lesions is the rule.

Magnitude of Teratogenic Risk

Teratogenic Effects: Minimal

Perinatal Infection: Small To Moderate

Quality and Quantity of Data

Teratogenic Effects: Good

Perinatal Infection: Good

Comment

1) This risk is for maternal infection when infection of the fetus is unknown. The risk is greater if fetal infection is demonstrated.

2) The risk of teratogenic effects is greatest with primary infection, especially in the third trimester.

3) The risk of perinatal infection is greatest with active genital lesions at the time of vaginal delivery.

Transplacental infection of the embryo or fetus rarely seems to occur with herpes simplex virus, but the consequences of such infection may be devastating. More than 20 and as many as 75 infants (depending on how intrauterine and neonatal infection are differentiated) with congenital anomalies associated with apparent transplacental herpes simplex infection have been reported (South et al., 1969; Florman et al., 1973; Montgomery et al., 1973; Hutto et al., 1987; Komorous et al., 1977; Karesh et al., 1983; Monif et al., 1985; Baldwin & Whitley, 1989; Parish, 1989; Fagnant & Monif, 1989; Rabalais et al., 1991; Jeffries, 1991). Typical skin lesions occur in almost all of the affected children at birth or shortly thereafter. Most cases are associated with type 2 virus, but some are associated with type 1. Frequent features include intrauterine growth retardation, microcephaly, chorioretinitis, and psychomotor re-

tardation. Hydranencephaly, hydrocephaly, porencephaly, intracranial calcification, microphthalmia, cutis aplasia, disseminated infection and neonatal death may occur. Similar abnormalities have been seen in infants born after either first-trimester or later maternal infection, suggesting that the lesions represent disruption rather than malformation.

Given the frequency of herpes simplex virus infection in pregnant women and the apparent rarity of herpes simplex embryopathy, transplacental infection must be uncommon (Jenista, 1984; Stagno & Whitley, 1985; Baldwin & Whitley, 1989; Jeffries, 1991). None of 160, 82, or 60 infants born to women with genital herpes infections in three studies had clinical features of congenital herpes (Grossman et al., 1981; Harger et al., 1983; Brown et al., 1985). The risk appears to be greater among the infants of pregnant women who have primary herpes simplex virus infections. In a series of 15 women who had primary type 2 herpes simplex virus infections during pregnancy, three of the five infants born after third trimester maternal infections had growth retardation and two of these five infants developed neonatal herpes; one of five women with first trimester infection miscarried (Brown et al., 1987).

Evidence of type 2 herpes simplex virus infection of the placenta has been observed with greater than expected frequency among spontaneous abortuses, and it has been suggested that this infection may be a common cause of miscarriage (Robb et al., 1986; Benirschke & Robb, 1987).

Neonatal herpes simplex due to ascending infection after rupture of the amnion or delivery through a contaminated birth canal is a well-recognized entity (Whitley et al., 1980; Jenista, 1984; Monif & Hardt, 1984; Stagno & Whitley, 1985; Whitley, 1990; Jeffries, 1991; Arvin & Prober, 1992). Many cases exhibit central nervous system and/or visceral lesions. Mortality without treatment is very high, and many of the survivors are left with serious sequelae. The risk appears greater if the infant is premature or if obvious genital lesions are present in the mother, but many mothers of affected infants are asymptomatic. The risk of neonatal disseminated infection has been estimated to be on the order of 5-25% if the mother has one or more genital herpes simplex lesions at the time of vaginal delivery (Monif & Hardt, Whittaker & Cho, 1991). The risk is clearly higher if the mother has an active primary genital infection at the time of delivery.

Experimental herpes simplex viremia in pregnant rabbits was associated with frequent fetal infection, death, and resorption in one uncontrolled study (Middlekamp et al., 1967). No teratogenic effect was observed in hamster or guinea pig embryos after maternal infection with herpes simplex virus (Ferm & Low, 1965; Chow & Hsiung, 1982).

Key References

Arvin AM, Prober CG: Herpes simplex virus infections: The genital tract and the newborn. Pediatr Rev 13(3):107-112, 1992. [R]

Baldwin S, Whitley RJ: Teratogen update: Intrauterine herpes simplex virus infection. Teratology 39:1-10, 1989. [R]

Benirschke K, Robb JA: Infectious causes of fetal death. Clin Obstet Gynecol 30(2):284-294, 1987. [R]

Brown ZA, Vontver LA, Benedetti J, et al.: Effects on infants of a first episode of genital herpes during pregnancy. N Engl J Med 317(20):1246-1251, 1987. [S]

Brown ZA, Vontver LA, Benedetti J, et al.: Genital herpes in pregnancy: Risk factors associated with recurrences and asymptomatic viral shedding. Am J Obstet Gynecol 153:24-30, 1985. [S]

Chow TC, Hsiung GD: Neonatal herpes simplex virus infection in guinea pigs (41459). Proc Soc Exp Biol Med 170:459-463, 1982. [A]

Fagnant RJ, Monif GRG: How rare is congenital herpes simplex? A literature review. J Reprod Med 34(6):417-422, 1989. [R]

Ferm VH, Low RJ: Herpes simplex virus infection in the pregnant hamster. J Pathol Bacteriol 89:295-300, 1965. [A]

Florman AL, Gershon AA, Blackett PR, Nahmias AJ: Intrauterine infection with herpes simplex virus. JAMA 225:129-139, 1973. [C]

Grossman JH, Wallen WC, Sever JL: Management of genital herpes simplex virus infection during pregnancy. Obstet Gynecol 58:1-4, 1981. [S]

Harger JH, Pazin GJ, Armstrong JA, et al.: Characteristics and management of pregnancy in women with genital herpes simplex virus infection. Am J Obstet Gynecol 145:784-791, 1983. [S]

Hutto C, Arvin A, Jacobs R, et al.: Intrauterine herpes simplex virus infections. J Pediatr 110:97-101, 1987. [S]

Jeffries DJ: Intra-uterine and neonatal herpes simplex virus infection. Scand J Infect Dis (Suppl 78):21-26, 1991. [R]

Jenista JA: Perinatal herpesvirus infections. In: Amstey MS (ed): Virus Infection in Pregnancy. New York: Grune and Stratton, 1984, pp 69-79. [R]

Karesh JW, Kapur S, MacDonald M: Herpes simplex virus and congenital malformations. South Med J 76:1561-1563, 1983. [C]

Komorous JM, Wheller CE, Briggaman RA, Caro I: Intrauterine herpes simplex infections. Arch Dermatol 113:918-922, 1977. [C]

Middlekamp JN, Reed CA, Patrizi G: Placental transfer of herpes simplex virus in pregnant rabbits. Proc Soc Exp Biol Med 125:757- 760, 1967. [A]

Monif GRG, Hardt NS: Management of herpetic vulvovaginitis in pregnancy. In: Amstey MS, ed. Virus Infection in Pregnancy. New York: Grune and Stratton, Inc., pp. 81-89, 1984. [R]

Monif GRG, Kellner KR, Donnelly WH Jr : Congenital herpes simplex type II infection. Am J Obstet Gynecol 152:1000-1002, 1985. [C]

Montgomery JR, Flanders RW, Yow MD: Congenital anomalies and herpes virus infection. Am J Dis Child 126:364-366, 1973. [C]

Parish WR: Intrauterine herpes simplex virus infection. Hydranencephaly and a nonvesicular rash in an infant. Int J Dermatol 28(6):397-401, 1989. [C]

Rabalais GP, Yusk JW, Wilkerson SA: Zosteriform denuded skin caused by intrauterine herpes simplex virus infection. Pediatr Infect Dis J 10(1):79-80, 1991. [C]

Robb JA, Benirschke K, Barmeyer R: Intrauterine latent herpes simplex virus infectiion: I. Spontaneous abortion. Hum Pathol 17:1196-1209, 1986. [E]

South MA, Tompkins WAF, Morris CR, Rawls WE: Congenital malformation of the central nervous system associated with genital type (type 2) herpes virus. J Pediatr 75:13-18, 1969. [C]

Stagno S, Whitley RJ: Herpes virus infections of pregnancy. Part II: Herpes simplex virus and varicella-zoster virus infections. N Engl J Med 313:1327-1330, 1985. [R]

Whitley RJ: Herpes simplex virus infections. In: Remington JS, Klein JO (eds). Infectious Diseases of the Fetus and Newborn Infant. Philadelphia: W.B. Saunders Co., 1990, pp 282-305. [R]

Whitley RJ, Nahmias AJ, Visintine AM, Fleming CL, et al.: The natural history of herpes simplex virus infection of mother and newborn. Pediatrics 66:489-494, 1980. [S]

Whittaker TJ, Cho CT: Prevention and management of neonatal herpes. Compr Ther 17(9):13-16, 1991. [R]

HESPERIDIN

Synonyms

Cirantin, Hesperidin Chalcone, Hesperidoside

Summary

Hesperidin is a flavinoid that has been used to treat capillary fragility.

Magnitude of Teratogenic Risk

Undetermined

Quality and Quantity of Data

None

Comment

None

No epidemiological studies of congenital anomalies among the infants of women who took hesperidin during pregnancy have been reported.

No animal teratology studies of hesperidin have been published.

Key References

None available.

HETASTARCH

Synonyms

Hespan, Hydroxyethyl Starch

Summary

Hetastarch is a plasma volume expander that is administered by infusion as an adjunct in the treatment of shock or other conditions associated with the loss of plasma proteins.

Magnitude of Teratogenic Risk

Undetermined

Quality and Quantity of Data

None To Poor

Comment

A small risk cannot be excluded, but a high risk of congenital anomalies in the children of women treated with hetastarch during pregnancy is unlikely.

No epidemiological studies of congenital anomalies in children born to women who were given hetastarch during pregnancy have been reported.

No teratogenic effects were observed in either rats or mice treated with up to 25,000 or 200,000 times the human equivalent dose of hetastarch during gestation, although embryotoxic effects occurred in rats at the highest dose used (Ivankovic et al., 1975).

Key References

Ivankovic S, Bulow I: Absence of teratogenic effect of the plasma expander hydroxyethyl starch in the rat and mouse. Anaesthesist 24:244-245, 1975. [A]

HEXACHLOROPHENE

Synonyms

Hexachlorophane, pHisoHex, Septisol

Summary

Hexachlorophene is a disinfectant that is used topically. It is absorbed through the skin.

Magnitude of Teratogenic Risk

None To Minimal

Quality and Quantity of Data

Poor To Fair

Comment

None

An increased frequency of a heterogenous group of congenital anomalies was reported among 460 children born to women medical personnel who very frequently washed with hexachlorophene-containing soaps during the first trimester of their pregnancies (Halling, 1979). This study has been severely criticized for its methodological deficiencies (Kallen, 1978), and could not be confirmed in a partially overlapping investigation of 3007 infants born to women who had worked in hospitals where hexachlorophene was used extensively (Baltzar et al., 1979). No association with maternal exposure to hexachlorophene during early pregnancy was observed in a case-control study involving 1047 children with various congenital anomalies (Hernberg et al., 1983).

Increased frequencies of ocular malformations, hydrocephalus, and other anomalies were observed among the offspring of rats treated intravaginally with 80-300 mg/kg/d or orally with 30 mg/kg/d of hexachlorophene during pregnancy (Kimmel et al., 1974; Kennedy et al., 1975). Similar results were observed in rabbits fed hexachlorophene in a dose 6 mg/kg/d (Kennedy et al., 1975). No teratogenic effects were seen after vaginal treatment with 20 mg/kg/d in rabbits. Maternal toxicity occurred with the high doses in both species.

Key References

Baltzar B, Ericson A, Kallen B: Pregnancy outcome among women working in Swedish hospitals. N Engl J Med 300:627-628, 1979. [E]

Halling H: Suspected link between exposure to hexachlorophene and malformed infants. Ann NY Acad Sci 320:426-436, 1979. [E]

Hernberg S, Kurppa K, Ojajarvi J, et al.: Congenital malformations and occupational exposure to disinfectants: A case-referent study. Scand J Work Environ Health 9:55, 1983. [E]

Kallen B: Hexachlorophene teratogenicity in humans disputed. JAMA 240(15):1585-1586, 1978. [O]

Kennedy Jr GL, Smith SH, Keplinger ML, Calandra JC: Evaluation of the teratological potential of hexachlorophene in rabbits and rats. Teratology 12:83-88, 1975. [A]

Kimmel CA, Moore Jr W, Hysell DK, Stara J: Teratogenicity of hexachlorophene in rats. Comparison of uptake following various routes of administration. Arch Environ Health 28:43-48, 1974. [A]

HEXOCYCLIUM METHYLSULFATE

Synonyms

Hexocyclum, Tral, Traline

Summary

Hexocyclium methylsulfate is an oral anticholinergic agent that inhibits gastric secretion and gastrointestinal motility. It is used as an adjunct in the treatment of peptic ulcers.

Magnitude of Teratogenic Risk

Undetermined

Quality and Quantity of Data

None

Comment

None

No epidemiological studies of congenital anomalies in infants born to women who were treated with hexocyclium methylsulfate during pregnancy have been reported.

No animal teratology studies of hexocyclium methylsulfate have been published.

Please see agent summary on atropine for information on a related agent that has been more thoroughly studied.

Key References

None available.

HEXOTHIOCAINE

Summary

Hexothiocaine is a local anesthetic that has been used topically.

Magnitude of Teratogenic Risk

Undetermined

Quality and Quantity of Data

None

Comment

None

No epidemiological studies of congenital anomalies in children born to women exposed to hexothiocaine during pregnancy have been reported.

No investigations of teratologic effects of hexothiocaine in experimental animals have been published.

Please see agent summary on procaine for information on a related agent that has been studied.

Key References

None available.

HEXYLCAINE

Synonyms

Cyclaine, Hexylcainium Chloride

Summary

Hexylcaine is a surface anesthetic of the ester class.

Magnitude of Teratogenic Risk

Undetermined

Quality and Quantity of Data

None

Comment

A small risk cannot be excluded, but there is no indication that the risk of congenital anomalies in the children of women treated with hexylcaine during pregnancy is likely to be great.

No epidemiological studies of congenital anomalies in children born to women exposed to hexylcaine during pregnancy have been reported.

No investigations of teratologic effects of hexylcaine in experimental animals have been published.

Please see agent summary on procaine for information on a related agent that has been studied.

Key References

None available.

HOMATROPINE

Synonyms

AK-Homatropine, I-Homatrine, Isopto Homatropine

Summary

Homatropine is an anticholinergic agent used in ophthalmic preparations as a mydriatic.

Magnitude of Teratogenic Risk

None To Minimal

Quality and Quantity of Data

Poor

Comment

None

The frequency of congenital anomalies was no greater than expected among the infants of 26 women treated with homatropine during the first four lunar months of pregnancy or of 86 women treated with this drug anytime during pregnancy in the Collaborative Perinatal Project (Heinonen et al., 1977).

No teratology studies of homatropine in experimental animals have been published.

Please see agent summary on atropine for information on a related agent that has been more thoroughly studied.

Key References

Heinonen OP, Slone D, Shapiro S: Birth Defects and Drugs in Pregnancy. Littleton, Mass.: John Wright-PSG, 1977, pp 346, 347, 439, 492. [E]

HUMAN IMMUNODEFICIENCY VIRUS

Synonyms

Acquired Immunodeficiency Syndrome Virus, AIDS, HIV

Summary

Human Immunodeficiency Virus (HIV) is the etiologic agent of AIDS and AIDS-related complex.

Magnitude of Teratogenic Risk

Congenital Infection: Moderate To High

Congenital Anomalies: None To Minimal

Quality and Quantity of Data

Congenital Infection: Excellent

Congenital Anomalies: Fair To Good

Comment

These risk assessments pertain to HIV itself and not to possible teratogenic effects of drugs used to treat HIV infection or its complications.

Many infants have been reported with AIDS symptoms including failure to thrive, interstitial pneumonia, recurrent bacterial and other infections, chronic diarrhea, and generalized lymphadenopathy (Scott et al., 1984; Falloon & Pizzo, 1990; Calvelli & Rubinstein, 1990; Novick, 1990; Abrams & Rogers, 1991). Growth retardation is common, and microcephaly, developmental delay, progressive encephalopathy, and other neurological abnormalities are often seen in HIV-infected children (Ryder et al., 1989; Calvelli & Rubinstein, 1990; Belman, 1990; Abrams & Rogers, 1991; Lepage et al., 1991; Brenneman et al., 1990). Children with AIDS usually die within a few years of diagnosis (Hira et al., 1989; Krasinski et al., 1989; European Collaborative Study, 1991).

Rates of HIV transmission from mother to fetus in various studies average 25-30% (Pizzo & Butler, 1991), but the United States and Europe have lower transmission rates while Africa has higher rates. Vertical transmission may be more likely if the mother's HIV infection is acquired during pregnancy, if she is symptomatic, or if the delivery is premature. Transplacental infection has been unequivocally demonstrated in some cases (Lewis et al., 1990; Lyman et al., 1990; Courgnaud et al., 1991; Ehrnst et al., 1991). First-born twins are infected more frequently than second-born twins, especially if delivered vaginally, suggesting that transmission to the fetus may also occur in the cervix and birth canal during labor (Goedert et al., 1991). Caesarean section may decrease the likelihood of maternal HIV transmission (Italian Multicentre Study, 1988; Blanche et al., 1989; Falloon & Pizzo, 1990; European Collaborative Study, 1992).

The frequency of congenital anomalies was no greater than expected in African cohort studies involving the infants of 466, 271, and 85 HIV-positive pregnant women, respectively (Embree et al., 1989; Ryder et al., 1989; Lepage et al., 1991). In an Italian cohort study, congenital anomalies were no more frequent than expected among the infants of 96 HIV-positive pregnant women, 74 of whom were drug addicts (Semprini et al., 1990).

A subtle dysmorphic syndrome has been described among young children with AIDS (Stevenson, 1986; Marion et al., 1986, 1987; Iosub et al., 1987), but this phenotype appears to reflect the ethnic origin of these children, their chronic illness, their mothers' drug abuse during pregnancy, or other confounding factors rather than a teratogenic effect of HIV (Cordero, 1988; European Collaborative Study, 1988). No difference in the frequency of such minor dysmorphic features was found between 30 children with perinatal HIV infection and 30 uninfected children matched for age, sex, and race in one investigation (Qazi et al., 1988). With the exception of growth retardation, the features of this syndrome were no more frequent among 85 infants of HIV-infected mothers than among the infants of HIV-negative mothers in an African cohort study (Embree et al., 1989). The syndrome was not observed among 600 children born to HIV-infected mothers in the European Collaborative Study (1991).

In utero HIV infection occurred in a chimpanzee born to a female that had been infected experimentally during pregnancy (Eichberg et al., 1988).

Key References

Abrams EJ, Rogers MF: Paediatric HIV infection. Bailliere's Clin Haematol 4(2):333-359, 1991. [R]

Belman AL: Central nervous system involvement in infants and children with symptomatic human immunodeficiency virus infection. Transplacental Disorders (Albany Birth Defects Symposium) 19:207-225, 1990. [S]

Blanche S, Rouzioux C, Guihard Moscato M-L, et al.: A prospective study of infants born to women seropositive for human immunodeficiency virus type 1. N Engl J Med 320:1043-1048, 1989. [E]

Brenneman DE, McCune Sk, Gozes I: Acquired immune deficiency syndrome and the developing nervous system. Int Rev Neurobiol 32:305-353, 1990. [R]

Calvelli TA, Rubinstein A: Pediatric HIV infection: A review. Immunodefic Rev 2(2):83-127, 1990. [R]

Cordero JF: Issues concerning AIDS embryopathy. AJDC 142:9, 1988. [O]

Courgnaud V, Laure F, Brossard A, et al.: Frequent and early in-utero HIV-1 Infection. AIDS Res Hum Retroviruses 7(3):337-341, 1991. [S]

Ehrnst A, Lindgren S, Dictor M, et al.: HIV in pregnant women and their offspring: Evidence for late transmission. Lancet 338:203-207, 1991. [S]

Eichberg JW, Lee DR, Allan JS, et al.: In utero infection of an infant chimpanzee with HIV. N Engl J Med 319:722-723, 1988. [A]

Embree JE, Braddick M, Datta P, et al.: Lack of correlation of maternal human immunodeficiency virus infection with neonatal malformations. Pediatr Infect Dis J 8:700-704, 1989. [E]

European Collaborative Study: Children born to women with HIV-1 infection: Natural history and risk of transmission. Lancet 337(8736):253-260, 1991. [S]

European Collaborative Study: Mother-to-child transmission of HIV infection. Lancet 2:1039-1043, 1988. [S]

European Collaborative Study: Risk factors for mother-to-child transmission of HIV-1. Lancet 339:1007-1012, 1992. [S]

Falloon J, Pizzo PA: Acquired immunodeficiency syndrome in the infant. In: Remington JS, Klein JO (eds). Infectious Diseases of the Fetus and Newborn Infant. Philadelphia: W.B. Saunders Co., 1990, pp. 306-324. [R]

Goedert JJ, Duliege A-M, Amos CI, et al.: High risk of HIV-1 infection for first-born twins. Lancet 338(8781):1471-1475, 1991. [S]

Hira SK, Kamanga J, Bhat GJ, et al.: Perinatal transmission of HIV-I in Zambia. Br Med J 299:1250-1252, 1989. [E]

Iosub S, Bamji M, Stone RK, et al.: More on human immunodeficiency virus embryopathy. Pediatrics 80(4):512-516, 1987. [S]

Italian Multicentre Study: Epidemiology, clinical features, and prognostic factors of paediatric HIV infection. Lancet 2:1043-1046, 1988. [S]

Krasinski K, Borkowsky W, Holzman RS: Prognosis of human immunodeficiency virus infection in children and adolescents. Pediatr Infect Dis J 8:216-220, 1989. [S]

Lepage P, Dabis F, Hitimana D-G, et al.: Perinatal transmission of HIV-1: Lack of impact of maternal HIV infection on characteristics of livebirths and on neonatal mortality in Kigali, Rwanda. AIDS 5:295-300, 1991. [E]

Lewis SH, Reynolds-Kohler C, Fox HE, et al.: HIV-1 in trophoblastic and villous Hofbauer cells, and haematological precursors in eight-week fetuses. Lancet 335:565-568, 1990. [S]

Lyman WD, Kress Y, Kure K, et al.: Detection of HIV in fetal central nervous system tissue. AIDS 4:917-920, 1990. [E]

Marion RW, Wiznia AA, Hutcheon RG, et al.: Fetal AIDS syndrome score. Correlation between severity of dysmorphism and age at diagnosis of immunodeficiency. Am J Dis Child 141:429-431, 1987. [S]

Marion RW, Wiznia AA, Hutcheon RG, et al.: Human T-cell lymphotropic virus Type III (HTLV-III) embryopathy. Am J Dis Child 140:638-640, 1986. [S]

Novick BE: The spectrum of HIV infection in children. Transplacental Disorders (Albany Birth Defects Symposium) 19:191-206, 1990. [R]

Pizzo PA, Butler KM: In the vertical transmission of HIV, timing may be everything. N Engl J Med 325(9):652-654, 1991. [O]

Qazi QH, Sheikh TM, Fikrig S, et al.: Lack of evidence for craniofacial dysmorphism in perinatal human immunodeficiency virus infection. J Pediatr 112(1):7-11, 1988. [E]

Ryder RW, Nsa W, Hassig SE, et al.: Perinatal transmission of the human immunodeficiency virus Type I to infants of seropositive women in Zaire. N Engl J Med 320:1637-1642, 1989. [E]

Scott GB, Buck BE, Leterman JG, et al.: Acquired immunodeficiency syndrome in infants. N Engl J Med 310(2):76-81, 1984. [S]

Semprini AE, Ravizza M, Bucceri A, et al.: Perinatal outcome in HIV-infected pregnant women. Gynecol Obstet Invest 30:15-18, 1990. [E]

Stevenson RE: Prenatal AIDS: A cause of postnatal progressive dysmorphism. Proc Greenwood Genetic Center 5:22-25, 1986. [R]

HYALURONIDASE

Synonyms

Hyason, Hyazyme, Jalovis, Kinaden, Lidase, Mucinase, Penetrase, Wydase

Summary

Hyaluronidase is an enzyme that reduces the viscosity of intracellular matrix. It is used therapeutically to facilitate absorption of fluids or medications administered subcutaneously or intramuscularly.

Magnitude of Teratogenic Risk

Undetermined

Quality and Quantity of Data

None

Comment

None

No epidemiological studies of congenital anomalies among infants born to women treated with hyaluronidase during pregnancy have been reported.

No mammalian teratology studies of hyaluronidase have been published.

Key References

None available.

HYDRALAZINE

Synonyms

Alphapress, Aprelazine, Apresolin, Apressin, Aprezolin, Cloridrato de Hidralazina, Hyperazin, Hyperex

Summary

Hydralazine is a peripheral vasodilator used to treat hypertension.

Magnitude of Teratogenic Risk

Undetermined

Quality and Quantity of Data

None To Poor

Comment

Transient neonatal thrombocytopenia and fetal distress have been reported in infants born to women treated with hydralazine late in pregnancy.

No adequate epidemiological studies of congenital anomalies in infants born to women treated with hydralazine during the first trimester of pregnancy have been reported. The frequency of congenital anomalies was not significantly increased among the children of 136 women treated with hydralazine anytime during pregnancy in the Collaborative Perinatal Project (Heinonen et al., 1977). Only eight of these women were treated during the first four lunar months.

Digital anomalies were observed with increased frequency among the offspring of rabbits treated during pregnancy with 12.5-25 times the human dose of hydralazine (Danielsson et al., 1989).

Fetal distress appears to be more common than expected among hypertensive pregnant women treated with hydralazine near term (Spinnato et al., 1986; Derham & Robinson, 1990; Kirshon et al., 1991). Transient neonatal thrombocytopenia has been noted in three infants born to women treated chronically with hydralazine for hypertension during the third trimester of pregnancy (Widerlov et al., 1980). Thrombocytopenia is a rare side effect of hydralazine therapy in adults, but no causal relationship can be inferred from these anecdotal observations regarding maternal hydralazine treatment and neonatal platelet deficiency.

Key References

Danielsson BRG, Reiland S, Rundqvist E, Danielson M: Digital defects induced by vasodilating agents: Relationship to reduction in uteroplacental blood flow. Teratology 40:351-358, 1989. [A]

Derham RJ, Robinson J: Severe preeclampsia: Is vasodilation therapy with hydralazine dangerous for the preterm fetus? Am J Perinatol 7(3):239-244, 1990. [R]

Heinonen OP, Slone D, Shapiro S: Birth Defects and Drugs in Pregnancy. Littleton, Mass.: John Wright-PSG, 1977, p 441. [E]

Kirshon B, Wasserstrum N, Cotton DB: Should continuous hydralazine infusions be utilized in severe pregnancy-induced hypertension? Am J Perinatol 8(3):206-208, 1991. [S]

Spinnato JA, Sibai BM, Anderson GD: Fetal distress after hydralazine therapy for severe pregnancy-induced hypertension. S Med J 79:559-562, 1986. [S]

Widerlov E, Karlman I, Storsater J: Hydralazine-induced neonatal thrombocytopenia. N Engl J Med 303:1235, 1980. [C]

HYDROCHLORO-THIAZIDE

Synonyms

Chlorzide, Dichlotride, Didral, Diuchlor H, Esidrix, Hydro-Z, HydroDIURIL, Natrimax, Neo-Codema, Novohydrazide, Oretic, Ro-Hydrazide, Thiuretic, Urozide

Summary

Hydrochlorothiazide is a widely used oral diuretic. It is most often employed in the treatment of edema, hypertension, and heart failure.

Magnitude of Teratogenic Risk

None To Minimal

Quality and Quantity of Data

Fair

Comment

Neonatal thrombocytopenia has been observed after maternal use of hydrochlorothiazide late in pregnancy (see below).

No increase in the frequency of congenital anomalies was observed among the infants of 107 women treated with hydrochlorothiazide during the first four lunar months of pregnancy in the Collaborative Perinatal Project or among the infants of between 50 and 99 women treated during the first trimester in the Boston Collaborative Drug Surveillance Program (Heinonen et al., 1977; Jick et al., 1981). Similarly, the frequency of congenital anomalies was no greater than expected among the children of 7575 women treated with hydrochlorothiazide anytime during pregnancy or of 506 women treated during the second half of gestation (Heinonen et al., 1977; Kraus et al., 1966).

No teratogenic effect was observed among the offspring of mice treated during pregnancy with 150-1500 times the usual human dose of hydrochlorothiazide during pregnancy (George

et al., 1984). No malformations were observed among a small group of rats born to animals treated during pregnancy with 125 times the usual human dose of hydrochlorothiazide (Maren & Ellison, 1972).

Neonatal thrombocytopenia has been observed after maternal use of hydrochlorothiazide and similar diuretics late in pregnancy (Rodriguez et al., 1964). The risk of this problem is unknown, but must be small, because symptomatic thrombocytopenia was not observed in any of the offspring of 506 treated pregnancies reported by Kraus et al. (1966).

Key References

George JD, Tyl RW, Price CJ, et al.: Teratologic evaluation of hydrochlorothiazide (CAS No. 58-93-5) administered to CD-1 mice on gestational days 6 through 15--Final Study Report. NTIS (National Technical Information Service) Report/PB 85-103570, 1984. [A]

Heinonen OP, Slone D, Shapiro S: Birth Defects and Drugs in Pregnancy. Littleton, Mass.: John Wright-PSG, 1977, pp 372-373, 441. [E]

Jick H, Holmes LB, Hunter JR, Madsen S, et al.: First-trimester drug use and congenital disorders. JAMA 246:343-346, 1981. [E]

Kraus GW, Marchese JR, Yen SSC: Prophylactic use of hydrochlorothiazide in pregnancy. JAMA 198:1150-1154, 1966. [E]

Maren TH, Ellison AC: The teratological effect of certain thiadiazoles related to acetazolamide, with a note on sulfanilamide and thiazide diuretics. John Hopkins Med J 130:95-104, 1972. [A]

Rodriguez SU, Leikin SL, Hiller MC: Neonatal thrombocytopenia associated with ante-partum administration of thiazide drugs. N Engl J Med 270:881-884, 1964. [S]

HYDROCODONE

Synonyms

Biocodone, Broncodid, Codone, Dicodid, Dihydrocodeinone, Hycon, Hydrokon, Nyodid, Robidone, Solucodan

Summary

Hydrocodone is a synthetic narcotic that is used as an analgesic and cough suppressant.

Magnitude of Teratogenic Risk

None To Minimal

Quality and Quantity of Data

Poor

Comment

None

The frequency of congenital anomalies was no greater than expected among the children of 60 women who took hydrocodone anytime during pregnancy in the Collaborative Perinatal Project; only 12 of these women used the drug in the first four lunar months of gestation (Heinonen et al., 1977).

The frequency of malformations was slightly increased among the offspring of hamsters treated during pregnancy with hydrocodone in a dose 100 times that used in humans (Geber & Schramm, 1975). The relevance of this observation to the use of this drug in human pregnancy is unknown.

Please see agent summary on codeine for information on a related agent that has been more thoroughly studied.

Key References

Geber WF, Schramm LC: Congenital malformations of the central nervous system produced by narcotic analgesics in the hamster. Am J Obstet Gynecol 123:705-713, 1975. [A]

Heinonen OP, Slone D, Shapiro S: Birth Defects and Drugs in Pregnancy. Littleton, Mass.: John Wright-PSG, 1977, pp 287, 434. [E]

HYDROCORTISONE

Synonyms

A-Hydrocort, CaldeCORT, Cetacort, Cortifoam, Cortisol, Efcortesol, Hycort, Hydrocortistab, Hydrocortone, Medicort, Solu-Cortef

Summary

Hydrocortisone is the primary glucocorticoid produced by the adrenal cortex. Hydrocortisone is a potent anti-inflammatory and immunosuppressive agent. It is also used in replacement therapy of adrenal insufficiency.

Magnitude of Teratogenic Risk

None To Minimal

Quality and Quantity of Data

Poor To Fair

Comment

None

The Collaborative Perinatal Project included 21 children whose mothers were treated with hydrocortisone during the first trimester of pregnancy and 74 children whose mothers were treated anytime during gestation (Heinonen et al., 1977). The frequency of congenital anomalies was no greater than expected in either group.

Hydrocortisone administration to pregnant mice and hamsters in doses respectively greater than 6 and 500 times those used clinically regularly produces cleft palate in the offspring (Rogoyski, 1969; Chaudhry & Shah, 1973; Shah & Travill, 1976; Harris, 1980; Roberts & Hendrickx, 1987). Typical stage-of-gestation and dose-dependence of the teratogenic effect has been demonstrated in hamsters. No malformations were seen with lower doses in some studies. The relevance of these observations to therapeutic use of hydrocortisone in human pregnancy is unknown.

Please see agent summary on prednisone for information on a related agent that has been more thoroughly studied.

Key References

Chaudhry AP, Shah RM: Estimation of hydrocortisone dose and optimal gestation period for cleft palate induction in golden hamsters. Teratology 8:139-142, 1973. [A]

Harris SB, Szczech GM, Stuckhardt JL, Kiley K, et al.: Evaluation of the Upj:TUC(ICR) strain of mice for use in teratology tests. J Toxicol Environ Health 6:155-165, 1980. [A]

Heinonen OP, Slone D, Shapiro S: Birth Defects and Drugs in Pregnancy. Littleton, Mass.: John-Wright-PSG, 1977, pp 389, 391, 443. [E]

Roberts LG, Hendrickx AG: Hydrocortisone-induced embryotoxicity and embryonic drug disposition in H-2 congenic mice. J Craniofac Genet Dev Biol 7:341-356, 1987. [A]

Rogoyski A: The influence of dianabol on fetuses in pregnant mice subjected to fasting or fasting and simultaneous damaging action of hydrocortisone acetate. Folia Morphologica 28:502-509, 1969. [A]

Shah RM, Travill AA: The teratogenic effects of hydrocortisone on palatal development in the hamster. J Embryol Exp Morphol 35:213-224, 1976. [A]

HYDROFLUMETHIAZIDE

Synonyms

Diucardin, Hydrenox, Saluron

Summary

Hydroflumethiazide is a thiazide diuretic and antihypertensive agent that is administered orally.

Magnitude of Teratogenic Risk

Undetermined

Quality and Quantity of Data

None

Comment

None

No epidemiological studies of congenital anomalies among the infants of women treated with hydroflumethiazide during pregnancy have been reported.

No animal teratology studies of hydroflumethiazide have been published.

Please see agent summary on chlorothiazide for information on a related agent that has been studied.

Key References

None available.

HYDROGEN PEROXIDE

Synonyms

Hioxyl, Hydrogen Dioxide, Peroxyl

Summary

Hydrogen peroxide is a strong oxidizing agent. Dilute solutions of hydrogen peroxide are used topically as disinfectants and deodorants. Hydrogen peroxide has many other uses: as a rocket fuel; in the chemical, plastics, textile, dye, and photographic industries; and in hair colorings. The 8-hour time-weighted average occupational exposure limit for hydrogen peroxide is 1 ppm (ACGIH, 1991).

Magnitude of Teratogenic Risk

Undetermined

Quality and Quantity of Data

Poor

Comment

A small risk cannot be excluded, but a high risk of congenital anomalies in the children of women

treated with hydrogen peroxide during pregnancy is unlikely.

No epidemiological studies of congenital anomalies among infants born to women exposed to large amounts of hydrogen peroxide during pregnancy have been reported.

No teratogenic effect was seen among the offspring of pregnant rats fed diets containing 0.02-2% hydrogen peroxide (Moriyama et al., 1982a, b). Decreased fetal and maternal weight were observed with diets containing 10% hydrogen peroxide. No teratogenic effect was found in rats treated with repeated cutaneous applications of hair dyes containing 3% hydrogen peroxide during pregnancy (Burnett et al., 1976).

Key References

ACGIH: 1991-1992 Threshold Limit Values for Chemical Substances and Physical Agents and Biological Exposure Indices. Cincinnati, Ohio: Am Conference Govt Ind Hyg, 1991, p 23. [O]

Burnett C, Goldenthal EI, Harris SB, Wazeter FX, et al.: Teratology and percutaneous toxicity studies on hair dyes. J Toxicol Environ Health 1:1027-1040, 1976. [A]

Moriyama I, Fujita M, Hiraoka K, Ichijo M, et al.: Effects of the food additive hydrogen peroxide on fetal development. Teratology 26(1):28A, 1982a. [A]

Moriyama I, Hiraoka K, Fujita M, Ichijo M, et al.: Effects of food additive hydrogen peroxide studied in fetal development. Acta Obstet Gynaecol Jpn 34:2149-2154, 1982b. [A]

HYDROMORPHONE

Synonyms

Dihydromorphinone, Dilaudid, Hidromorfona, Idromorfone, Laudicon

Summary

Hydromorphone is a narcotic that is used to alleviate pain and as a cough suppressant.

Magnitude of Teratogenic Risk

None To Minimal

Quality and Quantity of Data

Poor To Fair

Comment

None

The frequency of congenital anomalies was no greater than expected among the children of 61 women treated with hydromorphone anytime during pregnancy in the Collaborative Perinatal Project (Heinonen et al., 1977). Only 12 of these women were treated during the first four lunar months of gestation.

Increased frequencies of central nervous system and other malformations were observed among the offspring of hamsters treated with 40-540 but not 29 times the usual dose of hydromorphone during pregnancy (Geber & Schramm, 1975). Slightly increased frequencies of soft tissue anomalies (primarily undescended testes) and of skeletal variants were observed among the offspring of pregnant mice treated with continuous hydromorphone infusion in a daily dose 31-62 times that used in humans (Behm et al., 1985). Similar defects were seen after single administrations 10 times the human daily dose of hydromorphone. The relevance of these findings to the therapeutic use of hydromorphone in human pregnancy is unknown.

Symptoms of neonatal narcotic withdrawal including irritability, vomiting, and diarrhea have been reported in a child born to a woman who took hydromorphone in large doses throughout pregnancy (Cary, 1972).

Please see agent summary on heroin for information on a related agent that has been more thoroughly studied.

Key References

Behm MC, Stout-Caputi MV, Mahalik MP, et al.: Evaluation of the teratogenic potential of hydromorphone administered via a miniature implantable pump in mice. Res Commun Subst Abuse 6:165-177, 1985. [A]

Cary W: "Cold turkey" in the newborn. Med J Aust 1:361-363, 1972. [C]

Geber WF, Schramm LC: Congenital malformations of the central nervous system produced by narcotic analgesics in the hamster. Am J Obstet Gynecol 123(7):705-713, 1975. [A]

Heinonen OP, Slone D, Shapiro S: Birth Defects and Drugs in Pregnancy. Littleton, Mass.: John Wright-PSG, 1977, pp 287, 434. [E]

HYDROQUINONE

Synonyms

Benzoquinol, Eldopaque, Eldoquin, Phiaquin, Tecquinol, Tequinol

Summary

Hydroquinone is a derivative of benzene that is used in dermal and hair preparations to lighten color. Hydroquinone is also used industrially, especially in photographic developing.

Magnitude of Teratogenic Risk

Undetermined

Quality and Quantity of Data

None To Poor

Comment

A small risk cannot be excluded, but a high risk of congenital anomalies in the children of women who use dermal or hair preparations containing hydroquinone during pregnancy is unlikely.

No epidemiological studies of congenital anomalies among infants born to women treated with hydroquinone during pregnancy have been reported.

The frequency of malformations was not increased among the offspring of pregnant rats fed 15-300 mg/kg/d of hydroquinone (Blacker et al., 1991; Krasavage et al., 1991). Maternal toxicity and decreased fetal weight were noted at the highest dose. The frequency of fetal death was increased among rats fed 500 mg of hydroquinone during pregnancy (Telford et al., 1962). The frequency of malformations was not increased among the offspring of rabbits fed up to 150 mg/kg/d of hydroquinone, although maternal toxicity occurred in animals given 75 mg/kg or more per day (Murphy et al., 1991).

Key References

Blacker Am, Schroeder RE, English JC, et al.: A two-generation reproduction study with hydroquinone (HQ) in rats. Teratology 43(5):429, 1991. [A]

Krasavage WJ, Blacker AM, English JC, Murphy SJ: Hydroquinone: A developmental toxicity study in rats. Toxicologist 11(1):342, 1991. [A]

Murphy SJ, Schroeder RE, Blacker AM, et al.: Study of developmental toxicity of hydroquinone (HQ) in the rabbit. Toxicologist 11(1):343, 1991. [A]

Telford IR, Woodruff CS, Linford RH: Fetal resorption in the rat as influenced by certain antioxidants. Am J Anatomy 110:29-36, 1962. [A]

HYDROXOCOBALAMIN

Synonyms

AlphaRedisol, Hydrovit, Neo-Betalin, Neo-Cytamen, Vitamin B$_{12a}$

Summary

Hydroxocobalamin is an analogue of vitamin B-12 administered parenterally in the treatment of pernicious anemia and other vitamin B-12 deficiency states.

Magnitude of Teratogenic Risk

Undetermined

Quality and Quantity of Data

None

Comment

A small risk cannot be excluded, but a high risk of congenital anomalies in the children of women treated with hydroxocobalamin during pregnancy is unlikely.

No epidemiological studies of congenital anomalies in infants whose mothers were treated with hydroxocobalamin during pregnancy have been reported.

No teratogenic effect was observed among the offspring of mice treated during pregnancy with hydroxocobalamin in doses of 3000-12,000 times those used therapeutically in humans (Mitala et al., 1978).

Key References

Mitala JJ, Mann DE Jr, Gautieri RF: Influence of cobalt (dietary), cobalamins, and inorganic cobalt salts on phenytoin- and cortisone-induced teratogenesis in mice. J Pharmaceut Sci 67(3):377-380, 1978. [A]

HYDROXYAMPHETA-MINE

Summary

Hydroxyamphetamine is a sympathomimetic agent that is used topically as a mydriatic.

Magnitude of Teratogenic Risk

Undetermined

Quality and Quantity of Data

None To Poor

Comment

None

No epidemiological studies of congenital anomalies in infants whose mothers were treated with hydroxyamphetamine during pregnancy have been reported.

Mice treated systemically with 50-100 mg/kg/d of hydroxyamphetamine during pregnancy delivered "well formed but dead pups" in one study that has been reported as an abstract (Buttar et al., 1991).

Please see agent summary on ephedrine for information on a related agent that has been more thoroughly studied.

Key References

Buttar HS, Foster BC, Moffatt JH, Bura C: Developmental toxicity of 4-substituted amphetamines in mice. Teratology 43(5):434, 1991. [A]

HYDROXYCHLORO-QUINE

Synonyms

Plaquenil

Summary

Hydroxychloroquine is a 4-aminoquinoline compound that is used to treat malaria, systemic lupus erythematosus, and rheumatoid arthritis.

Magnitude of Teratogenic Risk

Undetermined

Quality and Quantity of Data

None

No epidemiological studies of congenital anomalies among the children of women treated with hydroxychloroquine during pregnancy have been reported.

No animal teratology studies of hydroxychloroquine have been published.

Please see agent summary on chloroquine for information on a related agent that has been studied.

Key References

None available.

HYDROXYDIONE

Synonyms

Viadril G

Summary

Hydroxydione is a steroid that has been used intravenously as a general anesthetic.

Magnitude of Teratogenic Risk

Undetermined

Quality and Quantity of Data

None

Comment

None

No epidemiological studies of congenital anomalies in children born to women exposed to hydroxydione during pregnancy have been reported.

No studies of teratologic effects of hydroxydione in experimental animals have been published.

Key References

None available.

HYDROXYETHYL-CELLULOSE

Synonyms

Cellobond HEC, Comfort Tears, Gelaser, Lyteers, Natrosol, Neo-Tears

Summary

Hydroxyethylcellulose is an emulsifying agent.

Magnitude of Teratogenic Risk

None

Quality and Quantity of Data

None To Poor

Comment

None

No epidemiological studies of congenital anomalies in infants born to women exposed to hydroxyethylcellulose during pregnancy have been reported.

The frequency of congenital anomalies was not significantly increased among the offspring of mice given intraperitoneal injections of 100-400 mg/kg of hydroxyethylcellulose during pregnancy (Guttner et al., 1980).

Key References

Guttner J, Klaus S, Heinecke H: Embryotoxicity of intraperitoneally administered hydroxyethylcellulose in mice. Anat Anz 149:282-285, 1980. [A]

HYDROXYPROPYL CELLULOSE

Synonyms

Klucel, Lacrisert

Summary

Hydroxypropyl cellulose is used as a stabilizer and coating agent in a variety of medicines. It is also employed in ophthalmic preparations to treat dry eyes.

Magnitude of Teratogenic Risk

None To Minimal

Quality and Quantity of Data

None To Poor

Comment

A small risk cannot be excluded, but a high risk of congenital anomalies in the children of women treated with hydroxypropyl cellulose during pregnancy is unlikely.

No epidemiological studies of congenital anomalies among infants born to women who took preparations containing hydroxypropyl cellulose during pregnancy have been reported.

The frequency of malformations was no greater than expected among the offspring of rabbits or rats fed hydroxypropyl cellulose during pregnancy in doses 8-200 times the WHO acceptable daily intake for humans (Kitagawa et al., 1978a, b).

Key References

Kitagawa H, Satoh T, Saito H, Katoh, et al.: Teratological study of hydroxypropylcellulose of low substitution (L-HPC) in rabbits. Oyo Yakuri (Pharmakometrics) 16:259-269, 1978a. [A]

Kitagawa H, Satoh T, Saito H, Katoh, et al.: Teratological study of hydroxypropylcellulose of low substitution (L-HPC) in rats. Oyo Yakuri (Pharmakometrics) 16:271-278, 1978b. [A]

HYDROXYUREA

Synonyms

Hydreia, Hydroxycarbamine, Litaler, Onco-Carbide

Summary

Hydroxyurea is administered orally in the treatment of malignant neoplasms. It acts by interfering with synthesis of DNA.

Magnitude of Teratogenic Risk

Undetermined

Quality and Quantity of Data

Poor To Fair

Comment

Although the risk of congenital anomalies in the children of women treated with hydroxyurea during pregnancy is unknown, it may be substantial because hydroxyurea inhibits DNA synthesis.

No epidemiological studies of congenital anomalies among the infants of women treated with hydroxyurea during pregnancy have been reported.

Hydroxyurea is teratogenic in experimental animals when administered in doses greater than those used clinically. Fetal death, fetal growth retardation, and increased frequencies of malformations of the central nervous system, eyes, heart, face, and limbs have been observed among the offspring of rats treated during pregnancy with 5-67 times the usual human dose of hydroxyurea (Murphy & Chaube, 1964; Chaube & Murphy, 1966; Wilson et al., 1975; Brunner et al., 1978; Aliverti et al., 1980; Barr & Beaudoin, 1981). Typical dependence of the teratogenic effect on dose and time of gestation have been demonstrated. Behavioral alterations have been observed among the offspring of rats treated during pregnancy with 12-67 times the usual human dose of hydroxyurea (Butcher et al., 1973, 1975; Brunner et al., 1979; Adlard et al., 1975; Vorhees et al., 1979). Studies in other species have been more limited, but increased frequencies of congenital anomalies have been reported among the offspring of rhesus monkeys, dogs, cats, rabbits, hamsters, and mice treated during pregnancy with hydroxyurea in doses 2-25 times those used in humans (Wilson, 1974; Earl et al., 1972; Ferm, 1966; DeSesso et al., 1977, 1990; Khera, 1979; Warner et al., 1983). Fetal growth retardation and a variety of congenital anomalies are seen in each species. Defects of the central nervous system, eyes, face, and limbs often occur.

Key References

Adlard BPF, Dobbing J: Maze learning by adult rats after inhibition of neuronal multiplication in utero. Pediat Res 9:139-142, 1975. [A]

Aliverti V, Bonanomi L, Giavini E: Hydroxyurea as a reference standard in teratological screening: Comparison of the embryotoxic and teratogenic effects following single intraperitoneal or repeated oral administrations to pregnant rats. Arch Toxicol Suppl 4:239-247, 1980. [A]

Barr Jr M, Beaudoin AR: An exploration of the role of hydroxyurea injection time in fetal growth and teratogenesis in rats. Teratology 24:163-167, 1981. [A]

Brunner RL, McLean M, Vorhees CV, Butcher RE: A comparison of behavioral and anatomical measures of hydroxyurea induced abnormalities. Teratology 18:379-384, 1978. [A]

Brunner RL, Vorhees CV, Kinney L, Butcher RE: Aspartame: Assessment of developmental psychotoxicity of a new artificial sweetener. Neurobehav Toxicol 1:79-86, 1979. [A]

Butcher RE, Scott WJ, Kazmaier K, Ritter EJ: Postnatal effects in rats of prenatal treatment with hydroxyurea. Teratology 7:161-166, 1973. [A]

Butcher RE, Hawver K, Kazmaier K, Scott W: Postnatal behavioral effects from prenatal exposure to teratogens. In: Marselli PL, Garattini S, Sereni F (eds). Basic and Therapeutic Aspects of Perinatal Pharmacology. New York: Raven Press, 1975, pp 171-176. [A]

Chaube S, Murphy ML: The effects of hydroxyurea and related compounds on the rat fetus. Cancer Res 26(1):1448-1457, 1966. [A]

DeSesso JM, Goeringer GC: Ethoxyquin and nordihydroguaiaretic acid reduce hydroxyurea developmental toxicity. Reprod Toxicol 4:267-275, 1990. [A]

DeSesso JM, Jordan RL: Drug-induced limb dysplasias in fetal rabbits. Teratology 15:199-212, 1977. [A]

Earl FL, Miller E, Van Loon EJ: Teratogenic research in beagle dogs and miniature swine. Lab Anim Drug Test Symp Int Comm Lab Anim 5:233-247, 1972. [A]

Ferm VH: Severe developmental malformations. Arch Path 81:174-177, 1966. [A]

Khera KS: A teratogenicity study on hydroxyurea and diphenylhydantoin in cats. Teratology 20:447-452, 1979. [A]

Murphy ML, Chaube S: Preliminary survey of hydroxyurea (NSC-32065) as a teratogen. Cancer Chemother Rep 40:1-7, 1964. [A]

Vorhees CV, Butcher RE, Brunner RL, Sobotka TJ: A developmental test battery for neurobehavioral toxicity in rats: A preliminary analysis using monosodium glutamate calcium carrageenan, and hydroxyurea. Toxicol Appl Pharmacol 50:267-282, 1979. [A]

Warner CW, Sadler TW, Shockey J, Smith MK: A comparison of the in vivo and in vitro response mammalian embryos to a teratogenic insult. Toxicology 28:271-282, 1983. [A]

Wilson JG: Teratologic causation in man and its evaluation in non-human primates. Excerpta Med Int Congr Ser 310:191-203, 1974. [A]

Wilson JG, Scott WJ, Ritter RJ, Fradkin R: Comparative distribution and embryotoxicity of hydroxyurea in pregnant rats and rhesus monkeys. Teratology 11:169-178, 1975. [A]

HYDROXYZINE

Synonyms

Atarax, Durrax, Multipax, Orgatrax, Pamazone, Quiess, Vistaril

Summary

Hydroxyzine is a piperazine antihistaminic agent. It is used as an anxiolytic, sedative, antipuritic, and antiemetic.

Magnitude of Teratogenic Risk

None To Minimal

Quality and Quantity of Data

Poor To Fair

Comment

None

The frequency of congenital anomalies was no greater than expected among the infants of 50 women treated with hydroxyzine during the first four lunar months of pregnancy or among the infants of 187 women so treated anytime during pregnancy in the Collaborative Perinatal Project (Heinonen et al., 1977). In a double-blind controlled trial of hydroxyzine treatment of gestational nausea and vomiting, the frequency of congenital anomalies was no greater than expected among 74 infants born to mothers who took hydroxyzine during the first two months of pregnancy (Erez et al., 1971).

The frequencies of fetal death and craniofacial and skeletal malformations were increased in a dose-dependent fashion among the offspring of rats treated with 8-25 but not 3-6 times the dose of hydroxyzine used in humans (King & Howell, 1966; Giurgea & Puigdevall, 1968).

Key References

Erez S, Schifrin BS, Dirim O: Double-blind evaluation of hydroxyzine as an antiemetic in pregnancy. J Reprod Med 7:35-37, 1971. [S]

Giurgia M, Puigdevall J: Maternal and foetal toxicity of some diphenylmethane piperazine derivatives. Proc Eur Soc Study Drug Toxic 9:134-143, 1968. [A]

Heinonen OP, Slone D, Shapiro S: Birth Defects and Drugs in Pregnancy. Littleton, Mass.: John Wright-PSG, 1977, pp 335-337, 438. [E]

King CTG, Howell J: Teratogenic effect of buclizine and hydroxyzine in the rat and chlorcyclizine in the mouse. Am J Obstet Gynecol 95:109-111, 1966. [A]

HYOSCYAMINE

Synonyms

Anaspaz, Cystospaz, Egazil, Levsin, Levsinex, Peptard

Summary

Hyoscyamine is an anticholinergic agent with central and peripheral action. It is used in gastrointestinal disorders, bronchial asthma, and whooping cough for its antispasmodic effects.

Magnitude of Teratogenic Risk

None

Quality and Quantity of Data

Fair

Comment

None

The frequencies of congenital anomalies, of major malformations, and of minor anomalies were no greater than expected among the children of 322 women treated with hyoscyamine during the first four lunar months of pregnancy in the Collaborative Perinatal Project (Heinonen et al., 1977). The frequency of congenital anomalies was not increased among the infants of 1067 women treated anytime during pregnancy in this study.

No experimental animal studies of the teratogenicity of hyoscyamine have been published.

Key References

Heinonen OP, Slone D, Shapiro S: Birth Defects and Drugs in Pregnancy. Littleton, Mass.: John-Wright-PSG, 1977, pp 346-347, 439. [E]

IBUPROFEN

Synonyms

Advil, Amersol, Haltran, Medipren, Motrin, Nuprin, Rufen, Trendar

Summary

Ibuprofen is an oral nonsteroidal anti-inflammatory agent that has analgesic and antipyretic actions.

Magnitude of Teratogenic Risk

None To Minimal

Quality and Quantity of Data

Poor To Fair

Comment

None

The frequency of congenital anomalies was no greater than expected among 51 infants whose mothers took ibuprofen during the first trimester of pregnancy in the Boston Collaborative Drug Surveillance Program (Aselton et al., 1985). The frequency and nature of anomalies was not unusual among the children of a small group of women who took ibuprofen at various times and at various doses during their pregnancies and whose experience was voluntarily reported to one manufacturer (Barry et al., 1984).

No teratogenic effect was observed among the offspring of rats and rabbits treated during pregnancy with ibuprofen in doses equivalent to or several times larger than those used in humans (Adams et al., 1969; Ono et al., 1982). Similarly, no teratogenic effect was observed among the offspring of pregnant mice treated with 390 times the human therapeutic dose of ibuprofen (Randall et al., 1991).

Ibuprofen is an inhibitor of prostaglandin synthesis. This class of drugs has been used therapeutically to produce closure of the ductus arteriosus and consequent changes in cardiovascular and pulmonary function in newborns with patent ductus arteriosus. Ibuprofen administration to near-term pregnant rats in doses similar to those used in humans has been shown to cause premature (in utero) closure of the ductus arteriosus in the fetuses (Momma & Takeuchi, 1983; Momma & Takao, 1990). The risk of a similar occurrence in humans after maternal exposure to ibuprofen late in pregnancy is unknown.

Several prostaglandin inhibitors, including ibuprofen, have been used as tocolytic agents in women with premature labor. The development of oligohydramnios has been associated with maternal ibuprofen treatment in such patients (Hendricks et al., 1990; Wiggins & Elliott, 1990).

Key References

Adams SS, Bough RG, Cliffe EE, Lessel B, et al.: Absorption, distribution and toxicity of ibuprofen. Toxicol Appl Pharmacol 15:310-330, 1969. [A]

Aselton P, Jick H, Milunsky A, Hunter JR, et al.: First-trimester drug use and congenital disorders. Obstet Gynecol 65:451-455, 1985. [S]

Barry WS, Meinzinger MM, Howse CR: Ibuprofen overdose and exposure in utero: Results from a postmarketing voluntary reporting system. Am J Med 77(1A):35-39, 1984. [S]

Hendricks SK, Smith JR, Moore DE, Brown ZA: Oligohydramnios associated with prostaglandin synthetase inhibitors in preterm labour. Br J Obstet Gynaecol 97:312-316, 1990. [E]

Momma K, Takao A: Transplacental cardiovascular effects of four popular analgesics in rats. Am J Obstet Gynecol 162(5):1304-1310, 1990. [A]

Momma K, Takeuchi H: Constriction of fetal ductus arteriosus by non-steroidal anti-inflammatory drugs. Prostaglandins 26:631-643, 1983. [A]

Ono M, Hoshida F, Nagase M, Asami K: Reproductive studies of ibuprofen by rectal administration (2). Teratogenicity study in rats. Oyo Yakuri 24:531-538, 1982. [A]

Powell JG, Cochrane RL: The effects of a number of non-steroidal anti-inflammatory compounds on parturition in the rat. Prostaglandins 23:469-488, 1982. [A]

Randall CL, Becker HC, Anton RF: Effect of ibuprofen on alcohol-induced teratogenesis in mice. Alcohol Clin Exp Res 15(4):673-677, 1991. [A]

Wiggins DA, Elliott JP: Oligohydramnios in each sac of a triplet gestation caused by Motrin - fulfilling Kock's postulates. Am J Obstet Gynecol 162:460-461; 1990. [C]

ICHTHAMMOL

Synonyms

Adnexol, Bitamon, Ichthalon, Ichthyol, Poudre Velours, Subitol

Summary

Ichthammol is a mild antiseptic agent used topically to treat skin disorders.

Magnitude of Teratogenic Risk

Undetermined

Quality and Quantity of Data

None

Comment

None

No epidemiological studies of congenital anomalies in infants whose mothers were treated with ichthammol during pregnancy have been reported.

No animal teratology studies of ichthammol have been published.

Key References

None available.

IDOXURIDINE

Synonyms

Cheratil, Herplex, Idoxene, Kerecid, Ophthalmadine, Stoxil

Summary

Idoxuridine is a DNA synthesis inhibitor that is used topically in the treatment of viral infections.

Magnitude of Teratogenic Risk

Undetermined

Quality and Quantity of Data

Poor

Comment

Although the risk of idoxuridine is undetermined, it may be substantial because it is a DNA synthesis inhibitor.

No epidemiological studies of congenital anomalies among the infants of women treated with idoxuridine during pregnancy have been reported.

Increased frequencies of central nervous system, palatal, and skeletal malformations were observed among the offspring of mice given extremely large doses of idoxuridine parenterally during pregnancy (Skalko & Packard, 1972). Typical dose and time dependence of this teratogenic effect were seen. Histological abnormalities of the brain and kidney were found among the offspring of rats and mice that received similar treatments late in pregnancy after embryogenesis was complete (Percy, 1975). Of most concern, however, is the observation that eye and skeletal malformations and fetal death occurred with increased frequency among the offspring of pregnant rabbits that had been administered idoxuridine solution topically to the eye in doses similar to those used in humans (Itoi et al., 1975).

Key References

Itoi M, Gefter JW, Kaneko N, Ishii U, et al.: Teratogenicities of ophthalmic drugs. I. Antiviral ophthalmic drugs. Arch Ophthalmol 93:46-51, 1975. [A]

Percy DH: Teratogenic effects of the pyrimidine analogues 5-iododeoxyuridine and cytosine arabinoside in late fetal mice and rats. Teratology 11:103-118, 1975. [A]

Skalko RG, Jacobs DA, Schottland J, McNee M: The ability of halogenated pyrimidines to produce cell death, inhibit DNA synthesis, and be embryotoxic agents in the mouse. Teratology 13:37A-38A, 1976. [A]

IMIPENEM

Synonyms

Imipemide, MK 0787, N-Formimidoylthien-amycin

Summary

Imipenem is a thienamycin antibiotic that is administered intravenously to treat serious infection.

Magnitude of Teratogenic Risk

Undetermined

Quality and Quantity of Data

None

Comment

None

No epidemiological studies of congenital anomalies in infants born to women treated with imipenem during pregnancy have been reported.

No animal teratology studies of imipenem have been published.

Key References

None available.

IMIPRAMINE

Synonyms

Antipress, Impril, Janimine, Novopramine, Praminil, Tofranil

Summary

Imipramine is a tricyclic antidepressant that has strong anticholinergic activity. It is used in the treatment of endogenous depression.

Magnitude of Teratogenic Risk

None To Minimal

Quality and Quantity of Data

Poor To Fair

Comment

None

Available studies of congenital anomalies among children born to women who used imipramine during the first trimester of pregnancy include too few cases to permit firm conclusions to be drawn (Scanlon, 1969; Banister et al., 1972; Crombie et al., 1972; Kuenssberg & Knox, 1972; Rachelefsky et al., 1972; Idanpaan-Heikkila & Saxen, 1973; Heinonen et al., 1977). None of these investigations includes more than 20 exposed pregnancies, but there is no indication of a major teratogenic effect. The suggestion, based on anecdotal observations, that maternal use of imipramine during pregnancy is associated with limb reduction defects in infants is probably incorrect (Morrow, 1972).

No malformations were observed among the offspring of 17 bonnet monkeys treated during pregnancy with imipramine in doses 7-70 times those used in humans (Hendrickx, 1975). Growth retardation and vertebral anomalies were observed among the offspring of a few rhesus monkeys treated during pregnancy with 4-5, but not 1-3, times the human dose of imipramine (Wilson, 1974). Increased frequencies of central nervous system and other malformations were observed among the offspring of mice, rabbits, and hamsters treated during pregnancy with imipramine in doses 31, 10, and 9-28 times those used in humans (Harper et al., 1965; Jurand, 1980; Guram et al., 1980). No increase in malformations was seen with lower doses in mice, rats, or rabbits (Harper et al., 1965; Larsen, 1963; Aoyama et al., 1970). Behavioral and developmental alterations have been reported among the offspring of rats treated with 1-5 times the usual human dose of imipramine during pregnancy (Coyle et al., 1975; Jason et al., 1981; Ali et al., 1986). The relevance of these observations to the therapeutic use of imipramine in human pregnancy is unknown.

Transient abnormalities of neonatal respiratory, circulatory, and neurological adaptation have been observed in three infants whose mothers had taken imipramine during pregnancy (Eggermont et al., 1972).

Key References

Ali SF, Buelke-Sam J, Newport GD, Slikker W: Early neurobehavioral and neurochemical alterations in rats prenatally exposed to imipramine. Neurotoxicol 7:365-380, 1986. [A]

Aoyama J, Nakai K, Ogura M, et al.: Acute toxicity and teratological studies on dimetacrine (Istonyl) in mice and rats. Oyo Yakuri (Pharmacometrics) 4:855-869, 1970. [A]

Banister P, Dafoe C, Smith ESO, Miller J: Possible teratogenicity of tricyclic antidepressants. Lancet 1:838-839, 1972. [E]

Coyle IR: Changes in developing behavior following prenatal administration of imipramine. Pharmacol Biochem Behav 3:799-807, 1975. [A]

Crombie DL, Pinsent RJFH, Fleming D: Imipramine in pregnancy. Br Med J 1:745, 1972. [E]

Eggermont E, Raveschot J, Deneve V, Casteels-Van Daele M: The adverse influence of imipramine on the adaptation of the newborn infant to extrauterine life. Acta Paediatr Belg 26:197-204, 1972. [C]

Guram MK, Gill TS, Geber WF: Teratogenicity of imipramine and amitriptyline in fetal hamsters. Res Commun Psychol Psychiatr Behav 5:275-282, 1980. [A]

Harper KH, Palmer AK, Davies RE: Effect of imipramine upon the pregnancy of laboratory animals. Arzneimittelforsch 15:1218-1221, 1965. [A]

Heinonen OP, Slone D, Shapiro S: Birth Defects and Drugs in Pregnancy. Littleton, Mass.: John Wright-PSG, 1977, p 336. [E]

Hendrickx AG: Teratologic evaluation of imipramine gydrochloride in bonnet (Macaca radiata) and rhesus monkeys (Macaca mulatta). Teratology 11:219-222, 1975. [A]

Idanpaan-Heikkila J, Saxen L: Possible teratogenicity of imipramine/chloropyramine. Lancet 2:282-284, 1973. [E]

Jason KM, Cooper TB, Friedman E: Prenatal exposure to imipramine alters early behavioral development and beta adrenergic receptors in rats. J Pharmacol Exp Ther 217:461-466, 1981. [A]

Jurand A: Malformations of the central nervous system induced by neurotropic drugs in mouse embryos. Dev Growth Differ 22:61-78, 1980. [A]

Kuenssberg EV, Knox JDE: Imipramine in pregnancy. Br Med J 2:292, 1972. [E]

Larsen V: The teratogenic effects of thalidomide, imipramine HCl and imipramine-N-oxide HCl on white Danish rabbits. Acta Pharmacol Toxicol 20:186-200, 1963. [A]

Morrow AW: Imipramine and congenital abnormalities. [Letter to the Editor.] N Zeal Med J 75:228-229, 1972. [O]

Rachelefsky GS, Flynt JW, Ebbin AJ, Wilson MG: Possible teratogenicity of tricyclic antidepressants. Lancet 1:838, 1972. [E]

Scanlon FJ: Use of antidepressant drugs during the first trimester. Med J Aust 2:1077, 1969. [S]

Wilson JG: Teratologic causation in man and its evaluation in non-human primates. Excerpta Med Int Congr Ser 310:191-203, 1974. [R]

INDOMETHACIN

Synonyms

Imbrilon, Indocin, Indoflex, Indolar, Indometacin, Indomod, Mobilan

Summary

Indomethacin is a prostaglandin synthetase inhibitor that is used as an analgesic, anti-inflammatory, and antipyretic agent. Indomethacin has also been used to arrest premature labor and to treat polyhydramnios.

Magnitude of Teratogenic Risk

Malformations: None To Minimal

Premature Closure Of The Ductus Arteriosus: Small To Moderate

Quality and Quantity of Data

Malformations: Poor To Fair

Premature Closure Of The Ductus Arteriosus: Fair To Good

Comment

Maternal treatment with indomethacin late in pregnancy may be associated with the development of fetal anuria, oligohydramnios, premature closure of the ductus arteriosus, and consequent problems in perinatal adaptation (see below).

In one cohort study of the offspring of 50 women who had been treated with indomethacin during the first trimester of pregnancy, the frequency of malformations was no greater than expected (Aselton et al., 1985).

Indomethacin may cause premature closure of the ductus arteriosus and persistent pulmonary hypertension (Manchester et al., 1976; Levin et al., 1978; Istkovitz et al., 1980; Mogilner et al., 1982; De Wit et al., 1988; van der Heijden et al., 1988b; Besinger et al., 1991). Indomethacin is used to induce closure of the ductus in premature infants (Douidar et al., 1988), and similar pharmacologic mechanisms are presumed to operate prenatally. Transient constriction of the fetal ductus arteriosus has been demonstrated by serial fetal echocardiography in women treated with indomethacin late in pregnancy (Moise et al., 1988; Mari et al., 1989; Kirshon et al., 1990a, 1990b; Eronen et al., 1991). Several perinatal deaths have been reported in the infants of women treated with indomethacin just prior to delivery (Levin et al., 1978; Rubaltelli et al., 1979; Itskovitz et al., 1980), but the occurrence of such events was not unusually frequent in clinical series of 30-170 infants born after maternal treatment with indomethacin (Atad et al., 1980; Dudley et al., 1985; Niebyl & Witter, 1986; Morales et al., 1989; Baerts et al., 1990; Gerson et al., 1990). In one series, hypoxic-ischemic cerebral lesions were more severe, but not more common, among small premature infants whose mothers had received indomethacin tocolysis (Baerts et al., 1990).

Fetal urinary output and amniotic fluid volume are decreased in women who are treated with indomethacin in the second or third trimester of pregnancy (Kirshon et al., 1988, 1990a; Lange et al., 1989; Hendricks et al., 1990; Kirshon et al., 1991; Uslu et al., 1992; Wiggins & Elliott, 1990). Oligohydramnios may occur as a result. The effect is usually reversible when therapy is stopped, but persistent renal dysfunction has been observed in infants born to women treated with indomethacin late in pregnancy (van der Heijden et al., 1988a, b; Vanhaesebrouck et al., 1988). Decreased renal function is a recognized complication of indomethacin therapy in premature infants (Douidar et al., 1988; Gal et al., 1990). Maternal indomethacin treatment has been used to decrease polyhydramnios (Lange et al., 1989; Kirshon et al., 1990a; Mamopoulos et al., 1990; Moise, 1991).

Uterine contractions can be reduced and parturition delayed by indomethacin treatment of women with premature labor in the late second or third trimester of pregnancy

(Zuckerman et al., 1974; Reiss et al., 1976; Grella & Zanor, 1978; van Kets et al., 1979; Morales et al., 1989). Similar effects have been observed in rhesus monkeys and rats (Novy, 1978; Powell & Cochrane, 1978).

Increased frequencies of fetal death and malformations have been observed when mice or rats were treated with 1-4 or 6-13 times the human dose of indomethacin during pregnancy (Persaud & Moore, 1974; Gavin et al., 1974; Persaud, 1975). Incomplete virilization of the external genitalia was reported in the male offspring of pregnant mice treated with indomethacin in doses similar to those used therapeutically in humans (Gupta & Goldman, 1986). In other studies, no increase in the frequency of malformations was observed among the offspring of mice or rats treated during pregnancy with indomethacin in doses, respectively, 1-100 times or 100 times those used in humans (Kalter, 1973; Klein et al., 1981; Randall et al., 1987; Kondoh et al., 1989).

Premature closure of the ductus arteriosus has been demonstrated in the fetuses of pregnant rats, sheep, and rabbits treated with indomethacin late in pregnancy in doses equivalent to or a few times greater than those used in humans (Levin et al., 1979; Harris, 1980; Harker et al., 1981; Momma & Takeuchi, 1983; Momma & Takao, 1989; Arishima et al., 1991). Oligohydramnios, fetal distress, and fetal death were observed in the offspring of rhesus monkeys treated orally with indomethacin in doses 5-7 times those used in humans late in pregnancy (Novy, 1978).

Key References

Aselton P, Jick H, Milunsky A, Hunter JR, et al.: First-trimester drug use and congenital disorders. Obstet Gynecol 65:451-455, 1985. [S]

Arishima K, Yamamoto M, Takizawa T, Ueda Y, et al.: Onset of the constrictive effect of indomethacin on the ductus arteriosus in fetal rats. Acta Anat 142:231-235, 1991. [A]

Atad J, David A, Moise J, Abramovici H: Classification of threatened premature labor related to treatment with a prostaglandin inhibitor: Indomethacin. Biol Neonate 37:291-296, 1980. [S]

Baerts W, Fetter WPF, Hop WCJ, Wallenburg HCS, et al.: Cerebral lesions in preterm infants after tocolytic indomethacin. Dev Med Child Neurol 32:910-918, 1990. (Erratum: Dev Med Child Neurol 32(11):1032, 1990.) [E]

Besinger RE, Niebyl JR, Keyes WG, Johnson TRB: Randomized comparative trial of indomethacin and ritodrine for the long-term treatment of preterm labor. Am J Obstet Gynecol 164:981-988, 1991. [E]

De Wit W, Mourik IV, Wiesenhaan PF: Prolonged maternal indomethacin therapy associated with oligohydramnios. Case reports. Br J Obstet Gynaecol 95:303-305, 1988. [C]

Douidar SM, Richardson J, Snodgrass WR: Role of Indomethacin in ductus closure: An update evaluation. Dev Pharmacol Ther 11:196-212, 1988. [R]

Dudley DKL, Hardie MJ: Fetal and neonatal effects of indomethacin used as a tocolytic agent. Am J Obstet Gynecol 151:181-184, 1985. [S]

Eronen M, Pesonen E, Kurki T, Ylikorkala O, et al.: The effects of indomethacin and a beta-sympathomimetic agent on the fetal ductus arteriosus during treatment of premature labor: A randomized double-blind study. Am J Obstet Gynecol 164:141-146, 1991. [E]

Gal P, Ransom JL, Schall S, Weaver RL, et al.: Indomethacin for patent ductus arteriosus closure. Application of serum concentrations and pharmacodynamics to improve response. J Perinatol 10:20-26, 1990. [E]

Gavin MA, Fernandez-Tejerina JCD, De Las Heras MFM, Maeso EV: [Effects of an inhibitor of prostaglandins biosynthesis (indomethacin) on the rat implantation.] Reproduccion 1:177-183, 1974. [A]

Gerson A, Abbasi S, Johnson A, Kalchbrenner M, et al.: Safety and efficacy of long-term tocolysis with indomethacin. Am J Perinatol 7:71-74, 1990. [E]

Grella P, Zanor P: Premature labor and indomethacin. Prostaglandins 16:1007-1017, 1978. [S]

Gupta C, Goldman A: The arachidonic acid cascade is involved in the masculinizing action of testosterone on embryonic external genitalia in mice. Proc Natl Acad Sci USA 83:4346-4349, 1986. [A]

Harker LC, Kirkpatrick SE, Friedman WF, Bloor CM: Effects of indomethacin on fetal rat lungs: A possible cause of persistent fetal circulation (PFC). Pediatr Res 15:147-151, 1981. [A]

Harris WH: The effects of repeated doses of indomethacin on fetal rabbit mortality and on the patency of the ductus arteriosus. Can J Physiol Pharmacol 58:212-216, 1980. [A]

Hendricks SK, Smith JR, Moore DE, Brown ZA: Oligohydramnios associated with prostaglandin synthetase inhibitors in preterm labour. Br J Obstet Gynaecol 97:312-316, 1990. [E]

Itskovitz J, Abramovici H, Brandes JM: Oligohydramnion, meconium death concurrent with indomethacin treatment in human pregnancy. J Reprod Med 24:137-140, 1980. [C]

Kalter H: Nonteratogenicity of indomethacin in mice. Teratology 7:A-19, 1973. [A]

Kirshon B, Mari G, Moise KJ Jr: Indomethacin therapy in the treatment of symptomatic polyhydramnios. Obstet Gynecol 75:202-205, 1990a. [E]

Kirshon B, Mari G, Moise KJ Jr, Wasserstrum N: Effect of indomethacin on the fetal ductus arteriosus during treatment of symptomatic polyhydramnios. J Reprod Med 35:529-532, 1990b. [S]

Kirshon B, Moise KJ Jr, Mari G, Willis R: Long-term indomethacin therapy decreases fetal urine output and results in oligohydramnios. Am J Perinatol 8(2):86-88, 1991. [S]

Kirshon B, Moise KJ Jr, Wasserstrum N, Ou C, et al.: Influence of short-term indomethacin therapy on fetal urine output. Obstet Gynecol 72:51-53, 1988. [E]

Klein KL, Scott WJ, Clark KE, Wilson JG: Indomethacin--Placental transfer, cytotoxicity, and teratology in the rat. Am J Obstet Gynecol 141:448-452, 1981. [A]

Kondoh S, Okada F, Goto K, Nishimura O, et al.: [Reproduction study of indometacin farnesil (II): Teratogenicity study in rats by oral administration.] Yakuri to Chiryo 17:63-85, 1989. [A]

Lange IR, Harman CR, Ash KM, Manning FA, et al.: Twin with hydramnios: Treating premature labor at source. Am J Obstet Gynecol 160:522-527, 1989. [E]

Levin DL, Fixler DE, Morriss FC, Tyson J: Morphologic analysis of the pulmonary vascular bed in infants exposed in utero to prostaglandin synthetase inhibitors. J Pediatr 92:478-483, 1978. [C]

Levin DL, Mills LJ, Parkey M, Garriott J, et al.: Constriction of the fetal ductus arteriosus after administration of indomethacin to the pregnant ewe. J Pediatr 94:647-650, 1979. [A]

Mamopoulos M, Assimakopoulos E, Reece A, Andreou A, et al.: Maternal indomethacin therapy in the treament of polyhydramnios. Am J Obstet Gynecol 162:1225-1229, 1990. [S]

Manchester D, Margolis HS, Sheldon RE: Possible association between maternal indomethacin therapy and primary pulmonary the newborn. Am J Obstet Gynecol 126:467-469, 1976. [C]

Mari G, Moise KJ Jr, Deter RL, Kirshon B, et al.: Doppler assessment of the pulsatility index of the middle cerebral artery during constriction of the fetal ductus arteriosus after indomethacin therapy. Am J Obstet Gynecol 161, 1528-1531, 1989. [E]

Mogilner BM, Ashkenazy M, Borenstein R, Lancet M: Hydrops fetalis caused by maternal indomethacin treatment. Acta Obstet Gynecol Scand 61:183-185, 1982. [C]

Moise KJ Jr: Indomethacin therapy in the treatment of symptomatic polyhydramnios. Clin Obstet Gynecol 34:310-318, 1991. [R]

Moise KJ Jr, Huhta JC, Sharif DS, et al.: Indomethacin in the treatment of premature labor: Effects on the fetal ductus arteriosus. N Engl J Med 319:327-331, 1988. [S]

Momma K, Takao A: Right ventricular concentric hypertrophy and left ventricular dilatation by ductal constriction in fetal rats. Circ Res 64:1137-1146, 1989. [A]

Momma K, Takeuchi H: Constriction of fetal ductus arteriosus by nonsteroidal antiinflammatory drugs. In: Samuelsson B et al., (eds). Advances in Prostaglandin, Thromboxane, and Leukotriene Research, Vol. 12. New York: Raven Press, 1983, pp 499-503. [A]

Morales WJ, Smith SG, Angel JL, O'Brien WF, et al.: Efficacy and safety of indomethacin versus ritodrine in the management of preterm labor: A randomized study. Obstet Gynecol 74:567-572, 1989. [E]

Niebyl JR, Witter FR: Neonatal outcome after indomethacin treatment for preterm labor. Am J Obstet Gynecol 155:747-749, 1986. [E]

Novy MJ: Effects of indomethacin on labor, fetal oxygenation, and fetal development in rhesus monkeys. Adv Prostaglandin Thromboxane Res 4:285-300, 1978. [A]

Persaud TVN: Prolongation of pregnancy and abnormal fetal development in rats treated with indomethacin. IRCS Med Sci Libr Compend 3:300, 1975. [A]

Persaud TVN, Moore KL: Inhibitors of prostaglandin synthesis during pregnancy. Anat Anz 136:349-353, 1974. [A]

Powell JG, Cochrane RL: The effects of the administration of fenoprofen or indomethacin to rat dams during late pregnancy, with special reference to the ductus arteriosus of the fetuses and neonates. Toxicol Appl Pharmacol 45:783-796, 1978. [A]

Randall CL, Anton RF, Becker HC: Effect of indomethacin on alcohol-induced morphological anomalies in mice. Life Sciences 41:361-369, 1987. [A]

Reiss U, Atad J, Rubinstein I, Zuckerman H: The effect of indomethacin in labour at term. Int J Gynaecol Obstet 14:369-374, 1976. [S]

Rubaltelli FF, Chiozza ML, Zanardo V, Cantarutti F, et al.: Effect on neonate of maternal treatment with indomethacin. J Pediatr 94:161, 1979. [C]

Uslu T, Ozcan FS, Aydin C: Oligohydramnios induced by maternal indomethacin therapy. Int J Clin Pharmacol Ther Toxicol 30(7):230-232, 1992. [E]

van der Heijden AJ, Provoost AP, Nauta J, Grose WA, et al.: Renal functional impairment in preterm neonates related to intrauterine indomethacin exposure. Pediatr Res 24:644-648, 1988b. [E]

van der Heijden AJ, Provoost AP, Nauta J, Wolff ED, et al.: Indomethacin as an inhibitor of preterm labor. Effect on postnatal renal function. Contr Nephrol 67:152-154, 1988a. [E]

van Kets H, Thiery M, Derom R, Van Egmond H, et al.: Perinatal hazards of chronic antenatal tocolysis with indomethacin. Prostaglandins 18:893-907, 1979. [S]

Vanhaesebrouck R, Thiery M, Leroy JG, Govaert P, et al.: Oligohydramnios, renal insufficiency, and ileal perforation in preterm infants after intrauterine exposure to indomethacin. J Pediatr 113:738-743, 1988. [C]

Wiggins DA, Elliott JP: Oligohydramnios in each sac of a triplet gestation caused by Motrin--Fulfilling Kock's postulates. Am J Obstet Gynecol 162:460-461, 1990. [C]

Zuckerman H, Reiss U, Rubinstein I: Inhibition of human premature labor by indomethacin. Obstet Gynecol 44:787-792, 1974. [S]

INFLUENZA VACCINE

Synonyms

Fluogen, Fluzone

Summary

Conventional influenza vaccine consists of whole or fractionated inactivated (i.e., killed) influenza virus that is administered by injection. An attenuated live influenza virus vaccine has been used by intranasal administration.

Magnitude of Teratogenic Risk

None

Quality and Quantity of Data

Fair

Comment

1) Live influenza virus vaccine is currently not in use in the united states. The formulation of influenza virus vaccine varies each year.

2) Since influenza is not known to be teratogenic and the vaccine used is inactivated, the risk of congenital anomalies in the children of women treated with influenza vaccine during pregnancy is probably small.

The frequencies of congenital anomalies in general, of major malformations, of minor anomalies, and of principal classes of malformations were no greater than expected among the children of 650 women who were treated with influenza virus vaccine during the first four lunar months of pregnancy in the Collaborative Perinatal Project (Heinonen et al., 1977). Similarly, the frequency of congenital anomalies was not increased among the children of 2283 women who had been given influenza virus vaccine anytime during pregnancy in this study. The frequency of congenital anomalies was no greater than expected among the infants of 39 women immunized with inactivated influenza virus vaccine during the first trimester of pregnancy or among the infants of 135 or 56 infants immunized with such vaccine during the last two trimesters in other studies (Deinard & Ogburn, 1981; Sumaya & Gibbs, 1979).

No animal teratology studies of inactivated influenza vaccine have been published. Intracerebral innoculation of live attenuated influenza virus into rhesus monkey fetuses has been shown to produce hydrocephalus (Krous & Altshuler, 1978), but these experimental conditions differ greatly from immunization of a pregnant woman with inactivated influenza vaccine.

Key References

Deinard AS, Ogburn P: A/NJ/8/76 influenza vaccination program: Effects on maternal health and pregnancy outcome. Am J Obstet Gynecol 140:240-245, 1981. [E]

Heinonen OP, Slone D, Shapiro S: Birth Defects and Drugs in Pregnancy. Littleton, Mass.: John Wright-PSG, 1977, pp 314-316, 318-319, 436, 474, 488. [E]

Krous HF, Altshuler G: Animal model: Congenital hydrocephalus produced by attenuated influenza A virus vaccine in rhesus monkeys. Am J Pathol 92:317-320, 1978. [A]

Sumaya CV, Gibbs RS: Immunization of pregnant women with influenza A/New Jersey/76 virus vaccine: Reactogenicity and immunogenicity in mother and infant. J Infect Dis 140:141-146, 1979. [E]

INOSITOL

Synonyms

Dambose, Hexopal, Linodil, Myoinositol, Palobex, Phaseomannitol

Summary

Inositol is an isomer of glucose, to which inositol is readily converted metabolically. Inositol is contained in the normal human diet and is sometimes taken as a nutritional supplement.

Magnitude of Teratogenic Risk

Undetermined

Quality and Quantity of Data

None To Poor

Comment

None

No epidemiological studies of congenital anomalies among the children of women who ingested unusually large amounts of inositol during pregnancy have been reported.

No gross abnormalities were observed among the offspring of rats fed diets containing 1% inositol during pregnancy (Ershoff, 1946).

Key References

Ershoff BH: Effects of massive doses of P-aminobenzoic acid and inositol on reproduction in the rat. Soc Exper Biol Med 63:479-480, 1946. [A]

INSULIN

Synonyms

Humulin, Iletin, Insulatard, Lentard, Monotard, Novolin, Protaphane, Ultralente, Velosulin

Summary

Insulin is a protein hormone produced by the pancreatic beta cells. Insulin regulates glucose metabolism and is involved in many other metabolic processes in the body. Insulin is administered parenterally in the treatment of diabetes mellitus.

Magnitude of Teratogenic Risk

None To Minimal

Many epidemiological studies have established that the risk of congenital anomalies is increased 2-4 fold among the children of women who have insulin-dependent diabetes during pregnancy (Dignan, 1981; Mills, 1982; Cousins, 1983; Reece & Hobbins, 1986). Since many metabolic alterations occur among insulin-dependent diabetics, and since diabetics who require insulin differ greatly from those who do not, neither pregnancies in normal women nor pregnancies in diabetic women who do not require insulin treatment can be used as a control to distinguish the effects of maternal insulin therapy from the effects of the underlying illness on embryogenesis in diabetic mothers. Recent evidence suggesting that congenital anomalies can be reduced by improved control of maternal diabetes very early in pregnancy is consistent with the interpretation that the increased risk of malformations among infants of diabetic mothers is largely a manifestion of the disease itself (Miller et al., 1981; Steel et al., 1982; Fuhrmann et al., 1984; Goldman et al., 1986; Reece & Hobbins, 1986; Miodovnik et al., 1988; Reece et al., 1988; Greene et al., 1989; Lucas et al., 1989). A high incidence of fetal death and congenital anomalies has been observed among the children of women treated in the first trimester of pregnancy with insulin-induced hypoglycemic coma for psychiatric illness (Impastato et al., 1964); this treatment induces an adverse metabolic reaction in the mother that may pose a substantial risk to the embryo.

Although central nervous system, skeletal, and other malformations can be produced among the offspring of mice, rats, and rabbits treated with insulin during pregnancy (Chomette, 1955; Cole & Trasler, 1980; Eriksson et al., 1982, 1989; Buchanan et al., 1986), such treatment also causes major alterations of maternal metabolic homeostasis. Thus, it is uncertain whether the teratogenic effects are due to insulin per se, to maternal metabolic derangement, or both. The observation that insulin treatment decreases the frequency of malformations among the offspring of diabetic rats and among mouse embryos cultured in diabetic rat serum suggests that maternal metabolic derangement is largely responsible for the teratogenic effects associated with the insulin treatment (Sadler & Horton, 1983; Eriksson et al., 1983, 1987, 1989; Wilson et al., 1985).

Key References

Buchanan TA, Schemmer JK, Freinkel N: Embryotoxic effects of brief maternal insulin-hypoglycemia during organogenesis in the rat. J Clin Invest 78:643-649, 1986. [A]

Chomette G: [Developmental disorders after insulin shock in pregnant rabbits.] Beitr Pathol Anat 115:439-451, 1955. [A]

Cole WA, Trasler DG: Gene-teratogen interaction in insulin-induced mouse exencephaly. Teratology 22:125-139, 1980. [A]

Cousins L: Congenital anomalies among infants of diabetic mothers. Etiology, prevention, prenatal diagnosis. Am J Obstet Gynecol 147:333-338, 1983. [R]

Dignan PSJ: Teratogenic risk and counseling in diabetes. Clin Obstet Gynecol 24:149-159, 1981. [R]

Eriksson JJ, Dahlstrom E, Hellerstrom C: Diabetes in pregnancy. Skeletal malformations in the offspring of diabetic rats after intermittent withdrawal of insulin in early gestation. Diabetes 32:1141-1145, 1983. [A]

Eriksson RSM, Thunberg L, Eriksson UJ: Effects of interrupted insulin treatment on fetal outcome of pregnant diabetic rats. Diabetes 38:764-772, 1989. [A]

Eriksson U, Dahlstrom E, Larsson KS, Hellerstrom C: Increased incidence of congenital malformations in the offspring of diabetic rats and their prevention by maternal insulin therapy. Diabetes 31:1-6, 1982. [A]

Eriksson UJ, Karlsson M-G, Styrud J: Mechanisms of congenital malformations in diabetic pregnancy. Biol Neonate 51:113-118, 1987. [R]

Fuhrmann K, Reiher H, Semmler K, Glockner E: The effect of intensified conventional insulin therapy before and during pregnancy on the malformation rate in offspring of diabetic mothers. Exp Clin Endocrinol 83:173-177, 1984. [S]

Goldman, JA, Dicker D, Feldberg D, et al.: Pregnancy outcome in patients with insulin-dependent diabetes mellitus with preconceptional diabetic control: A comparative study. Am J Obstet Gynecol 155:293-197, 1986. [E]

Greene MF, Hare JW, Cloherty JP, et al.: First-trimester hemoglobin A1 and risk for major malformation and spontaneous abortion in diabetic pregnancy. Teratology 39:225-231, 1989. [E]

Impastato DJ, Gabriel AR, Lardaro HH: Electric and insulin shock therapy during pregnancy. Dis Nerv Syst 25:542-546, 1964. [S]

Lucas MJ, Leveno KJ, Williams ML, et al.: Early pregnancy glycosylated hemoglobin, severity of diabetes, and fetal malformations. Am J Obstet Gynecol 161(2):426-431, 1989. [E]

Miller E, Hare JW, Cloherty JP, Dunn PJ, et al.: Elevated maternal hemoglobin A in early pregnancy and major congenital anomalies in infants of diabetic mothers. N Engl J Med 304:1331-1334, 1981. [S]

Mills JL: Malformations in infants of diabetic mothers. Teratology 25:385-394, 1982. [R]

Miodovnik M, Mimouni F, Dignan PSJ, et al.: Major malformations in infants of IDDM women. Vasculopathy and early first-trimester poor glycemic control. Diabetes Care 11(9):713-718, 1988. [E]

Reece EA, Gabrielli S, Abdalla M: The prevention of diabetes-associated birth defects. Semin Perinatol 12(4):292-301, 1988. [R]

Reece EA, Hobbins JC: Diabetic embryopathy: Pathogenesis, prenatal diagnosis and prevention. Obstet Gynecol Surv 41(6):325-335, 1986. [R]

Sadler TW, Horton WE: Effects of maternal diabetes on early embryogenesis. The role of insulin and insulin therapy. Diabetes 32:1070-1074, 1983. [A]

Steel JM, Johnstone FD, Smith AF, Duncan LJP: Five years' experience of a "prepregnancy" clinic for insulin-dependent diabetics. Br Med J 285:353-356, 1982. [S]

Wilson GN, Howe M, Stover JM: Delayed developmental sequences in rodent diabetic embryopathy. Pediatr Res 19(12):1337-1339, 1985. [A]

IODINATED GLYCEROL

Synonyms

Iophen, Organidin, R-Gen

Summary

Iodinated glycerol is a mixture of iodinated dimers of glycerol. Iodinated glycerol is taken orally as an expectorant.

Magnitude of Teratogenic Risk

Undetermined

Quality and Quantity of Data

None

Comment

Maternal use of iodinated glycerol following the 12th to the 14th week of pregnancy has the theoretical potential of inducing fetal goiter.

No epidemiological studies of congenital anomalies in infants born to mothers who took iodinated glycerol during pregnancy have been reported.

No animal teratology studies of iodinated glycerol have been published.

Key References

None available.

IODOQUINOL

Synonyms

Diiodohydroxyquin, Diodoquin, Floraquin, Moebiquin, Sebaquin, Yodoxin

Summary

Iodoquinol is administered orally in the treatment of intestinal parasites and acrodermatitis enteropathica. The drug is also used topically to treat a variety of dermatoses.

Magnitude of Teratogenic Risk

None To Minimal

Quality and Quantity of Data

Poor To Fair

Comment

None

The frequency of congenital anomalies was no greater than expected among the children of 169 women who took iodoquinol during the first four lunar months of pregnancy or of 172 women who took this drug anytime in pregnancy in the Collaborative Perinatal Project (Heinonen et al., 1977).

No animal teratology studies of iodoquinol have been reported.

Key References

Heinonen OP, Slone D, Shapiro S: Birth Defects and Drugs in Pregnancy. Littleton, Mass.: John Wright-PSG, 1977, pp 299, 302, 434, 435, 473, 486. [E]

IOHEXOL

Synonyms

Exypaque, Nycodenz, Omnigraf, Omnipaque, Omnitrast

Summary

Iohexol is an iodinated contrast medium used in radiographic studies.

Magnitude of Teratogenic Risk

Undetermined

Quality and Quantity of Data

None

Comment

None

No epidemiological studies of congenital anomalies among infants born to women who were treated with iohexol during pregnancy have been reported.

No animal teratology studies of iohexol have been published.

Key References

None available.

IPECAC

Synonyms

Ipecacuanha Tincture, Linituss, Pectomed

Summary

Ipecac is a mixture of alkaloids prepared from the dried root of Cephaelis ipecacuanha. It is used as an expectorant in cough medications and in larger doses as an emetic in poisonings.

Magnitude of Teratogenic Risk

None To Minimal

Quality and Quantity of Data

Poor To Fair

Comment

None

The frequency of congenital anomalies was no greater than expected among the infants of 68 women who took ipecac during the first four lunar months or among the infants of 379 women who used the drug anytime during pregnancy in the Collaborative Perinatal Project (Heinonen et al., 1977).

No animal teratology studies of ipecac have been published.

Key References

Heinonen OP, Slone D, Shapiro S: Birth Defects and Drugs in Pregnancy. Littleton, Mass.: John Wright-PSG, 1977, pp 378, 442. [E]

IRON

Synonyms

Ferrous Aspartate, Ferrous Carbonate, Ferrous Fumarate, Ferrous Gluconate, Ferrous Lactate, Ferrous Oxalate, Ferrous Succinate, Ferrous Sulfate, Ferrous Tartrate, Ferrum

Summary

Iron is an essential element of the diet. The body's iron requirements increase dramatically in pregnancy, and supplementation is often necessary to prevent development of anemia. The U.S. Recommended Dietary Allowance in pregnancy is 30 mg of elemental iron per day (NRC, 1989). Therapeutic doses are often 10 times as great.

Magnitude of Teratogenic Risk

None

Quality and Quantity of Data

Poor To Fair

Comment

This assessment refers to the risk associated with maternal use of iron in therapeutic doses.

The frequency of congenital anomalies was no higher than expected among the children of 66 women treated with parenteral iron during the first four lunar months of pregnancy or among 1864 women who received such treatment anytime during pregnancy in the Collaborative Perinatal Project (Heinonen et al., 1977). Similarly, no difference in the frequency of congenital anomalies was observed between the infants of 1336 women who received supplemental iron routinely in the second and third trimester of pregnancy and the infants of a similar number of women who received iron only if they were anemic (Hemminki & Rimpela, 1991). The perinatal mortality was significantly higher in pregnancies of the routinely supplemented women, but this did not appear to be related to the treatment.

In one clinical series, none of 19 infants born to women who had taken overdoses of iron in the second or third trimester of pregnancy sufficient to produce blood levels in the moderately or severely toxic range had abnormalities that could be attributed to the ingestion (McElhatton et al., 1991). No abnormalities have been reported in other infants born to women who ingested toxic doses of iron during pregnancy (Olenmark et al., 1987; Blanc et al., 1984; Tenenbein, 1989; Lacoste et al., 1992). A few spontaneous abortions have been reported among such women, and a direct or indirect toxic effect of the iron overdose is possible in these cases (Strom et al., 1976; McElhatton et al., 1991).

Animal teratology studies using iron have produced inconsistent results. No increase in the frequency of malformations was observed in the offspring of mice or rats treated during pregnancy in doses 1-100 times those used therapeutically in humans (Flodh et al., 1977; Tadokoro et al., 1979). In contrast, malformations have been observed in the offspring of rabbits treated with maternally toxic doses of iron during pregnancy (Flodh et al., 1977). Malformations were also observed in the offspring of treated mice in another investigation in which neither dose nor maternal toxicity was adequately measured (Kuchta, 1982). In both investigations, the most frequently observed fetal anomalies involved the central nervous system and skeleton. The relevance of these observations to the therapeutic use of iron in human pregnancy is unknown.

Key References

Blanc P, Hryhorczuk D, Danel I: Deferoxamine treatment of acute iron intoxication in pregnancy. Obstet Gynecol 64(3):12S-14S, 1984. [C] & [R]

Flodh H, Magnusson G, Malmfors T: Teratological, peri- and postnatal studies on Ferastral(R), an iron-poly (sorbitol-gluconic acid) complex. Scand J Haematol (Suppl)32:69-83, 1977. [A]

Heinonen OP, Slone D, Shapiro S: Birth Defects and Drugs in Pregnancy. Littleton, Mass.: John Wright-PSG, 1977, pp 402, 444. [E]

Hemminki E, Rimpela U: A randomized comparison of routine versus selective iron supplementation during pregnancy. J Am Coll Nutr 10(1):3-10, 1991. [E]

Kuchta B: Experiments and ultrastructural investigations on the mouse embryo during early teratogen-sensitive stages. Acta Anat 113:218-225, 1982. [A]

Lacoste H, Goyert GL, Goldman LS, et al.: Acute iron intoxication in pregnancy: Case report and review of the literature. Obstet Gynecol 80:500-501, 1992. [C] & [R]

McElhatton PR, Roberts JC, Sullivan FM: The consequences of iron overdose and its treatment with desferrioxamine in pregnancy. Hum Exp Toxicol 10:251-259, 1991. [S]

NRC (National Research Council): Recommended Dietary Allowances, 10th ed. Report of the Subcommittee on the Tenth Edition of the RDAs, Food and Nutrition Board, Commission on Life Sciences. Washington, D.C.: National Academy Press, 1989. [O]

Olenmark M, Biber B, Dottori O, et al.: Fatal iron intoxication in late pregnancy. Clin Toxicol 25(4):347-359, 1987. [C]

Strom RL, Schiler P, Seeds AE, et al: Fatal iron poisoning in a pregnant female: Case report. Minn Med 59:483-489, 1976. [C]

Tadokoro T, Miyaji T, Okumura M: Teratogenicity studies of slow-Fe in mice and rats. Oyo Yakuri (Pharmacology) 17:483-495, 1979. [A]

Tenenbein M: Iron overdose during pregnancy. Vet Hum Toxicol 31(4):346, 1989. [C]

ISOBUCAINE

Synonyms

2-Isobutylamino-2-methylpropyl benzoate hydrochloride

Summary

Isobucaine is a local anesthetic of the ester class that has been used in dentistry.

Magnitude of Teratogenic Risk

Undetermined

Quality and Quantity of Data

None

Comment

None

No epidemiological studies of congenital anomalies in children born to women exposed to isobucaine during pregnancy have been reported.

No investigations of teratologic effects of isobucaine in experimental animals have been published.

Please see agent summary on procaine for information on a related agent that has been studied.

Key References

None available.

ISOBUTAMBEN

Synonyms

Isobutyl para-Aminobenzoate

Summary

Isobutamben is a local anesthetic of the ester class.

Magnitude of Teratogenic Risk

Undetermined

Quality and Quantity of Data

None

Comment

None

No epidemiological studies of congenital anomalies in children born to women exposed to isobutamben during pregnancy have been reported.

No investigations of teratologic effects of isobutamben in experimental animals have been published.

Please see agent summary on procaine for information on a related agent that has been studied.

Key References

None available.

ISOETHARINE

Synonyms

Asthmalitan, Bronkometer, Bronkosol, Etyprenaline, Isoetarine, Numotac

Summary

Isoetharine is a sympathomimetic agent that is used orally or as an inhalant in the treatment of bronchospasms.

Magnitude of Teratogenic Risk

Undetermined

Quality and Quantity of Data

None

Comment

None

No epidemiological studies of congenital anomalies in infants whose mothers were treated with isoetharine during pregnancy have been reported.

No animal teratology studies of isoetharine have been published.

Please see agent summary on isoproterenol for information on a related agent that has been studied.

Key References

None available.

ISOFLURANE

Synonyms

Aerrane, Compound 469, Forane

Summary

Isoflurane is a general anesthetic that is administered by inhalation.

Magnitude of Teratogenic Risk

Undetermined

Quality and Quantity of Data

Poor

Comment

None

No epidemiological studies of congenital anomalies in children born to women exposed to isoflurane during pregnancy have been reported.

No adverse effect was noted among newborn infants delivered by Caesarean section to women who were anesthetized with isoflurane (Abboud et al., 1989).

Increased frequencies of cleft palate, skeletal variations, and fetal growth retardation were observed among the offspring of mice exposed repeatedly during pregnancy to light anesthetic doses of isoflurane (Mazze et al., 1985). No physical defects but alterations of neonatal behavior were seen among the offspring of animals treated with subanesthetic doses (Rice, 1986). In contrast, no teratogenic effect was observed among the offspring of rats or rabbits treated repeatedly during pregnancy with isoflurane in doses similar to or less than those used for full anesthesia in humans (Kennedy et al., 1978; Mazze et al., 1986; Fujinaga et al., 1987). The relevance of these observations to the teratogenic risk associated with isoflurane anesthesia in a pregnant woman is uncertain.

Key References

Abboud TK, D'Onofrio L, Reyes A, et al.: Isoflurane or halothane for cesarean section: Comparative maternal and neonatal effects. Acta Anaesthesiol Scand 33:578-581, 1989. [E]

Fujinaga M, Baden JM, Yhap EO, Mazze RI: Halothane and isoflurane prevent the teratogenic effects of nitrous oxide in rats, folinic acid does not. Anesthesiology 67(3A):A456, 1987. [A]

Kennedy GL, Smith SH, Keplinger ML, Calandra JC: Reproductive and teratologic studies with isoflurane. Drug Chem Toxicol 1:75-88, 1978. [A]

Mazze RI, Fujinaga M, Rice SA, et al.: Reproductive and teratogenic effects of nitrous oxide, halothane, isoflurane, and enflurane in Sprague-Dawley rats. Anesthesiology 64:339-344, 1986. [A]

Mazze RI, Wilson AI, Rice SA, Baden JM: Fetal development in mice exposed to isoflurane. Teratology 32:339-345, 1985. [A]

Rice SA: Behavioral effects of in utero isoflurane exposure in young SW mice. Teratology 33:100C, 1986. [A]

ISOMAZOLE

Summary

Isomazole is a cardiotonic drug.

Magnitude of Teratogenic Risk

Undetermined

Quality and Quantity of Data

None

Comment

None

No epidemiological studies of congenital anomalies in infants born to women who were treated with isomazole during pregnancy have been reported.

No animal teratology studies of isomazole have been published.

Key References

None available.

ISOMETHEPTENE

Synonyms

Isometepteno, Isomethepetene, Isonyl, Methylisooctenylamine, Methyloctenylamine, Octanil, Octine

Summary

Isometheptene is a sympathomimetic vasoconstrictor that is administered orally for the treatment of migraine headache.

Magnitude of Teratogenic Risk

Undetermined

No epidemiological studies of congenital anomalies in infants whose mothers were treated with isometheptene during pregnancy have been reported.

No animal teratology studies of iso-metheptene have been published.

Please see agent summary on epinephrine for information on a related agent that has been studied.

Key References

None available.

ISONIAZID

Synonyms

Hyzyd, Isonicotinylhydrazine, Isotamine, La-niazid, Nydrazid, Rimifon, Teebaconin

Summary

Isoniazid is a hydrazine derivative used to treat tuberculosis. It is usually administered orally but may be used parenterally in very serious illness.

Magnitude of Teratogenic Risk

Minimal

Quality and Quantity of Data

Poor To Fair

Comment

None

The frequency of congenital anomalies was not significantly increased among the children of 85 women treated with isoniazid during the first four lunar months of pregnancy or the children of 146 women treated with this drug anytime during gestation in the Collaborative Perinatal Project (Heinonen et al., 1977). In another cohort study, congenital anomalies were more frequent than expected among the children of 42 women treated with isoniazid and other medications during the first trimester of pregnancy, but there was no specificity to the kind of anomalies observed (Varpela, 1964). Several other investigations of congenital anomalies among infants born to women treated with antituberculous drugs during pregnancy have been reported (Warkany, 1979; Snider et al., 1980), but these studies are difficult to interpret because many patients are treated with more than one drug and individual agents are usually not considered separately. Moreover, the time and duration of therapy during pregnancy is variable and often incompletely documented, and underascertainment of congenital anomalies among the control infants seems likely. In general, however, no association between congenital anomalies and maternal use of isoniazid during pregnancy was apparent.

At least seven children with mental retardation, seizures, or other evidence of central nervous system dysfunction whose mothers took isoniazid and other antituberculous agents at various times during pregnancy have been reported (Varpela, 1964; Monnet et al., 1967). Available data are inadequate to determine whether or not this association is causal, but these reports are of concern because neurotoxicity is a recognized side-effect of isoniazid therapy in adults. Prophylactic administration of 50 mg/d of pyridoxine to pregnant women during isoniazid therapy has been recommended to prevent this complication (American Thoracic Society, 1986; Medchill & Gillum, 1989).

No increase in the frequency of malformations was observed among the offspring of mice treated with isoniazid during pregnancy in doses as high as 60 times those used in humans, despite considerable maternal toxicity at such doses (Kalter, 1972; Menon & Bhide, 1980).

No teratogenic effect was seen among the offspring of rabbits treated with isoniazid during pregnancy in doses equivalent to those used clinically, but in rats such treatment did increase the frequency of anomalies (mostly altered skeletal development) (Dluzniewski & Gastol-Lewinska, 1971).

An increased frequency of pulmonary adenocarcinomas has been observed among the offspring of mice treated with about 30 times the usual human dose of isoniazid during pregnancy and lactation (Menon & Bhide, 1983). The clinical relevance of this observation is uncertain, however. A study of 11,169 matched case-control pairs of children with cancer showed no apparent association with maternal isoniazid treatment during the mothers' pregnancies (Sanders & Draper, 1979). However, very few of the mothers in either group took this drug. In another investigation, no neoplasms were found among 660 one- to thirteen-year-old children born to women treated with isoniazid for various periods during their pregnancies (Hammond et al., 1967).

Key References

American Thoracic Society: Treatment of tuberculosis and tuberculosis infection in adults and children. Am Rev Respir Dis 134:355-363, 1986. [O]

Dluzniewski A, Gastol-Lewinska L: The search for teratogenic activity of some tuberculostatic drugs. Diss Pharm Pharmacol 23(4):383-392, 1971. [A]

Hammond EC, Selikoff IJ, Robitzek EH: Isoniazid therapy in relation to later occurrence of cancer in adults and in infants. Br Med J 2:792-795, 1967. [S]

Heinonen OP, Slone D, Shapiro S: Birth Defects and Drugs in Pregnancy. Littleton, Mass.: John Wright-PSG, 1977, pp 298-299, 302, 313, 435. [E]

Kalter H: Nonteratogenicity of isoniazid in mice. Teratology 5:259, 1972. [A]

Medchill MT, Gillum M: Diagnosis and management of tuberculosis during pregnancy. Obstet Gynecol Surv 44:81-84, 1989. [R]

Menon MM, Bhide SV: Perinatal carcinogenicity of isoniazid (INH) in Swiss Mice. J Cancer Res Clin Oncol 105:258-261, 1983. [A]

Menon MM, Bhide SV: Transplacental, biological and metabolic effects of isoniazid (INH) in Swiss mice. Indian J Exp Biol 18:1104-1106, 1980. [A]

Monnet P, Kalb JC, Pujol M: Harmful effects of isoniazid on the fetus and infants. Lyon Med 218:431-455, 1967. [C]

Sanders BM, Draper GJ: Childhood cancer and drugs in pregnancy. Br Med J 1:717-718, 1979. [E]

Snider DE Jr, Layde PM, Johnson MW, Lyle MA: Treatment of tuberculosis during pregnancy. Am Rev Respir Dis 122:65-79, 1980. [S]

Varpela E: On the effect exerted by the first-line tuberculosis medicines on the fetus. Acta Tuberc Scand 35:53-69, 1964. [E]

Warkany J: Antituberculous drugs. Teratology 20:133-138, 1979. [R]

ISOPROPAMIDE

Synonyms

Darbid, Isopropamide Iodide

Summary

Isopropamide is an anticholinergic agent used to treat gastric and duodenal ulcers and to relieve gastrointestinal spasms.

Magnitude of Teratogenic Risk

None To Minimal

Quality and Quantity of Data

Poor To Fair

Comment

None

The frequency of congenital anomalies was no greater than expected among 180 infants born to women who took isopropamide during the first four lunar months or among 1071 infants whose mothers took the drug anytime during pregnancy in the Collaborative Perinatal Project (Heinonen et al., 1977).

No animal teratology studies of isopropamide have been published.

Key References

Heinonen OP, Slone D, Shapiro S: Birth Defects and Drugs in Pregnancy. Littleton, Mass.: John Wright-PSG, 1977, pp 346, 439. [E]

ISOPROPYL MYRISTATE

Synonyms

Isomyst

Summary

Isopropyl myristate is a fatty acid ester used in many topical preparations as a solvent and emollient.

Magnitude of Teratogenic Risk

Undetermined

Quality and Quantity of Data

None

Comment

None

No epidemiological studies of congenital anomalies in infants whose mothers used isopropyl myristate during pregnancy have been reported.

No animal teratology studies of isopropyl myristate have been published.

Key References

None available.

ISOPROTERENOL

Synonyms

Aerolone, Isoprenaline, Isuprel, Medihaler Iso, Norisodrine, Vapo-Iso

Summary

Isoproterenol is a sympathomimetic agent that stimulates beta-adrenergic receptors. It is widely used in the treatment of asthma and cardiac dysfunction. Isoproterenol may be administered by several different routes; the dosage varies greatly according to route.

Magnitude of Teratogenic Risk

None To Minimal

Quality and Quantity of Data

Poor To Fair

Comment

None

The frequency of congenital anomalies was no greater than expected among the children of 31 women treated with isoproterenol during the first four lunar months of pregnancy in the Collaborative Perinatal Project (Heinonen et al., 1977).

No teratogenic effect was observed among the offspring of rats or rabbits treated with isoproterenol by inhalation in doses 5-15 times those used in humans (Vogin et al., 1970). Similarly, the frequency of malformations was not increased among the offspring of pregnant rats injected intraperitoneally with 6-22 times the maximal human oral dose of isoproterenol or of pregnant rabbits fed 4-14 times the maximal human dose (Jones-Price et al., 1982; Hollingsworth et al., 1971). In contrast, the frequency of central nervous system and other malformations was increased among the offspring of pregnant hamsters given isoproterenol in single subcutaneous injections 1250-8700 times those used in humans (Geber, 1969). Increased frequencies of congenital anomalies have also been reported among the offspring of pregnant mice given single isoproterenol injections about 720 times those used subcutaneously in humans (Sullivan & Robson, 1965). Alterations of cardiac muscle weight and histology, which appear to resolve with age, have been observed among the offspring of rats treated with daily subcutaneous injections of isoproterenol about 12 times greater than those used in humans (Iwasaki et al., 1990). The relevance of these observations to the therapeutic use of isoproterenol in humans is unknown.

Alterations in heart rate and blood pressure have been observed near term in the fetuses of rhesus monkeys given intravenous infusions of 2.5-20 times the usual human dose of isoproterenol (Myers et al, 1978).

Key References

Geber WF: Comparative teratogenicity of isoproterenol and trypan blue in the fetal hamster. Proc Soc Exp Biol Med 130:1168-1170, 1969. [A]

Heinonen OP, Slone D, Shapiro S: Birth Defects and Drugs in Pregnancy. Littleton, Mass.: John Wright-PSG, 1977, pp 346-347. [E]

Hollingsworth RL, Scott WJ, Woodard MW, Woodard G: Fetal rabbit ductus arteriosus assessed in a teratological study on isoproterenol and metaproterenol. Toxicol Appl Pharmacol 18:231-234, 1971. [A]

Iwasaki T, Takino Y, Suzuki T: Effects of isoproterenol on the developing heart in rats. Jpn Circ J 54:109-116, 1990. [A]

Jones-Price C, Ledoux TA, Reel JR, Wolkowski-Tyl R, Langhoff-Paschke L, et al: Teratologic evaluation of isoproterenol hydrochloride (CAS No. 51-30-9) in CD rats. NTIS (National Technical Information Service) Report/PB 83-153007, 1982. [A]

Myers RE, Joelsson I, Adamsons K: The effects of isoproterenol on fetal oxygenation. Acta Obstet Gynecol Scand 57:317-322, 1978. [A]

Sullivan FM, Robson JM: Discussion. In: Robson JM, Sullivan FM, Smith RL (eds). Embryopathic Activity of Drugs. Boston: Little Brown and Co., 1965, pp 110-115. [A]

Vogin EE, Goldhamer RE, Scheimberg J, Carson S: Teratology studies in rats and rabbits exposed to an isoproterenol aerosol. Toxicol Appl Pharmacol 16:374-381, 1970. [A]

ISOSORBIDE DINITRATE

Synonyms

Dilatrate-SR, Iso-Bid, Isordil, Isotrate Timecelles, Sorbide Nitrate, Sorbitrate

Summary

Isosorbide dinitrate is antianginal agent.

Magnitude of Teratogenic Risk

Undetermined

Quality and Quantity of Data

None

Comment

None

No epidemiological studies of congenital anomalies among infants born to women treated with isosorbide dinitrate during pregnancy have been reported.

The frequency of malformations was not increased among the offspring of pregnant rats or rabbits treated with <1-3 times the human therapeutic dose of isosorbide dinitrate (Mikami, 1985; Mochida, 1985).

Key References

Mikami T: Studies of intravenous administration of isosorbide dinitrate (ISDN) in rat fetuses during organogenesis. Kiso To Rinsho 19:5047-5064, 1985. [A]

Mochida H: Studies of intravenous administration of isorbide dinitrate (ISDN) in rabbit fetuses during organogenesis period. Kiso To Rinsho 19:5065-5074, 1985. [A]

ISOTRETINOIN

Synonyms

Accutane, 13-cis-Retinoic Acid

Summary

Isotretinoin (13-cis-retinoic acid) is a vitamin A congener used orally in the treatment of cystic acne and other dermatologic diseases.

Magnitude of Teratogenic Risk

High

Quality and Quantity of Data

Excellent

Comment

None

A very uncommon but strikingly similar pattern of anomalies has been observed in more than 80 children exposed to isotretinoin during embryonic development (Anonymous, 1983; Rosa, 1983; Anonymous, 1984; Lammer et al., 1985; Rosa et al., 1986; Strauss et al., 1988; Thomson & Cordero, 1989; Lynberg et al., 1990; Teratology Society, 1991). Characteristic features of this embryopathy include microtia/anotia, micrognathia, cleft palate, conotruncal heart and great vessel defects, thymic abnormalities, eye anomalies, and central nervous system (CNS) malformations. Limb reduction defects may occasionally occur (Rizzo et al., 1991). 62% of 233 pregnancies in women treated with isotretinoin during gestation and voluntarily reported to the manufacturer before outcome was known were electively aborted (Dai et al., 1992). Among the 115 pregnancies that were not terminated, 18% ended in spontaneous abortion. 28% of the 94 liveborn infants, almost all of whose mothers had been treated during the first trimester, had at least one major malformation. Typical malformations occurred in children born to women who took various

dosages of isotretinoin within the usual therapeutic range and in women who were treated for less than one week in the first trimester of pregnancy (Dai et al., 1992). In a follow-up study of 31 five-year-old children born to women who had been treated with isotretinoin during the first 60 days after conception, 52% performed in the subnormal range on standard intelligence tests (Adams, 1990; Adams et al., 1991; Adams & Lammer, 1992). Of 12 children who had major malformations, six (including four with major CNS anomalies) had IQ <70, four (including one with major CNS anomalies) had IQ 70-85, and two had IQ >85. Six of 19 children with no major malformations had IQ 70-85; the others had IQ >85.

The frequency of congenital anomalies does not appear to be increased among the children of women who discontinue isotretinoin therapy *prior to conception* (Dai et al., 1989). This finding is consistent with the 10- to 12-hour average serum half-life of isotretinoin in humans.

Isotretinoin produces a similar spectrum of malformations in experimental animals exposed during embryonic development. Teratogenic effects have been reported in monkeys, rabbits, hamsters, mice, and rats after administration of isotretinoin to pregnant females in doses several to many times greater than those used clinically (Kamm, 1982; Agnish et al., 1984; Kochhar et al., 1984; Willhite & Shealy, 1984; Willhite et al., 1986; Webster et al., 1986; Kochhar & Penner, 1987; Hummler et al., 1990; Kwasigroch & Bullen, 1991; Teratology Society, 1991). A typical dose-response relationship has been demonstrated in hamsters and mice (Willhite & Shealy, 1984; Kochhar & Penner, 1987; Kwasigroch & Bullen, 1991), and characteristic dependence on stage of embryogenesis has been shown in mice (Kochhar et al., 1984; Webster et al., 1986; Kwasigroch & Bullen, 1991).

Key References

Adams J: High incidence of intellectual deficits in 5 year old children exposed to isotretinoin "in utero". Teratology 41(5):614, 1990. [S]

Adams J, Lammer EJ: Relationship between dysmorphology and neuropsychological function in children exposed to isotretinoin "in utero". In: Fujii T, Boer GJ (eds). Functional Neuroteratology of Short Term Exposure to Drugs. Tokyo: Teikyo University Press (in press), 1992. [S]

Adams J, Lammer EJ, Holmes LB: A syndrome of cognitive dysfunctions following human embryonic exposure to isotretinoin. Teratology 43(5):497, 1991. [E]

Agnish ND, DiNardo B, Rusin G, Hoar RM: The effect of a teratogenic dose of isotretinoin on the subsequent pregnancy in the rat. J Am Acad Dermatol 11:665-666, 1984. [A]

Anonymous: Isotretinoin--A newly recognized human teratogen. MMWR 33:171-173, 1984. [R]

Anonymous: Update on isotretinoin (Accutane) for acne. Med Lett Drugs Ther 25:105-106, 1983. [R]

Dai WS, Hsu MA, Itri LM: Safety of pregnancy after discontinuation of isotretinoin. Arch Dermatol 125:362-365, 1989. [E]

Dai WS, LaBraico JM, Stern RS: Epidemiology of isotretinoin exposure during pregnancy. J Am Acad Dermatol 26:599-606, 1992. [S]

Hummler H, Korte R, Hendrickx AG: Induction of malformations in the cynomolgus monkey with 13-cis retinoic acid. Teratology 42;263-272, 1990. [A]

Kamm JJ: Toxicology, carcinogenicity, and teratogenicity of some orally administered retinoids. J Am Acad Dermatol 6:652-659, 1982. [R]

Kochhar DM, Penner JD: Developmental effects of isotretinoin and 4-oxo-isotretinoin: The role of metabolism in teratogenicity. Teratology 36:67-75, 1987. [A]

Kochhar DM, Penner JD, Tellone CI: Comparative teratogenic activities of two retinoids: Effects on palate and limb development. Teratogenesis Carcinog Mutagen 4:377-387, 1984. [A]

Kwasigroch TE, Bullen M: Effects of isotretinoin (13-cis-retinoic acid) on the development of mouse limbs in vivo and in vitro. Teratology 44:605-616, 1991. [A]

Lammer EJ, Chen DT, Hoar RM, Agnish ND, et al.: Retinoic acid embryopathy. N Engl J Med 313:837-841, 1985. [S]

Lynberg MC, Khoury MJ, Lammer EJ, et al.: Sensitivity, specificity, and positive predictive value of multiple malformations in isotretinoin em-

bryopathy surveillance. Teratology 42:513-519, 1990. [S]

Rizzo R, Lammer EJ, Parano E, et al.: Limb reduction defects in humans associated with prenatal isotretinoin exposure. Teratology 44:599-604, 1991. [C]

Rosa FW: Teratogenicity of isotretinoin. Lancet 2:513, 1983. [C]

Rosa FW, Wilk AL, Kelsey FO: Teratogen update: Vitamin A congeners. Teratology 33:355-364, 1986. [R]

Strauss JS, Cunningham WJ, Leyden JJ, et al.: Isotretinoin and teratogenicity. J Am Acad Dermatol 19:353-354, 1988. [O]

Teratology Society: Recommendations for isotretinoin use in women of childbearing potential. Teratology 44:1-6, 1991. [O]

Thomson EJ, Cordero JF: The new teratogens: Accutane and other vitamin-A analogs. MCN 14:244-248, 1989. [R]

Webster WS, Johnston MC, Lammer ED, et al.: Isotretinoin embryopathy and the cranial neural crest: An in vivo and in vitro study. J Craniofac Genet Dev Biol 6(3):211-222, 1986. [A]

Willhite CC, Hill RM, Irving DW: Isotretinoin-induced craniofacial malformations in humans and hamsters. J Craniofac Genet Dev Biol [Suppl]2:193-209, 1986. [A] & [C]

Willhite CC, Shealy YF: Amelioration of embryotoxicity by structural modification of the terminal group of cancer chemopreventive retinoids. J Natl Cancer Inst 72:689-695, 1984. [A]

ISOXSUPRINE

Synonyms

Duvadilan, Vasodilan

Summary

Isoxsuprine is a beta sympathomimetic vasodilator used in the treatment of vascular disease. Isoxsuprine is also used to inhibit premature labor.

None To Minimal

Quality and Quantity of Data

Poor

Comment

Neonatal death and abnormalities of perinatal adaptation including hypotension, hypocalcemia, and hypoglycemia, have been observed among infants born to women treated with isoxsuprine shortly before delivery (Brazy & Pupkin, 1979; Brazy et al., 1981).

The frequency of congenital anomalies was no greater than expected among the children of 54 women treated with isoxsuprine during the first four lunar months of pregnancy or among the children of 858 women treated with this agent anytime during pregnancy in the Collaborative Perinatal Project (Heinonen et al., 1977).

No difference in growth or development was observed in the first years of life among 201 children who had been born weighing 1500 g or less after their mothers had been treated with isoxsuprine or other beta-sympathomimetic agents in an attempt to prevent premature delivery (Laros et al., 1991). Six of nine clinically normal infants born to women who had been treated for more than 30 days with isoxsuprine to prevent premature delivery showed evidence of myocardial ischaemia on electrocardiograms during the first weeks of life (Gemelli et al., 1990).

No animal teratology studies of isoxsuprine have been published.

Key References

Brazy JE, Little V, Grimm J: Isoxsuprine in the perinatal period. 2. Relationships between neonatal symptoms, drug exposure, and drug concentration at the time of birth. J Pediatr 98:146-151, 1981. [E]

Brazy JE, Pupkin MJ: Effects of maternal isoxsuprine administration on preterm infants. J Pediatr 94:444-448, 1979. [E]

Gemelli M, DeLuca F, Manganaro R, et al.: Transient electrocardiographic changes suggesting myocardial ischaemia in newborn infants following tocolysis with beta-sympathomimetics. Eur J Pediatr 149:730-733, 1990. [E]

Heinonen OP, Slone D, Shapiro S: Birth Defects and Drugs in Pregnancy. Littleton, Mass.: John Wright-PSG, 1977, pp 346, 347, 439, 492. [E]

Laros RK, Kitterman JA, Heilbron DC, et al.: Outcome of very-low-birth-weight infants exposed to beta-sympathomimetics in utero. Am J Obstet Gynecol 164(6):1657-1665, 1991. [E]

KALAFUNGIN

Summary

Kalafungin is an antifungal agent.

Magnitude of Teratogenic Risk

Undetermined

Quality and Quantity of Data

None

Comment

None

No epidemiological studies of congenital anomalies in infants born to women who used kalafungin during pregnancy have been reported.

No animal teratology studies of kalafungin have been published.

Key References

None available.

KANAMYCIN

Synonyms

Anamid, Cantrex, Cristalomicina, Entero-kanacin, Kamycine, Kantrex, Klebcil

Summary

Kanamycin is an aminoglycoside antibiotic that is used parenterally to treat serious bacterial infections.

Magnitude of Teratogenic Risk

Ototoxicity: Small

Congenital Anomalies: None To Minimal

Quality and Quantity of Data

Ototoxicity: Fair

Congenital Anomalies: Poor

Comment

None

No epidemiological studies of congenital anomalies among infants born to women treated with kanamycin during pregnancy have been reported. Ototoxicity, a recognized complication of kanamycin therapy in adults, has been observed in a child whose mother was treated with kanamycin at about 28 weeks gestation and who herself developed deafness (Jones, 1973).

Increased frequencies of club feet were observed among the offspring of mice and increased frequencies of fetal death but not of malformations were observed among the offspring of rats treated during pregnancy with 9 times the human dose of kanamycin (Matsuzaki et al., 1975). No "gross malformations" were noted among the offspring of rats treated during pregnancy with 7 times the human therapeutic dose of kanamycin in another study (Bevelander & Cohlan, 1962). Histological and electrophysiological evidence of inner ear damage has been found among the offspring of guinea pigs treated during pregnancy with 7-27 times the human dose of kanamycin (Akiyoshi et al., 1977; Dumas & Charcon, 1982). Histological evidence of inner ear damage was not apparent in the offspring of pregnant rats treated with 27 times the human therapeutic dose of kanamycin, but such damage did occur when the infant rats themselves were treated (Onejeme & Khan, 1984).

Please see agent summary on streptomycin for information on a related agent that has been more thoroughly studied.

Key References

Akiyoshi M, Yano S, Tajima T: Ototoxic effect of BB-K8 administered to pregnant guinea pigs on development of inner ear of intrauterine litters. Jpn J Antibiot 30:185-196, 1977. [A]

Bevelander G, Cohlan SQ: The effect on the rat fetus of transplacentally acquired tetracycline. Biol Neonat 4:365-370, 1962. [A]

Dumas G, Charachon R: Ototoxicity of kanamycin in developing guinea pigs. An electrophysiological study. Acta Otolaryngol 94:203-212, 1982. [A]

Jones HC: Intrauterine ototoxicity. A case report and review of literature. J Natl Med Assoc 65(3):201-203, 1973. [C] & [R]

Matsuzaki M, Akutsu S, Mukogawa H, et al.: Teratological studies of amikacin (BB-K8) in mice and rats. Jpn J Antibiot 28:372-384, 1975. [A]

Onejeme AU, Khan KM: Morphologic study of effects of kanamycin on the developing cochlea of the rat. Teratology 29:57-71, 1984. [A]

KAOLIN

Synonyms

Kaopectate, Vanclay

Summary

Kaolin, a clay, is composed of hydrated aluminum silicate. It is used as an adsorbent, in dusting powders, and in poultices. It is administered orally in the treatment of diarrhea. Kaolin is practically insoluble.

Magnitude of Teratogenic Risk

Undetermined

Quality and Quantity of Data

None To Poor

Comment

A small risk cannot be excluded, but a high risk of congenital anomalies in the children of women treated with kaolin during pregnancy is unlikely.

No epidemiological studies of congenital anomalies among the children of women who took kaolin during pregnancy have been reported.

The frequency of malformations was not increased among the offspring of rats fed diets including 20% kaolin during pregnancy (Patterson & Staszak, 1977). Decreased weight was observed among the newborn pups, but this effect was reversed by supplementing the maternal diet with iron.

Key References

Patterson EC, Staszak DJ: Effects of geophagia (kaolin ingestion) on the maternal blood and embryonic development in the pregnant rat. J Nutr 107:2020-2025, 1977. [A]

KETAMINE

Synonyms

Ketalar

Summary

Ketamine is a dissociative anesthetic chemically related to the phencyclidine psychoactive agents. Ketamine is administered parenterally.

Magnitude of Teratogenic Risk

Undetermined

Quality and Quantity of Data

None To Poor

Comment

None

No epidemiological studies of congenital anomalies in children born to women anesthetized with ketamine during pregnancy have been reported.

The frequency of malformations was not increased among the offspring of rats treated during pregnancy with ketamine in doses 10-12 times greater than those used in humans (El-Karim & Benny, 1976; Llorente et al., 1979). Degenerative effects were seen on histopathological examination of various tissues in a study of the offspring of rats treated during pregnancy with 2.5-10 times the human dose of ketamine, but the biological and statistical significance of this finding is unclear (Kochhar et al., 1986).

Neonatal neurobehavioral alterations have been observed among infants delivered to women treated with ketamine during labor (Hodgkinson et al., 1978). The clinical significance of this observation is unknown. Profound neonatal respiratory depression has been reported in macaque monkeys born after maternal ketamine treatment near term (Eng et al., 1975).

Key References

El-Karim AHA, Benny R: Embryotoxic and teratogenic action of ketamine hydrochloride in rats. Ain Shams Med J 27:459-463, 1976. [A]

Eng M, Bonica JJ, Akamatsu TJ, Berges PU, et al.: Respiratory depression in newborn monkeys at caesarean section following ketamine administration. Br J Anaesth 47:917-921, 1975. [A]

Hodgkinson R, Bhatt M, Kim SS, Grewal G, et al.: Neonatal neurobehavioral tests following cesarean section under general and spinal anesthesia. Am J Obstet Gynecol 132:670-674, 1978. [S]

Kochhar MM, Aykac I, Davidson PP, et al.: Teratologic effects of d,1-2-(o-chlorophenyl)-2-(methylamino) cyclohexanone hydrochloride (ketamine hydrochloride) in rats. Res Commun Chem Pathol Pharmacol 54:413-415, 1986. [A]

Llorente R, Gomez-Capilla JL, Gelera CH: [Teratogenic activity of some anesthetics]. Rev Esp Anest Rean 26:137-144, 1979. [A]

KETOCONAZOLE

Synonyms

Fungarest, Fungo-Hubber, Fungoral, Keto-derm, Ketoisdin, Micoticum, Nizoral, Nizovules, Panfungal

Summary

Ketoconazole is an antifungal agent used to treat systemic mycotic infections.

Magnitude of Teratogenic Risk

Undetermined

Quality and Quantity of Data

Poor

Comment

A small risk cannot be excluded, but a high risk of congenital anomalies in the children of women treated with ketoconazole during pregnancy is unlikely.

No epidemiological studies of congenital anomalies in infants born to women who took ketoconazole during pregnancy have been reported.

The frequencies of fetal death and anomalies were increased among the offspring of rats treated during pregnancy with 2-4 times the human dose of ketoconazole (Nishikawa et al., 1984; Buttar et al., 1989). Ventricular septal

defect and cleft palate were among the most frequently observed anomalies. Increased frequencies of fetal death were also seen among the offspring of pregnant mice and rabbits treated with 1-2 and 1-4 times the human therapeutic dose of ketoconazole (Nishikawa et al., 1984; Buttar et al., 1989).

Key References

Buttar HS, Moffatt JH, Bura C: Pregnancy outcome in ketoconazole-treated rats and mice. Teratology 39(5):444, 1989. [A]

Nishikawa S, Hara T, Miyazaki H, Ohkuro T: Reproduction studies of KW-1414 in rats and rabbits. Clin Rep 18:1433-1448, 1984. [A]

LACTIC ACID (LACTATE)

Synonyms

2-Hydroxypropionic Acid, Milchsaure, Milk Acid, Phygiene, Tampovagan, Tonsillosan

Summary

Lactic acid is a product of normal carbohydrate metabolism. Lactic acid is administered intravenously in the treatment of acidosis and used locally to treat vaginal discharges.

Magnitude of Teratogenic Risk

Undetermined

Quality and Quantity of Data

None

Comment

A small risk cannot be excluded, but a high risk of congenital anomalies in the children of women treated with lactic acid (lactate) during pregnancy is unlikely.

No epidemiological studies of congenital anomalies among infants born to women

treated with large amounts of lactic acid during pregnancy have been reported.

No animal teratology studies of lactic acid have been published.

Key References

None available.

LACTULOSE

Synonyms

Cephulac, Cholac, Chronulac, Constilac, Constulose, Duphalac, Enulose, Generlac

Summary

Lactulose is a synthetic disaccharide used to treat constipation and hepatic encephalopathy. It is usually given orally and is absorbed very poorly from the gastrointestinal tract.

Magnitude of Teratogenic Risk

None

Quality and Quantity of Data

None To Poor

Comment

None

No epidemiological studies of congenital anomalies in infants whose mothers took lactulose during pregnancy have been reported.

The frequency of malformations was not increased among the offspring of rats or rabbits given lactulose during pregnancy in doses equal to or slightly greater than those used in humans during pregnancy (Baglioni & Dubini, 1976).

Key References

Baglioni A, Dubini F: Lattulosio: Valutazione tossicologica. Boll Chim Farm 115:596-606, 1976. [A]

LANATOSIDE C

Synonyms

Cedilanid, Ceglunate, Celanide, Digilanide C, Digilanogen C, Isolanide, Lanatigen C, Lanatosid C

Summary

Lanatoside C is a cardiac glycoside used to treat heart failure and dysrhythmias.

Magnitude of Teratogenic Risk

Undetermined

Quality and Quantity of Data

None

Comment

None

No epidemiological studies of congenital anomalies in infants born to mothers treated with lanatoside C during pregnancy have been reported.

No animal teratology studies of lanatoside C have been published.

Please see agent summary on digoxin for information on a related drug that has been studied.

Key References

None available.

LANOLIN

Synonyms

Acetadeps, Amerlate P, Aqualose, Golden Fleece, Lanogels, Modulan, Ohlan, Sebase, Wool Fat

Summary

Lanolin is prepared from wool fat. It is used as an emulsifying agent and emollient in skin creams. Lanolin can be absorbed through the skin.

Magnitude of Teratogenic Risk

None

Quality and Quantity of Data

None To Poor

Comment

None

No epidemiological studies of congenital anomalies among infants born to women who used preparations containing lanolin during pregnancy have been reported.

No teratogenic effect was observed among the offspring of pregnant rabbits fed a lanolin derivative (a C-12 alcohol ethoxylate) even in doses that were toxic to the mothers (up to 200 mg/kg/d) (Anonymous, 1982).

Key References

Anonymous: Final report on the safety assessment of laneth-10 acetate group. J Am Coll Toxicol 1(4):1-23, 1982. [A]

LECITHINS

Synonyms

Alcolec PG, Centrolex P, Centrophill IP, Emulthin M-35, Gliddex, Granulestin, Kelecin, Ovovitellin, Phospholutein, Unilex

Summary

Lecithins comprise a group of naturally-occurring phospholipids. The composition of a given preparation depends on the source and includes various amounts of phosphatidyl esters, triglycerides, fatty acids, and carbohydrates.

Magnitude of Teratogenic Risk

Undetermined

Quality and Quantity of Data

Poor

Comment

A small risk cannot be excluded, but a high risk of congenital anomalies in the children of women treated with lecithins during pregnancy is unlikely.

No epidemiological studies of congenital anomalies among infants born to women who ingested lecithins in unusually large amounts during pregnancy have been reported.

The frequency of malformations was not increased among the offspring of pregnant rats or rabbits given large doses of micelles composed largely of lecithin (Teelmann et al., 1984) or among the offspring of pregnant mice, rats, or rabbits given large doses of lecithins (Food and Drug Research Labs, 1974).

Key References

Food and Drug Research Labs: Teratologic evaluation of FDA 71-88 (Alcolec(R): Alcolec S Lecithin) in mice, rats and rabbits. NTIS (National Technical Information Service) Report/PB-234 874), 1974. [A]

Teelmann K, Schlappi B, Schupbach M, Kistler A: Preclinical safety evaluation of intravenously administered mixed micelles. *Arzneimittelforsch* 34(2):1517-1523, 1984. [A]

LEUCINOCAINE

Synonyms

Leucinocaine Mesylate

Summary

Leucinocaine is a local anesthetic of the ester class that has been used topically and by injection.

Magnitude of Teratogenic Risk

Undetermined

Quality and Quantity of Data

None

Comment

None

No epidemiological studies of congenital anomalies in children born to women exposed to leucinocaine during pregnancy have been reported.

No investigations of teratologic effects of leucinocaine in experimental animals have been published.

Please see agent summary on procaine for information on a related agent that has been studied.

Key References

None available.

LEUPROLIDE

Synonyms

Carcinil, Leuprorelin, Lucrin, Lupron, Procrin

Summary

Leuprolide is a synthetic peptide analog of luteinizing hormone-releasing hormone. Leuprolide is given intramuscularly as a depot injection to treat endometriosis. Leuprolide has also been used subcutaneously as part of a regimen for pharmacological stimulation of ovulation.

Magnitude of Teratogenic Risk

Undetermined

Quality and Quantity of Data

None To Poor

Comment

1) Multifetal pregnancies may be especially frequent in women who conceive after ovulation stimulation with leuprolide and gonadotropin (see below).

2) Multifetal gestation is associated with an increased risk of certain congenital anomalies (Myrianthopoulos, 1976; Schinzel et al., 1979).

3) 85-100% of an intramuscular dose of depot leuprolide is absorbed within four weeks following administration (AHFS Drug Information, 1991).

No epidemiological studies of congenital anomalies among infants born to women treated with leuprolide during pregnancy have been reported.

Multifetal pregnancies may be even more frequent in women who conceive after ovulation has been stimulated with leuprolide and gonadotropin than after other methods of ovulation stimulation (Jansen et al., 1990).

Fetal growth retardation was observed with increased frequency among the offspring of rats or rabbits treated during pregnancy with subcutaneous doses of leuprolide similar to those used in humans (Ooshima et al., 1990a, b). The frequency of malformations was not increased in either species, but fetal death was frequent after treatment of pregnant rats with the highest dose.

Key References

AHFS Drug Information--91. Bethesda, Md.: Board of Dir of Amer Soc of Hosp Pharmacists, 1991, pp 568-574. [O]

Jansen RPS, Anderson JC, Birrell WSR, et al.: Outpatient gamete intrafallopian transfer: A clinical anaylsis of 710 cases. Med J Aust 153:182-188, 1990. [S]

Myrianthopoulos NC: Congenital malformations in twins. Acta Genet Med Gemellol (Roma) 25:331-335, 1976. [E]

Ooshima Y, Negishi R, Yoshida T, et al.: [Teratological study of TAP-144-SR in rats]. Yakuri To Chiryo (Suppl) 18(3):S609-S623, 1990a. [A]

Ooshima Y, Nakamura H, Negishi R, et al.: [Teratological study of TAP-144-SR in rabbits]. Yakuri To Chiryo (Suppl) 18(3):S633-639, 1990b. [A]

Schinzel AAGL, Smith DW, Miller JR: Monozygotic twinning and structural defects. J Pediatr 95(6):921-930, 1979. [E]

LEVODOPA

Synonyms

Brocadopa, Dihydroxyphenylalanine, Dopa, Dopar, L-Dopa, Larodopa, Syndopa, Veldopa

Summary

Levodopa is a naturally occurring amino acid that is the immediate precursor of the neurotransmitter dopamine. Levodopa is used to treat Parkinson's disease and similar neurological disorders.

Magnitude of Teratogenic Risk

Undetermined

Quality and Quantity of Data

None To Poor

Comment

None

No studies of malformations in children born to women treated with levodopa during pregnancy have been reported.

The frequency of malformations was not increased among the offspring of mice or rats treated during pregnancy with levodopa in doses respectively 5-60 and 4-30 times those used clinically (Tanase et al., 1970). An increased frequency of cardiovascular anomalies was observed among the offspring of rabbits treated during pregnancy with levodopa in doses 25-50 times the usual human dose, but not at 12 times the usual human dose (Staples & Mattis, 1973). The relevance of this finding to the risks associated with therapeutic use of levodopa in human pregnancy is unknown.

Key References

Staples RE, Mattis PA: Teratology of L-DOPA. Teratology 8:238, 1973. [A]

Tanase H, Hirose K, Shimada K, Aoki K, et al.: The safety test of l-DOPA. II. Effect of l-DOPA on the development of pre- and post-natal offsprings of experimental animals. Sankyo Kenyusho Nempo 22:165-186, 1970. [A]

LEVONORDEFRIN

Synonyms

Cobefrin, Corbadrine, l-Nordefrin, Methylnoradrenaline, Neo-Cobefrin, Nordefrin

Summary

Levonordefrin is an adrenergic agent that is used as a vasoconstrictor in local anesthetic solutions, primarily during dental procedures.

Magnitude of Teratogenic Risk

None

Quality and Quantity of Data

None To Poor

Comment

None

The frequency of congenital anomalies was no greater than expected among the children of 26 women who had been given levonordefrin during the first four lunar months of pregnancy in the Collaborative Perinatal Project (Heinonen et al., 1977).

No animal teratology studies of levonordefrin have been published.

Please see epinephrine summary for information on a related agent that has been studied more thoroughly.

Key References

Heinonen OP, Slone D, Shapiro S: Birth Defects and Drugs in Pregnancy. Littleton, Mass.: John Wright-PSG, 1977, pp 345-347. [E]

LEVORPHANOL

Synonyms

Aromarone, Dromoran, Lemoran, Levo-Dromoran, Levorfanol, Levorphan Tartrate, Levorphanal

Summary

Levorphanol is a narcotic analgesic.

Magnitude of Teratogenic Risk

Undetermined

Quality and Quantity of Data

None To Poor

Comment

A small risk cannot be excluded, but a high risk of congenital anomalies in the children of women treated with levorphanol during pregnancy is unlikely.

No epidemiological studies of congenital anomalies among infants born to women treated with levorphanol during pregnancy have been reported.

The frequency of central nervous system and other anomalies was increased among the offspring of mice treated with levorphanol during pregnancy in doses 140 times those used clinically (Jurand, 1980).

Please see agent summary on morphine for information on a related agent that has been more thoroughly studied.

Key References

Jurand A: Malformations of the central nervous system induced by neurotropic drugs in mouse embryos. Dev Growth Differ 22:61-78, 1980. [A]

LEVOTHYROXINE

Synonyms

Choloxin, Eltroxine, Levothroid, L-Thyroxine Sodium, Sodium Thyroxine, Synthroid, T4

Summary

Levothyroxine (T4), a thyroid hormone, is used to treat goiter and thyroid deficiency states.

Magnitude of Teratogenic Risk

None

Quality and Quantity of Data

Fair

Comment

None

The frequencies of congenital anomalies, major malformations, minor anomalies, and major classes of anomalies were not increased among 537 children of women treated with levothyroxine or thyroid extract during the first four lunar months of pregnancy in the Collaborative Perinatal Project (Heinonen et al., 1977). Similarly, the frequency of congenital anomalies was no greater than expected among 1605 children of women treated with levothyroxine or thyroid extract anytime during pregnancy in this study.

The frequency of cleft palate was not increased among the offspring of mice treated with up to 300 times the usual human dose of levothyroxine during pregnancy (Lamb et al., 1986). No increase in malformations was seen among the offspring of pregnant rats treated with 25 times the usual human dose of levothyroxine during early pregnancy (Baksi, 1978), but at even higher doses, cataracts, permanent impairment of hypothalmo-pituitary-thyroid function, and fetal or neonatal death regularly occurred (Giroud & Rothschild, 1951; Lammers et al., 1978; Porterfield, 1985). The relevance, if any, of these findings with thyrotoxic doses to the therapeutic use of levothyroxine during human pregnancy is unknown.

In humans, direct fetal treatment with levothyroxine late in pregnancy has been used for fetal hypothyroidism and goitre (van Herle et al., 1975; Weiner et al., 1980). Intraamniotic instillation of levothyroxine has also been used to induce fetal lung maturity prior to premature delivery in the third trimester of pregnancy (Mashiach et al., 1978). Such therapy does not appear to have any adverse effect on the child (Barkai et al., 1988).

Key References

Baksi SN: Effect of dichlorvos on embryonal and fetal development in thyroparathyroidectomized, thyroxine-treated and euthyroid rats. Toxicol Lett 2:213-216, 1978. [A]

Barkai G, Zarfin Y, Ben-Harari M, et al.: In utero thyroxine therapy for the induction of fetal lung maturity: Long term effects. J Perinat Med 16:145-148, 1988. [E]

Giroud A, de Rothschild B: Effects of thyroxine on the fetal eye. C R Soc Biol 145:525-526, 1951. [S]

Heinonen OP, Slone D, Shapiro S: Birth Defects and Drugs in Pregnancy. Littleton, Mass.: John Wright-PSG, 1977, pp 397-398, 443. [E]

Lamb JC, Harris MW, McKinney JD, et al.: Effects of thyroid hormones on the induction of cleft palate by 2,3,7,8-tetrachlorodibenzo-p-dioxin (TCDD) in C57BL/6N mice. Toxicol Appl Pharmacol 84(1):115-124, 1986. [A]

Lammers M, von zur Muhlen A, Dohler U: Prenatal thyroxine treatment causes permanent impairment of hypothalamopituitary-thyroid function in rats. Acta Endocrinol (Copenh) 215:73-74, 1978. [A]

Mashiach S, Barkai G, Sack J, et al.: Enhancement of fetal lung maturity by intra-amniotic administration of thyroid hormone. Am J Obstet Gynecol 130(3):289-293, 1978. [S]

Porterfield SP: Prenatal exposure of the fetal rat to excessive L-thyroxine or 3,6-dimethyl-3'-isopropyl-thyronine produces persistent changes in the thyroid control system. Horm Metabol Res 17:655-659, 1985. [A]

van Herle Aj, Young RT, Fisher DA, et al.: Intra-uterine treatment of a hypothyroid fetus. J Clin Endocrinol Metab 40:474-477, 1975. [C]

Weiner S, Scharf JI, Bolognese RJ, et al.: Antenatal diagnosis and treatment of a fetal goiter. J Reprod Med 24:39-42, 1980. [C]

LEVOXADROL

Summary

Levoxadrol is a local anesthetic.

Magnitude of Teratogenic Risk

Undetermined

Quality and Quantity of Data

None

Comment

None

No epidemiological studies of congenital anomalies in children born to women exposed to levoxadrol during pregnancy have been reported.

No investigations of teratologic effects of levoxadrol in experimental animals have been published.

Key References

None available.

LIDOCAINE

Synonyms

Anestacon, Dalcaine, Democaine, LidoPen, Lignocaine, Xylocaine, Xylodase

Summary

Lidocaine is a local anesthetic of the amide class that is widely used by injection and topical application. Lidocaine is also used intravenously to treat cardiac arrhythmias.

Magnitude of Teratogenic Risk

None

Quality and Quantity of Data

Fair

Comment

This rating is for use of lidocaine as a local anesthetic. The risk for systemic use of this agent is undetermined.

The frequencies of congenital anomalies in general, of major malformations, of minor anomalies, and of major classes of congenital anomalies were not increased among the children of 293 women who had been treated with lidocaine as a local anesthetic during the first four lunar months of pregnancy in the Collaborative Perinatal Project (Heinonen et al., 1977). The frequency of congenital anomalies was no greater than expected among the children born to 947 women treated with lidocaine as a local anesthetic anytime during pregnancy in this study. No epidemiological investigations of congenital anomalies among children born to women treated with intravenous lidocaine for cardiac arrhythmia during pregnancy have been reported.

No teratogenic effect was observed among the offspring of rats treated continuously during pregnancy with lidocaine in doses 1-5 times those given by infusion in humans (Fujinaga & Mazze, 1986). In another study, no teratogenic effect was noted among the offspring of rats treated with single daily doses of lidocaine that were similar in magnitude to the total daily infusion dose used in humans (Ramazzotto et al., 1985). Increased frequencies of central nervous system (CNS) anomalies were observed among fetuses of pregnant mice given single injections of lidocaine 50-70% as great as those used daily by infusion in humans (Martin & Jurand, 1992). Alterations of neonatal behavior have been noted among the offspring of pregnant rats treated with single injections of lidocaine that are 1-2 times those used on an hourly basis in humans (Smith et al., 1986), but the effect on behavior later in life was variable (Teiling et al., 1987; Smith et al., 1989). The clinical significance of this observation is uncertain.

Transient alterations of perinatal cardio-pulmonary adaptation have been reported after maternal local or regional anesthesia with lidocaine (Shnider & Way, 1968; Liston et al., 1973; Baxi et al., 1979; Bozynski et al., 1987), but serious changes appear to be uncommon (Bratteby, 1981; Abboud et al., 1982; Kileff et al., 1982) except when inadvertent direct injection of drug into the fetus occurs during delivery (Kim et al., 1979; De Praeter et al., 1991). Alterations of brain stem auditory evoked responses have been observed in neonates born to women who had received regional anesthesia with lidocaine during delivery (Diaz et al., 1988; Bozynski et al., 1989). Changes in perinatal adaptation have also been reported in baboons and sheep after maternal administration of lidocaine late in pregnancy (Morishima et al., 1979, 1981; 1989).

Key References

Abboud TK, Khoo SS, Miller F, Doan R, et al.: Maternal, fetal, and neonatal responses after epidural anesthesia with bupivacaine, 2-chloroprocaine, or lidocaine. Anesth Analg 61:638-644, 1982. [E]

Baxi LV, Petrie RH, James LS: Human fetal oxygenation following paracervical block. Am J Obstet Gynecol 135:1109-1112, 1979. [E]

Bozynski MEA, Rubarth LB, Patel JA: Lidocaine toxicity after maternal pudendal anesthesia in a term infant with fetal distress. Am J Perinatol 4(2):164-166, 1987. [C]

Bozynski MEA, Schumacher RE, Deschner LS, Kileny P: Effect of prenatal lignocaine on auditory brain stem evoked response. Arch Dis Child 64:934-938, 1989. [E]

Bratteby LE: Effects on the infant of obstetric regional analgesia. J Perinat Med 9(Suppl 1):54-56, 1981. [E]

De Praeter C, Vanhaesebrouck P, De Praeter N, et al.: Episiotomy and neonatal lidocaine intoxication. Eur J Pediatr 150:685-686, 1991. [C]

Diaz M, Graff M, Hiatt M, et al.: Prenatal lidocaine and the auditory evoked responses in term infants. Am J Dis Child 142:160-161, 1988. [E]

Fujinaga M, Mazze RI: Reproductive and teratogenic effects of lidocaine in Sprague-Dawley rats. Anesthesiology 65:626-632, 1986. [A]

Heinonen OP, Slone D, Shapiro S: Birth Defects and Drugs in Pregnancy. Littleton, Mass.: John Wright-PSG, 1977, pp 358, 360, 477, 493. [E]

Kileff M, James FM III, Dewan D, et al.: Neonatal neurobehavioral responses after epidural anesthesia for cesarean section with lidocaine and bupivacaine. Anesthesiology 57(Suppl):A403, 1982. [S]

Kim WY, Pomerance JJ, Miller AA: Lidocaine intoxication in a newborn following local anesthesia for episiotomy. Pediatrics 64:643-645, 1979. [C]

Liston WA, Adjepon-Yamoah KK, Scott DB: Foetal and maternal lignocaine levels after paracervical block. Brit J Anaesth 45:750-754, 1973. [E]

Martin LVH, Jurand A: The absence of teratogenic effects of some analgesics used in anaesthesia. Additional evidence from a mouse model. Anaesthesia 47:473-476, 1992. [A]

Morishima HO, Covino BG, Yeh MN, Stark RI, et al.: Bradycardia in the fetal baboon following paracervical block anesthesia. Am J Obstet Gynecol 140:775-780, 1981. [A]

Morishima HO, Gutsche BG, Stark RI, Milliez JM, et al.: Relationship of fetal bradycardia to maternal administration of lidocaine in sheep. Am J Obstet Gynecol 134:289-296, 1979. [A]

Morishima HO, Pedersen H, Santos AC, et al.: Adverse effects of maternally administered lidocaine on the asphyxiated preterm fetal lamb. Anesthesiology 71:110-115, 1989. [A]

Ramazzotto LJ, Curro FA, Paterson JA, et al.: Toxicological assessment of lidocaine in the pregnant rat. J Dent Res 164:1214-1217, 1985. [A]

Shnider SM, WAy EL: Plasma levels of lidocaine (Xylocaine) in mother and newborn following obstetrical conduction anesthesia: Clinical applications. Anesthesiology 29:251-258, 1968. [E]

Smith RF, Kurkjian MF, Mattran KM, Kurtz SL: Behavioral effects of prenatal exposure to lidocaine in the rat: Effects of dosage and of gestational age at administration. Neurotoxicol Teratol 11:395-403, 1989. [A]

Smith RF, Wharton GG, Kurtz SL, et al.: Behavioral effects of mid-pregnancy administration of lidocaine and mepivacaine in the rat. Neurobehav Toxicol Teratol 8:61-68, 1986. [A]

Teiling AKY, Mohammed AK, Minor BG, et al.: Lack of effects of prenatal exposure to lidocaine on development of behavior in rats. Anesth Analg 66:533-541, 1987. [A]

LINDANE

Synonyms

Benzene Hexachloride, Gamma Hexachlor, Kwell, Lorexane, Quellada

Summary

Lindane is an organochlorine pesticide. It is used to control agricultural insects and house-flies. In medicine, topical application of lindane is employed in the treatment of lice and mites (scabies). The Threshold Limit Value for occupational exposure to lindane in air as an 8-hour time-weighted average is 0.5 mg/cu m (Hathaway et al., 1991). Lindane absorption may occur through the skin, lungs, or gastrointestinal tract.

Magnitude of Teratogenic Risk

Undetermined

Quality and Quantity of Data

Poor

Comment

1) A small risk cannot be excluded, but a high risk of congenital anomalies in the children of women exposed to lindane during pregnancy is unlikely.

2) This risk assessment is for occupational exposure within accepted limits. There may be a substantial risk with exposures that are toxic to a pregnant woman.

No epidemiological studies of congenital anomalies in infants whose mothers were exposed to lindane during pregnancy have been reported. Maternal and placental concentration of lindane and other organochloride insecticides were higher among 10 women with spontaneous abortion than among women with full-term pregnancies in one study (Saxena et al., 1981). This observation requires confirmation with control of the possible effect of gestational age.

No teratogenic effect was observed among the offspring of rats or rabbits fed up to 20 mg/kg/d or 5-15 mg/kg/d of lindane during pregnancy (Palmer et al., 1978; Khera et al., 1979; Saxena et al., 1986). Embryonic or fetal death occurred in pregnant rats, mice, hamsters, rabbits, and dogs fed lindane in one or more daily doses of 40-100 mg/kg, 6-11 mg/kg, 20-40 mg/kg, 20-60 mg/kg, 7.5-15 mg/kg, respectively (Earl et al., 1973; Dzierzawski, 1977; Palmer et al., 1978; Sicar & Lahiri, 1989).

Key References

Dzierzawski A: Embryotoxicity studies of lindane in the golden hamster, rat and rabbit. Bull Vet Inst Pulawy 21(3-4):85-93, 1977. [A]

Earl FL, Miller E, Van Loon EJ: Reproductive, teratogenic, and neonatal effects of some pesticides and related compounds in beagle dogs and miniature swine. Pestic Environ Pap Contin Controversy Inter-Am Conf Toxicol Occup Med 8th:253-266, 1973. [A]

Hathaway GJ, Proctor NH, Hughes JP, Fischman ML (eds): Proctor and Hughes' Chemical Hazards of the Workplace, 3rd ed. New York: Van Nostrand Reinhold, 1991, pp 359-360. [O]

Khera KS, Whalen C, Trivett G, Agners G: Assessment of the teratogenic potential of biphenyl, ethoxyquin, piperonyl butoxide, diuron, thiabendazole, phosalone, and lindane in rats. Toxicol Appl Pharmacol 48:A33, 1979. [A]

Palmer AK, Bottomley AM, Worden AN, et al.: Effect of lindane on pregnancy in the rabbit and rat. Toxicology 9:239-247, 1978. [A]

Palmer AK, Cozens DD, Spicer EJF, Worden AN: Effects of lindane upon reproductive function in a 3-generation study in rats. Toxicology 10:45-54, 1978. [A]

Saxena DK, Murthy RC, Chandra SV: Embryotoxic and teratogenic effects of interaction of cadmium and lindane in rats. Acta Pharmacol Toxicol 59:175-178, 1986. [A]

Saxena MC, Siddiqui MKJ, Seth TD, Murti CRK, et al.: Organochlorine pesticides in specimens from women undergoing spontaneous abortion, premature or full-term delivery. J Anal Toxicol 5:6-9, 1981. [S]

Sircar S, Lahiri P: Lindane (gamma-HCH) causes reproductive failure and fetotoxicity in mice. Toxicology 59:171-177, 1989. [A]

LITHIUM

Synonyms

Camcolit, Cibalith-S, Eskalith, Litarex, Lithane, Lithobid, Lithonate, Lithotabs, Phasal, Priadel

Summary

Lithium salts, especially lithium carbonate, are used for the prevention and treatment of affective mental illness.

Magnitude of Teratogenic Risk

Small

Quality and Quantity of Data

Fair To Good

Comment

None

An association has been observed between maternal treatment with lithium carbonate during pregnancy and the occurrence of cardiovascular malformations, especially Ebstein's anomaly, in children (Elia et al., 1987; Thiels, 1987; Warkany, 1988). Eighteen (8%) of 225 infants voluntarily reported to an international registry because they had been born to mothers treated with lithium salts during the first trimester of pregnancy had serious congenital cardiovascular anomalies (Weinstein, 1980). Six of the affected infants (2.7% of the total) had Ebstein's anomaly, a malformation that occurs with an expected incidence of only about 1/20,000. Non-cardiovascular malformations occurred in seven (3.1%) of the 225 infants, a frequency not much different from that expected. Because these cases were voluntarily reported and because no appropriate control data are available, it is not possible to use this registry to estimate the risk of congenital anomalies in children of women who take lithium salts during early pregnancy.

This risk appears to be relatively small on the basis of case-control and cohort studies, however. No instance of maternal lithium use during pregnancy was observed in case-control studies of 59, 40, or 34 children with Ebstein's anomaly or of 44 children with tricuspid atresia (Kallen, 1988; Zalzstein et al., 1990; Edmonds & Oakley, 1990).

The frequency of congenital anomalies was no greater than expected among the 105 liveborn infants whose mothers had taken lithium during all or part of the first trimester of pregnancy in a series ascertained through four teratogen information services (Jacobson et al., 1992). There was a total of 138 pregnancies with known outcome in this series; one fetus with Ebstein's anomaly was diagnosed prenatally and therapeutically aborted. The occurrence of this rare malformation in so small a series of patients is remarkable. In another cohort of children born to women with manic-depressive illness ascertained through a linked set of population-based registries, 59 infants were delivered by mothers who took lithium salts early in pregnancy (Kallen & Tanberg, 1983). Eleven (19%) of these infants had congenital anomalies and four (7%) had congenital heart disease. None had Ebstein's anomaly. The frequencies of congenital anomalies and of heart defects were significantly greater than among the children of manic-depressive women who had not been treated with lithium during pregnancy.

Prenatal diagnosis by fetal echocardiography has been recommended for pregnant women who have been treated with lithium early in pregnancy (Allan et al., 1982).

No differences were found between 60 children born of pregnancies in which the mother took lithium and their unexposed siblings in a postal survey of physical and mental developmental problems five or more years after birth (Schou, 1976).

Increased frequencies of cleft palate and fetal loss have been observed among the offspring of mice treated chronically during pregnancy with lithium carbonate in doses that produce blood levels within the human therapeutic range (Szabo, 1970; Smithberg & Dixit, 1982). Treatments of just a few days duration did not produce a teratogenic effect unless the dosage of lithium was increased six-fold. No teratogenic effect was noted among pregnant rats or rabbits treated with lithium carbonate in doses calculated to produce serum levels within the human therapeutic range (Gralla & McIlhenny, 1972). In another investigation, increased frequencies of eye and ear anomalies were observed in the offspring of pregnant rats given lithium chloride in doses that produced blood levels below the human therapeutic range but caused maternal toxicity (Wright et al., 1971).

Several other animal teratology studies have been done with lithium salts, but these investigations do not include measurements of serum levels and are therefore more difficult to interpret. Most involve treatment with lithium salts in doses one to several times those used in humans, and many of the studies are complicated by maternal toxicity. The results have been inconsistent. Increased frequencies of malformations or fetal death or both have been reported in swine (Kelley et al., 1978), and in rats or mice in some studies but not others (Trautner et al., 1958; Schluter, 1971; Marathe & Thomas, 1986; Jurand, 1988). No malformations were observed among seven rhesus monkeys born to mothers treated during pregnancy with lithium carbonate in a dose at the lower end of the human therapeutic range (Gralla & McIlhenny, 1972).

Lithium toxicity may occur in infants born to women who are receiving treatment with lithium salts near term. The abnormalities, which resemble those seen in adults with lithium toxicity, include neurological, cardiac, and hepatic dysfunction (Wilbanks et al., 1970; Woody et al., 1971; Stevens et al., 1974; Mizrahi et al., 1979; Arnon et al., 1981; Filtenborg, 1982; Morrell et al., 1983).

Key References

Allan LD, Desai G, Tynan MJ: Prenatal echocardiographic screening for Ebstein's anomaly for mothers on lithium therapy. Lancet 2:875-876, 1982. [S]

Arnon RG, Marin-Garcia J, Peeden JN: Tricuspid valve regurgitation and lithium carbonate toxicity in a newborn infant. Am J Dis Child 135:941-943, 1981. [C]

Edmonds LD, Oakley GP: Ebstein's anomaly and maternal lithium exposure during pregnancy. Teratology 41:551-552, 1990. [E]

Elia J, Katz IR, Simpson GM: Teratogenicity of psychotherapeutic medications. Psychopharmacol Bull 23(4):531-586, 1987. [R]

Filtenborg JA: Persistent pulmonary hypertension after lithium intoxication in the newborn. Eur J Pediatr 138:321-323, 1982. [C]

Gralla EJ, McIlhenny HM: Studies in pregnant rats, rabbits and monkeys with lithium carbonate. Toxicol Appl Pharmacol 21:428-433, 1972. [A]

Jacobson SJ, Jones K, Johnson K, et al.: Prospective multicentre study of pregnancy outcome after lithium exposure during first trimester. Lancet 339:530-533, 1992. [E]

Jurand A: Teratogenic activity of lithium carbonate: An experimental update. Teratology 38:101-111, 1988. [A]

Kallen B: Comments on teratogen update: Lithium. Teratology 38:597, 1988. [O]

Kallen B, Tanberg A: Lithium and pregnancy. A cohort study on manic-depressive women. Acta Psychiatr Scand 68:134-139, 1983. [E]

Kelley KW, McGlone JJ, Froseth JA: Lithium toxicity in pregnant swine. Proc Soc Exp Biol Med 158:123-127, 1978. [A]

Marathe MR, Thomas GP: Embryotoxicity and teratogenicity of lithium carbonate in Wistar rat. Toxicol Lett 34:115-120, 1986. [A]

Mizrahi EM, Hobbs JF, Goldsmith DI: Nephrogenic diabetes insipidus in transplacental lithium intoxication. J Pediatr 94:493-495, 1979. [C]

Morrell P, Sutherland GR, Buamah PK, Oo M, et al.: Lithium toxicity in a neonate. Arch Dis Child 58:539-541, 1983. [C]

Schluter G: Effects of lithium carmine and lithium carbonate on the prenatal development of mice. Naunyn Schmiedebergs Arch Pharmacol 270:56-64, 1971. [A]

Schou M: What happened later to the lithium babies? A follow-up study of children born without malformations. Acta Psychiat Scand 54:193-197, 1976. [E]

Smithberg M, Dixit PK: Teratogenic effects of lithium in mice. Teratology 26:239-246, 1982. [A]

Stevens D, Burman D, Midwinter A: Transplacental lithium poisoning. Lancet 2:595, 1974. [C]

Szabo KT: Teratogenic effect of lithium carbonate in the foetal mouse. Nature 225:73-75, 1970. [A]

Thiels C: Pharmacotherapy of psychiatric disorder in pregnancy and during breastfeeding: A Review. Pharmacopsychiat 20:133-146, 1987. [R]

Trautner EM, Pennycuik PR, Morris RJH, Gershon S, et al.: The effects of prolonged subtoxic lithium ingestion on pregnancy in rats. Austr J Exp Biol 36:305-322, 1958. [A]

Warkany J: Teratogen update: Lithium. Teratology 38:593-596, 1988. [R]

Weinstein MR: Lithium treatment of women during pregnancy and in the post-delivery period. In: Johnson FN (ed). Handbook of Lithium Therapy. Baltimore: Univ Park Press, 1980, pp 421-429. [R]

Wilbanks GD, Bressler B, Peete CH, et al.: Toxic effects of lithium carbonate in a mother and newborn infant. JAMA 213:865-967, 1970. [C]

Woody JN, London WL, Wilbanks GD: Lithium toxicity in a newborn. Pediatrics 47:94-96, 1971. [C]

Wright TL, Hoffman LH, Davies J: Teratogenic effects of lithium in rats. Teratology 4:151-156, 1971. [A]

Zalzstein E, Koren G, Einarson T, et al.: A case-control study on the association between first trimester exposure to lithium and Ebstein's Anomaly. Am J Cardiol 65:817-818, 1990. [E]

LOBELINE

Synonyms

Desista, Ethereal Lobelia Tincture, Habit-X, Inflatine, Lobatox, Lobidan, Lobnico, Nikoban, Refrane

Summary

Lobeline, an alkaloid from the plant Lobelia chinensis, is a stimulant of the central and peripheral nervous system. Lobeline is given orally to assist in smoking cessation and as an expectorant.

Magnitude of Teratogenic Risk

None To Minimal

Quality and Quantity of Data

Poor

Comment

None

The frequency of congenital anomalies was no greater than expected among the children of 38 women who took lobeline during the first four lunar months of pregnancy in the Collaborative Perinatal Project (Heinonen et al., 1977).

No animal teratology studies of lobeline have been published.

Key References

Heinonen OP, Slone D, Shapiro S: Birth Defects and Drugs in Pregnancy. Littleton, Mass.: John Wright-PSG, 1977, pp 358, 360. [E]

LOMOFUNGIN

Summary

Lomofungin is an antifungal agent.

Magnitude of Teratogenic Risk

Undetermined

Quality and Quantity of Data

None

Comment

None

No epidemiological studies of congenital anomalies in infants born to women who used lomofungin during pregnancy have been reported.

No animal teratology studies of lomofungin have been published.

Key References

None available.

LOMUSTINE

Synonyms

Belustine, Cecenu, Lucostine

Summary

Lomustine is a cytotoxic alkylating agent used to treat neoplastic disorders.

Magnitude of Teratogenic Risk

Undetermined

Quality and Quantity of Data

Poor

Comment

Although the risk of this agent is undetermined, it may be substantial because lomustine is a cytotoxic agent.

No epidemiological studies of congenital anomalies in infants born to women who were treated with lomustine during pregnancy have been reported.

The frequency of malformations was increased among the offspring of rats given 1 to 2 times the usual therapeutic dose of lomustine during pregnancy (Thompson et al., 1975).

Cardiovasular, ocular, central nervous system and other congenital anomalies were found with increased frequencies in a typical dose- and time-dependent fashion. The treatment was also toxic to the mothers.

Key References

Thompson DJ, Molello JA, Strebing RJ, Dyke IL: Reproduction and teratological studies with l-(2-chloroethyl)-3-cyclohexyl-l-nitrosourea (CCNU) in the rat and rabbit. Toxicol Appl Pharmacol 34:456-466, 1975. [A]

LOPERAMIDE

Synonyms

Arret, Blox, Colifilm, Dissenten, Elcoman, Fortasec, Gamanil, Imodium, Regulane, Suprasec

Summary

Loperamide is a smooth muscle relaxant that is used to treat diarrhea and in ileostomy management.

Magnitude of Teratogenic Risk

Undetermined

Quality and Quantity of Data

Poor

Comment

None

No epidemiological studies of congenital anomalies in children born to women who took loperamide during pregnancy have been reported.

The frequency of malformations was no greater than expected among the offspring of rats and rabbits treated with loperamide during pregnancy in doses, respectively, 8-110 and 16-

125 times those used in humans (Marsboom et al., 1974).

Key References

Marsboom R, Herin V, Verstraeten A, Vandesteene R, et al.: Loperamide (R 18553), a novel type of antidiarrheal agent. Part 4. Studies on subacute and chronic toxicity and the effect on reproductive processes in rats, dogs and rabbits. Arzneimittelforsch 24:1645-1649, 1974. [A]

LORAZEPAM

Synonyms

Alzapam, Ativan, Emotival, Novolorazem, Placinoral, Punktyl

Summary

Lorazepam is a member of the benzodiazepine class of minor tranquilizers. Its actions are anxiolytic and sedative.

Magnitude of Teratogenic Risk

Undetermined

Quality and Quantity of Data

None

Comment

None

No epidemiological studies of congenital anomalies in infants whose mothers used lorazepam during pregnancy have been reported.

No "gross dysmorphism" was seen, but decreased weight and increased activity were observed among the offspring of mice treated with 10 times the maximum human dose of lorazepam during pregnancy in one study (Chesley et al., 1991).

Neonatal hypotonia and feeding difficulties have been reported in infants born of women treated with lorazepam late in pregnancy, either chronically or just during labor (Whitelaw et al., 1981; McAuley et al., 1982; Sanchis et al., 1991). In one study of hypertensive gravidas, maternal intravenous lorazepam treatment was associated with low Apgar scores, hypothermia, poor feeding, and need for assisted ventilation in the neonates (Whitelaw et al., 1981). Preterm infants appeared to be especially susceptible to these adverse effects of lorazepam. Long-term effects of prenatal lorazepam exposure have not been studied.

Please see agent summary on diazepam for information on a related agent that has been studied.

Key References

Chesley S, Lumpkin M, Schatzki A, Galpern WR, et al.: Prenatal exposure to benzodiazepine--I. Prenatal exposure to lorazepam in mice alters open-field activity and GABAA receptor function. Neuropharmacology 30(1):53-58, 1991. [A]

McAuley DM, O'Neill MP, Moore J, et al.: Lorazepam premedication for labour. Br J Obstet Gynaecol 89:149-154, 1982. [E]

Sanchis A, Rosique D, Catala J: Adverse effects of maternal lorazepam on neonates. DICP 25(10):1137-1138, 1991. [C]

Whitelaw AGL, Cummings AJ, McFadyen IR: Effect of maternal lorazepam on the neonate. Br Med J 282:1106-1108, 1981. [E]

LOVASTATIN

Synonyms

Mevacor, Mevinacor, Mevinolin, Mevlor, Monacolin K

Summary

Lovastatin is a fungal product used in the treatment of hyper-cholesterolemia.

Magnitude of Teratogenic Risk

Undetermined

Quality and Quantity of Data

None To Poor

Comment

A small risk cannot be excluded, but a high risk of congenital anomalies in the children of women treated with lovastatin during pregnancy is unlikely.

No epidemiological studies of congenital anomalies among infants born to women treated with lovastatin during pregnancy have been reported.

An increased frequency of gastroschisis was observed among the offspring of rats treated during pregnancy with lovastatin in a dose 500 times that used in humans; no teratogenic effect was observed at doses 5-50 times those used clinically (Minsker et al., 1983). The relevance of this observation to the therapeutic use of lovastatin in human pregnancy is unknown.

Key References

Minsker DH, MacDonald JS, Robertson RT, Bokelman DL: Mevalonate supplementation in pregnant rats suppresses the teratogenicity of mevinolinic acid, an inhibitor of 3-hydroxy-3-methyl-glutaryl-coenzyme A reductase. Teratology 28:449-456, 1983. [A]

LYDIMYCIN

Summary

Lydimycin is an antifungal agent.

Magnitude of Teratogenic Risk

Undetermined

Quality and Quantity of Data

None

Comment

None

No epidemiological studies of congenital anomalies in infants born to women who used lydimycin during pregnancy have been reported.

No animal teratology studies of lydimycin have been published.

Key References

None available.

LYME DISEASE

Synonyms

B. burgdorferi, Borrelia burgdorferi, Lyme borrelia

Summary

Lyme disease is a recurrent multisystem condition caused by the tick-borne spirochete, Borrelia burgdorferi. Lyme disease is characterized by a distinctive rash that may be associated with arthritis and cardiac or neurological disturbances. Prompt penicillin treatment of women who develop Lyme disease during pregnancy has been recommended (Markowitz et al., 1986).

Magnitude of Teratogenic Risk

Minimal To Small

Quality and Quantity of Data

Poor To Fair

Comment

None

No recurrent pattern of congenital anomalies was observed among the infants of 19 women who developed symptomatic Lyme disease during pregnancy; eight of these women manifested Lyme diseases during the first 10 weeks of gestation (Markowtiz et al., 1986). Major congenital anomalies were no more frequent than expected among 30 infants with cord blood antibodies to B. bugdorferi in one cohort study (Williams et al., 1988). In a case-control study, specific antibodies to B. burgdorferi were detected in six of 49 women who had had spontaneous abortions compared to three of 49 women who had had normal babies in an area of Italy in which Lyme disease is endemic (Carlomango et al., 1988). This difference is not statistically significant. Serological studies of B. burgdorferi are not reliable indicators of previous infection (MacDonald, 1989).

Transplacental transmission of B. burgdorferi has been demonstrated in seven infants or fetuses with congenital heart disease (Schlesinger et al., 1985; MacDonald, 1989). The cardiac defects were ventricular septal defects in four children (one of whom also had meningomyelocele and omphalocele and a second of whom also had diaphragmatic hernia), coarctation of the aorta, atrial septal defect, and hypoplastic left heart. Six additional cases of transplacental transmission of B. burgdorferi have been documented in stillborn fetuses or infants who died in the newborn period (Lavoie et al., 1987; Weber et al., 1988; MacDonald, 1989). One fetus had hydrocephalus; no malformations were identified in the others. Two of three surviving infants with documented placental infection with B. burgdorferi developed neonatal sepsis; none had congenital anomalies (MacDonald, 1989).

No animal teratology studies of Lyme disease have been published.

Key References

Carlomagno G, Luksa V, Candussi G: Lyme borrelia positive serology associated with spontaneous abortion in an endemic Italian area. Acta Eur Fertil 19(5):279-281, 1988. [S]

Lavoie PE, Lattner BP, Duray PH, et al.: Culture positive, seronegative, transplacental Lyme borreliosis infant mortality. Arthritis Rheum 30(Suppl 4):S50, 1987. [C]

MacDonald AB: Gestational Lyme borreliosis. Implications for the fetus. Rheum Dis Clin North Am 15(4):657-677, 1989. [R] & [C]

Markowitz LE, Steere AC, Benach JL, Slade JD, et al.: Lyme disease during pregnancy. JAMA 255:3394-3396, 1986. [S]

Schlesinger PA, Duray PH, Burke BA, Steere AC, et al.: Maternal-fetal transmission of the Lyme disease spirochete, Borrelia burgdorferi. Ann Intern Med 103:67-69, 1985. [C]

Weber K, Bratzke H-J, Neubert U, et al.: Borrelia burgdorferi in a newborn despite oral penicillin for Lyme borreliosis during pregnancy. Pediatr Infect Dis J 7:286-289, 1988. [C]

Williams CL, Benach JL, Curran AS, et al.: Lyme disease during pregnancy. A cord blood serosurvey. Ann NY Acad Sci 539:504-506, 1988. [E]

LYNESTRENOL

Synonyms

Ethinylestrenol, Exlutena, Exluton, Linestrenol, Orgametril, Ovoresta M

Summary

Lynestrenol is a synthetic progestational hormone that is used alone or in combination with an estrogenic compound as an oral contraceptive and in treatment of menstrual disorders.

Magnitude of Teratogenic Risk

Undetermined

Quality and Quantity of Data

None

Comment

1) A small risk cannot be excluded, but there is no indication that the risk of congenital anomalies in

the children of women treated with lynestrenol during pregnancy is likely to be great.

2) There is a theoretical risk for virilization of female fetuses at high doses.

No epidemiological studies of congenital anomalies in infants born to women who took lynestrenol during pregnancy have been reported, but many investigations of children of women who took oral contraceptives or progestins during gestation are available.

Dose-dependent increases in the frequencies of fetal loss and central nervous system, skeletal, and other anomalies were observed among the offspring of rabbits treated with 2-10 times the usual human dose of lynestrenol during pregnancy; neurological dysfunction was seen among many of the liveborn offspring (Sannes et al., 1983; Hem et al., 1984).

An increased frequency of fetal loss occurred among rats treated with 200-800 times the usual human dose of lynestrenol during pregnancy (Overbeek et al., 1962). The clinical relevance of these observations is unknown.

Key References

Hem AL, Sannes E, Nafstad I, Nicolaissen B: Effects of oral lynestrenol administration on prenatal and postnatal progeny development in rabbits. NIPH Ann 7:41-45, 1984. [A]

Overbeek GA, Madjerek Z, de Visser J: The effect of lynestrenol on animal reproduction. Acta Endocrinol 41:351-370, 1962. [A]

Sannes E, Lyngset A, Nafstad I: Teratogenicity and embryotoxicity of orally administered lynestrenol in rabbits. Arch Toxicol 52:23-33, 1983. [A]

LYSERGIDE

Synonyms

Acid, Blotter Acid, LSD, Lysergic Acid Diethylamide, Windowpane

Summary

Lysergide is an amine alkaloid that is usually obtained by chemical syntheses. It has powerful hallucinogenic effects for which it is used "recreationally." Lysergide has been employed in treatment of psychiatric illness.

Magnitude of Teratogenic Risk

Undetermined

Quality and Quantity of Data

Poor

Comment

A small risk cannot be excluded, but there is no indication that the risk of congenital anomalies in the children of women who use lysergide during pregnancy is likely to be great.

Several case reports have been published describing children with a variety of congenital anomalies born to mothers who used lysergide before or during pregnancy (Long, 1972; Cohen & Shiloh, 1977). No consistent pattern of anomalies is apparent among these children, and many of them have anomalies or syndromes that are likely to have a cause unrelated to the mother's use of lysergide. Abnormalities of the limbs were noted most often among affected children, but the type of abnormality varied greatly and this probably represents a reporting bias.

No satisfactory epidemiological study of congenital anomalies among infants born to women who used lysergide during pregnancy has been published. In one series of 86 pregnancies in women who used lysergide at unspecified times during gestation, eight children were born with various congenital anomalies (Jacobson & Berlin, 1972). Five of these children had central nervous system defects, but only two were exposed to lysergide during the first trimester. The available data provide no convincing evidence that a mother's use of lysergide during pregnancy increases the risk of malformations in her children.

Results of animal teratology studies of lysergide have been inconsistent. Increased frequencies of fetal loss and central nervous system or eye anomalies have been reported in the offspring of rats, mice, and hamsters treated with lysergide in doses similar to those used in humans, but other studies, using similar doses or much larger ones, have not found these abnormalities (Long, 1972; Cohen & Shiloh, 1977). No teratogenic effect was observed in rabbits with doses 4-20 times those used by humans (Fabro & Sieber, 1968), and no malformations were observed among the offspring of six macaque monkeys treated during pregnancy with several times the usual human dose of lysergide (Wilson, 1969).

Some studies have shown an apparently increased frequency of chromosomal breakage in somatic tissues of individuals who used lysergide, in the children of women who used the drug, or in human cells treated with lysergide in pharmacological or greater doses in vitro (Long, 1972; Matsuyama & Jarvik, 1975; Cohen & Shiloh, 1977). Other studies have not found such effects. Even if these changes do occur in somatic cells, their relevance to the risk of congenital anomalies in children of parents who use lysergide is unknown. Meiotic chromosome studies in one man who had used lysergide were normal (Hulten et al., 1968). Cytogenetic studies in experimental animals have also yielded contradictory results (Matsuyama & Jarvik, 1975; Cohen & Shiloh, 1977).

Key References

Cohen MM, Shiloh Y: Genetic toxicology of lysergic acid diethylamide (LSE-25). Mutat Res 47:183-209, 1977/1978. [R]

Fabro S, Sieber SM: Is lysergide a teratogen? Lancet 1;639-640, 1968. [O]

Hulten M, Lindsten J, Lidberg L, Ekelund H: Studies on mitotic and meiotic chromosomes in subjects exposed to LSD. Ann Genet (Paris) 11:201-210, 1968. [C]

Jacobson CB, Berlin CM: Possible reproductive detriment in LSD users. JAMA 222:1367-1373, 1972. [S]

Long SY: Does LSD induce chromosomal damage and malformations? A review of the literature. Teratology 6:75-90, 1972. [R]

Matsuyama SS, Jarvik LF: Cytogenetic effects of psychoactive drugs. Mod Probl Pharmacopsych 10:99-132, 1975. [R]

Wilson JD: Teratological and reproductive studies in non-human primates. In: Nishimura H, Miller JR, Yasuda M (eds). Methods for Teratological Studies in Experimental Animals and Man. Tokyo: Igaku Soin Ltd. Medical Examination Publishing Co., 1969, pp 16-33. [A]

MAFENIDE

Synonyms

Homosulfamine, Malfamin, Maphenide, Marfanil, Sulfamylon

Summary

Mafenide is a sulfonamide antibacterial agent that is used topically to prevent infections in burns. Systemic absorption of mafenide from burned skin occurs.

Magnitude of Teratogenic Risk

Undetermined

Quality and Quantity of Data

None To Poor

Comment

A small risk cannot be excluded, but a high risk of congenital anomalies in the children of women treated with mafenide during pregnancy is unlikely.

No epidemiological studies of congenital anomalies among infants born to women treated with mafenide during pregnancy have been reported.

The frequency of malformations was no greater than expected among the offspring of rats or mice injected with mafenide in doses of

1-1000 mg/kg/d during pregnancy (Tokunaga et al., 1973). Decreased body weight was observed among the offspring of both species and decreased litter size among the offspring of rats treated with the largest doses.

Please see agent summary on sulfisoxazole for information on a related drug that has been more thoroughly studied.

Key References

Tokunaga Y, Kawada K, Nagano A, et al.: Influence of mafenide acetate on the offspring of rats and mice. Nichidai Igaku Zasshi 32:973-995, 1973. [A]

MAGALDRATE

Synonyms

Hydromagnesium Aluminate, Riopan

Summary

Magaldrate is used orally as an antacid to treat gastric hyperacidity.

Magnitude of Teratogenic Risk

Undetermined

Quality and Quantity of Data

None

Comment

None

No epidemiological studies of congenital anomalies in infants whose mothers were treated with magaldrate during pregnancy have been reported.

No animal teratology studies of magaldrate have been published.

Key References

None available.

MAGNESIUM SULFATE

Synonyms

Addex-Magnesium, Epsom Salts, Mg-Plus, Sal Amarum, Zinvit

Summary

Magnesium sulfate is administered parenterally to treat pregnancy-induced hypertension and premature labor. The drug is used orally as a purgative and topically in the treatment of skin infections.

Magnitude of Teratogenic Risk

None

Quality and Quantity of Data

Poor

Comment

None

The frequency of congenital anomalies was no greater than expected among the children of 141 women treated during pregnancy with magnesium sulfate parenterally in the Collaborative Perinatal Project (Heinonen et al., 1977). Only six of these women were treated during the first four lunar months of gestation.

No animal teratology studies of magnesium sulfate have been published.

Transient neurological depression has been observed in association with hypermagnesemia in newborn infants of women treated late in pregnancy for pre-eclampsia with magnesium sulfate (Lipsitz & English, 1967; Lipsitz, 1971; Brazy et al., 1982; Rasch et al., 1982). Osseous lesions of the metaphases, costochondral junctions, and skull have been been noted in infants born to women treated with continuous intravenous infusions of magnesium sulfate for several weeks prior to delivery (Lamm et al., 1988; Cumming & Thomas, 1989).

Key References

Brazy JE, Grimm JK, Little VA: Neonatal manifestations of severe maternal hypertension occurring before the thirty-sixth week of pregnancy. J Pediatr 100(2):265-271, 1982. [E]

Cumming WA, Thomas VJ: Hypermagnesemia: A cause of abnormal metaphyses in the neonate. AJR 152:1071-1072, 1989. [C]

Heinonen OP, Slone D, Shapiro S: Birth Defects and Drugs in Pregnancy. Littleton, Mass.: John Wright-PSG, 1977, pp 359, 440. [E]

Lamm CI, Norton KI, Murphy RJC, et al.: Congenital rickets associated with magnesium sulfate infusion for tocolysis. J Pediatr 113(6):1078-1082, 1988. [S]

Lipsitz PJ: The clinical and biochemical effects of excess magnesium in the newborn. Pediatrics 47(3):501-509, 1971. [S]

Lipsitz PJ, English IC: Hypermagnesemia in the newborn infant. Pediatrics 40(5):856-862, 1967. [C]

Rasch DK, Huber PA, Richardson CJ, et al.: Neurobehavioral effects of neonatal hypermagnesemia. J Pediatr 100(2):272-276, 1982. [E]

MALATHION

Synonyms

Carbofos, Cythion, Derbac-M, Forthion, Mercaptothion, Organoderm, Prioderm

Summary

Malathion is an organophosphorous insecticide. It is widely used in agriculture and is employed as a topical pediculicide in medicine. The U.S. permissible exposure limit for malathion is 15 mg/cu m of body surface area.

Magnitude of Teratogenic Risk

None To Minimal

Quality and Quantity of Data

Fair

Comment

1) Risk is likely to be dose related.

2) No information is available for exposures sufficient to produce maternal pharmacological response.

No consistent increase in the frequency of congenital anomalies was observed in a cohort of 22,465 infants born to women who lived in areas where aerial malathion spraying had occurred during the first trimester of pregnancy (Grether et al., 1987). Similarly, no biologically plausible association with potential malathion exposure was observed in a case-control study involving 474 spontaneous abortions, 163 infants with congenital anomalies, 78 infants with intrauterine growth retardation, or 37 stillbirths whose mothers lived in areas where spraying occurred during pregnancy (Thomas et al., 1990).

The frequency of malformations was not increased among the offspring of rats administered malathion during pregnancy in doses 1-60,000 times the acceptable daily intake for humans (Kimbrough & Gaines, 1968; Khera et al., 1978, Lechner & Abdel-Rahman, 1984). No teratogenic effect was observed among the offspring of pregnant rabbits treated with 220 times the human acceptable daily intake of malathion (Machin & McBride, 1989).

The frequency of chromosomal aberrations was not increased in the gametes of male mice injected with malathion at 12,000 times the acceptable daily human intake (Degraeve et al., 1984).

Key References

Degraeve N, Chollet MC, Moutschen J: Cytogenetic and genetic effects of subchronic treatments with organophosphorus insecticides. Arch Toxicol 56:66-67, 1984. [A]

Grether JK, Harris JA, Neutra R, Kizer KW: Exposure to aerial malathion application and the occurrence of congenital anomalies and low birthweight. Am J Public Health 77:1009-1010, 1987. [E]

Khera KS, Whalen C, Trivett G: Teratogenicity studies on linuron, malathion, and methoxychlor in rats. Toxicol Appl Pharmacol 45:435-444, 1978. [A]

Kimbrough RD, Gaines TB: Effect of organic phosphorus compounds and alkylating agents on the rat fetus. Arch Environ Health 16:805-808, 1968. [A]

Lechner DMW, Abdel-Rahman MS: A teratology study of carbaryl and malathion mixtures in rat. J Toxicol Environ Health 14:267-278, 1984. [A]

Machin MGA, McBride WG: Teratological study of malathion in the rabbit. J Toxicol Environ Health 26:249-253, 1989. [A]

Thomas D, Goldhaber M, Petitti D, et al.: Reproductive outcomes in women exposed to malathion. Am J Epidemiol 132:794-795, 1990. [E]

MANGANESE

Synonyms

Cutaval, Man-Gro, Mangan

Summary

Manganese is a metal used in making alloys. In trace amounts, it is an essential nutrient. Manganese salts are used therapeutically to increase the hematinic action of iron in anemia. The 1989 U.S. OSHA Permissible Exposure Limit for manganese fume is 1 mg/cu m as a time-weighted average for an 8-hour exposure.

Magnitude of Teratogenic Risk

Undetermined

Quality and Quantity of Data

None To Poor

Comment

None

No epidemiological studies of congenital anomalies among infants born to women exposed to large amounts of manganese during pregnancy have been reported. The frequency of congenital anomalies did not appear to be unusual among 293 Australian Aboriginal children born on an island with a high level of manganese contamination (Kilburn, 1987).

The frequencies of exencephaly, embryonic loss, and fetal growth retardation were increased among the offspring of mice treated once during pregnancy with 12.5-50 mg/kg (250-1000 times the human therapeutic dose) of manganese sulfate (Webster & Valios, 1987). Embryonic death was increased in pregnant hamsters given single doses of 20-35 mg/kg of manganese chloride during pregnancy, although the frequency of fetal malformations was not increased (Ferm, 1972). No teratogenic effect was observed in another study among the offspring of mice, rats, hamsters or rabbits treated during pregnancy with manganese sulfate in doses of 1.25-125 mg/kg/d, 0.783-783 mg/kg/d, 1.36-136 mg/kg/d, or 1.12-112 mg/kg/d, respectively (Barlow & Sullivan, 1982). Persistent alterations of behavior have been demonstrated among the offspring of pregnant mice exposed chronically to manganese oxide dust (49 mg/cu m for 7 h/d) (Massaro et al., 1980).

Key References

Barlow SM, Sullivan FM: Reproductive Hazards of Industrial Chemicals. An Evaluation of Animal and Human Data. London: Academic Press, 1982, pp 370-385. [R]

Ferm VH: The teratogenic effects of metals on mammalian embryos. Adv Teratol 5:51-75, 1972. [R]

Kilburn CJ: Manganese, malformations and motor disorders: Findings in a manganese-exposed population. Neurotoxicology 8(3):421-430, 1987. [E]

Massaro EJ, D'Agostino RB, Stineman CH, et al.: Alterations in behavior of adult offspring of female mice exposed to MnO2 dust during gestation. Fed Proc Fed Am Soc Exp Biol 39:623, 1980. [A]

Webster WS, Valois AA: Reproductive toxicology of manganese in rodents, including exposure during the postnatal period.   Neurotoxicology 8(3):437-444, 1987. [A]

MANNITOL

Synonyms

Cordycepic acid, Isotol, Manna Sugar, Osmitrol, Osmosal, Resectisol

Summary

Mannitol is an organic alcohol that is chemically related to the sugar mannose. Mannitol is used as an osmotic diuretic when given intravenously and as a urologic irrigant.

Magnitude of Teratogenic Risk

Undetermined

Quality and Quantity of Data

None To Poor

Comment

None

No epidemiological studies of congenital anomalies among infants born to women treated with mannitol during pregnancy have been reported.

A high frequency of hemorrhagic lesions of the extremities was noted among the fetuses of rats that had been administered hypertonic mannitol intravenously in a dose about 3 times that used in humans (Petter, 1967). This treatment produced profound (15%) dehydration in the mothers. No teratogenic effect was observed among the offspring of pregnant rats, mice, or rabbits given mannitol orally in doses of 16-1600 mg/kg/d or among the offspring of hamsters treated in this way with 12-1200 mg/kg/d (Food and Drug Research Labs, 1972, 1974). These doses all are less than that usually given intravenously in humans to induce osmotic diuresis.

Key References

Food and Drug Research Labs: I. Teratologic Evaluation of FDA 71-32 (Mannitol).   NTIS (National Technical Information Service) Report/PB-221 781, 1972. [A]

Food and Drug Research Labs: I. Teratologic Evaluation of Compound FDA 71-32, Mannitol, in rabbits.   NTIS (National Technical Information Service) Report/PB-267 197, 1974. [A]

Petter C: Lesions of the extremities provoked in the fetus of the rat by intravenous injection of hypertonic mannitol into the mother. C R Soc Biol 161:1010-1014, 1967. [A]

MAPROTILINE

Synonyms

Ludiomil

Summary

Maprotiline is a tetracyclic antidepressant with sedative action.

Magnitude of Teratogenic Risk

Undetermined

Quality and Quantity of Data

None To Poor

Comment

None

No epidemiological studies of congenital anomalies in infants born to mothers treated with maprotiline during pregnancy have been published.

The frequency of malformations was not increased among the offspring of mice or rats given 5-10 times the usual human dose (Esaki et al., 1976), or among the offspring of rabbits treated with 1-13 times the usual human dose of maprotiline during pregnancy (Hirooka et al., 1978).

Please see agent summary on amitriptyline for information on a related drug.

Key References

Esaki K, Tanioka Y, Tsukada M, Izumiyama K: Teratogenicity of maprotiline tested by oral administration in mice and rats. Jitchuken Zenrinsho Kenkyuho 2:69-77, 1976. [A]

Hirooka T, Morimoto K, Tadokoro T, Takahashi S, et al.: Teratogenicity test on maprotiline (CIBA 34, 276-Ba) in rabbits. Oyo Yakuri (Pharmacometrics) 15:555-565, 1978. [A]

MARIJUANA

Synonyms

Cannabis, Guaza, Hash, Joints, Mariquita, Pot, Tetrahydrocannabinol, Weed

Summary

Marijuana is widely used as a "recreational" drug. It is usually smoked or eaten. The active ingredient is delta-9-tetrahydrocannabinol (THC). Marijuana is used medically in treatment of glaucoma and as an antiemetic during cancer chemotherapy.

Magnitude of Teratogenic Risk

None To Minimal

Quality and Quantity of Data

Fair

Comment

Behavioral alterations have been observed among the infants of women who smoked marijuana during pregnancy (see below).

Most published epidemiological studies of infants of women who smoked marijuana dur-

ing pregnancy are compromised by poor or absent information on the magnitude, duration, and gestational timing of exposures (Day & Richardson, 1991). Moreover, many of these studies may be confounded by correlated factors such as alcohol and tobacco use, race, and socioeconomic status among the mothers.

The frequency of major malformations was no greater than expected among the children born of 1246 pregnancies in which the mother smoked marijuana in one cohort study (Linn et al., 1983). A similar result was obtained when only the children of 137 women who smoked marijuana daily were considered. In three other studies, the frequency of congenital anomalies was no greater than expected among 392, 331, or 417 infants of women who reported marijuana use during pregnancy (Gibson et al., 1983; Zuckerman et al., 1989; Witter & Niebyl, 1990). Five infants with intrauterine growth retardation and minor dysmorphic features have been reported whose mothers smoked two to 14 joints of marijuana daily during pregnancy (Qazi et al., 1985). The prevalence of this exposure in the general population and the nonspecificity of the anomalies in the infants preclude any causal inference. The frequency of minor physical anomalies was no greater than expected among the children of women who smoked marijuana during pregnancy in other studies (Tennes & Blackard, 1980; Linn et al., 1983; O'Connell & Fried, 1984; Zuckerman et al., 1989; Day et al., 1991).

Birth weight and length do not appear to be associated with maternal marijuana smoking during pregnancy in most well-controlled studies when the effects of confounding variables are eliminated (Fried, 1980; Tennes & Blackard, 1980; Linn et al., 1983; Greenland et al., 1983; Gibson et al., 1983; Fried et al., 1984; Tennes et al., 1985; Fried & O'Connell, 1987). A few investigations have found such an association, but even within these studies the observations are often inconsistent (Hingson et al., 1982; Hatch & Bracken, 1986; Kline et al., 1987; Zuckerman et al., 1989; Day et al., 1991). No association with marijuana use during pregnancy was observed among the mothers of either 567 chromosomally normal or 393 chromosomally abnormal spontaneous abortuses (Kline et al., 1991).

Behavioral abnormalities have been observed among the infants of women who used marijuana during pregnancy (Fried, 1980, 1982, 1991; Fried et al., 1987; Fried & Makin, 1987; Lester & Dreher, 1989; Parker et al., 1990). Neurobehavioral alterations have also been found among older children who had been born to mothers who used marijuana during pregnancy in some studies (Fried & Watkinson, 1989; Fried, 1991), but postnatal environmental conditions appear to exert increasingly important effects on these assessments as children grow older (O'Connell & Fried, 1991).

Many teratologic studies of marijuana and THC have been performed in rats, mice, hamsters, and rabbits (Abel, 1980, 1985b; Schardein, 1985). Various anomalies have been reported among the offspring of animals treated during pregnancy with marijuana in doses many times greater than those usually encountered in humans. Most animal teratology studies of marijuana have been negative, however, especially if dosing is more comparable to the human situation in magnitude and route. Fetal growth retardation and embryo or fetal mortality are frequently seen at high doses. These effects may be more marked in pregnant animals treated with both marijuana and alcohol concomitantly (Abel, 1985a; Abel & Dintcheff, 1986). People often use this combination of agents together, and there is some evidence that intrauterine growth retardation occurs more commonly in human pregnancies exposed to both substances than in pregnancies exposed to either alone (Hingson et al., 1982).

A number of behavioral alterations have been observed among the offspring of rats given large doses of marijuana or THC during gestation (Abel, 1980, 1985b; Brown & Fishman, 1984).

The observation of an association of maternal marijuana use in the year before conception, during pregnancy, or during nursing in a case-control study of 204 children with acute nonlymphoblastic leukemia (RR=10, p=0.005) requires independent confirmation before its biological significance can be determined (Robison et al., 1989).

Studies of cytogenetic alterations in somatic cells of humans and somatic or germinal cells of experimental animals exposed to marijuana in vivo or in vitro have yielded inconsistent results (Zimmerman & Zimmerman, 1990). The relationship of such findings to human disease or congenital anomalies is uncertain, in any case.

Key References

Abel EL: Alcohol enhancement of marijuana-induced fetotoxicity. Teratology 31:35-40, 1985a. [A]

Abel EL: Effects of prenatal exposure to cannabinoids. Natl Inst Drug Abuse Res Monogr Ser 59:20-35, 1985b. [R]

Abel EL: Prenatal exposure to cannabis: A critical review of effects on growth, development, and behavior. Behav Neural Biol 29:137-156, 1980. [R]

Abel EL, Dintcheff BA: Increased marihuana-induced fetotoxicity by a low dose of concomitant alcohol administration. J Stud Alcohol 47:440-443, 1986. [A]

Brown RM, Fishman RHB: An overview and summary of the behavioral and neural consequences of perinatal exposure to psychotropic drugs. In: Yanai J (ed). Neurobehavioral Teratology. Amsterdam: Elsevier Science Publishers BV, 1984, pp 3-53. [R]

Day NL, Richardson GA: Prenatal marijuana use: Epidemiology, methodologic issues, and infant outcome. Clin Perinatol 18(1):77-92, 1991. [R]

Day N, Sambamoorthi U, Taylor P, et al.: Prenatal marijuana use and neonatal outcome. Neurotoxicol Teratol 13(3):329-334, 1991. [E]

Fried PA: Marihuana use by pregnant women and effects on offspring: An update. Neurobehav Toxicol Teratol 4:451-454, 1982. [E]

Fried PA: Marihuana use by pregnant women: Neurobehavioral effects in neonates. Drug Alcohol Depend 6:415-424, 1980. [S]

Fried PA: Marijuana use during pregnancy: Consequences for the offspring. Semin Perinatol 15(4):280-287, 1991. [E]

Fried PA, Makin JE: Neonatal behavioural correlates of prenatal exposure to marihuana, cigarettes and alcohol in a low risk population. Neurotoxicol Teratol 9(1):1-7, 1987. [E]

Fried PA, O'Connell CM: A comparison of the effects of prenatal exposure to tobacco, alcohol, cannabis and caffeine on birth size and subsequent growth. Neurotoxicol Teratol 9:79-85, 1987. [E]

Fried PA, Watkinson B: 36- and 48-month neurobehavioral follow-up of children prenatally exposed to marijuana, cigarettes, and alcohol. J Dev Behav Pediatr 11:49-58, 1990. [E]

Fried PA, Watkinson B, Dillon RF, Dulberg CS: Neonatal neurological status in a low-risk population after prenatal exposure to cigarettes, marijuana, and alcohol. J Dev Behav Pediatr 8:318-326, 1987. [E]

Fried PA, Watkinson B, Willan A: Marijuana use during pregnancy and decreased length of gestation. Am J Obstet Gynecol 150:23-27, 1984. [E]

Gibson GT, Baghurst PA, Colley DP: Maternal alcohol, tobacco and cannabis consumption and the outcome of pregnancy. Aust NZ J Obstet Gynaecol 23:15-19, 1983. [E]

Greenland S, Richwald GA, Honda GD: The effects of marijuana use during pregnancy. II. A study in a low-risk home-delivery population. Drug Alcohol Depend 11:359-366, 1983. [S]

Hatch EE, Bracken MB: Effect of marijuana use in pregnancy on fetal growth. Am J Epidemiol 124:986-993, 1986. [E]

Hingson R, Alpert JJ, Day N, Dooling E, et al.: Effects of maternal drinking and marijuana use on fetal growth and development. Pediatrics 70:539-546, 1982. [S]

Kline J, Hutzler M, Levin B, et al.: Marijuana and spontaneous abortion of known karyotype. Paediatr Perinat Epidemiol 5:320-332, 1991. [E]

Kline J, Stein Z, Hutzler M: Cigarettes, alcohol and marijuana: Varying associations with birthweight. Int J Epidemiol 16:44-51, 1987. [E]

Lester BM, Dreher M: Effects of marijuana use during pregnancy on newborn cry. Child Dev 60:765-771, 1989. [E]

Linn S, Schoenbaum SC, Monson RR, Rosner R, et al.: The association of marijuana use with outcome of pregnancy. Am J Public Health 73:1161-1164, 1983. [E]

O'Connell CM, Fried PA: An investigation of prenatal cannabis exposure and minor physical anomalies in a low risk population. Neurobehav Toxicol Teratol 6:345-350, 1984. [E]

O'Connell CM, Fried PA: Prenatal exposure to cannabis: A preliminary report of postnatal consequences in school-age children. Neurotoxicol Teratol 13(6):631-639, 1991. [E]

Parker S, Zuckerman B, Bauchner H, et al.: Jitteriness in full-term neonates: Prevalence and correlates. Pediatrics 85(1):17-23, 1990. [E]

Qazi QH, Mariano E, Milman DH, Beller E, et al.: Abnormalities in offspring associated with prenatal marihuana exposure. Dev Pharmacol Ther 8:141-148, 1985. [S]

Robison LL, Buckley JD, Daigle AE, et al.: Maternal drug use and risk of childhood nonlymphoblastic leukemia among offspring: An epidemiologic investigation implicating marijuana. (A report from the Childrens Cancer Study Group). Cancer 63:1904-1911, 1989. [E]

Schardein JL: Chemically Induced Birth Defects. New York: Marcel Dekker, 1985, pp 774-775. [R]

Tennes K, Blackard C: Maternal alcohol consumption, birth weight, and minor physical anomalies. Am J Obstet Gynecol 138:774-780, 1980. [E]

Tennes K, Avitable N, Blackard C, Boyles C, et al.: Marijuana: Prenatal and postnatal exposure in the human. Natl Inst Drug Abuse Res Monogr Ser 59:48-59, 1985. [E]

Witter FR, Niebyl JR: Marijuana use in pregnancy and pregnancy outcome. Am J Perinatol 7(1):36-38, 1990. [E]

Zimmerman S, Zimmerman AM: Genetic effects of marijuana. Int J Addict 25(1A):19-33, 1990-91. [R]

Zuckerman B, Frank DA, Hingson R, et al.: Effects of maternal marijuana and cocaine use on fetal growth. N Engl J Med 320:762-768, 1989. [E]

MAZINDOL

Synonyms

Afilan, Dimagrir, Magrilan, Mazanor, Mazildene, Samonter, Sanorex, Sanoux, Teronac

Summary

Mazindol is a sympathomimetic agent that is administered orally in the treatment of obesity.

Magnitude of Teratogenic Risk

Undetermined

Quality and Quantity of Data

None

Comment

None

No epidemiological studies of congenital anomalies in infants whose mothers were treated with mazindol during pregnancy have been reported.

No animal teratology studies of mazindol have been published.

Please see agent summary on dextroamphetamine for information on a related agent that has been studied.

Key References

None available.

MEASLES VACCINE, LIVE

Synonyms

Attenuvax, More Attenuated Enders Strain, Rubeola Vaccine

Summary

Live measles vaccine contains living attenuated measles virus. It is administered subcutaneously to elicit immunity to measles (rubeola).

Magnitude of Teratogenic Risk

None To Minimal

Quality and Quantity of Data

Poor

Comment

None

No malformations were observed among the children of 37 women immunized with live measles vaccine during the first four lunar months of pregnancy in the Collaborative Perinatal Project (Heinonen et al., 1977).

No animal teratology studies of live measles vaccine have been published.

Key References

Heinonen OP, Slone D, Shapiro S: Birth Defects and Drugs in Pregnancy. Littleton, Mass.: John Wright-PSG, 1977, pp 315-316. [E]

MEBENDAZOLE

Synonyms

Medazole, Nemasole, Vermox, Wormox, Zadomen

Summary

Mebendazole is an antihelmintic administered orally to treat a variety of parasitic infections. It is poorly absorbed from the gastrointestinal tract.

Magnitude of Teratogenic Risk

Undetermined

Quality and Quantity of Data

None To Poor

Comment

None

No epidemiological studies of congenital anomalies in infants whose mothers took mebendazole during pregnancy have been reported.

A very high frequency of congenital malformations including hydrocephalus, neural tube defects, and limb anomalies was observed among the offspring of rats treated with 4-8 times the usual human dose of mebendazole during pregnancy (Delatour & Richard, 1976). The relevance of this observation to the clinical use of mebendazole in human pregnancy is unknown.

Key References

Delatour P, Richard Y: Embryotoxic and antimitotic properties of some benzimidazole related compounds. Therapie 31:505-515, 1976. [A]

MECAMYLAMINE

Synonyms

Inversine, Mecamilamina, Mecamine, Mekamine, Mevasine, Revertina, Versamine

Summary

Mecamylamine is an autonomic ganglionic blocking agent that is administered orally in the management of hypertension.

Magnitude of Teratogenic Risk

Undetermined

Quality and Quantity of Data

None

Comment

None

No epidemiological studies of congenital anomalies in infants born to women who were treated with mecamylamine during pregnancy have been reported.

No animal teratology studies of mecamylamine have been published.

Mecamylamine has the theoretical potential of producing meconium ileus in the fetus.

Key References

None available.

MECHLORETHAMINE

Synonyms

Caryolysine, Chlorethazine, Chlormethine, Cloramin, Clormetina, Erasol, HN2, Mustargen, Mustine, Nitrogen Mustard Oxide

Summary

Mechlorethamine (nitrogen mustard) is an alkylating agent that is administered parenterally in the treatment of neoplastic disease.

Magnitude of Teratogenic Risk

Small To Moderate

Quality and Quantity of Data

Poor To Fair

Comment

None

No congenital anomalies were observed among the children of seven women treated with mechlorethamine and other antineoplastic agents during pregnancy in one series (Aviles et al., 1991); only two of these women were treated in the first trimester. A few fetal anomalies have been observed after first trimester maternal chemotherapy with various drug combinations including mechlorethamine. The cases include a fetus with hypoplastic and malpositioned kidneys (Mennuti et al., 1975), a fetus with oligodactyly (Thomas & Andes, 1982), and a dysmature infant with atrial septal defect who died on the second day of life

357

(Thomas & Peckham, 1976). No causal relationship can be inferred from these anecdotes with respect to either the maternal chemotherapy in general or the mechlorethamine treatment in particular.

Parental chemotherapy with mechlorethamine and other drugs completed prior to conception did not appear to alter the frequency of congenital anomalies among more than 50 infants substantially (Schilsky et al., 1981, Andrieu & Ochoa-Molina, 1983; Whitehead et al., 1983; Green et al., 1991; Zuazu et al., 1991).

Increased frequencies of fetal death and of fetal craniofacial, limb and other malformations have been observed after treatment of pregnant rats, mice, ferrets, and rabbits with mechlorethamine in doses 1 to 2 or more times that used therapeutically in humans (Haskin, 1948; Danforth & Center, 1954; Murphy & Karnofsky, 1956; Murphy et al., 1957; Nishimura & Takagaki, 1959; Gottschewski, 1964; Beck et al., 1976). Typical dependence of the teratogenic effect on time of gestation during exposure has been demonstrated in rats and ferrets (Murphy & Karnofsky, 1956; Beck et al., 1976).

An increased frequency of dividing cells with abnormal metaphases and chromosomal damage has been observed in embryos removed from pregnant rats or mice shortly after treatment with teratogenic doses of mechlorethamine (Soukup et al., 1967; Meyne & Legator, 1983). The clinical relevance of this observation is unknown.

Key References

Andrieu JM, Ochoa-Molina ME: Menstrual cycle, pregnancies and offspring before and after MOPP therapy for Hodgkin's disease. Cancer 52:435-438, 1983. [S]

Aviles A, Diaz-Maqueo JC, Talavera A, et al.: Growth and development of children of mothers treated with chemotherapy during pregnancy: Current status of 43 children. Am J Hematol 36:243-248, 1991. [S]

Beck F, Schon H, Mould G, Swidzinska P, et al.: Comparison of the teratogenic effects of mustine hydrochloride in rats and ferrets. The value of the ferret as an experimental animal in teratology. Teratology 13:151-160, 1976. [A]

Danforth CH, Center E: Nitrogen mustard as a teratogenic agent in the mouse. Proc Soc Exp Biol Med 86:705-707, 1954. [A]

Gottschewski GHM: Mammalian blastopathies due to drugs. Nature 201:1232-1233, 1964. [A]

Green DM, Zevon MA, Lowrie G, et al.: Congenital anomalies in children of patients who received chemotherapy for cancer in childhood and adolescence. N Engl J Med 325:141-146, 1991. [S]

Haskin D: Some effects of nitrogen mustard on the development of external body form in the fetal rat. Anat Res 102:493-511, 1948. [A]

Mennuti MT, Shepard TH, Mellman WJ: Fetal renal malformation following treatment of Hodgkin's disease during pregnancy. Obstet Gynecol 46:194-196, 1975. [C]

Meyne J, Legator MS: Clastogenic effects of transplacental exposure of mouse embryos to nitrogen mustard or cyclophosphamide. Teratogenesis Carcinog Mutagen 3:281-287, 1983. [A]

Murphy ML, Dagg CP, Karnofsky DA: Comparison of teratogenic chemicals in the rat and chick embryos. Pediatrics 19:701-714, 1957. [A]

Murphy ML, Karnofsky DA: Effect of azaserine and other growth-inhibiting agents on fetal development of the rat. Cancer 9:955-962, 1956. [A]

Nishimura H, Takagaki S: Congenital malformations in mice induced by nitrogen mustard. Acta Sch Med Univ Kioto 36:20-26, 1959. [A]

Schilsky RL, Sherins RJ, Hubbard SM, Wesley MN, et al.: Long-term follow-up of ovarian function in women treated with MOPP chemotherapy for Hodgkin's disease. Am J Med 71:552-556, 1981. [S]

Soukup S, Takacs E, Warkany J: Chromosome changes in embryos treated with various teratogens. J Embryol Exp Morph 18:215-226, 1967. [A]

Thomas L, Andes WA: Fetal anomaly associated with successful chemotherapy for Hodgkin's disease during the first trimester of pregnancy. Clin Res 30:424A, 1982. [C]

Thomas PRM, Peckham MJ: The investigation and management of Hodgkin's disease in the pregnant patient. Cancer 38:1443-1451, 1976. [S]

Whitehead E, Shalet SM, Blackledge G, Todd I, et al.: The effect of combination chemotherapy on ovarian function in women treated for Hodgkin's disease. Cancer 52:988-993, 1983. [S]

Zuazu J, Julia A, Sierra J, et al.: Pregnancy outcome in hematologic malignancies. Cancer 67:703-709, 1991. [S]

MECLIZINE

Synonyms

Antivert, Bonamine, Bonine, Ru-Vert-M

Summary

Meclizine is an antihistamine used primarily as an antiemetic.

Magnitude of Teratogenic Risk

None To Minimal

Quality and Quantity of Data

Good

Comment

None

The frequencies of congenital anomalies in general, of major malformations, and of minor anomalies were no greater than expected among the children of 1014 women who took meclizine during the first four lunar months of pregnancy in the Collaborative Perinatal Project (Heinonen et al., 1977). A weak association was seen between maternal use of meclizine in the first four lunar months of pregnancy and congenital anomalies of the ear or eye among the infants, but the biological significance of this association is uncertain. No association was seen with any other anatomical class of malformations. The frequency of congenital anomalies was no greater than expected among the children of 613 women treated with meclizine during the first trimester of pregnancy in another cohort study (Milkovich & van den Berg, 1976). Similarly, in three case-control studies involving respectively 266, 175, and 836 infants with various malformations, the frequency of maternal use of meclizine during the first trimester of pregnancy was no greater than among normal control infants (Mellin, 1964; Nelson & Forfar, 1971; Greenberg et al., 1977). Congenital anomalies were no more frequent than expected among children of 1463 women who used meclizine anytime during pregnancy in the Collaborative Perinatal Project (Heinonen et al., 1977).

No teratogenic effect was observed among the offspring of 14 macaque monkeys treated with 10 times the usual human dose of meclizine during early pregnancy (Wilson & Gavan, 1967; Courtney & Valerio, 1968). In rats, a variety of craniofacial and skeletal malformations were induced in the offspring by maternal treatment with meclizine in doses more than 175 times greater than those used clinically, but not usually in doses 25-125 those used in humans (King, 1963). The relevance, if any, of these observations to therapeutic use of meclizine by pregnant women is unknown.

Key References

Courtney KD, Valerio DA: Teratology in the Macaca mulatta. Teratology 1:163-172, 1968. [A]

Greenberg G, Inman WHW, Weatherall JAC, et al.: Maternal drug histories and congenital abnormalities. Br Med J 2:853-6, 1977. [E]

Heinonen OP, Slone D, Shapiro S: Birth Defects and Drugs in Pregnancy. Littleton, Mass.: John Wright-PSG, 1977, pp 323-324, 437. [E]

King CTG: Teratogenic effects of meclizine hydrochloride on the rat. Science 141:353-355, 1963. [A]

Mellin GW: Drugs in the first trimester of pregnancy and the fetal life of Homo sapiens. Am J Obstet Gynecol 90:1169-1180, 1964. [E]

Milkovich L, van den Berg, BJ: An evaluation of the teratogenicity of certain antinauseant drugs. Am J Obstet Gynecol 125:244-248, 1976. [E]

Nelson MM, Forfar JO: Associations between drugs administered during pregnancy and congenital abnormalities of the fetus. Br Med J 1:523-527, 1971. [E]

Wilson JG, Gavan JA: Congenital malformations in nonhuman primates: Spontaneous and experimentally induced. Anat Rec 158:99-109, 1967. [A]

MECLOCYCLINE

Synonyms

Meclan, Meclociclina, Mecloderm, Meclutin Semplice, Selexid, Traumatociclina

Summary

Meclocycline is a tetracycline used topically in the treatment of acne. It is very poorly absorbed through the skin.

Magnitude of Teratogenic Risk

Undetermined

Quality and Quantity of Data

None

Comment

A small risk cannot be excluded, but a high risk of congenital anomalies in the children of women treated with meclocycline during pregnancy is unlikely.

No epidemiological studies of congenital anomalies in infants whose mothers were treated with meclocycline during pregnancy have been reported.

No animal teratology studies of meclocycline have been published.

Please see agent summary on tetracycline for information on a related agent that has been studied.

Key References

None available.

MECLOFENAMATE

Synonyms

Meclomen

Summary

Meclofenamate is a nonsteroidal anti-inflammatory agent that has analgesic and antipyretic actions. It is used to treat rheumatic disorders.

Magnitude of Teratogenic Risk

Undetermined

Quality and Quantity of Data

None To Poor

Comment

None

No epidemiological studies of malformations in the infants of women treated with meclofenamate during pregnancy have been reported.

The frequency of malformations was not increased among the offspring of pregnant rats treated with 0.4-2.5 times the maximal human dose of meclofenamate (Schardein et al., 1969; Patrere et al., 1985). No teratogenic effect was observed among the offspring of rabbits treated with meclofenamate during pregnancy in a dose 0.4 times that used in humans (Schardein et al., 1969).

Please see agent summary on indomethacin for information on a related agent that has been more thoroughly studied.

Key References

Patrere JA, Humphrey RR, Anderson JA, et al.: Studies on reproduction in rats with meclofenamate sodium, a nonsteroidal anti-inflammatory agent. Fundam Appl Toxicol 5:665-671, 1985. [A]

Schardein JL, Blatz AT, Woosley ET, Kaump DH: Reproduction studies on sodium meclofenamate in comparison to aspirin and phenylbuta-zone. Toxicol Appl Pharmacol 15:46-55, 1969. [A]

MEDROXYPROGEST-ERONE

Synonyms

Amen, Curretab, Cycrin, Depo-Provera, DMPA, Farlutin, MPA, Provera

Summary

Medroxyprogesterone is a long-acting progestin that is used in the treatment of menstrual disorders and, in smaller doses, as an injectable contraceptive. In much larger doses, medroxyprogesterone is used in the treatment of cancer.

Magnitude of Teratogenic Risk

None To Minimal

Quality and Quantity of Data

Fair To Good

Comment

A minimal risk for virilization of the genitalia in a female fetus may exist with maternal use of large doses of this agent during pregnancy. Assessment of this risk is based primarily on studies involving use of progestational hormones at doses much greater than those used for contraception (Schardein, 1993).

The frequency of congenital anomalies was slightly increased among the children of 130 women treated with medroxyprogesterone during the first four lunar months of pregnancy in the Collaborative Perinatal Project, but this increase was due entirely to a difference in the frequency of mild anomalies that had non-uniform rates at participating institutions (Heinonen et al., 1977). The frequency of congenital anomalies among the infants of 217 women treated with medroxyprogesterone anytime during pregnancy was no greater than expected in this study. Congenital anomalies were seen with a frequency no greater than expected in a cohort of 366 infants whose mothers were treated with medroxyprogesterone during the first trimester of pregnancy for recurrent or threatened abortion (Yovich et al., 1988). In another cohort study, the frequency of polysyndactyly and of chromosomal abnormalities was increased among the children of 1229 women who had used medroxyprogesterone as an injectable contraceptive prior to or during pregnancy, but these associations were not seen if only the 724 women who had received an injection of medroxyprogesterone within six months of conception were considered (Pardthaisong et al., 1988).

Ambiguity of the external genitalia has been reported among both sons and daughters of women who were treated with medroxyprogesterone to prevent miscarriage during pregnancy, but genital abnormalities among these infants are uncommon (Shardein, 1993; Yovich et al., 1988).

Increased frequencies of perinatal death (odds ratio 1.8, 95% confidence interval 1.3-2.4) and low birth weight (odds ratio 1.5, 95% confidence interval 1.2-1.9) were observed in a cohort study of 1431 infants whose mothers had received depot medroxyprogesterone injections for contraception around the time of conception (Pardthaisong & Gray, 1991; Gray & Pardthaisong, 1991). Substantial differences existed between the exposed and control groups in this study, and these differences may account for the associations observed. No major adverse effects on growth or pubertal development were observed among children up to 17 years of age (Pardthaisong et al., 1992). Similarly, no alteration of growth, general health, sexual maturation, or sexually dimorphic behavior was found among 74 teenage boys or 98 teenage girls who had been exposed to medroxyprogesterone in utero in another study (Jaffe et al., 1989, 1990).

The frequency of nongenital malformations was not obviously increased among the offspring of baboons and cynomologus monkeys treated during pregnancy with me-

361

droxyprogesterone at 1-40 and 10-40 times the single 3-monthly contraceptive dose used in humans (Tarara, 1984; Prahalada et al., 1985a, b). The frequency of nongenital malformations was no greater than expected among the offspring of rats or mice treated during pregnancy with medroxyprogesterone in doses hundreds of times larger than those used in women, although growth retardation and fetal death were sometimes seen (Andrew & Staples, 1977; Carbone et al., 1990). In another study, a slightly increased frequency of cleft palate and other malformations was observed among the offspring of rats treated with medroxyprogesterone in 2-300 times the single contraceptive dose during pregnancy, but the effect was not clearly dose-related (Eibs et al., 1982). A dose-dependent increase was observed in the frequency of malformations, mostly cleft palates, among the offspring of rabbits treated with repeated injections of medroxyprogesterone in doses 1-10 times the single contraceptive dose used in women (Andrew & Staples, 1977).

Genital ambiguity has been observed among the offspring of baboons, cynomolgus monkeys, guinea pigs, and rats treated during pregnancy with medroxyprogesterone in doses greater than those used in humans (Lerner et al., 1962; Foote et al., 1968; Kawashima et al., 1977; Prahalada et al., 1985a, b).

Key References

Andrew FD, Staples RE: Prenatal toxicity of medroxyprogesterone acetate in rabbits, rats, and mice. Teratology 15:25-32, 1977. [A]

Carbone JP, Figurska K, Buck S, Brent RL: Effect of gestational sex steroid exposure on limb development and endochondral ossification in the pregnant C57B1/6J mouse: I. Medroxyprogesterone acetate. Teratology 42(2):121-130, 1990. [A]

Eibs HG, Spielmann H, Hagele M: Teratogenic effects of cyproterone acetate and medroxyprogesterone treatment during the pre- and postimplantation period of mouse embryos. I. Teratology 25:27-36, 1982. [A]

Foote WD, Foote WC, Foote LH: Influence of certain natural and synthetic steroids on genital development in guinea pigs. Fertil Steril 19:606-615, 1968. [A]

Gray RH, Pardthaisong T: In utero exposure to steroid contraceptives and survival during infancy. Am J Epidemiol 134(8):804-811, 1991. [E]

Heinonen OP, Slone D, Shapiro S: Birth Defects and Drugs in Pregnancy. Littleton, Mass.: John Wright-PSG, 1977, pp 389-391, 443. [E]

Jaffe B, Shye D, Harlap S, et al.: Aggression, physical activity levels and sex role identity in teenagers exposed in utero to MPA. Contraception 40:351-363, 1989. [E]

Jaffe B, Shye D, Harlap S, et al.: Health, growth and sexual development of teenagers exposed in utero to medroxyprogesterone acetate. Paediatr Perinat Epidemiol 4(2):184-195, 1990. [E]

Kawashima K, Nakaura S, Nagao S, Tanaka S, et al.: Virilizing activities of various steroids in female rat fetuses. Endocrinol Japon 24:77-81, 1977. [A]

Lerner LJ, DePhillipo M, Yiacas E, Brennan D, et al.: Comparison of the acetophenone derivative of 16alpha, 17alpha-dihydroxyprogesterone with other progestational steroids for masculinization of the rat fetus. Endocrinology 71:448-451, 1962. [A]

Pardthaisong T, Gray RH: In utero exposure to steroid contraceptives and outcome of pregnancy. Am J Epidemiol 134(8):795-803, 1991. [E]

Pardthaisong T, Gray RH, McDaniel EB, et al.: Steroid contraceptive use and pregnancy outcome. Teratology 38:51-58, 1988. [E]

Pardthaisong T, Yenchit C, Gray R: The long-term growth and development of children exposed to depo-provera during pregnancy or lactation. Contraception 45(4):313-324, 1992. [E]

Prahalada S, Carroad E, Cukierski M, Hendrickx AG: Embryotoxicity of a single dose of medroxyprogesterone acetate (MPA) and maternal serum MPA concentrations in cynomolgus monkey (Macaca fascicularis). Teratology 32:421-432, 1985a. [A]

Prahalada S, Carroad E, Hendrickx AG: Embryotoxicity and maternal serum concentrations of medroxyprogesterone acetate (MPA) in baboons (Papio cynocephalus). Contraception 32:497-515, 1985b. [A]

Schardein JL: Chemically Induced Birth Defects. New York: Marcel Dekker, 1993, pp 284-301, 1993. [R]

Tarara R: The effect of medroxyprogesterone acetate (Depo- Provera) on prenatal development in the baboon (Papio anubis): A preliminary study. Teratology 30:181-185, 1984. [A]

Yovich JL, Turner SR, Draper R: Medroxyprogesterone acetate therapy in early pregnancy has no apparent fetal effects. Teratology 38:135-144, 1988. [E]

MEFENAMIC ACID

Synonyms

Ponstel

Summary

Mefenamic acid is an oral nonsteroidal anti-inflammatory agent that has analgesic and antipyretic actions.

Magnitude of Teratogenic Risk

Undetermined

Quality and Quantity of Data

None To Poor

Comment

Maternal mefenamic acid treatment late in pregnancy may be associated with premature closure of the fetal ductus arteriosus (see below).

No epidemiological studies of congenital anomalies in infants born to women who were treated with mefenamic acid during pregnancy have been reported.

An increased frequency of cleft palate has been observed among the offspring of mice treated with less than the usual human dose of mefenamic acid during pregnancy (Montenegro & Palomino, 1990). The relevance of this observation to the use of mefenamic acid in pregnant women is unknown.

Mefenamic acid is an inhibitor of prostaglandin synthesis. This class of drugs has been used therapeutically to produce closure of the ductus arteriosus and consequent changes in cardiovascular and pulmonary function in newborns with patent ductus arteriosus. Mefenamic acid administration to near-term pregnant rats in doses similar to those used in humans has been shown to cause premature (in utero) closure of the ductus arteriosus in the fetuses (Momma & Takeuchi, 1983). The risk of a similar occurrence in humans after maternal exposure to mefenamic acid late in pregnancy is unknown.

Please see agent summary on indomethacin for information on a related agent.

Key References

Momma K, Takeuchi H: Constriction of fetal ductus arteriosus by non-steroidal anti-inflammatory drugs. Prostaglandins 26:631-643, 1983. [A]

Montenegro MA, Palomino H: Induction of cleft palate in mice by inhibitors of prostaglandin synthesis. J Craniofac Genet Dev Biol 10:83-94, 1990. [A]

MEFLOQUINE

Synonyms

Lariam

Summary

Mefloquine is used in the prophylaxis and treatment of malaria.

Magnitude of Teratogenic Risk

Undetermined

Quality and Quantity of Data

None To Poor

Comment

None

No epidemiological studies of congenital anomalies among infants born to women

treated with mefloquine during pregnancy have been reported.

According to one abstract, "some anomalies were observed" among the offspring of mice and rats treated during pregnancy with mefloquine in doses 4 times those used in humans (Minor et al., 1976). This observation cannot be assessed on the basis of the limited published information.

Key References

Minor JL, Short RD, Heiffer MH, et al.: Reproductive effects of mefloquine HCl (MFQ) in rats and mice. Pharmacologist 18:171, 1976. [A]

MEGESTROL

Synonyms

Megace, Niagestin, Ovaban, Primobolan

Summary

Megestrol is an oral progestational agent used in the treatment of breast and uterine cancer.

Magnitude of Teratogenic Risk

None To Minimal

Quality and Quantity of Data

None To Poor

Comment

A minimal risk for virilization of the genitalia in female fetuses may exist with maternal use of megestrol in large doses during pregnancy (Katz et al., 1985).

No epidemiological studies of congenital anomalies among infants born to women treated with megestrol during pregnancy have been reported.

Virilization of the external genitalia was observed among the female offspring of rats treated during pregnancy with megestrol in doses six times those used to treat breast cancer in humans (Kawashima et al., 1977).

Please see agent summary on medroxyprogesterone for information on a related drug that has been more thoroughly studied.

Key References

Katz Z, Lancet M, Skornik J, Chemke J, et al.: Teratogenicity of progestogens given during the first trimester of pregnancy. Obstet Gynecol 65:775-780, 1985. [R]

Kawashima K, Nakaura S, Nagao S, Tanaka S, et al.: Virilizing activities of various steroids in female rat fetuses. Endocrinol Jpn 24(1):77-81, 1977. [A]

MELPHALAN

Synonyms

Alkeran, L-PAM, L-Sarcolysin, Levofalan, Phenylalanine Mustard, Sarcolysin

Summary

Melphalan is a derivative of nitrogen mustard that is used as an antineoplastic agent.

Magnitude of Teratogenic Risk

Undetermined

Quality and Quantity of Data

None

Comment

Although the risk of this agent is undetermined, it may be substantial because it is a cancer chemotherapeutic agent.

No epidemiological studies of congenital anomalies in infants born to women who were treated with melphalan during pregnancy have been reported.

No animal teratology studies of melphalan have been published.

Please see agent summary on mechlorethamine for information on a related agent that has been studied.

Key References

None available.

MENADIOL

Synonyms

Aquamephyton, Dihydrovitamin K_3, Kappadione, Konakion, Mephyton, Naphthidone, Phytonadione Tablets, Synkavit, Vitamin K_3

Summary

Menadiol is a synthetic water-soluble derivative of vitamin K-3, to which menadiol is converted in the body. Menadiol is used to treat hypoprothrombinemia and hemorrhagic disorders.

Magnitude of Teratogenic Risk

Undetermined

Quality and Quantity of Data

None To Poor

Comment

A small risk cannot be excluded, but a high risk of congenital anomalies in the children of women treated with menadiol during pregnancy is unlikely.

No epidemiological studies of congenital anomalies in infants whose mothers were treated with menadiol during pregnancy have been reported.

No teratogenic effect was observed among the offspring of mice treated during pregnancy with menadiol in a dose 200 times that used therapeutically in humans (Packer et al., 1970).

Key References

Packer AD, Fozzard JAF, Woollam DHM: The effect of synkavit on the teratogenic activity of X radiation--A preliminary report. Br J Radiol 43:36-39, 1970. [A]

MENINGOCOCCAL POLYSACCHARIDE VACCINE

Synonyms

Menomune-A/C/Y/W-135

Summary

Meningococcal polysaccharide vaccine is used for immunization against meningococcal disease.

Magnitude of Teratogenic Risk

Undetermined

Quality and Quantity of Data

None

Comment

A small risk cannot be excluded, but a high risk of congenital anomalies in the children of women treated with meningococcal polysaccharide vaccine during pregnancy is unlikely.

No epidemiological studies of congenital anomalies in infants whose mothers were given meningococcal polysaccharide vaccine during pregnancy have been reported.

No animal teratology studies of meningococcal polysaccharide vaccine have been published.

Key References

None available.

MENTHOL

Synonyms

Hexahydrothymol, Icy Hot Cream

Summary

Menthol, an alcohol found in peppermint oil, is used topically to prevent itching and as a mild anesthetic. Menthol is taken orally as an antitussive or antiflatulent agent. Menthol is also used to impart its peppermint taste or odor to liqueurs, confections, perfumes, and cigarettes. The WHO estimated acceptable daily intake of menthol is up to 0.2 mg/kg.

Magnitude of Teratogenic Risk

Undetermined

Quality and Quantity of Data

None To Poor

Comment

A small risk cannot be excluded, but a high risk of congenital anomalies in the children of women treated with menthol during pregnancy is unlikely.

No epidemiological studies of congenital anomalies among infants born to women treated with menthol during pregnancy have been reported.

No teratogenic effect was observed among the offspring of mice, rats, hamsters, or rabbits treated during pregnancy with menthol in doses respectively 9-900, 11-1100, 20-2000, or 21-2100 times the estimated acceptable daily intake of menthol for humans (Food and Drug Research Labs, 1973).

Key References

Food and Drug Research Labs: Teratologic Evaluation of FDA 71-57 (Menthol natural, Brazillian). NTIS(National Technical Information Service) Report/PB 223-815, 1973. [A]

MEPARTRICIN

Synonyms

Tricandil

Summary

Mepartricin is an antifungal and antiprotozoal. It is used topically to treat vaginal infection.

Magnitude of Teratogenic Risk

Undetermined

Quality and Quantity of Data

None

Comment

None

No epidemiological studies of congenital anomalies in infants born to women who used mepartricin during pregnancy have been reported.

No animal teratology studies of mepartricin have been published.

Key References

None available.

MEPENZOLATE

Synonyms

Cantil, Cantril, Colibantil, Eftoron, Gastro-pidil, Glycophenylate, Tralanta

Summary

Mepenzolate is an anticholinergic agent that is administered orally in the treatment of visceral spasms or peptic ulcer.

Magnitude of Teratogenic Risk

Undetermined

Quality and Quantity of Data

None To Poor

Comment

None

No epidemiological studies of congenital anomalies in infants whose mothers were treated with mepenzolate during pregnancy have been reported.

No animal teratology studies of mepenzolate have been published.

Please see agent summary on atropine for information on a related agent that has been more thoroughly studied.

Key References

None available.

MEPERIDINE

Synonyms

Demerol, Isonipecaine Hydrochloride, Peth-adol, Pethidine Hydrochloride

Summary

Meperidine is a widely used synthetic narcotic analgesic.

Magnitude of Teratogenic Risk

None To Minimal

Quality and Quantity of Data

Fair

Comment

Respiratory depression and behavioral alterations occur with increased frequency among infants born within a few hours of maternal treatment with meperidine.

The frequency of congenital anomalies was no greater than expected among the infants of 268 women who were treated with meperidine during the first four lunar months of pregnancy or of 1100 women who were treated with the drug anytime during pregnancy in the Collaborative Perinatal Project (Heinonen et al., 1977). No association was observed between maternal use of meperidine during the first trimester of pregnancy and congenital anomalies in more than 50 infants in another cohort study (Jick et al., 1981).

A dose-dependent increase in the frequency of central nervous system and other anomalies was observed in the offspring of hamsters treated with meperidine during pregnancy in doses 8-29 times those used in humans (Geber & Schramm, 1975). The frequency of malformations was not significantly increased among the offspring of pregnant mice given single doses of meperidine 40-50 times those used in humans (Martin & Jurand, 1992). Alterations of neonatal behavior were seen among infant rhesus monkeys born to mothers that had received meperidine during labor in a dose similar to that used in humans (Golub et al., 1988). The relevance of these observations to the clinical use of meperidine in human pregnancy is unknown.

Maternal treatment with meperidine within a few hours of delivery may cause transient respiratory depression in newborn infants (Shnider & Moya, 1964; Koch & Wendel, 1968; Morrison et al., 1973; Hamza et al., 1992). Behavioral alterations have also been observed among such infants in the newborn period (Belsey et al., 1981; Hodgkinson et al., 1982; Busacca et al., 1982), but no physical or psychological deficit was apparent at ages five to 10 years in one series of 70 children born to mothers treated with meperidine within two hours of birth (Buck, 1975).

Key References

Belsey EM, Rosenblatt DB, Lieberman BA, Redshaw M, et al.: The influence of maternal analgesia on neonatal behaviour: I. Pethidine. Br J Obstet Gynaecol 88:398-406, 1981. [E]

Buck C: Drugs in pregnancy. Can Med Assoc J 112:1285, 1975. [O]

Busacca M, Gementi P, Gambini E, et al.: Neonatal effects of the administration of meperidine and promethazine to the mother in labor. Double blind study. J Perinat Med 10:48-53, 1982. [E]

Geber WF, Schramm LC: Congenital malformations of the central nervous system produced by narcotic analgesics in the hamster. Am J Obstet Gynecol 123:705-713, 1975. [A]

Golub MS, Eisele JH, Donald JM: Obstetric analgesia and infant outcome in monkeys. Am J Obstet Gynecol 158:1219-1225, 1988. [A]

Hamza J, Benlabed M, Orhant E, Escourrou P, et al.: Neonatal pattern of breathing during active and quiet sleep after maternal administration of meperidine. Pediatr Res 32:412-416, 1992. [E]

Heinonen OP, Slone D, Shapiro S: Birth Defects and Drugs in Pregnancy. Littleton, Mass.: John Wright-PSG, 1977, pp 287, 288, 434, 471, 484. [E]

Hodgkinson R, Husain FJ: The duration of effect of maternally administered meperidine on neonatal neurobehavior. Anesthesiology 56(1):51-52, 1982. [E]

Jick H, Holmes LB, Hunter JR, Madsen S, et al.: First-trimester drug use and congenital disorders. JAMA 246:343-346, 1981. [S]

Koch G, Wendel H: The effect of pethidine on the postnatal adjustment of respiration and acid base balance. Acta Obstet Gynecol Scand 47:27-37, 1968. [E]

Martin LVH, Jurand A: The absence of teratogenic effects of some analgesics used in anaesthesia. Anaesthesia 47:473-476, 1992. [A]

Morrison JC, Wiser WL, Rosser SI, Gayden JO, et al.: Metabolites of meperidine related to fetal depression. Am J Obstet Gynecol 115:1132-1137, 1973. [S]

Shnider SM, Moya F: Effects of meperidine on the newborn infant. Am J Obstet Gynecol 89:1009-1014, 1964. [S]

MEPHENESIN

Synonyms

Cresoxydiol, Cresoxypropanediol, Decontractyl, Glykresin, Mefenesina, Myanesin, Relaxar

Summary

Mephenesin is a centrally acting skeletal muscle relaxant.

Magnitude of Teratogenic Risk

Undetermined

Quality and Quantity of Data

None

Comment

None

No epidemiological studies of congenital anomalies in the infants of women who took mephenesin during pregnancy have been reported.

No teratology studies of mephenesin in experimental animals have been published.

Key References

None available.

MEPHENYTOIN

Synonyms

Mesantoin, Mesontoin, Methoin, Phenantoin, Sedantoinal

Summary

Mephenytoin is a hydantoin anticonvulsant.

Magnitude of Teratogenic Risk

Minimal To Small

Quality and Quantity of Data

Poor To Fair

Comment

None

Maternal use of mephenytoin for treatment of seizure disorder during pregnancy was not seen significantly more often than expected (odds ratio = 3.5, 95% confidence interval 0.7-32.3) among 10,698 infants with congenital anomalies in an Hungarian case-control study (Czeizel et al., 1992). Maternal anticonvulsant polytherapy that included mephenytoin was associated with congenital anomalies in this study (odds ratio = 10.1, 95% confidence interval 1.8-57.1). The anomalies seen in affected children, which were similar to those reported among infants of epileptic women treated with other anticonvulsants, included congenital heart disease, facial clefts, and other malformations.

A characteristic pattern of congenital anomalies called the "fetal hydantoin syndrome" has been observed among the children of epileptic women who were treated with hydantoin anticonvulsants during pregnancy (Speidel & Meadow, 1972; Hanson et al., 1976). Some of the features of this syndrome may be due to the maternal epilepsy per se rather than to the anticonvulsant therapy (Shapiro et al., 1976; Dieterich et al., 1980; Kelly, 1984; Kelly et al., 1984a, 1984b). Although most children with the fetal hydantoin syndrome are born to women who have taken phenytoin during pregnancy, a few affected children have been born to women treated with mephenytoin (Hanson & Smith, 1975; Schinzel, 1979).

The frequency of malformations was not increased among the offspring of mice treated during pregnancy with mephenytoin in doses 4 to 12 times those used clinically, although fetal weight was reduced with the higher doses (Brown et al., 1982; Wells et al., 1982). Decreased weight was observed both before and after weaning among the offspring of rats treated during pregnancy with about four times the human dose of mephenytoin, a dose which produces a blood level in rats that would be considered to be subtherapeutic in humans (Minck et al., 1991). Some behavioral alterations were observed in the treated pups in the first three weeks of life in this study, but the effects were much less than those seen with phenytoin.

Please see agent summary on phenytoin for information on a similar drug that has been more thoroughly studied.

Key References

Brown NA, Shull G, Kao J, Goulding EH, et al.: Teratogenicity and lethality of hydantoin derivatives in the mouse: Structure--toxicity relationships. Toxicol Appl Pharmacol 64:271-288, 1982. [A]

Czeizel AE, Bod M, Halasz P: Evaluation of anticonvulsant drugs during pregnancy in a population-based Hungarian study. Eur J Epidemiol 8(1):122-127, 1992. [E]

Dieterich E, Steveling A, Lukas A, Seyfeddinipur N, et al.: Congenital anomalies in children of epileptic mothers and fathers. Neuropediatrics 11:274-283, 1980. [S]

Hanson JW, Myrianthopoulos NC, Harvey MAS, Smith DW: Risks to the offspring of women treated with hydantoin anticonvulsants, with emphasis on the fetal hydantoin syndrome. J Pediatr 89:662-668, 1976. [S]

Hanson JW, Smith DW: The fetal hydantoin syndrome. J Pediatr 87:285-290, 1975. [C]

Kelly TE: Teratogenicity of anticonvulsant drugs. I: Review of the literature. Am J Med Genet 19:413-434, 1984. [R]

Kelly TE, Edwards P, Rein M, Miller JQ, et al.: Teratogenicity of anticonvulsant drugs. II: A prospective study. Am J Med Genet 19:435-443, 1984a. [S]

Kelly TE, Rein M, Edwards P: Teratogenicity of anticonvulsant drugs. IV: The association of clefting and epilepsy. Am J Med Genet 19:451-458, 1984b. [S]

Minck DR, Acuff-Smith KD, Vorhees CV: Comparison of the behavioral teratogenic potential of phenytoin, mephenytoin, ethotoin, and hydantoin in rats. Teratology 43:279-293, 1991. [A]

Schinzel A: [Fetal hydantoin-syndrome in siblings.] Schweiz Med Wochenschr 109:68-72, 1979. [A]

Shapiro S, Slone D, Hartz SC, Rosenberg L, et al.: Anticonvulsants and parental epilepsy in the development of birth defects. Lancet 1:272-275, 1976. [E]

Speidel BD, Meadow SR: Maternal epilepsy and abnormalities of the fetus and newborn. Lancet 2:839-843, 1972. [E]

Wells PG, Kupfer A, Lawson JA, et al.: Relation of in vivo drug metabolism to stereoselective fetal hydantoin toxicology in mouse: Evaluation of mephenytoin and its metabolite, Nirvanol. J Pharmacol Exp Ther 221:228-234, 1982. [A]

MEPHOBARBITAL

Synonyms

Mebaral, Methylphenobarbital

Summary

Mephobarbital is a barbiturate used as an anticonvulsant and sedative.

Magnitude of Teratogenic Risk

None To Minimal

Quality and Quantity of Data

Poor To Fair

Comment

None

The frequency of congenital anomalies was no greater among a cohort of 111 children born to epileptic mothers who were treated with mephobarbital during the first trimester of pregnancy than among the children of epileptic mothers that were treated in other ways in a Japanese multi-institutional study (Nakane et al., 1980). Similarly, congenital anomalies were no more frequent among the infants of 17 epileptic women who received mephobarbital treatment during the first trimester of pregnancy than among the infants of untreated epileptic women in another study (Annegers et al., 1974).

No animal teratology studies of mephobarbital have been published.

Please see agent summary on phenobarbital for information on a closely related agent that is also a major metabolite of mephobarbital.

Key References

Annegers JF, Elveback LR, Hauser WA, Kurland LT: Do anticonvulsants have a teratogenic effect? Arch Neurol 31:364-373, 1974. [E]

Nakane Y, Okuma T, Takahashi R, Sato Y, et al.: Multi-institutional study on the teratogenicity and fetal toxicity of antiepileptic drugs: A report of a collaborative study group in Japan. Epilepsia 21:663-680, 1980. [E]

MEPIVACAINE

Synonyms

Carbocaine, Chlorocain, Meaverin, Mepivastesin, Scandicaine

Summary

Mepivacaine is a local anesthetic of the amide class.

Magnitude of Teratogenic Risk

None To Minimal

Quality and Quantity of Data

Poor

Comment

None

A 2.5-fold increase in the frequency of congenital anomalies was observed among the children of 82 women treated with mepivacaine during the first four lunar months of pregnancy in the Collaborative Perinatal Project, a large cohort study (Heinonen et al., 1977). This association was not observed for any of the structurally similar local anesthetics evaluated in this study, and no other epidemiological investigations of congenital anomalies in children of women treated with mepivacaine during pregnancy are available. The frequency of congenital anomalies was no greater than expected among the children of 224 women treated with mepivacaine anytime during pregnancy in the Collaborative Perinatal Project.

Alterations of neonatal behavior have been observed among the offspring of rats treated systemically with 6 mg/kg of mepivacaine during pregnancy (Smith et al., 1986).

Transient fetal bradycardia has been noted in some studies of women who had epidural or regional anesthesia with mepivacaine during labor (Gordon, 1968; Teramo, 1971; Goins, 1992).

Please see agent summary on lidocaine for information on a related agent that has been more thoroughly studied.

Key References

Goins JR: Experience with mepivacaine paracervical block in an obstetric private practice. Am J Obstet Gynecol 167:342-345, 1992. [E]

Gordon HR: Fetal bradycardia after paracervical block. Correlation with fetal and maternal blood levels of local anesthetic (Mepivacaine). N Engl J Med 279:910-914, 1968. [S]

Heinonen OP, Slone D, Shapiro S: Birth Defects and Drugs in Pregnancy. Littleton, Mass.: John Wright-PSG, 1977, pp 358, 360, 440. [E]

Smith RF, Wharton GG, Kurtz SL, et al.: Behavioral effects of mid-pregnancy administration of lidocaine and mepivacaine in the rat. Neurobehav Toxicol Teratol 8:61-68, 1986. [A]

Teramo K: Effects of obstetrical paracervical blockade on the fetus. Acta Obstet Gynecol Scand Suppl 16:1-55, 1971. [R]

MEPROBAMATE

Synonyms

Equanil, Meprospan, Miltown, Neuramate

Summary

Meprobamate is a carbamate tranquilizer used to treat anxiety.

Magnitude of Teratogenic Risk

Minimal

Quality and Quantity of Data

Fair To Good

Comment

None

Human epidemiological studies regarding possible teratogenic effects of meprobamate are inconsistent. Weak associations have been reported between maternal use of meprobamate early in pregnancy and a variety of malformations in children, but no two studies have found an association with the same malformation. An increased frequency of congenital anomalies (principally cardiac defects) was observed among infants of 66 women who were prescribed meprobamate in the first 42 days after their last menstrual period in one cohort study

(Milkovich & van den Berg, 1974), an increased frequency of hypospadias among 186 male infants after maternal use of meprobamate during the first four lunar months of pregnancy in another study (Heinonen et al., 1977), and an "unexpectedly high" frequency of serious malformations among the children of more than 50 women who were prescribed meprobamate during the first trimester in a third study (Jick et al., 1981). In a case-control study, an increased frequency of maternal use of antianxiety agents, including meprobamate, during the first, but not the second or third, trimester of pregnancy was found among 232 children with cleft palate and among 232 with cleft lip or without cleft palate (Saxen, 1975). In contrast, frequencies of congenital anomalies in general, major malformations, minor anomalies, and major classes of malformations were no greater than expected among the children of 356 women treated with meprobamate during the first four lunar months of pregnancy in the Collaborative Perinatal Project (Heinonen et al., 1977). Another cohort study of congenital anomalies among children of 207 women treated with meprobamate during the first trimester of pregnancy also found no association, but the frequency of malformations in both the exposed and the control groups was so low that underascertainment of defects is very likely (Belafsky et al., 1969). The inconsistency of the findings does not permit a conclusion that maternal use of meprobamate early in pregnancy increases the risk of congenital anomalies in the offspring, but the available data are not sufficient to rule out a small increase in the risk.

No alteration of the frequency of malformations was observed among the offspring of mice, rats, or rabbits treated during pregnancy with meprobamate in doses 8-16, 2.5, and 4-16 times those used in humans, respectively (Brar, 1969; Clavert, 1963; Werboff & Dembicki, 1962). However, increased fetal and neonatal loss were observed in rabbits after maternal doses 16 times those used in humans and in rats after maternal doses 2.5 or 20 times the usual human dose of meprobamate during pregnancy (Bertrand, 1960; Clavert, 1963; Werboff and Kesner, 1963). Behavioral alterations that persist into adulthood have been observed among the offspring of rats treated with 2.5 times the usual human dose of meprobamate during pregnancy (Werboff and Kesner, 1963; Murai, 1966; Hoffeld et al, 1968. The clinical importance of these findings is unclear. No difference was found in mental and motor status scores at eight months of age or in IQ scores at four years of age between controls and 851 children born to women who had taken meprobamate during pregnancy (Hartz et al., 1975).

No malformations were observed in an infant whose mother took an overdose of meprobamate in the first trimester of pregnancy (Czeizel et al., 1984, 1988).

Key References

Belafsky HA, Breslow S, Hirsch LM, Shangold JE, et al.: Meprobamate during pregnancy. Obstet Gynecol 34:378-386, 1969. [E]

Bertrand M: Effect of meprobamate on rat pregnancy. C R Soc Biol 154:2309-2312, 1960. [A]

Brar BS: The effect of meprobamate on fertility, gestation and offspring viability and development of mice. Arch Int Pharmacodyn 177:416-422, 1969. [A]

Clavert J: Effect of meprobamate on embryogenesis. C R Soc Biol 157:1481-1482, 1963. [A]

Czeizel A, Szentesi I, Szekeres I, Glauber A, et al.: Pregnancy outcome and health conditions of offspring of self-poisoned pregnant women. Acta Paediatr Hung 25(3):209-236, 1984. [S]

Czeizel A, Szentesi I, Szekeres I, Molnar G, et al.: A study of adverse effects on the progeny after intoxication during pregnancy. Arch Toxicol 62:1-7, 1988. [S]

Hartz SC, Heinonen OP, Sharpiro S, Siskind V, et al.: Antenatal exposure to meprobamate and chlordiazepoxide in relation to malformations, mental development, and childhood mortality. N Engl J Med 292:726-728, 1975. [S]

Heinonen OP, Slone D, Shapiro S: Birth Defects and Drugs in Pregnancy. Littleton, Mass.: John Wright-PSG, 1977, pp 336-337. [E]

Hoffeld DR, McNew J, Webster RL: Effect of tranquilizing drugs during pregnancy on activity of offspring. Nature 218:357-358, 1968. [A]

Jick H, Holmes LB, Hunter JR, Madsen S, et al.: First trimester drug use and congenital defects. JAMA 246:343-346, 1981. [E]

Milkovich L, van den Berg BJ: Effects of prenatal meprobamate and chlordiazepoxide hydrochloride on human embryonic and fetal development. N Eng J Med 291:1268-1271, 1974. [E]

Murai N: Effect of maternal medication during pregnancy upon behavioral development of offspring. Tohoku J Exp Med 89:265-272, 1966. [A]

Saxen I: Associations between oral clefts and drugs taken during pregnancy. Int J Epidemiol 4:37-44, 1975. [E]

Werboff J, Dembicki EL: Toxic effects of tranquilizers administered to gravid rats. J Neuropsychiatry 4:87-91, 1962. [A]

Werboff J, Kesner R: Learning deficits of offspring after administration of tranquilizing drugs to the mothers. Nature 197:106-107, 1963. [A]

MEPRYLCAINE

Synonyms

Meprylcaini Chloridum

Summary

Meprylcaine is a local anesthetic of the ester class that is used in dentistry.

Magnitude of Teratogenic Risk

Undetermined

Quality and Quantity of Data

None

Comment

None

No epidemiological studies of congenital anomalies in children born to women exposed to meprylcaine during pregnancy have been reported.

No investigations of teratologic effects of meprylcaine in experimental animals have been published.

Please see agent summary on procaine for information on a related agent that has been studied.

Key References

None available.

MERCAPTOPURINE

Synonyms

Ismipur, Leupurin, Mercaleukin, Mercapurin, Purinethol

Summary

Mercaptopurine is a purine analog that interferes with nucleic acid synthesis. Mercaptopurine is administered orally in the treatment of neoplastic disease.

Magnitude of Teratogenic Risk

Small To Moderate

Quality and Quantity of Data

Poor To Fair

Comment

1) Transient neonatal anemia and pancytopenia have been observed among the infants of women treated with mercaptopurine and other chemotherapeutic agents during pregnancy (McConnell et al., 1973; Okun et al., 1979; Pizzuto et al., 1980).

2) Teratogenic risks associated with maternal polydrug therapy that includes mercaptopurine may be greater than those associated with maternal mercaptopurine monotherapy.

No congenital anomalies were observed among the infants of eight women treated with mercaptopurine and other antineoplastic agents during pregnancy in one series (Aviles et al., 1991); five of these patients were treated during the first trimester. Several anomalies, including microphthalmia and cleft palate in one instance and hypospadias in another, have been observed among infants born to women treated with mercaptopurine and other antineoplastic agents early in pregnancy (Diamond et al., 1960; Sosa Munoz et al., 1983). However, more than 50 women treated with mercaptopurine during various stages of pregnancy have been reported to have had children without major malformations (Nicholson, 1968; Moloney, 1964; Pizzuto et al., 1980; Catanzarite & Ferguson, 1984; Feliu et al., 1988; Zuazu et al., 1991; Aviles et al., 1991). Low birth weight may be unusually frequent among such infants.

Mercaptopurine is teratogenic in experimental animals at doses similar to or greater than those used in humans. Increased frequencies of fetal death and of central nervous system, facial and limb anomalies have been observed among the offspring of pregnant rats, mice, and rabbits treated with <1 to many times the human therapeutic dose of mercaptopurine (Mercier-Parot & Duplessis, 1967; Puget et al., 1975). Similar teratogenic effects were seen among the offspring of hamsters and Afghan pikas treated with mercaptopurine during pregnancy in doses 11-65 or 2-12 times that used in humans (Shah & Burdett, 1979; Puget et al., 1975). Typical dependence of the teratogenic effect on dose and time of gestation at exposure was observed in some of these experiments.

Decreased fertility and an increased frequency of fetal loss were found among adult female mice that had been born to mothers treated with mercaptopurine during pregnancy in doses similar to those used in humans (Reimers & Sluss, 1978; Reimers et al., 1980).

Key References

Aviles A, Diaz-Maqueo JC, Talavera A, et al.: Growth and development of children of mothers treated with chemotherapy during pregnancy: Current status of 43 children. Am J Hematol 36:243-248, 1991. [S]

Catanzarite VA, Ferguson JE II: Acute leukemia and pregnancy: A review of management and outcome, 1972-1982. Obstet Gynecol Survey 39(11):663-678, 1984. [C] & [R]

Diamond I, Anderson MM, McCreadie SR: Transplacental transmission of busulfan (MyleranR) in a mother with leukemia. Pediatrics 25:85-90, 1960. [C]

Feliu J, Juarez S, Ordonez A, et al.: Acute leukemia and pregnancy. Cancer 61:580-584, 1988. [S] & [R]

McConnell JB, Bhoola R: A neonatal complication of maternal leukaemia treated with 6-mercaptopurine. Postgrad Med J 49:211-213, 1973. [C]

Mercier-Parot L, Tuchmann-Duplessis H: Limb malformations induced by 6-mercaptopurine in the rabbit, rat and mouse. C R Soc Biol 161:762-768, 1967. [A]

Moloney WC: Management of leukemia in pregnancy. Ann NY Acad Sci 114:857-867, 1964. [R]

Nicholson OH: Cytotoxic drugs in pregnancy. J Obstet Gynaecol Br Commonw 75:307-312, 1968. [R]

Okun DB, Groncy PK, Sieger L, Tanaka KR: Acute leukemia in pregnancy: Transient neonatal myelosuppression after combination chemotherapy in the mother. Med Pediatr Oncol 7:315-319, 1979. [C]

Pizzuto J, Aviles A, Noriega L, Niz J, et al.: Treatment of acute leukemia during pregnancy: Presentation of nine cases. Cancer Treat Rep 64:679-683, 1980. [S]

Puget A, Cros S, Oreglia J, Tollon Y: A study of the embryonic sensitivity of the Afghan pika (ochotona rufescens-rufescens) to two teratogenous agents, azathioprin and 6-mercaptopurine. Zentrabl Veterinarmed Reihe A 22:38-56, 1975. [A]

Reimers TJ, Sluss PM: 6-mercaptopurine treatment of pregnant mice: Effects on second and third generations. Science 201:65-67, 1978. [A]

Reimers TJ, Sluss PM, Godwin J, Seidel GE: Bi-generational effects of 6-mercaptopurine on reproduction in mice. Biol Reprod 22:367-375, 1980. [A]

Shah RM, Burdett DN: Developmental abnormalities induced by 6-mercaptopurine in the hamster. Can J Physiol Pharmacol, 1979, 57:53-58, 1979. [A]

Sosa Munoz JL, Perez Santana MT, Sosa Sanchez R, Labardini JR: Acute leukemia and pregnancy. Rev Invest Clin 35:55-58, 1983. [C]

Zuazu J, Julia A, Sierra J, et al.: Pregnancy outcome in hematologic malignancies. Cancer 67:703-709, 1991. [S]

MERCURY (ELEMENTAL)

Synonyms

Metallic Mercury, Phenylmercuric Acetate, Quick Silver

Summary

Elemental mercury occurs as a liquid metal or vapor at room temperature. Mercury is used in dentistry, in making thermometers, switches, and fluorescent lamps, and in the metals, chemical, and pharmaceutical industries. Liquid mercury is poorly absorbed but mercury vapor is readily absorbed through the lungs, intact skin, and gastrointestinal tract. Acute and chronic mercury toxicity is well recognized (Clarkson & Marsh, 1982; Hathaway et al., 1991). The acceptable limit for occupational exposure to mercury vapor is 0.05 mg/cu m as an 8-hour time- weighted average (Hathaway et al., 1991).

Magnitude of Teratogenic Risk

None

Quality and Quantity of Data

Fair

Comment

Absorption of mercury from dental amalgams has been found to be very low (Mandel, 1991).

The frequencies of congenital anomalies and miscarriage reported in a postal survey of 3212 pregnancies in dental assistants who prepared more than 40 mercury amalgams per week were no greater than the frequencies in dental assistants with less exposure to mercury (Brodsky et al., 1985). Similarly, the frequency of congenital anomalies in general and of major classes of congenital anomalies did not appear unusual among 8157 infants born to women who worked during pregnancy as dentists, dental assistants, or dental technicians (Ericson & Kallen, 1989). No significant increase in the frequencies of congenital anomalies or spontaneous abortions was observed among 120 pregnancies in women who were occupationally exposed to mercury vapor in a lamp factory (de Rosis et al., 1985). The frequency of spontaneous abortion was not increased in 305 pregnancies of dental assistants who were occupationally exposed to mercury in another cohort study (Heidam, 1984) or among more than 1000 pregnancies of woman dentists, dental assistants and dental technicians (Ericson & Kallen, 1989). Adverse outcomes (spontaneous abortion, stillbirth, or malformation) were observed more often than expected in 117 pregnancies of female dentists and dental assistants who were occupationally exposed to mercury in one other study (Sikorski et al., 1987), and five of the six infants with congenital anomalies born to exposed women had neural tube defects. None of 220 infants with neural tube defects in one series were born to women who were dentists; the expectation was 0.5 (Ericson & Kallen, 1989).

Placental abruption with fetal death occurred in a woman who was acutely exposed to toxic amounts of mercury vapor at 32 weeks gestation (Ortiz et al., 1989). No adverse effect was observed in the child of a woman chronically exposed to toxic levels of mercury vapor throughout the first 17 weeks of pregnancy (Thorp et al., 1992).

An increased frequency of embryo/fetal death was observed among the offspring of pregnant rats continually exposed to mercury vapors in concentrations 4-20 times the human occupational exposure limit (Rao et al., 1983; Steffek et al., 1987). No significant increase in malformations was observed, but such doses did produce maternal toxicity. No adverse effect was observed among the offspring of pregnant rats continually exposed to mercury vapor in a concentration twice the human occupational exposure limit (Rao et al., 1982; Steffek et al., 1987).

Key References

Brodsky JB, Cohen EN, Whitcher C, et al.: Occupational exposure to mercury in dentistry and pregnancy outcome. J Am Dent Assoc 111:779-780, 1985. [E]

Clarkson TW, Marsh DO: Mercury toxicity in man. In: Prasad AS (ed). Current Topics in Nutrition and Disease. Vol. 6. Clinical, Biochemical, and Nutritional Aspects of Trace Elements. New York: Alan R. Liss, 1982, pp 549-568. [R]

de Rosis F, Anastasio SP, Selvaggi L, et al.: Female reproductive health in two lamp factories: Effects of exposure to inorganic mercury vapour and stress factors. Br J Ind Med 42:488-494, 1985. [E]

Ericson A, Kallen B: Pregnancy outcome in women working as dentists, dental assistants or dental technicians. Int Arch Occup Environ Health 61:329-333, 1989. [E]

Hathaway GJ, Proctor NH, Hughes JP, Fischman ML (eds). Proctor and Hughes' Chemical Hazards of the Workplace, 3rd ed. New York: Van Nostrand Reinhold, 1991, pp 367-369. [O]

Heidam LZ: Spontaneous abortions among dental assistants, factory workers, painters, and gardening workers: A follow up study. J Epidemiol Community Health 38:149-155, 1984. [E]

Mandel ID: Amalgam Hazards. An assessment of research. J Am Dent Assoc 122:62-65, 1991. [R]

Ortiz Esqueda G, Vazquez Rosales J, de Dios Maldonado Alvarado J, et al.: [Mercury poisoning in pregnancy. A case report and review of the literature]. Ginecol Obstet Mex 57:274-276, 1989. [C] & [R]

Rao GS, Radchenko V, Tong YS: Reproductive effects of elemental mercury vapor in pregnant Wistar rats. J Dent Res 62(Spec Iss):232, 1983. [A]

Rao GS, Tong YS, Radchenko V, Verrusio AC: Toxicity of dental mercury: Effect on developing embryos in pregnant rats. J Dent Res 61(Spec Iss):202, 1982. [A]

Sikorski R, Juszkiewicz T, Paszkowski T, Szprengier-Juszkiewicz T: Women in dental surgeries: Reproductive hazards in occupational exposure to metallic mercury. Int Arch Occup Environ Health 59:551-557, 1987. [E]

Steffek AJ, Clayton R, Siew C, Verrusio AC: Effects of elemental mercury vapor exposure on pregnant Sprague-Dawley rats. Teratology 35:59A, 1987. [A]

Thorp JM Jr: Elemental mercury exposure in early pregnancy. Obstet Gynecol 79:874-876, 1992. [C] & [R]

MESALAMINE

Synonyms

Asacol, Asacolitin, Claversal, Fisalamine, Mesalazine, Pentasa, Rowasa, Salofalk

Summary

Mesalamine is a salicylate (5-amino-salicylic acid) that is administered orally or rectally in the treatment of inflammatory bowel disease.

Magnitude of Teratogenic Risk

Undetermined

Quality and Quantity of Data

None

Comment

None

No epidemiological studies of congenital anomalies among infants born to women treated with mesalamine during pregnancy have been reported.

No animal teratology studies of mesalamine have been published.

Please see agent summaries on sulfasalazine, which produces mesalamine on breakdown in the bowel, and aspirin, a related agent which has been more thoroughly studied.

Key References

None available.

MESCALINE

Synonyms

Mescal Buttons, Peyote, Peyote Buttons, Peyote Cactus, Peyotl, 3,4,5-trimethoxyphenethylamine

Summary

Mescaline is an hallucinogenic alkaloid that occurs in the peyote cactus, Lophophora williamsii. The flattened seed pods ("buttons") are also called peyote and are ingested "recreationally" and in Native American rituals. Natural mescaline is contaminated with strychnine; mescaline may also be obtained through chemical synthesis.

Magnitude of Teratogenic Risk

Undetermined

Quality and Quantity of Data

None To Poor

Comment

None

No epidemiological studies of malformations in infants born to mothers who ingested mescaline during pregnancy have been reported.

An increased frequency of neural tube malformations was observed in the offspring of hamsters administered 0.1-0.6 times the usual human dose of mescaline during pregnancy in one study (Geber, 1967). However, the effect was not dose-related and no such abnormalities were seen in another study in which doses 3-6 times those used by humans were employed (Hirsch & Fritz, 1981). An increased rate of fetal loss was seen among the offspring of exposed animals in both investigations.

Key References

Geber WF: Congenital malformations induced by mescaline, lysergic acid diethylamide, and bromolysergic acid in the hamster. Science 158:265-267, 1967. [A]

Hirsch KS, Fritz HI: Teratogenic effects of mescaline, epinephrine, and norepinephrine in the hamster. Teratology 23:287-291, 1981. [A]

MESORIDAZINE

Synonyms

Lidanar, Lidanil, Serentil

Summary

Mesoridazine is a phenothiazine used as an antipsychotic agent.

Magnitude of Teratogenic Risk

Undetermined

Quality and Quantity of Data

None To Poor

Comment

A small risk cannot be excluded, but a high risk of congenital anomalies in the children of women treated with mesoridazine during pregnancy is unlikely.

No epidemiological studies of congenital anomalies in infants whose mothers were treated with mesoridazine during pregnancy have been reported.

No teratogenic effect is said to have been observed among the offspring of rats or rabbits treated during pregnancy with up to 12 times the usual human dose of mesoridazine (Van

Ryzin et al., 1971). Unfortunately, these experiments are reported only in a brief abstract and cannot be evaluated independently.

Please see agent summary on chlorpromazine for information on a related agent that has been studied.

Key References

Van Ryzin RJ, Carson SE, Hartman HA, Trapold JH: Animal safety evaluation studies on the antipsychotic phenothiazine, mesoridazine. Toxicol Appl Pharmacol 19:363, 1961. [A]

MESTRANOL

Synonyms

Ethinyloestradiol-3-methyl Ether

Summary

Mestranol is an estrogenic agent that is widely used, generally in combination with a progestin, in oral contraception and in treatment of menstrual disorders.

Magnitude of Teratogenic Risk

None

Quality and Quantity of Data

Fair

Comment

None

The frequency of congenital anomalies was no greater than expected among the infants of 179 women who had taken mestranol during the first four lunar months of pregnancy or of 206 women who had taken this drug anytime in pregnancy in the Collaborative Perinatal Project (Heinonen et al., 1977).

The frequency of malformations was not increased among the offspring of mice or rats treated during pregnancy with mestranol combined with a progestin in doses respectively 10-200 and 10-100 times those used in human contraception (Takano et al., 1966; Saunders & Elton, 1967). Fetal loss occurred with increased frequency in both species at the higher doses. No increase in malformations was observed among the offspring of rabbits treated during pregnancy with mestranol alone or in combination with progestins in doses 5-100 times those used clinically in humans (Takano et al., 1966; Saunders & Elton, 1967).

Increased aggressive behavior was observed among the male (but not the female) offspring of mice treated during pregnancy with mestranol combined with norethynodrel (a progestin) in a dose about 50 times greater than that used in human contraception (Abbatiello & Scudder, 1970). Decreased serum testosterone concentrations were found in adult male rats born to mothers that had been treated with 50 times the human dose of mestranol in another study (Varma & Bloch, 1987). The clinical relevance of these observations is unknown.

Key References

Abbatiello E, Scudder CL: The effect of norethynodrel with mestranol treatment of pregnant mice on the isolation-induced aggression of their male offspring. Int J Fert 15:182-189, 1970. [A]

Heinonen OP, Slone D, Shapiro S: Birth Defects and Drugs in Pregnancy. Littleton, Mass.: John Wright-PSG, 1977, pp 389-391, 443. [E]

Saunders FJ, Elton RL: Effects of ethynodiol diacetate and mestranol in rats and rabbits, on conception, on the outcome of pregnancy and on the offspring. Toxicol Appl Pharmacol 11:229-244, 1967. [A]

Takano K, Yamamura H, Suzuki M, et al.: Teratogenic effect of chlormadinone acetate in mice and rabbits. Proc Soc Exp Biol Med 121:455-457, 1966. [A]

Varma SK, Bloch E: Effects of prenatal administration of mestranol and two progestins on testosterone synthesis and reproductive tract development in male rats. Acta Endocrinol (Copenh) 116:193-199, 1987. [A]

METABUTETHAMINE

Summary

Metabutethamine is a local anesthetic of the ester class that has been used in dentistry.

Magnitude of Teratogenic Risk

Undetermined

Quality and Quantity of Data

None

Comment

None

No epidemiological studies of congenital anomalies in children born to women exposed to metabutethamine during pregnancy have been reported.

No investigations of teratologic effects of metabutethamine in experimental animals have been published.

Key References

None available.

METABUTOXYCAINE

Summary

Metabutoxycaine is a local anesthetic that has been used in dentistry.

Magnitude of Teratogenic Risk

Undetermined

Quality and Quantity of Data

None

Comment

None

No epidemiological studies of congenital anomalies in children born to women exposed to metabutoxycaine during pregnancy have been reported.

No investigations of teratologic effects of metabutoxycaine in experimental animals have been published.

Please see agent summary on procaine for information on a related agent that has been studied.

Key References

None available.

METAPROTERENOL

Synonyms

Alupent, Dosalupent, Metaprel, Novasmasol, Orciprenaline Sulfate

Summary

Metaproterenol is a beta-2 selective adrenergic receptor blocking agent. It is used in treatment of bronchospasm and in management of premature labor.

Magnitude of Teratogenic Risk

Undetermined

Quality and Quantity of Data

Poor

Comment

None

No epidemiological studies of congenital anomalies among the children of women treated with metaproterenol during pregnancy have been reported.

No increase in the frequency of malformations was apparent among the offspring of 12 rhesus monkeys treated with about three times the usual human dose of metaproterenol during pregnancy (Banerjee & Woodard, 1971). The frequency of malformations was no greater than expected among the offspring of rabbits given 2-25 times the usual human dose of metaproterenol during pregnancy (Hollingsworth et al., 1971; Matsuo et al., 1982). An increased frequency of cleft palate was observed among the offspring of mice treated during pregnancy with 25-250 but not 2.5 times the usual human dose of metaproterenol (Iida et al., 1988). Increased fetal death and maternal cardiotoxicity occurred at the highest dose.

Key References

Banerjee BN, Woodard G: Teratologic evaluation of metaproterenol in the rhesus monkey (Macaca mulatta). Toxicol Appl Pharmacol 20:562-564, 1971. [A]

Hollingsworth RL, Scott WJ, Woodard MW, Woodard G: Fetal rabbit ductus arteriosus assessed in a teratological study on isoproterenol and metaproterenol. Toxicol Appl Pharmacol 18:231-234, 1971. [A]

Iida H, Kast A, Tsunenari Y, Asakura M: Corticosterone induction of cleft palate in mice dosed with orciprenaline sulfate. Teratology 38:15-27, 1988. [A]

Matsuo A, Kast A, Tsunenari Y: Teratology study with orciprenaline sulfate in rabbits. Arzneimittelforsch 32:808-810, 1982. [A]

METARAMINOL

Synonyms

Aramine, Hydroxynorephedrine, Icoral B, Levicor, Metaradrine, Pressonex, Select-A-Jet Metaraminol

Summary

Metaraminol is a sympathomimetic amine that is administered parenterally in the treatment of acute hypotension.

Magnitude of Teratogenic Risk

Undetermined

Quality and Quantity of Data

None

Comment

None

No epidemiological studies of congenital anomalies among infants born to women treated with metaraminol during pregnancy have been reported.

No animal teratology studies of metaraminol have been published.

Key References

None available.

METAXALONE

Synonyms

Metassalone, Skelaxin, Zorane

Summary

Metaxalone is a skeletal muscle relaxant that is administered orally for the relief of painful muscular spasms.

Magnitude of Teratogenic Risk

Undetermined

Quality and Quantity of Data

None

None

No epidemiological studies of congenital anomalies in infants whose mothers were given metaxalone during pregnancy have been reported.

No animal teratology studies of metaxalone have been published.

Key References

None available.

METHACRYLATES

Synonyms

2-Methylacrylic Acid, Acrylic Acid, Butyl Acrylate

Summary

Methacrylates are a series of organic esters used to make plastics, resins, and adhesives. Methacrylates are widely used in dentistry and in other occupational settings. The current occupational exposure limit for methyl methacrylate vapor is 100 ppm as an 8-hour time-weighted average (OSHA, 1971).

Magnitude of Teratogenic Risk

Undetermined

Quality and Quantity of Data

Poor

Comment

Teratogenic risk is probably greater if the exposure is sufficient to cause maternal toxicity.

No epidemiological studies of congenital anomalies among infants born to women ex-

posed to methacrylates during pregnancy have been reported.

No malformations were observed among the offspring of mice exposed to methylmethacrylate vapors at a dose of 1330 ppm repeatedly during pregnancy (McLaughlin et al., 1978). Increased frequencies of hematomas and skeletal anomalies were observed among the offspring of pregnant rats injected with one of five different methacrylates in doses equivalent to one-tenth to one-third the adult LD50 (Singh et al., 1972). (The LD50 is the dose of an agent that will kill 50% of the exposed animals). The effect was dose-related and associated with increased frequencies of fetal death in some cases. Similar fetal abnormalities occurred among the offspring of rats exposed by inhalation to methyl methacrylate in doses that were toxic to the mothers (Nicholas et al., 1979). The relevance of these findings to usual human occupational exposures to methacrylates is unknown.

Key References

McLaughlin RE, Reger SI, Barkalow JA, et al.: Methylmethacrylate: A study of teratogenicity and fetal toxicity of the vapor in the mouse. J Bone Joint Surg 60-A(3):355-358, 1978. [A]

Nicholas CA, Lawrence WH, Autian J: Embryotoxicity and fetotoxicity from maternal inhalation of methyl methacrylate monomer in rats. Toxicol Appl Pharmacol 50(3):451-458, 1979. [A]

Singh AR, Lawrence WH, Autian J: Embryonic-fetal toxicity and teratogenic effects of a group of methacrylate esters in rats. J Dent Res 51(6):1632-1638, 1972. [A]

METHACYCLINE

Synonyms

Benciclina, Bialatan, Metaciclina, Metacycline, Optimycine, Physiomycine, Plurigram, Rondomycin

Summary

Methacycline is an oral tetracycline used to treat a variety of infections.

Magnitude of Teratogenic Risk

Undetermined

Quality and Quantity of Data

None

Comment

Because it is a tetracycline, caution should be used with regard to methacycline's potential for dental staining.

No epidemiological studies of congenital anomalies in infants whose mothers were treated with methacycline during pregnancy have been reported.

No animal teratology studies of methacycline have been published.

Please see agent summary on tetracycline agent for information on a related agent that has been studied.

Key References

None available.

METHADONE

Synonyms

Dolophine, Methadose

Summary

Methadone is a strong narcotic analgesic that can be administered orally as well as parenterally. It is used for the treatment of pain and narcotic addiction.

Magnitude of Teratogenic Risk

None To Minimal

Quality and Quantity of Data

Poor To Fair

Comment

Neonatal withdrawal symptoms may occur in newborn infants of women who take methadone during pregnancy (see below).

Although many epidemiological studies of the children of women who took methadone during pregnancy have been reported, interpretation of these investigations with respect to the teratogenic effects of methadone is difficult. The studies deal with narcotic addicts who participated in methadone-treatment programs during pregnancy. Such women often use other illicit drugs and suffer from a variety of adverse nutritional, infectious, and psychosocial factors (Finnegan et al., 1977; Aylward, 1982). Selection of an appropriate comparison group is, therefore, problematical; many of the studies do not even include a control group. Most of the investigations provide only limited information regarding the duration of methadone treatment in the women; many appear not to have taken methadone until after the first trimester of pregnancy.

The frequency of malformations was no greater than expected in cohort studies of 150, 39, and 31 infants born to women who were treated with methadone during all or part of their pregnancies (Kandall et al., 1977; Wilson et al., 1981; Stimmel & Adamsons, 1976). Similarly, the frequency of malformations did not appear to be unusually great in several uncontrolled series of between 50 and 220 children of women who took methadone during part or all of their pregnancies (Blinick et al., 1973; Harper et al., 1974; Lipsitz & Blatman, 1974; Finnegan et al., 1977; Suffet & Brotman, 1984).

Cohort studies of infants born to narcotic-addicted women treated with methadone during all or part of pregnancy have usually found decreased fetal growth as indicated by reduced birth weight, length, and head circumference compared to controls (Harper et al., 1974; Kandall et al., 1976; Finnegan, 1978; Chasnoff et al., 1986). It is difficult to know if this effect is due to the methadone directly or to an associated factor. The observation that birth weight appears to be positively correlated with maternal methadone dose during the first trimester (Kandall et al., 1976) suggests that associated factors are of primary importance. The growth deficit in infants of women treated with methadone during pregnancy does not appear to persist into later childhood (Wilson et al., 1981; Lifschitz et al., 1983).

Neonatal narcotic withdrawal symptoms occur in most infants born to women treated with methadone late in pregnancy (Newman et al., 1975; Kandall et al., 1977; Finnegan, 1978; Stimmel et al., 1982; Suffet & Brotman, 1984; Besunder & Blumer, 1990). The features are variable and include hypertonicity, tremor, irritability, diarrhea, and vomiting. Onset is usually in the first days after birth but may be delayed for two to four weeks (Kandall & Gartner, 1974).

Mild deficits in performance on psychometric and behavioral tests have been demonstrated in children born to women treated with methadone during pregnancy (Hutchings, 1982; Kaltenbach & Finnegan, 1984; Rosen & Johnson, 1985; Davis & Templer, 1988; Kaltenbach & Finnegan, 1989; Hans, 1989; Ward et al., 1989; Sandberg et al., 1990).

Increased frequencies of central nervous system and other malformations have been observed among the offspring of hamsters and mice treated during pregnancy with methadone in doses equivalent to 13-77 or 10 times the maximum dose used in humans (Geber & Schramm, 1975; Jurand, 1973). A typical dose-response effect was demonstrated in the hamsters. No increase in malformations was observed among the offspring of rats or rabbits treated with 8-17 times the maximum human dose of methadone during pregnancy (Markham et al., 1971; Chandler et al., 1975), but an increased frequency of fetal death was seen in pregnant rats treated with 2-23 times the maximum human dose of methadone

(Buchenauer et al., 1974, Chandler et al., 1975; Hutchings et al., 1976; Bui et al., 1986). Decreased fetal weight has been noted among the offspring of rats treated during pregnancy with methadone in doses equal to or greater than the maximum used in humans (Field et al., 1977; Buchenauer et al., 1974; Biu et al., 1986). Persistent alterations of behavior occur among the offspring of rats treated with methadone during pregnancy in doses a few times greater than those used in humans (Hutchings, 1982; Zagon & McLaughlin, 1983; Enters et al., 1991).

Key References

Aylward GP: Methadone outcome studies: Is it more than the methadone? J Pediatr 101:214-215, 1982. [O]

Besunder JB, Blumer JF: Neonatal drug withdrawal syndromes. In: G. Koren (ed). Maternal-fetal toxicology. A clinician's guide. New York: Marcel Dekker, 1990, pp 161-190. [R]

Blinick G, Jerez E, Wallach RC: Methadone maintenance, pregnancy, and progeny. J Am Med Assoc 225:477-479, 1973. [S]

Buchenauer D, Turnbow M, Peters MA: Effect of chronic methadone administration on pregnant rats and their offspring. J Pharmacol Exp Ther 189:66-71, 1974. [A]

Bui QQ, Tran MB, West WL: A comparative study of the reproductive effects of methadone and benzo[a]pyrene in the pregnant and pseudopregnant rat. Toxicology 42:195-204, 1986. [A]

Chandler JM, Robie PW, Schoolar JC, Desmond MM: The effects of methadone on maternal-fetal interactions in the rat. J Pharmacol Exp Ther 192:549-554, 1975. [A]

Chasnoff IJ, Burns KA, Burns WJ, Schnoll SH: Prenatal drug exposure: Effects on neonatal and infant growth and development. Neurobehav Toxicol Teratol 8:357-362, 1986. [E]

Davis DD, Templer DI: Neurobehavioral functioning in children exposed to narcotics in utero. Addict Behav 13:275-283, 1988. [E]

Enters EK, Guo H, Pandey U, et al.: The effect of prenatal methadone exposure on development and nociception during the early postnatal period of the rat. Neurotoxicol Teratol 13:161-166, 1991. [A]

Field T, McNelly A, Sadava D: Effect of maternal methadone addiction on offspring in rats. Arch Int Pharmacodyn 228:300-303, 1977. [A]

Finnegan LP: Management of pregnant drug-dependent women. Ann NY Acad Sci 811:135-146, 1978. [E]

Finnegan LP, Reeser DS, Connaughton JF: The effects of maternal drug dependence on neonatal mortality. Drug Alcohol Depend 2:131-140, 1977. [S]

Geber WF, Schramm LC: Congenital malformations of the central nervous system produced by narcotic analgesics in the hamster. Am J Obstet Gynecol 123:705-713, 1975. [A]

Hans SY: Developmental consequences of prenatal exposure to methadone. Ann NY Acad Sci 562:195-207, 1989. [E]

Harper RG, Solish GI, Purow HM, Sang E: The effect of a methadone treatment program upon pregnant heroin addicts and their newborn infants. Pediatrics 54:300-305, 1974. [E]

Hutchings DE: Methadone and heroin during pregnancy: A review of behavioral effects in human and animal offspring. Neurobehav Toxicol Teratol 4:429-434, 1982. [R]

Hutchings DE, Hunt HF, Towey JP, Rosen TS, et al.: Methadone during pregnancy in the rat: Dose level effects on maternal and perinatal mortality and growth in the offspring. J Pharmacol Exp Ther 197:171-179, 1976. [A]

Jurand A: Teratogenic activity of methadone hydrochloride in mouse and chick embryos. J Embryol Exp Morphol 30:449-458, 1973. [A]

Kaltenbach K, Finnegan LP: Developmental outcome of children born to methadone maintained women: A review of longitudinal studies. Neurobehav Toxicol Teratol 6:271-275, 1984. [R]

Kaltenbach KA, Finnegan LP: Prenatal narcotic exposure: Perinatal and developmental effects. Neurotoxicology 10:597-604, 1989. [R]

Kandall SR, Albin S, Gartner LM, Lee K-S, et al.: The narcotic-dependent mother: Fetal and neonatal consequences. Early Hum Dev 1:159-169, 1977. [E]

Kandall SR, Albin S, Lowinson J, Berle B, et al.: Differential effects of maternal heroin and methadone use on birthweight. Pediatrics 58:681-685, 1976. [E]

Kandall SR, Gartner LM: Late presentation of drug withdrawal symptoms in newborns. Am J Dis Chil 127:58-61, 1974. [C]

Lifschitz MH, Wilson GS, Smith EO, Desmond MM: Fetal and postnatal growth of children born to narcotic-dependent women. J Pediatr 102:686-691, 1983. [E]

Lipsitz PJ, Blatman S: Newborn infants of mothers on methadone maintenance. NY State J Med 74:994-999, 1974. [S]

Markham JK, Emmerson JL, Owen NV: Teratogenicity studies of methadone HCl in rats and rabbits. Nature 233:342-343, 1971. [A]

Newman RG, Bashkow S, Calko D: Results of 313 consecutive live births of infants delivered to patients in the New York City Methadone Maintenance Treatment Program. Am J Obstet Gynecol 121:233-237, 1975. [S]

Rosen TS, Johnson HL: Long-term effects of prenatal methadone maintenance. Natl Inst Drug Abuse Res Monogr Ser 59:73-83, 1985. [E]

Sandberg DE, Meyer-Bahlburg HFL, Rosen TS, Johnson HL: Effects of prenatal methadone exposure on sex-dimorphic behavior in early school-age children. Psychoneuroendocrinology 15(1):77-82, 1990. [E]

Stimmel B, Adamsons K: Narcotic dependency in pregnancy. J Am Med Assoc 235:1121-1124, 1976. [E]

Stimmel B, Goldberg J, Reisman A, Murphy RJ, et al.: Fetal outcome in narcotic-dependent women: The importance of the type of maternal narcotic used. Am J Drug Alcohol Abuse 9:383-395, 1982. [E]

Suffet F, Brotman R: A comprehensive care program for pregnant addicts: Obstetrical, neonatal, and child development outcomes. Int J Addict 19:199-219, 1984. [S]

Ward OB, Kopertowski DM, Finnegan LP, Sandberg DE: Gender-identity variations in boys prenatally exposed to opiates. Ann NY Acad Sci 562:365-366, 1989. [E]

Wilson GS, Desmond MM, Wait RB: Follow-up of methadone-treated and untreated narcotic-dependent women and their infants: Health, developmental, and social implications. J Pediatr 98:716-722, 1981. [E]

Zagon IS, McLaughlin PJ: Behavioral effects of prenatal exposure to opiates. Monogr Neural Sci 9:159-168, 1983. [A] & [R]

METHAMPHETAMINE

Synonyms

Desoxyephedrine, Desoxyn, Methampex, Methedrine, Norodin, Syndrox

Summary

Methamphetamine is a sympathomimetic agent and a potent central nervous system stimulant. It is used to promote weight loss and in the treatment of narcolepsy and childhood hyperkinetic states. Methamphetamine is a popular "recreational drug." It is also used illicitly to "cut" or dilute other drugs.

Magnitude of Teratogenic Risk

Therapeutic Use: None To Minimal

Abuse: Small

Quality and Quantity of Data

Therapeutic Use: Poor To Fair

Abuse: Fair

Comment

None

The frequency of congenital anomalies was no greater than expected among the children of 89 women treated with methamphetamine during the first four lunar months of pregnancy or among the infants of 320 women treated anytime during pregnancy in the Collaborative Perinatal Project (Heinonen et al., 1977). In a study of 52 infants born to women who abused methamphetamine intravenously throughout pregnancy, the frequency of congenital anomalies was no greater than expected, but birth weight, length, and head circumference were decreased (Little et al., 1988). Abnormal echoencephalograms with evidence of intracranial hemorrhage were observed in nine of 24 infants of mothers who abused methamphetamine during pregnancy in another investigation (Dixon & Bejar, 1989).

No malformations were found among the offspring of five macaque monkeys treated during pregnancy with methamphetamine in doses similar to those used in humans (Courtney & Valerio, 1968). Increased frequencies of fetal death, growth retardation, and brain and eye malformations were observed among the offspring of rabbits and mice treated during pregnancy with methamphetamine in doses respectively 2 and 16-42 times those used clinically (Kasirsky & Tansy, 1971; Yamamoto et al., 1992). Typical dose-dependence of this teratogenic effect was observed in mice (Yamamoto et al., 1992). High frequencies of anophthalmia were seen among the offspring of pregnant rats treated with 200 times the human therapeutic dose of methamphetamine (Vorhees & Acuff-Smith, 1990). Persistently decreased weight and long-lasting behavioral alterations were noted in the offspring of rats treated during pregnancy with methamphetamine in doses 4-16 times those used clinically (Martin, 1975; Martin et al., 1976; Sato & Fujiwara, 1986; Cho et al., 1991). The relevance of these observations to the risks associated with therapeutic or recreational use of methamphetamine in human pregnancy is unknown.

Please see agent summary on dextroamphetamine for information on a related agent that has been more thoroughly studied.

Key References

Cho D-H, Lyu H-M, Lee H-B, Kim P-Y, et al.: Behavioral teratogenicity of methamphetamine. J Toxicol Sci 16(Suppl 1):37-49, 1991. [A]

Courtney KD, Valerio DA: Teratology in the Macaca mulatta. Teratology 1:163-172, 1968. [A]

Dixon SD, Bejar R: Echoencephalographic findings in neonates associated with maternal cocaine and methamphetamine use: Incidence and clinical correlates. J Pediatr 115:770-778, 1989. [E]

Heinonen OP, Slone D, Shapiro S: Birth Defects and Drugs in Pregnancy. Littleton, Mass.: John Wright-PSG, 1977, pp 346-347, 439. [E]

Kasirsky G, Tansy MF: Teratogenic effects of methamphetamine in mice and rabbits. Teratology 4:131-134, 1971. [A]

Little BB, Snell LM, Gilstrap LC: Methamphetamine abuse during pregnancy: Outcome and fetal effects. Obstet Gynecol 72(4):541-544, 1988. [E]

Martin JC: Effects on offspring of chronic maternal methamphetamine exposure. Dev Psychobiol 8:397-404, 1975. [A]

Martin JC, Martin DC, Radow B, Sigman G: Growth, development and activity in rat offspring following maternal drug exposure. Exp Aging Res 2:235-251, 1976. [A]

Sato M, Fujiwara Y: Behavioral and neurochemical changes in pups prenatally exposed to methamphetamine. Brain Dev 8:390-396, 1986. [A]

Vorhees CV, Acuff-Smith KD: Prenatal methamphetamine-induced anophthalmia in rats. (Letter) Neurotoxicol Teratol 12:409, 1990. [A]

Yamamoto Y, Yamamoto K, Fukui Y, Kurishita A: Teratogenic effects of methamphetamine in mice. Nippon Hoigaku Zasshi [Jpn J Legal Med] 46(2):126-131, 1992. [A]

METHARBITAL

Synonyms

Endiemal, Gemonil, Gemonit, Metarbital, Metharbitone

Summary

Metharbital is a barbiturate that is used orally to treat seizure disorders.

Magnitude of Teratogenic Risk

None To Minimal

Quality and Quantity of Data

Poor

Comment

Risk assessment is for the chronic use of metharbital.

No adequate epidemiological studies of congenital anomalies among infants born to women treated with metharbital during pregnancy have been reported. Two of six infants born to women treated with metharbital for epilepsy during the first trimester of pregnancy had malformations in one study (Nakane et al., 1980). One child had cleft lip and palate and the other had a ventricular septal defect.

No animal teratology studies of metharbital have been published.

Please see agent summary on phenobarbital for information on a related agent that has been more thoroughly studied.

Key References

Nakane Y, Okuma T, Takahashi R, Sato Y, et al.: Multi-institutional study on the teratogenicity and fetal toxicity of antiepileptic drugs: A report of a collaborative study group in Japan. Epilepsia 21:663-680, 1980. [E]

METHAZOLAMIDE

Synonyms

Neptazane

Summary

Methazolamide is a sulfonamide derivative that acts as an inhibitor of carbonic anhydrase. Methazolamide is administered orally in the treatment of glaucoma.

Magnitude of Teratogenic Risk

Undetermined

Quality and Quantity of Data

None To Poor

Comment

A small risk cannot be excluded, but a high risk of congenital anomalies in the children of women treated with methazolamide during pregnancy is unlikely.

No epidemiological studies of congenital anomalies among children born to women treated with methazolamide during pregnancy have been reported.

No abnormalities were observed among the embryos of pregnant rabbits treated with 20 times the human therapeutic dose of methazolamide prior to implantation (Adams et al., 1961).

Please see agent summary on acetazolamide for information on a related agent that has been more thoroughly studied.

Key References

Adams CE, Hay MF, Lutwak-Mann C: The action of various agents upon the rabbit embryo. J Embryol Exp Morph 9(3):468-491, 1961. [A]

METHDILAZINE

Synonyms

Disyncran, Metodilazina, Tacaryl, Tacryl

Summary

Methdilazine is a phenothiazine derivative with antihistaminic properties. It is administered orally to treat pruritus in various allergic conditions.

Magnitude of Teratogenic Risk

Undetermined

Quality and Quantity of Data

None

Comment

None

No adequate epidemiological studies of congenital anomalies among the infants of women treated with methdilazine during pregnancy have been reported.

No animal teratology studies of methdilazine have been published.

Please see agent summary on promethazine for information on a related agent that has been studied.

Key References

None available.

METHENAMINE

Synonyms

Hexamethylenamine, Hexamethylenetetramine, Hexamine, Hiprex, Mandelamine, Uritone

Summary

Methenamine is taken orally as a urinary antimicrobial agent. It acts by releasing formaldehyde in the urine.

Magnitude of Teratogenic Risk

Minimal To Small

Quality and Quantity of Data

Poor To Fair

Comment

None

The frequency of congenital anomalies was not increased among the children of 49 women treated with methenamine during the first four lunar months of pregnancy in the

Collaborative Perinatal Project (Heinonen et al., 1977). A small but statistically significant increase in the rate of anomalies was found among the infants of 299 women treated with methenamine anytime during pregnancy in this study. No mention was made of whether any specificity of the anomalies was observed.

No increase in the frequency of malformations was noted among the offspring of pregnant rats or dogs fed methenamine in doses similar to those used clinically (Hurni & Ohder, 1973; WHO, 1974).

Please see agent summary on formaldehyde for information on this chemical which is produced from methenamine in the urine.

Key References

Heinonen OP, Slone D, Shapiro S: Birth Defects and Drugs in Pregnancy. Littleton, Mass.: John Wright-PSG, 1977, pp 299, 302, 434-435. [E]

Hurni H, Ohder H: Reproduction study with formaldehyde and hexamethylenetetramine in beagle dogs. Fd Cosmet Toxicol 2(3):459-462, 1973. [A]

WHO (World Health Organization): Antimicrobials. Hexamethylenetetramine. In: Toxicological evaluation of some food additives including anticaking agents, antimicrobials, antioxidants, emulsifiers and thickening agents. Geneva: World Health Organization, 1974, pp 63-74. [A]

METHIONINE

Synonyms

Antamon, Cymethion, Lobamine, Methnine, Pedameth, Uracid, Uranap

Summary

Methionine is an amino acid that is required in the diet. Methionine has been used to acidify the urine and in the treatment of acetaminophen poisoning.

Magnitude of Teratogenic Risk

Undetermined

Quality and Quantity of Data

Poor

Comment

A small risk cannot be excluded, but a high risk of congenital anomalies in the children of women treated with conventional therapeutic doses of methionine during pregnancy is unlikely.

No epidemiological studies of congenital anomalies among infants born to women who ingested unusually large amounts of methionine during pregnancy have been reported.

Increased frequencies of fetal loss and decreased fetal and maternal weight gain have been observed in some studies among pregnant rats fed diets supplemented with 1.6-6% methionine (Viau & Leathem, 1973; Kaemmerer & Aly, 1975; Chandrashekar & Leathem, 1977; Matsueda & Niiyama, 1982).

Key References

Chandrashekar V, Leathem JH: Effect of excess dietary methionine on rat pregnancy: Influence on ovarian delta5-3beta-hydroxysteroid dehydrogenase activity. Fertil Steril 28(5):590-593, 1977. [A]

Kaemmerer VK, Aly ZH: Investigations on the effect of high doses of amino acids on the fetal development of rats. Dtsch Tierarztl Wochenschr 82:429-472, 1975. [A]

Matsueda S, Niiyama Y: The effects of excess amino acids on maintenance of pregnancy and fetal growth in rats. J Nutr Sci Vitaminol 28:557-573, 1982. [A]

Viau AT, Leathem JH: Excess dietary methionine and pregnancy in the rat. J Reprod Fert 33:109-111, 1973. [A]

METHIXENE

Synonyms

Methyloxan, Tremaril, Tremarit, Tremonil, Tremoquil, Trest

Summary

Methixene is an anticholinergic agent used to treat peptic ulcers and in the management of parkinsonism.

Magnitude of Teratogenic Risk

Undetermined

Quality and Quantity of Data

None

Comment

None

No epidemiological studies of congenital anomalies in infants born to women who used methixene during pregnancy have been reported.

No animal teratology studies of methixene have been published.

Please see agent summary on atropine for information on a related drug that is more thoroughly studied.

Key References

None available.

METHOCARBAMOL

Synonyms

Guaiphenesin Carbamate, Methocabal, Relax Llano, Robaxan

Summary

Methocarbamol is a muscle relaxant used in the treatment of acute painful musculoskeletal disorders.

Magnitude of Teratogenic Risk

None To Minimal

Quality and Quantity of Data

Poor

Comment

None

The frequency of congenital anomalies was no greater than expected among the offspring of 22 women who were treated with methocarbamol during the first four lunar months of pregnancy in the Collaborative Perinatal Project (Heinonen et al., 1977).

No animal teratology studies of methocarbamol have been published.

Arthrogryposis was observed in one child who had been exposed to methocarbamol and propoxyphene for three days during embryogenesis. The clinical significance of this is unknown since no other cases have been reported (Hall & Reed, 1982).

Key References

Hall JG, Reed SD: Teratogens associated with congenital contractures in humans and in animals. Teratology 25:173-191, 1982. [C] & [R]

Heinonen OP, Slone D, Shapiro S: Birth Defects and Drugs in Pregnancy. Littleton, Mass.: John Wright-PSG, 1977, pp 358, 360, 493. [E]

METHOHEXITAL

Synonyms

Brevimytal Natrium, Brevital Sodium, Brietal, Enallynymalnatrium, Methohexitone

Summary

Methohexital is a short-acting barbiturate that is used as a general anesthetic. It is usually administered intravenously.

Magnitude of Teratogenic Risk

None To Minimal

Quality and Quantity of Data

Poor

Comment

None

The frequency of congenital anomalies was no greater than expected among the children of 41 women treated with methohexital during the first four lunar months of pregnancy in the Collaborative Perinatal Project (Heinonen et al., 1977).

No studies of teratologic effects of methohexital in experimental animals have been published.

Please see agent summary on thiopental for information on a related agent that has been more thoroughly studied.

Key References

Heinonen OP, Slone D, Shapiro S: Birth Defects and Drugs in Pregnancy. Littleton, Mass.: John Wright-PSG, 1977, pp 336-337. [E]

METHOSERPIDINE

Synonyms

Deaserpyl, Decaserpil, Decaserpine, Decaserpyl, Decoserpyl, Metoserpidina, Minoran

Summary

Methoserpidine is a Rauwolfia derivative administered orally in the treatment of hypertension.

Magnitude of Teratogenic Risk

Undetermined

Quality and Quantity of Data

None

Comment

None

No epidemiological studies of congenital anomalies among the children of women who were treated with methoserpidine during pregnancy have been reported.

No animal teratology studies of methoserpidine have been published.

Please see the agent summary on reserpine for information on a related agent that has been studied.

Key References

None available.

METHOTREXATE

Synonyms

alpha-Methopterin, Amethopterin, Dichloromethotrexate, Emtexate, Folex, Ledertrexate, Maxtrex, Methylaminopterin, Metotrexato, Mexate

Summary

Methotrexate is a folic-acid antagonist. It is used in the treatment of neoplastic and rheumatic diseases. The dose employed varies substantially and is generally lower in rheumatic than in malignant disease.

Magnitude of Teratogenic Risk

Moderate To High

Quality and Quantity of Data

Fair To Good

Comment

1) Maternal doses of methotrexate as small as 2.5 mg per day (less than the usual therapeutic range) during the first trimester of pregnancy have been associated with a characteristic pattern of congenital anomalies in infants.

2) The effect on the fetus of maternal treatment with methotrexate during the second or third trimester of pregnancy is unknown.

At least four children with a very uncommon and characteristic pattern of congenital anomalies have been born to women treated with methotrexate during the first trimester of pregnancy (Milunsky et al., 1968; Powell & Ekert, 1971; Diniz et al., 1978; Sosa Munoz et al., 1983). These children exhibited abnormal head shape, large fontanelles, craniosynostosis, ocular hypertelorism, and skeletal defects. The pattern of anomalies is strikingly similar to that seen in children born to women who took aminopterin, a closely-related agent, early in pregnancy (Warkany, 1978). The frequency of malformations among infants of women treated with methotrexate during pregnancy does not appear to be extremely high and is probably dose-related (Roubenoff et al., 1988; Kozlowski et al., 1990; Aviles et al., 1991).

Fetal death occurs with increased frequency in pregnant mice, rats, cats, and rabbits treated with methotrexate in doses equivalent to or greater than those used in humans (Jordan et al., 1977; Skalko & Gold, 1974; Khera, 1976; DeSesso & Goeringer, 1991, 1992). Somewhat higher doses are required to produce this effect in pregnant rhesus monkeys (Wilson et al., 1979). Dose-dependent increases in the frequency of malformations were observed among the offspring of rats and rabbits treated during pregnancy with methotrexate in doses equivalent to those used in humans, but such defects were not found in rhesus monkeys at this or a 5-fold greater dose level or in mice until the dose was increased to about 4 times that used therapeutically (Skalko & Gold, 1974; Jordan et al., 1977; Wilson et al., 1979). Cleft palate and limb malformations were the anomalies observed most often. Increased frequencies of median facial clefts and other anomalies were observed among the offspring of mice treated during pregnancy with about 8 times the usual human dose of methotrexate (Darab et al., 1987).

A higher-than-expected frequency of acquired chromosomal aberrations has been found in the somatic cells of adult humans, in cultured human cells, and in mouse embryonic oogonia exposed to methotrexate (Voorhees et al., 1969; Hansmann, 1974; Jensen & Nyfors, 1979; Mondello et al., 1984). Various acquired cytogenetic abnormalities were also observed in lymphocytes of an infant whose mother was treated with methotrexate and other cytotoxic drugs during the second and third trimesters of pregnancy (Schleuning & Clemm, 1987). The relevance, if any, of these findings to the reproductive risks of patients treated with methotrexate prior to conception is unknown.

No increase in the incidence of congenital anomalies was apparent in over 375 pregnancies in women who had previously been treated with methotrexate for gestational or other neoplasms (van Thiel et al., 1970; Rustin et al., 1984; Hsieh et al., 1985; Green et al., 1991).

Please see agent summary on aminopterin for information on a related agent.

Key References

Aviles A, Diaz-Macqueo JC, Talavera A, Guzman T, et al.: Growth and development of children of mothers treated with chemotherapy during pregnancy: Current status of 43 children. Am J Hematol 36:243-248, 1991. [S]

Darab DJ, Minkoff R, Sciote J, et al.: Pathogenesis of median facial clefts in mice treated with methotrexate. Teratology 36:77-88, 1987. [A]

DeSesso JM, Goeringer GC: Amelioration by leucovorin of methotrexate developmental toxicity of rabbits. Teratology 43:201-215, 1991. [A]

DeSesso JM, Goeringer GC: Methotrexate-induced developmental toxicity in rabbits is ameliorated by 1-(p-tosyl)-3,4,4-trimethylimidazolidine, a functional analog for tetrahydrofolate-mediated one-carbon transfer. Teratology 45:271-283, 1992. [A]

Diniz EMA, Corradini HB, Ramos JL, et al.: The effects of methotrexate on the developing fetus. Rev Hosp Clin Fac Med Univ Sao Paulo 33:286-290, 1978. [C]

Green DM, Zevon MA, Lowrie G, Seigelstein N, et al.: Congenital anomalies in children of patients who received chemotherapy for cancer in childhood and adolescence. N Engl J Med 325:141-146, 1991. [E]

Hansmann I: Chromosome aberrations in metaphase II-oocytes stage sensitivity in the mouse oogenesis to amethopterin and cyclophosphamide. Mutat Res 22:175-191, 1974. [A]

Hsieh F-J, Chen T-CG, Cheng Y-T, Huang S-C, et al.: The outcome of pregnancy after chemotherapy for gestational trophoblastic disease. Biol Res Pregnancy Perinatol 6(4):177-180, 1985. [S]

Jensen MK, Nyfors A: Cytogenetic effect of methotrexate on human cells in vivo. Comparison between results obtained by chromosome studies on bone-marrow cells and blood lymphocytes and by the micronucleus test. Mutat Res 64:339-343, 1979. [O]

Jordan RL, Wilson JG, Schumacher HJ: Embryotoxicity of the folate antagonist methotrexate in rats and rabbits. Teratology 15:73-80, 1977. [A]

Khera KS: Teratogenicity studies with methotrexate, aminopterin, and acetylsalicylic acid in domestic cats. Teratology 14:21-28, 1976. [A]

Kozlowski RD, Steinbrunner JV, MacKenzie AH, et al.: Outcome of first-trimester exposure to low-dose methotrexate in eight patients with rheumatic disease. Am J Med 88(6):589-592, 1990. [S]

Milunsky A, Graef JW, Gaynor MF: Methotrexate-induced congenital malformations. J Pediatr 72:790-795, 1968. [C]

Mondello C, Giorgi R, Nuzzo F: Chromosomal effects of methotrexate on cultured human lymphocytes. Mutat Res 139:67-70, 1984. [O]

Powell HR, Ekert H: Methotrexate-induced congenital malformations. Med J Aust 2:1076-1077, 1971. [C]

Roubenoff R, Hoyt J, Petri M, et al.: Effects of antiinflammatory immunosuppressive drugs on pregnancy and fertility. Semin Arthritis Rheum 18(2):88-110, 1988. [R]

Rustin GJS, Booth M, Dent J, et al.: Pregnancy after cytotoxic chemotherapy for gestational trophoblastic tumours. Br Med J 288:103-106, 1984. [E]

Schleuning M, Clemm C: Chromosomal aberrations in a newborn whose mother received cytotoxic treatment during pregnancy. N Engl J Med 317:1666-1667, 1987. [C]

Skalko RG, Gold MP: Teratogenicity of methotrexate in mice. Teratology 9:159-164, 1974. [A]

Sosa Munoz JL, Perez Santana MT, Sosa Sanchez R, et al.: Acute leukemia and pregnancy. Rev Invest Clin (Mex) 35:55-58, 1983. [C]

van Thiel DH, Ross GT, Lipsett MB: Pregnancies after chemotherapy of trophoblastic neoplasms. Science 169:1326-1327, 1970. [S]

Voorhees JJ, Janzen MK, Harrell ER, Chakrabarti SG: Cytogenetic evaluation of methotrexate-treated psoriatic patients. Arch Derm 100:269-274, 1969. [O]

Warkany J: Aminopterin and methotrexate: Folic acid deficiency. Teratology 17:353-358, 1978. [R]

Wilson JG, Scott WJ, Ritter EJ, Fradkin R: Comparative distribution and embryotoxicity of methotrexate in pregnant rats and rhesus monkeys. Teratology 19:71-80, 1979. [A]

METHOXAMINE

Synonyms

Idasol, Methoxamedrine, Metossamina, Vasoxine Hydrochloride, Vasoxyl

Summary

Methoxamine is an alpha-adrenergic sympathomimetic agent. It is administered parenterally in the prophylaxis and treatment of acute hypotension.

Magnitude of Teratogenic Risk

Undetermined

Quality and Quantity of Data

None

Comment

Maternal treatment with methoxamine in the perinatal period may impair fetal metabolic adaptation (see below).

No epidemiological studies of congenital anomalies among infants born to women treated with methoxamine during pregnancy have been reported.

No animal teratology studies of methoxamine have been published.

Increased uterine contraction was observed in women treated with methoxamine late in pregnancy (Senties et al., 1970). Increased hypoxia, hypercarbia, and metabolic acidosis occurred in the fetuses of near-term pregnant ewes after treatment with methoxamine in doses sufficient to correct maternal hypotension produced by spinal anesthesia (Shnider et al., 1970).

Please see agent summary on phenylephrine for information on a related agent that has been more thoroughly studied.

Key References

Senties L, Arellano G, Casellas A, Ontiveros E, et al.: Effects of some vasopressor drugs upon uterine contractility in pregnant women. Am J Obstet Gynecol 107(6):892-897, 1970. [S]

Shnider SM, deLorimier AA, Asling JH, Morishima HO: Vasopressors in obstetrics. II. Fetal hazards of methoxamine administration during obstetric spinal anesthesia. Am J Obstet Gynecol 106(5):680-686, 1970. [A]

METHOXSALEN

Synonyms

Ammoidin, Deltasoralen Tablets, Geroxalen, Meladinin, Meladoxen, 8-MOP, Oxsoralen, Oxypsoralen, Psoralen

Summary

Methoxsalen is a psoralen that is administered orally in combination with ultraviolet radiation (PUVA) to treat psoriasis and other chronic skin disorders. Methoxsalen has also been used topically to treat vitiligo.

Magnitude of Teratogenic Risk

Undetermined

Quality and Quantity of Data

None

Comment

None

No congenital anomalies were observed among 17 infants born to women treated with oral methoxsalen photochemotherapy (PUVA) at the time of conception or during early pregnancy in one series (Stern et al., 1991).

No animal teratology studies of methoxsalen have been published.

Key References

Stern RS, Lange R: Outcomes of pregnancies among women and partners of men with a history of exposure to methoxsalen photochemotherapy (PUVA) for the treatment of psoriasis. Arch Dermatol 127:347-350, 1991. [E]

METHOXYFLURANE

Synonyms

Analgizer, Anecotan, Ingalan, Inhalan, Methoflurane, Methoxane, Metofane, Penthrane, Pentrane

Summary

Methoxyflurane is a general anesthetic that is administered by inhalation.

Magnitude of Teratogenic Risk

Undetermined

Quality and Quantity of Data

Poor

Comment

None

No epidemiological studies of congenital anomalies in children born to women exposed to methoxyflurane during pregnancy have been reported.

The frequency of malformations was not increased among the offspring of mice repeatedly exposed to anesthetic doses of methoxyflurane in pregnancy in one study, although fetal growth retardation and delayed skeletal development occurred (Wharton et al., 1980). No increase in the frequency of congenital anomalies was observed among the offspring of mice or rats exposed repeatedly during pregnancy to methoxyflurane in subanesthetic doses similar to or greater than those associated with occupational exposure in humans (Wharton et al., 1980; Pope et al., 1978).

Key References

Pope WDB, et al.: Fetotoxicity in rats following chronic exposure to halothane, nitrogen oxide or methoxyflurane. Anesthesiology 48:11-16, 1978. [A]

Wharton RS, et al.: Developmental toxicity of methoxyflurane in mice. Anesth Analg 59:421-425, 1980. [A]

METHSUXIMIDE

Synonyms

Celontin, Mesuximide, Metosuccimmide, Metsuccimide, Petinutin

Summary

Methsuximide is a succinimide anticonvulsant that is administered orally in the treatment of petit mal and psychomotor epilepsy.

Magnitude of Teratogenic Risk

Undetermined

Quality and Quantity of Data

Poor

Comment

Although the risk of this agent is undetermined, it may be substantial because it is an anticonvulsant.

No adequate epidemiological study of congenital anomalies among the infants of women treated with methsuximide during pregnancy has been reported.

An increased frequency of skeletal and cardiovascular malformations was observed among the offspring of mice treated with 14 times the human therapeutic dose of methsuximide during pregnancy in one study (Kao et al., 1979).

Fatal neonatal hemorrhage has been reported in the infant of a woman treated with methsuximide throughout pregnancy (Bleyer & Skinner, 1976). This complication has been observed among infants of women treated during pregnancy with other anticonvulsants.

Please see agent summary on ethosuximide for information on a related agent that has been more thoroughly studied.

Key References

Bleyer WA, Skinner AL: Fatal neonatal hemorrhage after maternal anticonvulsant therapy. JAMA 235:626-627, 1976. [C]

Kao J, Brown NA, Shull G, Fabro S: Chemical structure and teratogenicity of anticonvulsants. Fed Pro Fed Am Soc Exp Biol 38:438, 1979. [A]

METHYCLOTHIAZIDE

Synonyms

Aquatensen, Duretic, Enduron, Methylchlorothiazide, Methylcyclothiazide, Meticlotiazide, Naturon, Thiazidil, Urimor

Summary

Methyclothiazide is a thiazide diuretic. It is used to relieve edema and in the treatment of hypertension.

Magnitude of Teratogenic Risk

Minimal

Quality and Quantity of Data

Poor To Fair

Comment

None

The Collaborative Perinatal Project included 942 pregnancies exposed to methyclothiazide anytime during pregnancy, but only three pregnancies exposed during the first trimester (Heinonen et al., 1977). The frequency of patent ductus arteriosus appeared higher than expected among the children of women who took this drug late in pregnancy, but the statistical (as well as the biological) significance of this observation is uncertain.

No animal teratology studies of methyclothiazide have been published.

Neonatal thrombocytopenic purpura was observed in one infant whose mother was treated with methyclothiazide during pregnancy (Rodriguez et al., 1964). Thrombocytopenia has also been reported among the newborn infants of women treated during pregnancy with other thiazide diuretics, but it appears to be very uncommon under such circumstances (Finnerty & Assali, 1964).

Please see agent summary on chlorothiazide for information on a closely related drug that has been more thoroughly studied.

Key References

Finnerty FA, Assali NS: Thiazide and neonatal thrombocytopenia. N Engl J Med 271:160-161, 1964. [O]

Heinonen OP, Slone D, Shapiro S: Birth Defects and Drugs in Pregnancy. Littleton, Mass.: John Wright-PSG, 1977, pp 372, 495. [E]

Rodriguez SU, Leikin SL, Hiller MC: Neonatal thrombocytopenia associated with ante-partum administration of thiazide drugs. N Engl J Med 270:881-884, 1964. [C]

METHYL MERCAPTAN

Summary

Methyl mercaptan is an intermediate in the production of jet fuels, pesticides, fungicides and plastics, and occurs as a byproduct in pulp mills and oil refineries. It is also used as an odorant for natural gas and in the synthesis of methionine. The 8-hour time-weighted threshold limit value for occupational exposure is 0.5 ppm (1 mg/cu m) (HSDB, 1993).

Magnitude of Teratogenic Risk

Undetermined

Quality and Quantity of Data

None

Comment

None

No epidemiological studies of congenital anomalies among infants whose mothers were exposed to methyl mercaptan during pregnancy have been reported.

No animal teratology studies of methyl mercaptan have been published.

Key References

HSDB [database online]. Bethesda, Md: National Library of Medicine; 1985- [updated 1993 April 30]. Available from: National Library of Medicine; BRS Information Technologies, McLean Va. [O]

METHYLBENZE-THONIUM

Synonyms

Delavan, Diaparene

Summary

Methylbenzethonium is a quaternary ammonium disinfectant that is used in deodorants and applied topically to treat ammonia dermatitis.

Magnitude of Teratogenic Risk

Undetermined

Quality and Quantity of Data

None

Comment

A small risk cannot be excluded, but a high risk of congenital anomalies in the children of women treated with methylbenzethonium during pregnancy is unlikely.

No epidemiological studies of congenital anomalies in infants born to women who used methylbenzethonium during pregnancy have been reported.

No animal teratology studies of methylbenzethonium have been published.

Key References

None available.

METHYLDOPA

Synonyms

Aldomet, Dopamet, Medomet, Novomedopa, Presinol, Sembrina

Summary

Methyldopa is an antihypertensive agent used frequently in pregnancy.

Magnitude of Teratogenic Risk

Undetermined

Quality and Quantity of Data

Poor

Comment

A small risk cannot be excluded, but a greatly increased risk of congenital anomalies in children of women treated with methyldopa during pregnancy is unlikely.

No epidemiological studies of malformations in children born to women treated with methyldopa early in pregnancy have been reported.

No consistent adverse effect has been observed among children born to women treated with methyldopa late in pregnancy (La Selve et al., 1968; Redman et al., 1976; Cockburn et al., 1982; Fidler et al., 1983). In one well-controlled study involving about 100 children born to women treated with methyldopa during pregnancy, a small but statistically significant decrease in head circumference was observed at birth and four years of age among males whose mothers' treatment had begun between 16 and 20 weeks gestation (Redman et al., 1976; Moar et al., 1978; Ounsted et al., 1980). This effect was not seen in the boys at 7.5 years of age, was not seen in girls, was not associated with any functional deficits, and was not observed in an independent study (Moar et al., 1978; Ounsted et al., 1980; Cockburn et al., 1982; Fidler et al., 1983).

Transient neonatal tremor, irritability, and mildly decreased systolic blood pressure have been noted in infants of mothers treated chronically with methyldopa late in pregnancy (Whitelaw, 1981; Bodis et al., 1982; Sulyok et al., 1991). No clinically significant problems have been associated with these findings, however.

No teratogenic effect was observed in mice, rats, or rabbits treated with methyldopa throughout pregnancy in doses 2 or more times greater than those used in humans (Peck et al., 1965).

Treatment of rabbits late in pregnancy with methyldopa in doses similar to those used in humans caused transient depression of cardiac norepinephrine stores in the neonates (Hoskins & Friedman, 1980). The clinical relevance of this observation is unknown.

Key References

Bodis J, Sulyok E, Ertl T, Varga L, et al.: Methyldopa in pregnancy hypertension and the newborn. Lancet 2:498-499, 1982. [C]

Cockburn J, Moar VA, Ounsted M, Redman CWG: Final report of study on hypertension during pregnancy: The effects of specific treatment on the growth and development of the children. Lancet 2:647-648, 1982. [E]

Fidler J, Smith V, Fayers P, De Swiet M: Randomised controlled comparative study of methyldopa and oxprenolol in treatment of hypertension in pregnancy. Br Med J 286:1927-1930, 1983. [E]

Hoskins EJ, Friedman WF: Influence of maternal alpha-methyldopa on sympathetic innervation in the newborn rabbit heart. Am J Obstet Gynecol 137:496-498, 1980. [A]

La Selve A, Berger R, Vial JY, Gaillard MF: [Alpha-methyl-dopa (aldomet) and reserpin (serpasil) treatments of gravid high blood pressure.] J Med Lyon:1369-1375, 1968. [S]

Moar VA, Jefferies MA, Mutch LMM, Ounsted MK, et al.: Neonatal head circumference and the treatment of maternal hypertension. Br J Obstet Gynaecol 85:933-937, 1978. [E]

Ounsted MK, Moar VA, Good FJ, Redman CWG: Hypertension during pregnancy with and without specific treatment; the development of the children at the age of four years. Br J Obstet Gynaecol 87:19-24, 1980. [E]

Peck HM, Mattis PA, Zawoiski EJ: The evaluation of drugs for their effects on reproduction and fetal development. Excerpta Med Int Congr Serv 85:19-29, 1965. [A]

Redman CWG, Beilin LJ, Bonnar J, Ounsted MK: Fetal outcome in trial of antihypertensive treatment in pregnancy. Lancet 2:753-756, 1976. [E]

Sulyok E, Bodis J, Hartman G, Ertl T: Neonatal effects of methyldopa therapy in pregnancy hypertension. Acta Paediatr Hung 31(1):53-63, 1991. [E]

Whitelaw A: Maternal methyldopa treatment and neonatal blood pressure. Br Med J 283:471, 1981. [E]

METHYLENE BLUE

Synonyms

Desmoid Piller, Desmoidpillen, Methylthionine Chloride, Methylthioninium Chloride, Panatone, Urolene Blue, Vitableu

Summary

Methylene blue is used in the treatment of methemoglobinemia and as a marker after injection into amniotic fluid. Methylene blue is also used as a bacteriological stain, as a skin or tissue marker, and as a chemical indicator.

Magnitude of Teratogenic Risk

Minimal To Small

Quality and Quantity of Data

Poor To Fair

Comment

1) Hemolytic anemia and jaundice may occur among newborn infants of women given intra-amniotic injection of methylene blue late in pregnancy (see below).

2) Risk assessment is for intra-amniotic injection of methylene blue.

3) Risk related to the topical use of methylene blue is unknown but unlikely to be great.

4) Risk related to intravenous use is unknown.

The frequency of congenital anomalies was not significantly increased among the children of 46 women who had been treated with methylene blue during pregnancy in the Collaborative Perinatal Project (Heinonen et al., 1977). Only nine of these women received this treatment during the first trimester. No anomalies were noted in an infant born following inadvertent intrauterine injection of methylene blue to his mother about three and one-half weeks after conception (Katz & Lancet, 1981).

Multiple intestinal atresias have been observed among several infants born of twin pregnancies in which methylene blue had been injected into the amniotic cavity at about 16 weeks during amniocentesis (Nicolini & Monni, 1990; Moorman-Voestermans et al., 1990). It is unclear, however, whether these defects are related to the methylene blue or to the generally increased risk of congenital anomalies associated with twin pregnancies, or are just coincidental (Dolk, 1991).

Neonatal hemolytic anemia and jaundice have been observed in several infants born after intra-amniotic injection of methylene blue late in pregnancy (Plunkett, 1973; Cowett et al., 1976; Serota et al., 1979; Spahr et al., 1980; Crooks, 1982; McEnerney & McEnerney, 1983; Vincer et al., 1987). Hemolytic anemia is a recognized complication of methylene blue therapy in children.

An increased frequency of fetal loss was noted among pregnant rats fed a diet containing methylene blue in an amount sufficient to inhibit maternal weight gain (Telford et al., 1962). Increased frequencies of fetal death were observed in pregnant rats after intra-amniotic injection of methylene blue in an amount proportionally similar to that used in humans (Piersma et al., 1991).

Key References

Cowett RM, Hakanson DO, Kocon RW, Oh W: Untoward neonatal effect of intraamniotic administration of methylene blue. Obstet Gynecol 48(Suppl):745-755, 1976. [C]

Crooks J: Haemolytic jaundice in a neonate after intra-amniotic injection of methylene blue. Arch Dis Child 57:872-886, 1982. [C]

Dolk H: Methylene blue and atresia or stenosis of ileum and jejunum. Lancet 338:1021-1022, 1991. [S]

Heinonen OP, Slone D, Shapiro S: Birth Defects and Drugs in Pregnancy. Littleton, Mass.: John Wright-PSG, 1977, pp 299, 434, 455. [E]

Katz Z, Lancet M: Inadvertent intrauterine injection of methylene blue in early pregnancy. N Engl J Med 304:1427, 1981. [C]

McEnerney JK, McEnerney LN: Unfavorable neonatal outcome after intraamniotic injection of methylene blue. Obstet Gynecol 61:35S-37S, 1983. [C]

Moorman-Voestermans CGM, Heig HA, Vos A: Jejunal atresia in twins. J Pediatr Surg 25:638-639, 1990. [C]

Nicolini U, Monni G: Intestinal obstruction in babies exposed in utero to methylene blue. Lancet 336:1258-1259, 1990. [S]

Piersma AH, Verhoef A, De Liefde A, et al.: Embryotoxicity of methylene blue in the rat. Teratology 43(5):458-459, 1991. [A]

Plunkett GD: Neonatal complications. Obstet Gynecol 41:476-477, 1973. [C]

Serota FT, Bernbaum JC, Schwartz E: The methylene blue baby. Lancet 2:1142-1143, 1979. [C]

Spahr RC, Salsburey DJ, Krissberg A, Prin W: Intraamniotic injection of methylene blue leading to methemoglobinemia in one of twins. Int J Gynaecol Obstet 17:477-478, 1980. [C]

Telford IR, Woodruff CS, Linford RH: Fetal resorption in the rat as influenced by certain antioxidants. Am J Anat 110:29-36, 1962. [A]

Vincer MJ, Allen AC, Evans JR, et al.: Methylene-blue-induced hemolytic anemia in a neonate. Can Med Assoc J 136:503-504, 1987. [C]

METHYLERGONOVINE

Synonyms

Methergin, Methylergobasine Maleate, Methylergometrine Maleate

Summary

Methylergonovine is an ergot derivative used to stimulate uterine contraction in the treatment of missed abortion or postpartum hemorrhage.

Magnitude of Teratogenic Risk

Undetermined

Quality and Quantity of Data

None

Comment

Administration of methylergonovine to a pregnant woman near term can cause uterine tetany, fetal hypoxia, and their sequellae (Moise & Carpenter, 1988).

No epidemiological studies of congenital anomalies among the infants of women treated with methylergonovine during pregnancy have been reported.

No teratological studies of methylergonovine in experimental animals have been published.

Key References

Moise KJ Jr, Carpenter RJ Jr: Methylergonovine-induced hypertonus in term pregnancy. A case report. J Reprod Med 33(9):771-773, 1988. [C]

METHYLPARABEN

Synonyms

Methyl Chemosept, Methyl 4-Hydroxybenzoate, Methyl Parasept

Summary

Methylparaben is a methyl ester of hydroxybenzoic acid. It is used a preservative in foods, beverages, and cosmetics.

Magnitude of Teratogenic Risk

Undetermined

Quality and Quantity of Data

None

Comment

None

No epidemiological studies of congenital anomalies among infants born to women exposed to large amounts of methylparaben during pregnancy have been reported.

No animal teratology studies of methylparaben have been published.

Key References

None available.

METHYLPHENIDATE

Synonyms

Methidate, Rilatine, Ritalin, Ritaline, Rubifen

Summary

Methylphenidate is a sympathomimetic agent that is given orally to treat narcolepsy. It is also employed in the management of attention deficit disorders in children. Methylphenidate is used "socially" as a stimulant, sometimes by the intravenous route.

Magnitude of Teratogenic Risk

Undetermined

Quality and Quantity of Data

None To Poor

Comment

None

No epidemiological studies of congenital anomalies among infants born to women treated with methylphenidate during pregnancy have been reported.

An increased frequency of fetal death was observed after treatment of pregnant mice with methylphenidate in a dose 200 times that used in humans; such treatment also produced maternal toxicity (Takano et al., 1963). The clinical importance of this observation is unknown.

Please see agent summary on dextroamphetamine for information on a related agent that has been more thoroughly studied.

Key References

Takano K, Tanimura T, Nishimura H: Effects of some psychoactive drugs administered to pregnant mice upon the development of their offspring. Congen Anom 3:2-3, 1963. [A]

METHYLPRED-NISOLONE

Synonyms

A-Methapred, depMedalone, Depo-Medrol, Depo-Medrone, Medrol, Mepred, Metilcort, Metilprednilone, Neo-Medrol, Solu-Medrol

Summary

Methylprednisolone is a synthetic glucocorticoid used for its anti-inflammatory and immunosuppressive properties.

Magnitude of Teratogenic Risk

None To Minimal

Quality and Quantity of Data

None To Poor

Comment

None

No epidemiological studies of congenital anomalies in infants born to women treated with methylprednisolone during pregnancy have been reported.

An increased frequency of cleft palate was observed among the offspring of mice treated during pregnancy with methylprednisolone in doses similar to those used therapeutically in humans (Walker, 1971). A typical dose-response relationship was seen. An increased frequency of cardiovascular defects and decreased body weight were observed among the offspring of pregnant rats treated with methylprednisolone in a dose that was similar to that used in humans but was toxic to the rat dams (Kageyama et al., 1991). In contrast, no teratogenic effect was noted in rats with doses <1-18 times those used clinically in another study (Walker, 1971). High frequencies of fetal death and a variety of central nervous system and skeletal anomalies were reported in the offspring of pregnant rabbits treated with methylprednisolone in doses less than those used in humans (Walker, 1967; Langhoff et al., 1979). The relevance of these findings to the risk of malformations in human infants born to mothers treated with methylprednisolone early in pregnancy is unknown.

Please see the agent summary on prednisone for information on a closely related drug that has been more thoroughly studied.

Key References

Kageyama A, Kato K, Urabe K, et al.: [Toxicity study of methylprednisolone aceponate (Zk 91 588) (V) -- teratogenicity study in rats]. Yakuri To Chiryo 19(8):91-106, 1991. [A]

Langhoff LM, Rudiger HF, Hoar RM: Teratology of methylprednisolone acetate (Depo-MedrolR) in rabbits. Anat Rec 193:598, 1979. [A]

Walker BE: Induction of cleft palate in rabbits by several glucocorticoids. Proc Soc Exp Biol Med 125:1281-1284, 1967. [A]

Walker BE: Induction of cleft palate in rats with antiinflammatory drugs. Teratology 4:39-42, 1971. [A]

METHYLTESTOS-TERONE

Synonyms

Android, Metandren, Oreton-M, Testred, Virilon

Summary

Methyltestosterone is an androgen used to treat postpartum breast engorgement and breast cancer. The buccal preparation is twice as potent as the oral.

Magnitude of Teratogenic Risk

Virilization Of Female Fetus: Moderate

Congenital Anomalies: Undetermined

Quality and Quantity of Data

Virilization Of Female Fetus: Good

Congenital Anomalies: Poor

Comment

A small risk cannot be excluded, but a high risk of congenital anomalies in the children of women treated with methyltestosterone during pregnancy is unlikely.

Virilization of the external genitalia has been observed in more than a dozen girls born to women who had been treated with methyltestosterone during pregnancy (Grumbach & Ducharme, 1960; Schardein, 1985). Affected girls have varying degrees of phallic enlargement and labioscrotal fusion. Phallic enlargement may be produced by exposure to methyltestosterone anytime after the genitalia have developed; labioscrotal fusion is only seen with exposure between the eighth and thirteenth weeks of gestation. In general, the degree of virilization is greater with exposure to larger doses of methyltestosterone. Surgical correction of the genital defect is available, but often is unnecessary. Normal female maturation can be anticipated at puberty in affected girls.

Dose-dependent virilization of the external genitalia has been observed among female offspring of pregnant rats treated with methyltestosterone in doses equivalent to those used in humans (Neumann & Junkmann, 1963; Kawashima et al., 1975). Similar effects have been observed in dogs and rabbits (Jost, 1947; Shane et al., 1969).

Key References

Grumbach MM, Ducharme JR: The effects of androgens on fetal sexual development. Androgen-induced female pseudohermaphrodism. Fertil Steril 11:157-180, 1960. [R]

Jost A: Studies about the sexual differentiation of the rabbit embryo. 2. Effect of synthetic androgens on genital histogenesis. Arch Anat Microsc Morphol Exp 36:242-270, 1947. [A]

Kawashima K, Nakaura S, Nagao S, Tanaka S, et al.: Quantitative evaluation of virilizing activity of steroids by measuring morphological changes in uro-genital region of rats. Endocrinol Jpn 22:439-444, 1975. [A]

Neumann F, Junkmann K: A new method for determination of virilizing properties of steroids on the fetus. Endocrinol 73:33-37, 1963. [A]

Schardein JL: Chemically Induced Birth Defects. New York: Marcel Dekker, 1985, pp 260-338. [R]

Shane BS, Dunn HO, Kenney RM, Hansel W, et al.: Methyl testosterone-induced female pseudo-hermaphroditism in dogs. Biol Reprod 1:41-48, 1969. [A]

METHYPRYLON

Synonyms

Methyprylone, Noludar

Summary

Methyprylon is a piperidinedione derivative administered orally as a sedative and hypnotic.

Magnitude of Teratogenic Risk

Undetermined

Quality and Quantity of Data

None

Comment

None

No epidemiological studies of congenital anomalies in infants born to women who took methyprylon during pregnancy have been reported.

No animal teratology studies of methyprylon have been published.

Please see the agent summary on glutethimide for information on a chemically related agent that has been studied.

Key References

None available.

METHYSERGIDE

Synonyms

Deseril, Desernil, Desernyl, Deserril, Deseryl, Metisergide, Metisergido, Sansert

Summary

Methysergide is a semi-synthetic ergot alkaloid derivative used to treat migraine.

Magnitude of Teratogenic Risk

Undetermined

Quality and Quantity of Data

None

Comment

None

No epidemiological studies of congenital anomalies in infants born to mothers who took methysergide during pregnancy have been reported.

No animal teratology studies of methysergide have been published.

Key References

None available.

METOCLOPRAMIDE

Synonyms

Ananda, Maxeran, Maxolon, Metox, Octamide, Parmid, Primperan, Reglan

Summary

Metoclopramide is used to treat disorders of gastrointestinal motility and as an antiemetic.

Magnitude of Teratogenic Risk

None To Minimal

Quality and Quantity of Data

Poor To Fair

Comment

None

No malformations were observed among the children of about 25 women treated with metoclopramide during the first trimester of pregnancy in one study (Sidhu & Lean, 1970).

The frequency of malformations was no greater than expected among the offspring of mice, rats, or rabbits treated during pregnancy with metoclopramide in doses, respectively, 17-330, 17-330, and 3-17 times those used clinically in humans (Watanabe et al., 1968).

Key References

Sidhu MS, Lean TH: The use of metoclopramide (Maxolon) in hyperemesis gravidarum. Proc Obstet Gynaecol Soc Singapore 1:43-46, 1970. [E]

Watanabe N, Iwanami K, Nakahara N: Teratogenicity of metoclopramide. Yukagaku Kenkyu (Jpn J Pharmacy Chem) 39:92-106, 1968. [A]

METOCURINE

Synonyms

Dimethylchondrocurarine, Metubine Iodide

Summary

Metocurine is a skeletal muscle relaxant that is administered intravenously.

Magnitude of Teratogenic Risk

Undetermined

Quality and Quantity of Data

None

Comment

None

No epidemiological studies of congenital anomalies in infants whose mothers were administered metocurine during pregnancy have been reported.

No animal teratology studies of metocurine have been published.

Please see agent summary on tubocurarine for information on a related agent that has been studied.

Key References

None available.

METOLAZONE

Synonyms

Diulo, Mykrox, Zaroxolyn

Summary

Metolazone is a diuretic used to treat hypertension and edema.

Magnitude of Teratogenic Risk

Undetermined

Quality and Quantity of Data

None To Poor

Comment

None

No epidemiological studies of congenital anomalies in infants born to women who took metolazone during pregnancy have been reported.

No consistent increase in malformations was observed among the offspring of mice or rats treated during pregnancy with metolazone in doses 10-1250 times those used in humans (Nakajima et al., 1978a, 1978b).

No adverse effects attributable to metolazone were noted in babies born to 35 women treated with this drug in the third trimester for pregnancy-induced hypertension in one study (Duffy et al., 1972).

Key References

Duffy GJ, O'Dwyer WF, Martin F: The effects of a new diuretic (Metolazone) on pre-eclamptic toxaemia of pregnancy. J Ir Med Assoc 65:615-619, 1972. [S]

Nakajima T, Ishisaka K, Taylor P, Matsuda S: Effects of metolazone on reproduction of rabbits. Teratogenicity test. Clin Rep 12:3417-3421, 1978b. [A]

Nakajima T, Ishisaka K, Taylor P, Matsuda S: Effects of metolazone on the reproduction function of rats. 2. Teratogenicity test. Clin Rep 12:3394-3406, 1978a. [A]

METOPROLOL

Synonyms

Betaloc, Lopressor, Meteros, Prelis

Summary

Metoprolol is a beta-adrenergic receptor blocking agent used in the treatment of hypertension, angina, and cardiac arrythmias.

Magnitude of Teratogenic Risk

Undetermined

Quality and Quantity of Data

Poor

Comment

A small risk cannot be excluded, but there is no indication that the risk of congenital anomalies in the children of women treated with metoprolol during pregnancy is likely to be great.

No epidemiological studies of congenital anomalies among infants born to women treated with metoprolol during pregnancy have been reported.

The frequency of malformations was no greater than expected among the offspring of rats or rabbits treated during pregnancy with metoprolol in doses respectively 1-25 or 1-3 times those used in humans (Bodin et al., 1975). Impaired adaptive response to severe asphyxia was observed in the exteriorized fetuses of sheep that had received continuous intravenous infusions with 10 mg/hr of metoprolol (Dagbjartsson et al., 1985).

In a series of 184 infants born to women with hypertension who were treated with metoprolol and other agents after the first trimester, the only adverse effect noted was mild fetal growth retardation (Sandstrom, 1982). This may have been due to the maternal hypertension rather than to its treatment. No significant difference in birth weight, head circumference, or neonatal complications was observed among 69 infants born to women treated with metoprolol and hydralazine for hypertension during the second and third trimesters of pregnancy when compared to control infants in another study (Hogstedt et al., 1985).

Please see agent summary on propranolol for information on a closely related drug that has been more thoroughly studied.

Key References

Bodin NO, Flodh H, Magnusson G, Malmfors T, et al.: Toxicological studies on metoprolol. Acta Pharmacol Toxicol 36(Suppl V):96-103, 1975. [A]

Dagbjartsson A, Karlsson K, Kjellmer I, Rosen KG: Maternal treatment with a cardioselective beta-blocking agent--Consequences for the ovine fetus during intermittent asphyxia. J Dev Physiol 7:387-396, 1985. [A]

Hogstedt S, Lindeberg S, Axelsson O, et al.: A prospective controlled trial of metoprolol-hydralazine treatment in hypertension during pregnancy. Acta Obstet Gynecol Scand 64:505-510, 1985. [E]

Sandstrom B: Adrenergic beta-receptor blockers in hypertension of pregnancy. Clin Exp Hypertens [B] B1:127-141, 1982. [E]

METRONIDAZOLE

Synonyms

Elyzol, Flagyl, Metric 21, Metrogel, Metrolyl, Nidazol, Protostat, Vaginyl, Zadstat

Summary

Metronidazole is an imidazole that is widely used in the treatment of vaginal trichomoniasis. It is also employed in the therapy of amebiasis and other parasitic and anaerobic bacterial infections.

Magnitude of Teratogenic Risk

None To Minimal

Quality and Quantity of Data

Fair

Comment

None

The frequency of maternal treatment with metronidazole during the first four lunar months of pregnancy was no greater than expected among 4264 spontaneous abortions or among 6564 infants with various birth defects, 984 infants with cardiovascular defects, 122 infants with oral clefts, or 56 infants with spina bifida in a Michigan Medicaid record linkage study (Rosa et al., 1987). No increase in the frequency of congenital anomalies was seen among the children of more than 200 women treated with metronidazole during the first trimester of pregnancy in two cohorts of the Boston Collaborative Drug Surveillance Program (Jick et al., 1981; Aselton et al., 1985). No significant increase in the frequency of congenital anomalies was observed among the children of 62 or 31 women treated with metronidazole during the first trimester of pregnancy in two other cohort studies (Morgan 1978; Heinonen et al., 1977).

Most studies in mice, rats, guinea pigs, and rabbits have shown no increase in the frequency of malformations among the offspring of animals treated during pregnancy with metronidazole, even in doses many times greater than those used clinically (Bost, 1977; Roe, 1985). However, one study found an increased frequency of fetal anomalies among the offspring of pregnant mice, rats, and guinea pigs treated with metronidazole in doses equivalent to those used in humans (Ivanov, 1969), and similar findings were reported by other investigators in mice (Giknis & Damjanov, 1983). The relevance of these observations to metronidazole therapy in human pregnancy is unknown.

Metronidazole is mutagenic in bacterial systems, but the drug has not been found to cause gene mutations or chromosomal damage in most studies in mammals (Goldman, 1980; Roe, 1983, 1985; Drinkwater, 1987).

Key References

Aselton P, Jick H, Milunsky A, et al.: First-trimester drug use and congenital disorders. Obstet Gynecol 65:451-455, 1985. [S]

Bost RG: Metronidazole: Toxicology and teratology. In: Finegold SM (ed). Metronidazole: Proceedings of the International Metronidazole Conference, 1976. New York: Excerpta Medica, 1977, pp 112-118. [A]

Drinkwater P: Metronidazole. Aust NZ J Obstet Gynaecol 27:228-230, 1987. [R]

Giknis MLA, Damjanov I: The transplacental effects of ethanol and metronidazole in Swiss Webster mice. Toxicol Lett 19:37-42, 1983. [A]

Goldman P: Metronidazole. N Engl J Med 303:1212-1218, 1980. [R]

Heinonen Op, Slone D, Shapiro S: Birth Defects and Drugs in Pregnancy. Littleton, Mass.: John Wright-PSG, 1977, pp 298-299, 302. [E]

Ivanov I: The effect of the preparation "trichomonacid" on pregnancy in experimental animals. Akush Ginekol (Sofiia) 8:241-244, 1969. [A]

Jick H, Holmes LB, Hunter JR, et al.: First-trimester drug use and congenital disorders. JAMA 246:343-346, 1981. [S]

Morgan I: Metronidazole treatment in pregnancy. Int J Gynecol Obstet 15:501-502, 1978. [E]

Roe FJC: Safety of nitroimidazoles. Scand J infect Dis Suppl 46:72-81, 1985. [R]

Roe FJC: Toxicologic evaluation of metronidazole with particular reference to carcinogenic, mutagenic, and teratogenic potential. Surgery 93:158-164, 1983. [R]

Rosa FW, Baum C, Shaw M: Pregnancy outcomes after first-trimester vaginitis drug therapy. Obstet Gynecol 69:751-755, 1987. [E]

METYRAPONE

Synonyms

Methopyrone, Metopirone

Summary

Metyrapone is an inhibitor of the enzyme 11-beta-hydroxylase that is necessary for synthesis of cortisone and hydrocortisone in the adrenal gland. Metyrapone is used to test pituitary function and in the treatment of Cushing's syndrome.

Magnitude of Teratogenic Risk

Undetermined

Quality and Quantity of Data

None To Poor

Comment

1) A small risk cannot be excluded, but a high risk of congenital anomalies in the children of women who received a single test for hypothalamo-pituitary function during pregnancy is unlikely.

2) The risk for virilization of female fetuses is probably substantial with chronic use of metyrapone.

No epidemiological studies of congenital anomalies among infants born to women treated with metyrapone during pregnancy have been reported.

Adrenal hyperplasia and clitoral hypertrophy were observed among the offspring of rats treated with metyrapone repeatedly during late pregnancy in doses sufficient to produce maternal adrenal hyperfunction (Goldman, 1967). The effects are analogous to those seen in congenital virilizing adrenal hyperplasia in humans, a condition caused by a genetic deficiency of 11-beta-hydroxylase.

No teratogenic effect was observed among the offspring of pregnant mice or rats given metyrapone in doses similar to those used to treat Cushing's syndrome (but less than those used to test pituitary function) in humans (Bird et al., 1970; Saito et al., 1981).

Key References

Bird CC, Crawford AM, Currie AR, Stirling BF: Protection from the embryopathic effects of 7-hydroxymethyl-12-methylbenz(a)anthracene by 2-methyl-1, 2-bis-(3-pyridyl)-1-propanone(metopirone, CIBA) and beta-diethylaminoethyldiphenyl-n-propyl acetate (SKF 525-A). Br J Cancer 24:548-553, 1970. [A]

Goldman AS: Experimental model of congenital adrenal cortical hyperplasia produced in utero with an inhibitor of 11-beta-steroid hydroxylase. J Clin Endocrinol Metab 27(10):1390-1394, 1967. [A]

Saito H, Naminohira S, Sakai T, Ueno K, et al.: Drug metabolism and fetal toxicity: Changes in fetal toxicity of aminopyrine by variation of drug metabolizing enzyme activity in mice. Res Commun Chem Pathol Pharmacol 34 (1):141-144, 1981. [A]

METYROSINE

Synonyms

AMPT, Demser, OGMT

Summary

Metyrosine is a competitive tyrosine hydroxylase inhibitor that is administered orally, often concomitantly with alpha- and beta-adrenergic blocking agents, in the management of hypertension and the treatment of metastatic pheochromocytoma.

Magnitude of Teratogenic Risk

Undetermined

Quality and Quantity of Data

None

Comment

None

No epidemiological studies of congenital anomalies in infants born to women who had been treated with metyrosine during pregnancy have been reported.

No animal teratology studies of metyrosine have been published.

Key References

None available.

MEXILETINE

Synonyms

Mexitil, Mexitilen

Summary

Mexiletine is a local anesthetic used to treat cardiac arrhythmias.

Magnitude of Teratogenic Risk

Undetermined

Quality and Quantity of Data

Poor

Comment

None

No epidemiological studies of congenital anomalies among infants born to women treated with mexiletine during pregnancy have been reported (Timmis et al., 1980; Lownes & Ives, 1987; Gregg & Tomich, 1988).

No teratogenic effect was observed among the offspring of rats or rabbits treated during pregnancy with mexiletine in doses <1-7.5 or <1-4 times those used in humans (Matsuo et al., 1983; Nishimura et al., 1983)

Please see agent summary on lidocaine for information on a related agent that has been studied.

Key References

Gregg AR, Tomich PG: Mexilitene use in pregnancy. J Perinatol 8:33-34, 1988. [C]

Lownes HE, Ives TJ: Mexiletine use in pregnancy and lactation. Am J Obstet Gynecol 157(2):446-447, 1987. [C]

Matsuo A, Kast A, Tsunenari Y: Reproduction studies of mexiletine hydrochloride by oral administration. Fertility, teratogenicity and perinatal and postnatal testing in rats, and teratogenicity testing in rabbits. Iyakuhin Kenkyu 14:527-549, 1983. [A]

Nishimura M, Kast A, Tsunenari Y: Reproduction studies of mexiletine hydrochloride by intravenous administration. Fertility, teratogenicity and perinatal and postnatal testing in rats, and teratogenicity testing in rabbits. Iyakuhin Kenkyu 14:550-570, 1983. [A]

Timmis AD, Jackson G, Holt DW: Mexiletine for control of ventricular dysrhythmias in pregnancy. Lancet 2:647-648, 1980. [C]

MEZLOCILLIN

Synonyms

Mezlin

Summary

Mezlocillin is a semisynthetic penicillin that is administered parenterally as a broad spectrum antibiotic.

Magnitude of Teratogenic Risk

Undetermined

Quality and Quantity of Data

None To Poor

Comment

A small risk cannot be excluded, but a high risk of congenital anomalies in the children of women treated with mezlocillin during pregnancy is unlikely.

No epidemiological studies of congenital anomalies among infants born to women treated with mezlocillin during pregnancy have been reported.

No teratogenic effect was observed among the offspring of pregnant rhesus monkeys or rats treated with mezlocillin in doses respectively, <1 or 1-3 times those used in humans (Tanioka & Koizumi, 1978; Hamada & Imanishi, 1978).

Key References

Hamada Y, Imanishi M: Reproduction study of mezlocillin in rats. 2. Teratogenicity study. Iyakuhin Kenkyu 9:986-996, 1978. [A]

Tanioka Y, Koizumi H: Influence of sodium mezlocillin on fetuses of rhesus monkeys. Jitchuken Zenrinsho Kenkyu 4:11-22, 1978. [A]

MICONAZOLE

Synonyms

Daktarin, Dermonistat, Gyno-Daktarin, Gyno-Monistat, Micatin, Monistat

Summary

Miconazole is an imidazole antifungal agent. It is used intravenously to treat severe systemic mycotic infections and orally, vaginally, and topically to treat local mycoses. The local preparations are poorly absorbed.

Magnitude of Teratogenic Risk

Systemic: Undetermined

Topical: None To Minimal

Quality and Quantity of Data

Systemic: Poor

Topical: Fair To Good

Comment

None

The frequency of congenital anomalies was not increased among 360 infants of women treated during the first trimester of pregnancy with miconazole in one cohort study (Jick et al., 1981). In a case-control study performed by record linkage on Michigan Medicaid data, Rosa et al. (1987) observed no association with maternal use of vaginal miconazole during the first trimester of pregnancy among 6564 infants with congenital anomalies, 122 infants with oral clefts, 984 infants with congenital cardiovascular defects, or 56 infants with spina bifida. Similarly, the rate of congenital anomalies did not appear unusual among the children of 43 women treated with miconazole vaginal cream in the first trimester or the infants of 248 women treated later in pregnancy in another investigation (McNellis et al., 1977). No epidemiological studies of congenital anomalies among infants born to women treated with systemic miconazole during pregnancy have been reported. A study of vaginal miconazole use and spontaneous abortion based on Medicare records (Rosa et al., 1987) is difficult to interpret because of uncertainty regarding the exposures.

The frequency of malformations was not increased among the offspring of rats or rabbits treated with (1-2.5 times the systemic human dose of miconazole during pregnancy (Ito et al., 1976a, b). Increased fetal loss occurred in both species at the high dose which was also toxic to the mother. Similar findings were reported briefly by other workers (Sawyer et al., 1975).

Key References

Ito C, Shibutani Y, Inoue K, et al.: Toxicological studies of miconazole. II. Teratological studies of miconazole in rats. Iyakuhin Kenkyu 7:367-376, 1976a. [A]

Ito C, Shibutani Y, Taya K, et al.: Toxicological studies of miconazole. III. Teratological studies of miconazole in rabbits. Iyakuhin Kenkyu 7:377-381, 1976b. [A]

Jick H, Holmes LB, Hunter JR, Madsen S, et al.: First-trimester drug use and congenital disorders. JAMA 246:343-346, 1981. [S]

McNellis D, McLeod M, Lawson J, Pasquale SA: Treatment of vulvovaginal candidiasis in pregnancy. Obstet Gynecol 50:674-678, 1977. [E]

Rosa FW, Baum C, Shaw M: Pregnancy outcomes after first-trimester vaginitis drug therapy. Obstet Gynecol 69(5):751-755, 1987. [E]

Sawyer PR, Brogden RN, Pinder RM, et al.: Miconazole: A review of its antifungal activity and therapeutic efficacy. Drugs 9:406-423, 1975. [A] & [R]

MIDAZOLAM

Synonyms

Versed

Summary

Midazolam is a benzodiazepine tranquilizer used parenterally for the induction of anesthesia.

Magnitude of Teratogenic Risk

Undetermined

Quality and Quantity of Data

None

Comment

A small risk cannot be excluded, but there is no indication that the risk of congenital anomalies in the children of women treated with midazolam during pregnancy is likely to be great.

No epidemiological studies of congenital anomalies in children born to women treated with midazolam during pregnancy have been reported.

Decreased postnatal weight gain and behavioral alterations were observed among the offspring of pregnant rats treated daily with 4-8 times the maximum human anesthetic dose of midazolam (Pankaj & Brain, 1991).

Please see agent summary on diazepam for information on a related agent that has been studied.

Key References

Pankaj V, Brain PF: Effects of prenatal exposure to benzodiazepine-related drugs on early development and adult social behaviour in Swiss mice--I. Agonists. Gen Pharmacol 22(1):33-41, 1991. [A]

MIFEPRISTONE (RU-486)

Synonyms

Mifegyne, R 38486, RU-486

Summary

Mifepristone, a chemical derivative of norethisterone, is a strong blocker of progestational hormones and a less-potent antigluco-corticoid and antiandrogen. Mifepristone is given orally as an abortifacient in early pregnancy.

Magnitude of Teratogenic Risk

Undetermined

Quality and Quantity of Data

None To Poor

Comment

A small risk cannot be excluded, but a high risk of congenital anomalies in the children of women treated with mifepristone (RU-486) during pregnancy is unlikely.

The abortifacient activity of mifepristone is incomplete. The treatment is unsuccessful in inducing termination of pregnancy in 10-20% of women treated with mifepristone alone in the first two to three weeks after conception and in a smaller proportion of women treated with mifepristone in combination with prostaglandin during this period (Ulmann, 1987; Couzinet & Schaison, 1988; Dubois et al., 1989). No epidemiological studies have been reported of congenital anomalies among infants born to women in whom treatment with mifepristone had been unsuccessful in terminating pregnancy, but four normal infants and one with sirenomelia and cleft palate have been reported after such treatment (Lim et al., 1990; Pons et al., 1991). No causal inference can be made on the basis of this anecdotal observation.

No malformations were observed among seven offspring of cynomolgus monkeys that remained pregnant despite treatment with mifepristone in doses similar to those used in humans (Wolf et al., 1989). Most of the treated monkeys did abort unless they received simultaneous treatment with progesterone as well. Fetal growth retardation, neural tube defects, and other anomalies were frequently observed among the offspring of rabbits that had been treated with mifepristone in early pregnancy but that did not abort completely (Jost, 1986). The dose of mifepristone used in these studies was much smaller than that employed in humans but produced complete abortion in about half of the treated rabbits.

Key References

Couzinet B, Schaison G: Mifegyne (mifepristone), a new antiprogestagen with potential therapeutic use in human fertility control. Drugs 35:187-191, 1988. [R]

Dubois C, Silvestre L, Ulmann A: Mifepristone for termination of early pregnancy. The French experience. Presse Med 15:757-760, 1989. [S]

Jost A: Animal reproduction. C R Acad Sci Ser III 303:281-284, 1986. [A]

Lim BH, Lees DAR, Bjornsson S, et al.: Normal development after exposure to mifepristone in early pregnancy. Lancet 336:257-258, 1990. [C]

Pons J-C, Imbert M-C, Elefant E, et al.: Development after exposure to mifepristone in early pregnancy. Lancet 338(8769):763, 1991. [C]

Ulmann A: Uses of RU 486 for contragestion: An update. Contraception 36(Suppl):27-31, 1987. [S]

Wolf JP, Chillik CF, Dubois C, et al.: Tolerance of perinidatory primate embryos to RU 486 exposure in vitro and in vivo. Contraception 41(1):85-92, 1990. [A]

MILRINONE

Synonyms

WIN 47203

Summary

Milrinone is a cardiotonic drug.

Magnitude of Teratogenic Risk

Undetermined

Quality and Quantity of Data

None

Comment

None

No epidemiological studies of congenital anomalies in infants born to women treated with milrinone during pregnancy have been reported.

No animal teratology studies of milrinone have been published.

Key References

None available.

MINAXOLONE

Synonyms

CCI-12923

Summary

Minaxolone has been used as an intravenous general anesthetic.

Magnitude of Teratogenic Risk

Undetermined

Quality and Quantity of Data

None

Comment

None

No epidemiological studies of congenital anomalies in children born to women exposed to minaxolone during pregnancy have been reported.

No investigations of teratologic effects of minaxolone in experimental animals have been published.

Key References

None available.

MINERAL OIL

Synonyms

Agarol, Kondremul, Liquid Paraffin, Neo-Cultol, Paraffin Oil, Petrolatum, Liquid, Vaseline Oil, White Mineral Oil

Summary

Mineral oil is a mixture of liquid hydrocarbons. It is taken orally and rectally as a stool lubricant and used topically as an emollient and ointment base. Mineral oil may be slightly absorbed from the gastrointestinal tract.

Magnitude of Teratogenic Risk

Undetermined

Quality and Quantity of Data

None

Comment

A small risk cannot be excluded, but a high risk of congenital anomalies in the children of women treated with mineral oil during pregnancy is unlikely.

No epidemiological studies of congenital anomalies in infants whose mothers took mineral oil during pregnancy have been reported.

No animal teratology studies of mineral oil have been published.

Key References

None available.

MINOCYCLINE

Synonyms

Klinomycin, Minociclina, Minocine, Minomycin, Mynocine, Ultramycin, Vectrin

Summary

Minocycline is a broad-spectrum antibiotic agent which is chemically related to tetracycline. It is used in a wide range of infections.

Magnitude of Teratogenic Risk

Undetermined

Quality and Quantity of Data

None To Poor

Comment

None

No epidemiological studies of children born after maternal minocycline use during pregnancy have been published.

No teratogenic effect was apparent among the offspring of pregnant macaques given 1-4 times the usual human dose of minocycline during embryogenesis (Jackson et al., 1975).

Tetracycline causes staining of the primary dentition in fetuses exposed during the second or third trimesters of pregnancy *(See tetracycline agent summary)*; it is not known whether or not minocycline produces similar problems.

Key References

Jackson BA, Rodwell DE, Kanegis LA, Noble JF: Effect of maternally administered minocycline on embryonic and fetal development in the rhesus monkey (Macaca mulatta). Toxicol Appl Pharmacol 33:156, 1975. [A]

MINOXIDIL

Synonyms

Loniten, Minodyl, Rogaine

Summary

Minoxidil is an arteriolar vasodilator that is used as an oral antihypertensive agent. It is also used topically to promote hair growth in male-pattern baldness.

Magnitude of Teratogenic Risk

Undetermined

Quality and Quantity of Data

Poor

Comment

Transient hypertrichosis has been observed in infants born to women treated with minoxidil during pregnancy (see below).

No epidemiological studies of congenital anomalies among infants born to women treated with minoxidil during pregnancy have been published. Two infants with hypertrichosis whose mothers took minoxidil during pregnancy have been reported; one of these infants also had multiple congenital anomalies (Kaler et al., 1987; Rosa et al., 1987). Since hypertrichosis is a frequent side effect of minoxidil treatment in adults, a causal relationship to the excess hair growth seems likely. In both cases, the hypertrichosis disappeared within a few months.

The frequency of malformations was no greater than expected among the offspring of pregnant rats or rabbits treated with minoxidil in doses 4-12 times those conventionally used in humans (Carlson & Feenstra, 1977). An increased rate of fetal death was observed among the rabbits at the higher dose.

Key References

Carlson RG, Feenstra ES: Toxicologic studies with the hypotensive agent minoxidil. Toxicol Appl Pharmacol 39:1-11, 1977. [A]

Kaler SG, Patrinos ME, Lambert GH, Myers TF, et al.: Hypertrichosis and congenital anomalies associated with maternal use of minoxidil. Pediatr 79(3):434-436, 1987. [C]

Rosa FW, Idanpaan-Heikkila J, Asanti R: Fetal minoxidil exposure. Pediatr 80(1):120, 1987. [C]

MITOMYCIN

Synonyms

Ametycine, Mitocin-C, Mutamycin

Summary

Mitomycin is an antibiotic that acts as an inhibitor of DNA synthesis and as an alkylating agent. It is administered parenterally in the treatment of solid tumors.

Magnitude of Teratogenic Risk

Undetermined

Quality and Quantity of Data

Poor

Comment

Although undetermined, the teratogenic risk associated with mitomycin may be substantial because this agent is cytotoxic.

No epidemiological studies of congenital anomalies in infants born to women treated with mitomycin during pregnancy have been reported.

Increased frequencies of skeletal, eye, and other malformations and of fetal death have been observed among the offspring of mice treated during pregnancy with mitomycin in doses three or more times those used in humans (Tanimura, 1968; Snow & Tam, 1979; Fujii & Nakatsuka, 1983; Gregg & Snow, 1983; Inouye & Kajiwara, 1988). The frequency of malformations was not increased among the offspring of rats treated with 4-5 times the human dose of mitomycin during pregnancy, although both maternal and fetal death frequently occurred with this dose (Chaube & Murphy, 1968).

Dose-dependent increases in frequencies of chromosomal breaks and rearrangements have been demonstrated in fetal somatic cells from mice treated during pregnancy with mitomycin in doses 3 or more times those used therapeutically in humans (Basler, 1982; Adler, 1983; Sharma et al., 1985; Muller 1988). Similar chromosomal abnormalities can be induced in cultured human lymphocytes by treatment with mitomycin (Evans, 1982). The relevance of these observations to the clinical use of mitomycin in human pregnancy is unknown.

Key References

Adler ID: New approaches to mutagenicity studies in animals for carcinogenic and mutagenic agents. II. Clastogenic effects determined in transplacentally treated mouse embryos. Teratogen Carcinogen Mutagen 3:321-334, 1983. [A]

Basler A: Transplacental cytogenetic effects of chemical mutagens. Sister-Chromatid-Exch Test Workshop Ges Umwelt-Mutationforsch, 1980:45-52, 1982. [A]

Chaube S, Murphy ML: The teratogenic effects of the recent drugs active in cancer chemotherapy. Adv Teratol 3:181-237, 1968. [R]

Evans HJ, Newton V, Newton MS: The response of cells from patients with Huntington's chorea to mutagen-induced chromosome damage. Ann Hum Genet 46:177-185, 1982. [E]

Fujii T, Nakatsuka T: Potentiating effects of caffeine on teratogenicity of alkylating agents in mice. Teratology 28:29-33, 1983. [A]

Gregg BC, Snow MHL: Axial abnormalities following disturbed growth in mitomycin C-treated mouse embryos. J Embryol Exp Morphol 73:135-149, 1983. [A]

413

Inouye M, Kajiwara Y: Teratogenic interactions between methylmercury and mitomycin-C in mice. Arch Toxicol 61:192-195, 1988. [A]

Muller L: Stage-related induction of chromosomal aberrations and SCE in mouse embryos treated transplacentally during organogenesis with MMC and DMBA. Teratogenesis, Carcinogenesis and Mutagenesis 8:95-105, 1988. [A]

Sharma RK, Jacobson-Kram D, Lemmon M, Bakke J, et al.: Sister-chromatid exchange and cell replication kinetics in fetal and maternal cells after treatment with chemical teratogens. Mutat Res 158:217-231, 1985. [A]

Snow MHL, Tam PPL: Is compensatory growth a complicating factor in mouse teratology? Nature 279:555-557, 1979. [A]

Tanimura T: Effects of mitomycin C administered at various stages of pregnancy upon mouse fetuses. Okajimas Fol Anat Jap 44:337-355, 1968. [A]

MITOTANE

Synonyms

Chloditan, Chlodithane, Lysodren

Summary

Mitotane is an inhibitor of the adrenal cortex. It is administered orally in the treatment of adrenal carcinoma.

Magnitude of Teratogenic Risk

Undetermined

Quality and Quantity of Data

None To Poor

Comment

Although the risk of mitotane is unknown, it may be substantial because of its ability to inhibit adrenal cortex activity.

No epidemiological studies of congenital anomalies among infants born to women treated with mitotane during pregnancy have been reported. Histological abnormalities of the adrenal anlage but no malformations were apparent in an embryo that was therapeutically aborted at 42 days gestation because the mother became pregnant while being treated with mitotane for Cushing's disease (Leiba et al., 1989).

An increased frequency of ocular, central nervous system, and other anomalies was observed among the offspring of mice treated with less than the usual human dose of mitotane during pregnancy in one study (Anonymous, 1968).

Key References

Anonymous: Evaluation of carcinogenic, teratogenic, and mutagenic activities of selected pesticides and industrial chemicals. Volume II. Teratogenic study in mice and rats. NTIS (National Technical Information Service) Report/PB-223 160, 1968. [A]

Leiba S, Weinstein R, Shindel B, et al.: The protracted effect of o,p'-DDD in Cushing's disease and its impact on adrenal morphogenesis of young human embryo. Annales d'Endocrinologie (Paris) 50:49-53, 1989. [C]

MOLINDONE

Synonyms

Moban

Summary

Molindone is an indole derivative that is used as an antipsychotic agent. It is chemically unrelated to other commonly used antipsychotics.

Magnitude of Teratogenic Risk

Undetermined

Quality and Quantity of Data

None

Comment

If used topically, a small risk cannot be excluded, but a high risk of congenital anomalies in the children of women treated with molindone during pregnancy is unlikely.

No epidemiological studies of congenital anomalies in infants born to women who were treated with molindone during pregnancy have been reported.

No animal teratology studies of molindone have been published.

Please see agent summary on chlorpromazine for information on a more thoroughly studied agent with similar properties.

Key References

None available.

MOLYBDENUM

Synonyms

Disodium Molybdate, Molybdate, Molybdic Acid, Natriummolybdat, Sodium Molybdate

Summary

Molybdenum is an essential trace metal in the human diet and acts as an antagonist of copper. It is used in industry to make steel and nonferrous alloys.

Magnitude of Teratogenic Risk

Undetermined

Quality and Quantity of Data

Poor

Comment

None

No association was observed between the occurrence of 468 cases of anencephaly and community drinking water concentrations of molybdenum (Elwood & Coldman, 1981). No other epidemiological studies of congenital anomalies among infants born to women exposed to unusually high concentrations of molybdenum during pregnancy have been reported.

No teratogenic effect was observed among the offspring of golden hamsters injected with 40-100 mg/kg of sodium molybdate during pregnancy (Ferm, 1972). The frequency of congenital anomalies was no greater than expected among the offspring of pregnant mice injected with 100 mg/kg of sodium molybdate, but decreased fetal weight and delayed skeletal maturation were observed (Wide, 1984). Fetal resorption was increased among pregnant rats fed diets containing sodium molybdate in concentrations great enough to inhibit maternal weight gain (Fungwe et al., 1990).

Key References

Elwood JM, Coldman AJ: Water composition in the etiology of anencephalus. Am J Epidemiol 113:681-690, 1981. [E]

Ferm VH: The teratogenic effects of metals on mammalian embryos. Adv Teratol 5:51-75, 1972. [A]

Fungwe TV, Buddingh F, Demick DS, et al.: The role of dietary molybdenum on estrous activity, fertility, reproduction and molybdenum and copper enzyme activities of female rats. Nutr Res 10:515-524, 1990. [A]

Wide M: Effect of short-term exposure to five industrial metals on the embryonic and fetal development of the mouse. Environ Res 33:47-53, 1984. [E]

MOMETASONE FUROATE

Synonyms

Elocon

Summary

Mometasone furoate is a synthetic adrenocorticoid that is used topically to treat various dermatoses. Systemic absorption occurs following topical application of mometasone furoate.

Magnitude of Teratogenic Risk

Undetermined

Quality and Quantity of Data

Poor

Comment

A small risk cannot be exluded when mometasone furoate is used topically, but a high risk of congenital anomalies in the children of women treated with mometasone furoate during pregnancy is unlikely.

No epidemiological studies of congenital anomalies among infants born to women who were treated with mometasone furoate during pregnancy have been reported.

The frequency of malformations was not increased among the offspring of rats treated with 0.0012-0.03 mg/kg/d of mometasone furoate during pregnancy (Morita et al., 1990). Congenital anomalies, especially cleft palate and ventricular septal defect, were seen with increased frequency among the offspring of rabbits treated with 1.0 mg/kg/d but not lower doses of mometasone furoate during pregnancy (Wada et al., 1990).

Please see agent summary on beclomethasone for information on a related agent that has been studied.

Key References

Morita Y, Ota T, Watanabe C, et al.: [Teratogenicity study of mometasone furoate in rats]. Kiso To Rinsho 24(5):271-297, 1990. [A]

Wada K, Hashimoto Y, Mizutani M, et al.: [Teratogenicity study of mometasone furoate in rabbits]. Kiso To Rinsho 24(5):299-309, 1990. [A]

MONENSIN

Synonyms

Coban, Elancoban, Monelan, Monensic Acid, Romensin, Rumensin

Summary

Monensin is an antibiotic used in veterinary medicine and agriculture.

Magnitude of Teratogenic Risk

Undetermined

Quality and Quantity of Data

None To Poor

Comment

None

No epidemiological studies of congenital anomalies in infants whose mothers were exposed to monensin during pregnancy have been reported.

Fetal death and growth retardation were observed among the offspring of pregnant rats treated with subtherapeutic doses of monensin, but no increase in malformations was seen (Atef et al., 1986). After treatment with therapeutic doses in rats (3.50 mg/kg/d), no viable fetuses were delivered.

Key References

Atef M, Shalaby MA, El-Sayed MGA, El-Din S, Youssef AH, El-Sayed MAI: Influence of monensin on fertility in rats. Clin Exper Pharm Physiol 13:113-121, 1986. [A]

MONOBENZONE

Synonyms

Agerite, Aloquin, Benoquin, Benzoquin, Depigman, Dermochinona, Leucodinine

Summary

Monobenzone is a depigmenting agent which lightens hyperpigmented skin by inhibiting the melanin-forming enzyme tyrosinase. It is applied topically in the form of an ointment.

Magnitude of Teratogenic Risk

Undetermined

Quality and Quantity of Data

None

Comment

A small risk cannot be excluded when monobenzone is used topically, but a high risk of congenital anomalies in the children of women treated with monobenzone during pregnancy is unlikely.

No epidemiological studies of congenital anomalies in infants born to women who used monobenzone during pregnancy have been reported.

No adequate animal teratology studies of monobenzone have been published.

Key References

None available.

MORPHINE

Synonyms

Astramorph, Duromorph, Morfina, MS Contin, MSIR, Nepenthe, White Stuff

Summary

Morphine is a narcotic analgesic. It is used as a pain reliever, particularly in the treatment of myocardial infarction and cardiac failure. Morphine is also used as an antitussive.

Magnitude of Teratogenic Risk

Congenital Anomalies: None To Minimal

Neonatal Neurobehavioral Effects: Moderate

Quality and Quantity of Data

Congenital Anomalies: Fair To Good

Neonatal Neurobehavioral Effects: Fair To Good

Comment

Neonatal withdrawal symptoms often occur among infants born to women who regularly use morphine during pregnancy.

The frequency of congenital anomalies was no greater than expected among the children of 70 women who were treated with morphine during the first four lunar months of pregnancy or of 448 women treated with this drug anytime during pregnancy in the Collaborative Perinatal Project (Heinonen et al., 1977).

No malformations were observed in the infant of a woman who attempted suicide by taking an overdose of morphine and other medication during the first trimester of pregnancy (Czeizel et al., 1988).

The frequency of malformations was no greater than expected among the offspring of mice or rats treated during pregnancy with morphine in doses 2-17 times those used clinically (Yamamoto et al., 1972; Fujinaga &

Mazze, 1988), but fetal growth retardation and increased frequencies of central nervous system and other anomalies were seen among the offspring of pregnant mice treated with doses 40-200 times those used in humans (Harpel & Gautieri, 1968). Similar anomalies were observed among the offspring of hamsters treated with 15-130 but not 10 times the human dose of morphine during pregnancy (Geber & Schramm, 1975; Geber, 1977). Fetal growth retardation was also seen among the offspring of pregnant rabbits or rats treated with morphine at 20-40 or 5-60 times the human dose (Raye et al., 1977; Zagon & McLaughlin, 1977; Eriksson & Ronnback, 1989). Increased rates of fetal and neonatal death were observed after treatment of pregnant rats with morphine in doses 5 or more times those used clinically (Fujinaga & Mazze, 1988; Eriksson & Ronnback, 1989).

Long-lasting behavioral alterations have been observed among the offspring of mice, rats, and hamsters treated with large doses of morphine during pregnancy (Davis & Lin, 1972; Zimmerberg et al., 1974; Sobrian, 1977; Vathy et al., 1985; Zagon et al., 1989; Johnston et al., 1992; Vathy & Katay, 1992).

Neonatal withdrawal symptoms similar to those seen in the infants of heroin addicts have been observed in the infants of morphine-addicted women (Perlstein, 1947; Cobrinik et al., 1959). These symptoms include tremors, irritability, sneezing, diarrhea, vomiting, and occasionally seizures.

Key References

Cobrinik RW, Hood RT, Chusid E: The effect of maternal narcotic addiction on the newborn infant. Pediatrics 24:288-304, 1959. [R] & [C]

Czeizel A, Szentesi I, Szekeres I, Molnar G, et al.: A study of adverse effects on the progeny after intoxication during pregnancy. Arch Toxciol 62:1-7, 1988. [E]

Davis WM, Lin CH: Prenatal morphine effects on survival and behavior of rat offspring. Res Commun Chem Pathol Pharmacol 3:205-214, 1972. [A]

Eriksson PS, Ronnback L: Effects of prenatal morphine treatment of rats on mortality, bodyweight and analgesic response in the offspring. Drug Alcohol Depend 24:187-194, 1989. [A]

Fujinaga M, Mazze RI: Teratogenic and postnatal developmental studies of morphine in Sprague-Dawley rats. Teratology 38:401-410, 1988. [A]

Geber WF: Effects of central nervous system active and nonactive drugs on the fetal central nervous system. Neurotoxicology 1:585-593, 1977. [A]

Geber WF, Schramm LC: Congenital malformations of the central nervous system produced by narcotic analgesics in the hamster. Amer J Obstet Gynecol 123:705-713, 1975. [A]

Harpel HS, Gautieri RF: Morphine-induced fetal malformations. I. Exencephaly and axial skeletal fusions. J Pharmaceut Sci 57:1590-1597, 1968. [A]

Heinonen OP, Slone D, Shapiro S: Birth Defects and Drugs in Pregnancy. Littleton, Mass.: John Wright-PSG, 1977, pp 287-288, 434, 484. [E]

Johnston HM, Payne AP, Gilmore DP: Perinatal exposure to morphine affects adult sexual behavior of the male golden hamster. Pharmacol Biochem Behav 42(1):41-44, 1992. [A]

Perlstein MA: Congenital morphinism. J Amer Med Assoc 10:633, 1947. [C]

Raye JR, Dubin JW, Blechner JN. Fetal growth retardation following maternal morphine administration: Nutritional or drug effect? Biol Neonate 32:222-228, 1977. [A]

Sobrian SK: Prenatal morphine administration alters behavioral development in the rat. Pharmacol Biochem Behav 7:285-288, 1977. [A]

Vathy I, Katay L: Effects of prenatal morphine on adult sexual behavior and brain catecholamines in rats. Brain Res Dev Brain Res 68(1):125-131, 1992. [A]

Vathy IU, Etgen AM, Barfield RJ: Effects of prenatal exposure to morphine on the development of sexual behavior in rats. Pharmacol Biochem Behav 22:227-232, 1985. [A]

Yamamoto H, Kuchii M, Hayano T, Nishino H: Study on teratogenicity of both CG-315 and morphine in mice and rats. Oyo Yakuri (Pharmacometrics) 6:1055-1069, 1972. [A]

Zagon IS, McLaughlin PJ: Effects of chronic morphine administration on pregnant rats and their offspring. Pharmacology 15:302-310, 1977. [A]

Zagon IS, Zagon E, McLaughlin PJ: Opioids and the developing organism: A comprehensive bibliography, 1984-1988. Neurosci Biobehav Rev 13:207-235, 1989. [R]

Zimmerberg B, Charap AD, Glick SD: Behavioural effects of in utero administration of morphine. Nature 247:376-377, 1974. [A]

MORRHUATE

Synonyms

Scleromate

Summary

Morrhuate is comprised of the fatty acids of cod-liver oil. Morrhuate is used as a sclerosant to treat varicose veins.

Magnitude of Teratogenic Risk

Undetermined

Quality and Quantity of Data

None

Comment

None

No epidemiological studies of congenital anomalies in infants whose mothers were treated with morrhuate during pregnancy have been reported.

No animal teratology studies of morrhuate have been published.

Key References

None available.

MOXALACTAM

Synonyms

Lamoxactam, Latamoxef, Latamoxefum, Moxam

Summary

Moxalactam is a beta-lactam antibiotic. It is used parenterally to treat serious infections.

Magnitude of Teratogenic Risk

Undetermined

Quality and Quantity of Data

None To Poor

Comment

A small risk cannot be excluded, but there is no indication that the risk of congenital anomalies in the children of women treated with moxalactam during pregnancy is likely to be great.

No epidemiological studies of congenital anomalies in infants born to women treated with moxalactam during pregnancy have been reported.

The frequency of congenital anomalies was no greater than expected among the offspring of mice or rats treated with moxalactam during pregnancy in doses respectively 3-12.5 and 6-25 times those used in humans (Harada et al., 1982). An increased frequency of abortion occurred in rabbits treated with moxalactam at doses <1-3 times those used in humans, but such doses were toxic to the mothers (Harada et al., 1982).

Key References

Harada Y, Kobayashi F, Muraoka Y, Hasegawa Y, et al.: An evaluation of the toxicity of moxalactam in laboratory animals. Rev Infect Dis 4(Suppl):S536-S545, 1982. [A]

MUMPS SKIN TEST ANTIGEN

Synonyms

MSTA

Summary

Mumps skin test antigen is a suspension of formaldehyde-inactivated mumps virus prepared from the allantoic fluid of virus-infected chick embryos. It is used intradermally to evaluate immunocompetence.

Magnitude of Teratogenic Risk

Undetermined

Quality and Quantity of Data

Poor

Comment

A small risk cannot be excluded, but a high risk of congenital anomalies in the children of women treated with mumps skin test antigen during pregnancy is unlikely.

No epidemiological studies of congenital anomalies in infants whose mothers were given mumps skin test antigen during pregnancy have been reported.

No animal teratology studies of mumps skin test antigen have been published.

Key References

None available.

MUMPS VIRUS

Summary

Mumps virus, the causative agent of mumps, is an RNA-containing paramyxovirus.

Magnitude of Teratogenic Risk

Minimal

Quality and Quantity of Data

Fair

Comment

None

The frequency of malformations was no greater than expected among the children of 117 women with documented histories of mumps during pregnancy (Siegel & Fuerst, 1966). In 24 of these cases the disease is said to have occurred in the first trimester. Similarly, the frequency of major congenital anomalies did not appear unusual among the children of 19 women with serological evidence of mumps virus infection during pregnancy, but at least 18 of these infections occurred during the second or third trimester (Korones et al., 1970). Only one congenital anomaly was found among 29 infants born to women reported to have had mumps during pregnancy in another series; 16 of these cases involved first trimester maternal disease (Hill et al., 1958). Various congenital anomalies have been observed in individual cases of infants born to women who had mumps during pregnancy, but no recurrent pattern of anomalies is apparent in these anecdotal reports (Gershon, 1990).

An association appears to exist between maternal mumps infection in the first four months of pregnancy and miscarriage (Gershon, 1990). Among 33 pregnancies prospectively identified because of maternal mumps during the first trimester, there were nine fetal deaths (27%), a rate significantly greater than expected (Siegel et al., 1966). Most of the fetal deaths occurred within two weeks of onset of the maternal disease. In a case in which miscarriage occurred at ten weeks gestation, four days after the development of mumps in the mother, mumps virus was isolated from the fetus (Kurtz et al., 1982).

An association between the occurrence of mumps virus infection during pregnancy and congenital myocardiopathy has been suggested on the basis of the observation of an increased frequency of positive skin test reactivity to mumps antigen among children with clinically diagnosed endocardial fibroelastosis (Noren et al., 1963; Sellers et al., 1964; Vosburgh et al., 1965; Shone et al., 1966; St. Geme et al., 1966; Gershon, 1990). This association was not found in other studies (Gersony et al., 1966; Nahmias & Armstrong, 1966) and no history of maternal mumps during pregnancy is usually elicitable in children with endocardial fibroelastosis who exhibit skin test sensitivity to mumps antigen. No cases of endocardial fibroelastosis were identified among the infants of 31 women with serologically proven mumps infection during pregnancy (Korones et al., 1970; Aase et al., 1972). It appears that if the association between maternal mumps during pregnancy and endocardial fibroelastosis is real, the risk is small, probably no more than a few percent (St. Geme et al., 1974).

Fetal infection has been produced after intra-amniotic or intravenous inoculation of rhesus monkeys with mumps virus during pregnancy (St. Geme & Van Pelt, 1974; Moreland et al., 1979). Obstructive hydrocephalus can be caused by inoculation of mumps virus into the cerebral ventricles of weanling hamsters or the amniotic sacs of fetal hamsters (Johnson & Johnson, 1967, 1968; Kilham & Margolis, 1975). Neonatal myocarditis has been observed in chicks inoculated in ovo with mumps virus (St. Geme et al., 1971). The relevance of these experimental manipulations to natural mumps infection in human pregnancy is uncertain.

Key References

Aase JM, Noren GR, Reddy DV, St. Geme JW: Mumps-virus infection in pregnant women and the immunologic response of their offspring. N Engl J Med 286:1379-1382, 1972. [E]

Gershon AA: Chickenpox, measles, and mumps. In: Remington JS, Klein JO (eds). Infectious Diseases of the Fetus and Newborn Infant. Philadelphia: W.B. Saunders Co., 1990, pp 395-445. [O]

Gersoney WM, Katz SL, Nadas AS: Endocardial fibroelastosis and the mumps virus. Pediatrics 37:430-434, 1966. [S]

Hill AB, Doll R, Galloway TM, Hughes JPW: Virus diseases in pregnancy and congenital defects. Br J Prev Soc Med 12:1-7, 1958. [S]

Johnson RT, Johnson KP: Hydrocephalus following viral infection: The pathology of aqueductal stenosis developing after experimental mumps virus infection. J Neuropathol Exp Neurol 27:591-606, 1968. [A]

Johnson RT, Johnson KP, Edmonds CJ: Virus-induced hydrocephalus: Development of aqueductal stenosis in hamsters after mumps infection. Science 157:1066-1067, 1967. [A]

Kilham L, Margolis G: Induction of congenital hydrocephalus in hamsters with attenuated and natural strains of mumps virus. J Infect Dis 132:462-466, 1972. [A]

Korones SB, Todaro J, Roane JA, Sever JL: Maternal virus infection after the first trimester of pregnancy and status of offspring to 4 years of age in a predominantly Negro population. J Pediatr 77:245-251, 1970. [E]

Kurtz JB, Tomlinson AH, Pearson J: Mumps virus isolated from a fetus. Br Med J 284:471, 1982. [C]

Moreland AF, Gaskin JM, Schimpff RD, Woodard JC, et al.: Effects of influenza, mumps, and western equine encephalitis viruses on fetal rhesus monkeys (Macaca mulatta). Teratology 20:53-64, 1979. [A]

Nahmias AJ, Armstrong G: Mumps virus and endocardial fibroelastosis. N Engl J Med 275:1448-1449, 1966. [S]

Noren GR, Adams P, Anderson RC: Positive skin reactivity to mumps virus antigen in endocardial fibroelastosis. J Pediatr 62:604-606, 1963. [S]

Sellers FJ, Keith JD, Manning JA: The diagnosis of primary endocardial fibroelastosis. Circulation 29:49-59, 1964. [S]

Shone JD, Armas SM, Manning JA, Keith JD: The mumps antigen skin test in endocardial fibroelastosis. Pediatrics 37:423-429, 1966. [E]

Siegel M, Fuerst HT: Low birth weight and maternal virus diseases. JAMA 197:680-684, 1966. [E]

Siegel M, Fuerst HT, Peress NS: Comparative fetal mortality in maternal virus diseases. N Engl J Med 274:768-771, 1966. [E]

St. Geme JW, Davis CWC, Noren GR: An overview of primary endocardial fibroelastosis and chronic viral cardiomyopathy. Perspect Biol Med pp 495-505, 1974. [O]

St. Geme JW, Noren GR, Adams P: Proposed embryopathic relation between mumps virus and primary endocardial fibroelastosis. N Engl J Med 275:339-347, 1966. [E]

St. Geme JW, Peralta H, Farias E, Davis CWC: Experimental gestational mumps virus infection and endocardial fibroelastosis. Pediatrics 48:821-826, 1971. [A]

St. Geme JW, Van Pelt LF: Fetal and postnatal growth retardation associated with gestational mumps virus infection of the rhesus monkey. Lab Anim Sci 24:895-899, 1974. [A]

Vosburgh JB, Diehl AM, Chien L, Lauer RM, et al.: Relationship of mumps to endocardial fibroelastosis. Amer J Dis Child 109:69-73, 1965. [E]

MUMPS VIRUS VACCINE

Synonyms

Mumpsvax

Summary

Mumps virus vaccine is a live attenuated virus vaccine that is used for immunization against mumps.

Magnitude of Teratogenic Risk

Undetermined

Quality and Quantity of Data

None

Comment

A small risk cannot be excluded, but a high risk of congenital anomalies in the children of women treated with mumps virus vaccine during pregnancy is unlikely.

No epidemiological studies of congenital anomalies in infants born to women who were inoculated with mumps virus vaccine during pregnancy have been reported.

No animal teratology studies of mumps virus vaccine have been published.

Please see agent summary on mumps virus.

Key References

None available.

MUPIROCIN

Synonyms

Bactroban, Pseudomonic Acid A

Summary

Mupirocin is an antibiotic that is used topically to treat bacterial skin infections. Mupirocin is poorly absorbed after topical application.

Magnitude of Teratogenic Risk

Undetermined

Quality and Quantity of Data

None

Comment

A small risk cannot be excluded, but a high risk of congenital anomalies in the children of women treated with mupirocin during pregnancy is unlikely.

No epidemiological studies of congenital anomalies in infants whose mothers were treated with mupirocin during pregnancy have been reported.

No animal teratology studies of mupirocin have been published.

Key References

None available.

MUROMONAB-CD3

Synonyms

Murine Monoclonal Antibody, OKT3, Orthoclone OKT3

Summary

Muromonab-CD3 is a murine monoclonal IgG2a antibody that reacts with the CD3, or T3, molecular complex of T-lymphocytes. It is administered intravenously in renal transplant patients to suppress acute allograft rejection.

Magnitude of Teratogenic Risk

Undetermined

Quality and Quantity of Data

None

Comment

None

No epidemiological studies of congenital anomalies among infants of women who were treated with muromonab-CD3 during pregnancy have been reported.

No animal teratology studies of muromonab-CD3 have been published.

Key References

None available.

NABILONE

Synonyms

Cesamet

Summary

Nabilone is a synthetic cannabinoid that is taken orally as an antiemetic during cancer chemotherapy.

Magnitude of Teratogenic Risk

Undetermined

Quality and Quantity of Data

None To Poor

Comment

A small risk cannot be excluded, but a high risk of congenital anomalies in the children of women treated with nabilone during pregnancy is unlikely.

No epidemiological studies of congenital anomalies among infants born to women treated with nabilone during pregnancy have been reported.

No teratogenic effect was observed among the offspring of rats or rabbits treated respectively with 10-120 or 7-33 times the usual human dose of nabilone during pregnancy (Markham et al., 1979). Dose-dependent decreases in liveborn litter size were observed in both species, however. The clinical significance of this observation is unknown.

Please see agent summary on marijuana for information on a related agent that has been studied.

Key References

Markham JK, Hanasono GK, Adams ER, Owen NV: Reproduction studies on nabilone, a synthetic 9-keto-cannabinoid. Toxicol Appl Pharmacol 48:A119, 1979. [A]

NADOLOL

Synonyms

Corgard

Summary

Nadolol is a beta-adrenergic receptor blocking agent used in the treatment of hypertension and angina pectoris

Magnitude of Teratogenic Risk

Undetermined

Quality and Quantity of Data

None To Poor

Comment

None

No epidemiological studies of congenital anomalies among infants born to women treated with nadolol during pregnancy have been reported.

The frequency of malformations was no greater than expected among the offspring of rats, hamsters, or rabbits treated during pregnancy with nadolol in doses respectively 16-160, 16-47, and 16-78 times those used in humans (Sibley et al., 1978; Saegusa et al., 1983; Stevens et al., 1984). Fetal growth retardation was observed among the rats and fetal death among the rabbits at the higher doses.

One infant with cardiorespiratory depression, hypoglycemia, and growth retardation born to a woman treated with nadolol throughout pregnancy had been reported (Fox et al., 1985). Similar neonatal effects have been observed among infants whose mothers were treated with propranolol during pregnancy.

Please see agent summary on propranolol for information on this closely related agent that has been more thoroughly studied.

Key References

Fox RE, Marx C, Stark AR: Neonatal effects of maternal nadolol therapy. Am J Obstet Gynecol 152:1045-1046, 1985. [C]

Saegusa T, Suzuki T, Narama I: Reproduction studies of nadolol a new beta-adrenergic blocking agent. Yakuri to Chiryo 11:5119-5138, 1983. [A]

Sibley PL, Peim GR, Kulesza JS, Murphy BF, et al.: Preclinical toxicologic evaluation of nadolol, a new beta-adrenergic antagonist. Toxicol Appl Pharmacol 44:379-389, 1978. [A]

Stevens AC, Keysser CH, Kulesza JS, Miller MM: Preclinical safety evaluations of the nadolol/bendroflumethiazide combination in mice, rats and dogs. Fund Appl Toxicol 4:360-369, 1984. [A]

NAFCILLIN

Synonyms

Nafcil, Naftopen, Nallpen, Naphthicillin, Unipen

Summary

Nafcillin is an antibiotic used to treat penicillin resistant staphylococcal infections.

Magnitude of Teratogenic Risk

Undetermined

Quality and Quantity of Data

None To Poor

Comment

A small risk cannot be excluded, but there is no indication that the risk of congenital anomalies in the children of women treated with nafcillin during pregnancy is likely to be great.

No epidemiological studies of congenital anomalies in infants born to women treated with nafcillin during pregnancy have been reported.

No teratogenic effect was observed among the offspring of mice or rats treated during pregnancy with 5-20 or 5-40 times the usual human dose of nafcillin (Mizutani et al., 1970).

Please see agent summary on penicillin for information on a closely related drug that has been more thoroughly studied.

Key References

Mizutani M, Ihara T, Kanamori H, Takatani O, et al.: [Influence of sodium nafcillin upon the developing fetuses of mice and rats]. J Takeda Res Lab 29:283-296, 1970. [A]

NAFTIFINE

Synonyms

Naftin

Summary

Naftifine is an antifungal agent.

Magnitude of Teratogenic Risk

Undetermined

Quality and Quantity of Data

None

Comment

None

No epidemiological studies of congenital anomalies in infants born to women treated with naftifine during pregnancy have been reported.

No animal teratology studies of naftifine have been published.

Key References

None available.

NALBUPHINE

Synonyms

Nubain

Summary

Nalbuphine is a narcotic analgesic used parenterally.

Magnitude of Teratogenic Risk

Undetermined

Quality and Quantity of Data

None

Comment

None

No epidemiological studies of congenital anomalies in infants born to women who took nalbuphine during pregnancy have been reported.

No animal teratology studies of nalbuphine have been published.

Transient neonatal respiratory depression has been observed among infants born to women treated with nalbuphine shortly before delivery (Guillonneau et al., 1990; Sgro et al., 1990).

Please see agent summary on codeine for information on a related drug that has been more thoroughly studied.

Key References

Guillonneau M, Jacqz-Aigrain E, de Crepy A, et al.: Perinatal adverse effects of nalbuphine given during parturition. Lancet 335:1588, 1990. [C]

Sgro C, Escousse A, Tennenbaum D, et al.: Perinatal adverse effects of nalbuphine given during labor. Lancet 336:1070, 1990. [C]

NALIDIXIC ACID

Synonyms

Betaxina, Mictral, Nalidixinic acid, Nalidixol, Nalurin, Neg-Gram, NegGram, Uriben, Wintomylon

Summary

Nalidixic acid is an antibacterial agent of the 4-quinolone class. It is administered orally in the treatment of urinary tract infections.

Magnitude of Teratogenic Risk

None To Minimal

Quality and Quantity of Data

Poor To Fair

Comment

None

No epidemiological studies of congenital anomalies among infants born to women treated with nalidixic acid during pregnancy have been reported. No adverse effects were noted among the children of 63 women treated with nalidixic acid during pregnancy in one clinical series (Murray, 1981). Treatment occurred during the first trimester in six of these cases, during the second trimester in 26, and during the third trimester in 31.

The frequency of congenital anomalies was no greater than expected among the offspring of rabbits treated during pregnancy with nalidixic acid in doses <1-1.5 those used in humans; fetal growth retardation was seen with the higher dose (Pagnini et al., 1971). Similarly, no increase in the frequency of congenital anomalies was observed among the offspring of pregnant rats treated with <1 to almost 4 times the usual human dose of nalidixic acid (Pagnini et al., 1971; Sato et al., 1980a, b). Stillbirth and neonatal death were unusually frequent at the highest dose.

Intracranial hypertension, which has been reported in children given nalidixic acid, is a theoretical risk in infants born to women treated with this agent late in pregnancy.

Key References

Murray EDS: Nalidixic acid in pregnancy. Br Med J 282:224, 1981. [S]
Pagnini G, Pelagalli GV, Di Carlo F: Effect of nalidixic acid on the chick embryo and on pregnancy and embryonic development in rabbits and rats. Atti Soc Ital Sci Vet 25:137-140, 1971. [A]
Sato T, Kaneko Y, Saegusa T: Reproduction studies of cinoxacin in rats. Chemotherapy 28(Suppl 4):484-507, 1980. [A]
Sato T, Kobayashi F: Teratological study on cinoxacin in rabbits. Chemotherapy 28(Suppl 4):508-515, 1980. [A]

NALOXONE

Synonyms

Nalonee, Nalossone, Narcan

Summary

Naloxone is a narcotic antagonist. It is given parenterally in the treatment of respiratory depression and toxicity due to narcotics.

Magnitude of Teratogenic Risk

Undetermined

Quality and Quantity of Data

Poor

Comment

A small risk cannot be excluded, but a high risk of congenital anomalies in the children of women treated with naloxone during pregnancy is unlikely.

No epidemiological studies of congenital anomalies among infants born to women

treated with naloxone during pregnancy have been reported.

No teratogenic effect was observed among the offspring of mice or hamsters treated during pregnancy with naloxone in doses 2500-20,000 times or 9200-28,800 times those used as single injections in humans (Geber & Schramm, 1975; Jurand, 1985). Behavioral alterations were seen among the offspring of rats treated during pregnancy with naloxone in doses of 100-2000 times those used as a single injection in humans (Vorhees, 1981; Shepanek et al., 1989). The clinical significance of this observation is unknown.

Naloxone has been used to reverse neonatal respiratory depression related to maternal narcotic analgesia during delivery (Clark et al., 1976).

Key References

Clark RB, Beard AG, Greifenstein FE, Barclay DL: Naloxone in the parturient and her infant. South Med J 69:570-575, 1976. [E]

Geber WF, Schramm LC: Congenital malformations of the central nervous system produced by narcotic analgesics in the hamster. Am J Obstet Gynecol 123:705-713, 1975. [A]

Jurand A: The interference of naloxone hydrochloride in the teratogenic activity of opiates. Teratology 31:235-240, 1985. [A]

Shepanek NA, Smith RF, Tyer ZE, et al.: Behavioral and neuroanatomical sequelae of prenatal naloxone administration in the rat. Neurotoxicol Teratol 11:441-446, 1989. [A]

Vorhees CV: Effects of prenatal naloxone exposure on postnatal behavioral development of rats. Neurobehav Toxicol Teratol 3:295-301, 1981. [A]

NALTREXONE

Synonyms

Trexan

Summary

Naltrexone is a narcotic antagonist that is adminstered orally in the treatment of opioid dependence.

Magnitude of Teratogenic Risk

Undetermined

Quality and Quantity of Data

None To Poor

Comment

None

No epidemiological studies of congenital anomalies among infants born to women treated with naltrexone during pregnancy have been reported.

The frequency of malformations was not increased among the offspring of rats or rabbits treated with 20-200 times the usual human dose of naltrexone during pregnancy (Nuite et al., 1975; Christian, 1984). Long-lasting behavioral alterations were noted among the offspring of mice treated with 1-4 times the usual human dose of naltrexone during pregnancy (D'Amato et al., 1988).

Key References

Christian MS: Reproductive toxicity and teratology evaluations of naltrexone. J Clin Psychiatry 45:7-10, 1984. [A]

D'Amato FR, Castellano C, Ammassari-Teule M, Oliverio A: Prenatal antagonism of stress by naltrexone administration: Early and long-lasting effects on emotional behaviors in mice. Dev Psychobiol 21(3):283-292, 1988. [A]

Nuite JA, Kennedy GL, Smith S, Keplinger ML, et al.: Reproductive and teratogenic studies with naltrexone in rats and rabbits. Toxicol Appl Pharmacol 33:173-174, 1975. [A]

NANDROLONE

Synonyms

Androlone, Deca-Durabolin, Durabolin, Dyn-abolon, Hybolin Decanoate, Nandrobolic, Nortestosterone Decanoate

Summary

Nandrolone is an androgenic and anabolic steroid. It is administered parenterally in the treatment of metastatic breast cancer and ure-mic anemia. It has also been used to attempt to enhance athletic performance.

Magnitude of Teratogenic Risk

Undetermined

Quality and Quantity of Data

None To Poor

Comment

1) The androgenic effect of nandrolone would be expected to cause virilization of the genitalia in female fetuses.

2) Although the risk of this agent is unknown, it may be substantial because of its androgenic effect.

No epidemiological studies of congenital anomalies among infants born to women treated with nandrolone during pregnancy have been reported.

Increased frequencies of fetal loss were observed in pregnant rats treated daily with 0.5-2.5 times the usual human dose of nandrolone (Naqvi & Warren, 1971).

Key References

Naqvi RH, Warren JC: Interceptives: Drugs interrupting pregnancy after implantation. Steroids 18:731-739, 1971. [A]

NAPHAZOLINE

Synonyms

Albalon, Comfort Eye Drops, Degest-2, Na-phcon, Privine, Vasoclear, Vasocon

Summary

Naphazoline is a sympathomimetic vasocon-strictor used by nasal instillation to treat rhinitis and sinusitis and in an ophthalmic solution as a conjunctival decongestant. Systemic absorp-tion can occur following topical application of naphazoline.

Magnitude of Teratogenic Risk

Undetermined

Quality and Quantity of Data

None

Comment

A small risk cannot be excluded, but a high risk of congenital anomalies in the children of women treated with naphazoline during pregnancy is unlikely.

No epidemiological studies of congenital anomalies among infants born to women who used naphazoline during pregnancy have been reported.

No animal teratology studies of napha-zoline have been published.

Please see agent summary on ephedrine for information on a related agent.

Key References

None available.

NAPROXEN

Synonyms

Anaprox, Naprosyn, Naprosyne, Proxine, Synflex

Summary

Naproxen is a non-steroidal anti-inflammatory agent with analgesic and antipyretic actions.

Magnitude of Teratogenic Risk

Undetermined

Quality and Quantity of Data

Poor

Comment

1) A small risk cannot be excluded, but there is no indication that the risk of congenital anomalies in the children of women treated with naproxen during pregnancy is likely to be great.

2) Maternal use of naproxen just before delivery may be associated with abnormalities of neonatal cardiovascular adaptation (see below).

No epidemiological studies of congenital anomalies among infants born to women treated with naproxen during pregnancy have been reported.

Dose-dependent increases in the frequencies of cleft palate and fetal death were observed among the offspring of pregnant mice treated with naproxen in doses similar to those used in humans (Montenegro & Palomino, 1990). No such effect was seen with similar doses in mice or rats in another study (Kuramoto et al., 1973). Increased frequencies of fetal death but not of congenital anomalies were observed among the offspring of pregnant mice and rabbits treated with naproxen in doses at or just above the maximum used in humans in a study that has not been reported in detail (Hallesy et al., 1973).

Naproxen is an inhibitor of prostaglandin synthesis. This class of drugs has been used therapeutically to produce closure of the ductus arteriosus and consequent changes in cardiovascular and pulmonary function in newborns with patent ductus arteriosus. Persistent pulmonary hypertension and premature closure of the ductus arteriosus have been reported in infants whose mothers took naproxen just before delivery (Wilkinson et al., 1979, Wilkinson, 1980). Constriction of the ductus arteriosus was observed among the offspring of pregnant rats treated at term with naproxen in doses similar to those used in humans (Momma & Takeuchi, 1983).

Several prostaglandin inhibitors, including naproxen, have been shown to delay labor in rats and hamsters (Vickery, 1979). A similar action appears to occur in humans with naproxen (Csapo et al., 1974) and pharmacologically related drugs (Grella & Zanor, 1978).

Please see agent summary on indomethacin for information on a related agent that has been more thoroughly studied.

Key References

Csapo AI, Henzl MR, Kaihola HL, Kivikoski A, et al.: Suppression of uterine activity and abortion by inhibition of prostaglandin synthesis. Prostaglandins 7:39-47, 1974. [E]

Grella P, Zanor P: Premature labor and indomethacin. Prostaglandins 16:1007-1017, 1978. [S]

Hallesy DW, Shott LD, Hill R: Comparative toxicology of naproxen. Scand J Rheumatol (Suppl 2):20-28, 1973. [A]

Kuramoto M, Ishimura Y, Daikoku S, Hashimoto T: Studies on teratogenicity of naproxen on mice and rats. Shikoku Igaku Zasshi 29:465-470, 1973. [A]

Momma K, Takeuchi H: Constriction of fetal ductus arteriosus by non-steroidal anti-inflammatory drugs. Prostaglandins 26:631-643, 1983. [A]

Montenegro MA, Palomino H: Induction of cleft palate in mice by inhibitors of prostaglandin synthesis. J Craniofac Genet Dev Biol 10:83-94, 1990. [A]

Vickery B: Prolongation of gestation in the rat and hamster by naproxen. Prostaglandins Med 2:325-335, 1979. [A]

Wilkinson AR: Naproxen levels in preterm infants after maternal treatment. Lancet 2:591-592, 1980. [C]

Wilkinson AR, Aynsley-Green A, Mitchell MD: Persistent pulmonary hypertension and abnormal prostaglandin E levels in preterm infants after maternal treatment with naproxen. Arch Dis Child 54:942-945, 1979. [C]

NARCOBARBITAL

Synonyms

Enibomal

Summary

Narcobarbital is a barbiturate that has been used as an intravenous general anesthetic.

Magnitude of Teratogenic Risk

Undetermined

Quality and Quantity of Data

None

Comment

None

No epidemiological studies of congenital anomalies in children born to women exposed to narcobarbital during pregnancy have been reported.

No investigations of teratologic effects of narcobarbital in experimental animals have been published.

Please see agent summary on thiopental for information on a related agent that has been more thoroughly studied.

Key References

None available.

NEOMYCIN

Synonyms

Burn-Gel, Fradiomycin Sulphate, Mycifradin Sterile Powder, Myciguent Ointment, Neocin

Summary

Neomycin is a broad-spectrum antibiotic used topically in a variety of skin and mucous membrane infections. An oral preparation, which is poorly absorbed, is used to kill bowel flora in preparation for surgery or in treatment of hepatic coma.

Magnitude of Teratogenic Risk

None

Quality and Quantity of Data

Poor To Fair

Comment

None

The Collaborative Perinatal Project included 30 pregnancies exposed to neomycin during the first trimester. The frequency of malformations among the offspring of these pregnancies was no greater than expected (Heinonen et al., 1977).

The frequency of malformations was not increased among the offspring of pregnant mice given drinking water containing 4 g/l of neomycin (Skalko & Gold, 1974). No teratogenic effect was observed among the offspring of pregnant rats given twice the human dose of neomycin orally (Takeno & Sakai, 1991). Decreased hearing was seen among the offspring of pregnant rats given intramuscular injections of neomycin in a dose similar to that used orally in humans (Kameyama et al., 1982).

Key References

Heinonen OP, Slone D, Shapiro S: Birth Defects and Drugs in Pregnancy. Littleton, Mass.: John Wright-PSG, 1977, p 297. [S]

Kameyama T, Nabeshima T, Itoh J: Measurement of an auditory impairment induced by prenatal administration of aminoglycosides using a shuttle box method. Folia Pharmacol Jpn 80:525-535, 1982. [A]

Skalko RG, Gold MP: Teratogenicity of methotrexate in mice. Teratology 9:159-164, 1974. [A]

Takeno S, Sakai T: Involvement of the intestinal microflora in nitrazepam-induced teratogenicity in rats and its relationship to nitroreduction. Teratology 44:209-214, 1991. [A]

NEOSTIGMINE

Synonyms

Intrastigmina, Juvastigmin, Proserinum, Prostigmin, Synstigmine Bromide

Summary

Neostigmine is a parasympathomimetic agent that is used in the diagnosis and treatment of myasthenia gravis. Neostigmine is also used to relieve paralytic ileus and postoperative urinary retention.

Magnitude of Teratogenic Risk

None To Minimal

Quality and Quantity of Data

Poor To Fair

Comment

None

The frequency of congenital anomalies was no greater than expected among the children of 22 women treated with neostigmine during the first trimester of pregnancy in the Collaborative Perinatal Project (Heinonen et al., 1977).

Malformations were found no more often than expected among the offspring of rats treated with 16-166 times the usual human dose of neostigmine during pregnancy (Brock et al., 1967).

Key References

Brock VN, Lenke D, Abel HH: On the pharmacology and toxicology of the spasmolytic B-Diethylaminoethyl-(alpha-methyl-2,5-endomethylene delta3-tetrahydrobenzohydryl)-ether-brommethylate. Arzneimittelforsch 17:1005-1112, 1967. [S]

Heinonen OP, Slone D, Shapiro S: Birth Defects and Drugs in Pregnancy. Littleton, Mass.: John Wright-PSG, 1977, pp 346-347. [E]

NETILMICIN

Synonyms

Certomycin, Netillin, Netilyn, Netrocin, Netromicine, Netromycin, Nettacin, Zetamicin

Summary

Netilmicin is an aminoglycoside antibiotic that is given parenterally to treat bacterial infections.

Magnitude of Teratogenic Risk

Undetermined

Quality and Quantity of Data

Poor

A small risk cannot be excluded, but a high risk of congenital anomalies in the children of women treated with netilmicin during pregnancy is unlikely.

No epidemiological studies of congenital anomalies among infants born to women treated with netilmicin during pregnancy have been reported.

The frequency of malformations was no greater than expected among the offspring of rats or rabbits treated during pregnancy with netilmicin in doses 5-20 times those usually employed in humans (Bamonte et al., 1979; Weinberg et al., 1981). Nephrotoxicity was observed among the offspring of pregnant rats treated with 12 times the usual human dose of netilmicin. The clinical significance of this observation is unknown.

Please see agent summary on streptomycin for information on a related agent that has been more thoroughly studied.

Key References

Bamonte F, Albiero L, Ongini E: Reproductive and teratological studies with a new aminoglycoside: Netilmicin (Sch 20569). Acta Pharmacol et Toxicol 45:145-151, 1979. [A]

Weinberg EH, Field, WE, Gray WD, Klein MF, et al.: Preclinical toxicologic studies of netilmicin. Arzneimittelforsch 31:816-822, 1981. [A]

NIACIN

Synonyms

Nico-400, Nicobid, Nicolar, Nicotinex, Nicotinic Acid

Summary

Niacin is a vitamin of the B complex. It occurs naturally in many foods. Niacin is used in doses 200-400 times the recommended daily allowance to treat hyperlipidemia.

Magnitude of Teratogenic Risk

Undetermined

Quality and Quantity of Data

None

Comment

A small risk cannot be excluded, but there is no indication that the risk of congenital anomalies in the children of women treated with niacin during pregnancy is likely to be great.

No epidemiological studies of congenital anomalies in infants born to mothers who took niacin in pharmacological doses have been reported.

No studies of the teratogenicity of therapeutic or greater doses of niacin in mammals have been published. Fetal resorption occurred in pregnant rats maintained on a niacin-deficient diet (Fratta et al., 1964; Fratta, 1969).

Key References

Fratta ID: Nicotinamide deficiency and thalidomide: Potential teratogenic disturbances in Long-Evans rats. Lab Anim Care 19(5):727-732, 1969. [A]

Fratta I, Zak SB, Greengard P, et al.: Fetal death from nicotinamide-deficient diet and its prevention by chlorpromazine and imipramine. Science 145:1429-1430, 1964. [A]

NIACINAMIDE

Synonyms

Nicotinamide, Nicotinic Acid Amide, Nicotylamide, Vitamin PP

Summary

Niacinamide is a water-soluble vitamin of the B complex that occurs naturally in many foods.

Doses of more than 30 times the recommended daily allowance are used to treat pellagra.

Magnitude of Teratogenic Risk

Undetermined

Quality and Quantity of Data

Poor

Comment

None

The frequency of maternal use of vitamin supplements containing niacinamide during the first 56 days of pregnancy was greater than expected among 458 infants with congenital anomalies in a retrospective case-control study (Nelson & Forfar, 1971); but this result may be spurious because it may have arisen from multiple comparisons in the study.

No teratogenic effect was observed among the offspring of rats or mice treated during pregnancy with 25 or 45 times the human therapeutic dose of niacinamide (Beaudoin, 1973; Smithberg & Runner, 1963).

Key References

Beaudoin AR: Teratogenic activity of 2-amino-1,3,4-thiadiazole hydrochloride in Wistar rats and the protection afforded by nicotinamide. Teratology 7:65-72, 1973. [A]

Fratta ID: Nicotinamide deficiency and thalidomide: Potential teratogenic disturbances in Long-Evans rats. Lab Anim Care 19(5):727-732, 1969. [A]

Fratta I, Zak SB, Greengard P, et al.: Fetal death from nicotinamide-deficient diet and its prevention by chlorpromazine and imipramine. Science 145:1429-1430, 1964. [A]

Nelson MM, Forfar JO: Associations between drugs administered during pregnancy and congenital abnormalities of the fetus. Br Med J 1:523-527, 1971. [E]

Smithberg M, Runner MN: Teratogenic effects of hypoglycemic treatments in inbred strains of mice. Am J Anat 113:479-489, 1963. [A]

NICLOSAMIDE

Synonyms

Cestocida, Niclocide, Sulqui, Tredemine, Vermitid, Yomesan

Summary

Niclosamide is an anthelmintic agent that is administered orally in the treatment of tapeworms. Niclosamide is not appreciably absorbed from the gastrointestinal tract.

Magnitude of Teratogenic Risk

Undetermined

Quality and Quantity of Data

None

Comment

None

No epidemiological studies of congenital anomalies in infants born to women who were treated with niclosamide during pregnancy have been reported.

No animal teratology studies of niclosamide have been published.

Key References

None available.

NIFEDIPINE

Synonyms

Adalate, Felodipine, Hydialazine, Nifedipinum, Nifelat, Nitroendipine, Procardia

Summary

Nifedipine is a calcium channel-blocking agent used as a vasodilator in the treatment of hypertension and angina pectoris. Nifedipine has also been used to arrest premature labor.

Magnitude of Teratogenic Risk

Undetermined

Quality and Quantity of Data

None To Poor

Comment

None

No epidemiological studies of congenital anomalies among infants born to women treated with nifedipine during pregnancy have been reported.

No treatment-related adverse effect was observed among the infants of women treated in the second or third trimester of gestation with nifedipine for preterm labor or pregnancy-induced hypertension (Read & Wellby, 1986; Ferguson et al., 1990; Meyer et al., 1990; Bracero et al., 1991; Fenakel et al., 1991).

Increased frequencies of skeletal and cardiovascular malformations have been seen among the offspring of rats treated with nifedipine during pregnancy in doses 9-62 times those used in humans (Cabov & Palka, 1984; Yoshida et al., 1988). Distal digital hypoplasia was observed with increased frequency among the offspring of rabbits treated with 3.5-14 times the human therapeutic dose of nifedipine during pregnancy (Danielsson et al., 1989, 1992).

Delayed parturition occurs in rats treated during labor with nifedipine in doses similar to those used in humans (Hahn et al., 1984; Tracy & Black, 1992). Evidence of dose-dependent cardiac failure was observed among the offspring of pregnant rats treated just prior to delivery with <1-4 times the human dose of nifedipine (Momma & Takao, 1989). Decreased fetal and placental weight were ob-

served among the offspring of rats treated during late pregnancy with 4-10 times the human dose of nifedipine (Furuhashi et al., 1991).

Key References

Bracero LA, Leikin E, Kirshenbaum N, Tejani N: Comparison of nifedipine and ritodrine for the treatment of preterm labor. Am J Perinatol 8(6):365-369, 1991. [E]

Cabov AN, Palka E: Some effects of Cordipin (nifedipine) administered during pregnancy in the rats. Teratology 29(3):21A, 1984. [A]

Danielsson BRG, Danielson M, Rundqvist E, Reiland S: Identical phalangeal defects induced by phenytoin and nifedipine suggest fetal hypoxia and vascular disruption behind phenytoin teratogenicity. Teratology 45:247-258, 1992. [A]

Danielsson BRG, Reiland S, Rundqvist E, Danielson M: Digital defects induced by vasodilating agents: Relationship to reduction in uteroplacental blood flow. Teratology 40:351-358, 1989. [A]

Fenakel K, Fenakel G, Appelman ZVI, et al.: Nifedipine in the treatment of severe preeclampsia. Obstet Gynecol 77:331-337, 1991. [E]

Ferguson JE, Dyson DC, Schutz T, Stevenson DK: A comparison of tocolysis with nifedipine or ritodrine: Analysis of efficacy and maternal, fetal, and neonatal outcome. Am J Obstet Gynecol 163:105-111, 1990. [E]

Furuhashi N, Tsujiei M, Kimura H, Yajima A: Effects of nifedipine on normotensive rat placental blood flow, placental weight and fetal weight. Gynecol Obstet Invest 32:1-3, 1991. [A]

Hahn DW, McGuire JL, Vanderhoof M, et al.: Evaluation of drugs for arrest of premature labor in a new animal model. Am J Obstet Gynecol 148:775-778, 1984. [A]

Meyer WR, Randall HW, Graves WL: Nifedipine versus ritodrine for suppressing preterm labor. J Reprod Med 35:649-653, 1990. [E]

Momma K, Takao A: Fetal cardiovascular effects of nifedipine in rats. Pediatr Res 26(5):442-447, 1989. [A]

Read MD, Wellby DE: The use of a calcium antagonist (nifedipine) to suppress preterm labour. Br J Obstet Gynaecol 93:933-937, 1986. [E]

Tracy TS, Black CD: Ability of nifedipine to prolong parturition in rats. J Reprod Fert 95:139-144, 1992. [A]

Yoshida T, Kanamori S, Hasegawa Y: Hyperphalangeal bones induced in rat pups by maternal treatment with nifedipine. Toxicol Lett 40:127-132, 1988. [A]

NIFURATEL

Synonyms

Macmiror, Magmilor, Methylmercadone, Nifuratel, Polmiror, Tydantil

Summary

Nifuratel is an antimicrobial agent used to treat candidal and trichomonal infections of the genitourinary tract.

Magnitude of Teratogenic Risk

None To Minimal

Quality and Quantity of Data

None To Poor

Comment

None

No epidemiological studies of congenital anomalies in infants whose mothers were treated with nifuratel during pregnancy have been reported.

The frequency of malformations was not greater than expected among the offspring of mice, rats, or rabbits treated respectively with 13, 13, and 7 times the usual human dose of nifuratel during pregnancy (Scuri, 1966).

Key References

Scuri R: [Toxicological study of methylmercadone n(nitro-5'furfurylidene-2') amino-3 methylmercaptomethyl-5 oxazolidinone-2. Chim Ther March-April:181-189, 1966. [A]

NIFURMERONE

Synonyms

Metofurone, NF-71

Summary

Nifurmerone is an antifungal.

Magnitude of Teratogenic Risk

Undetermined

Quality and Quantity of Data

None

Comment

None

No epidemiological studies of congenital anomalies in infants born to women who used nifurmerone during pregnancy have been reported.

No animal teratology studies of nifurmerone have been published.

Key References

None available.

NIKETHAMIDE

Synonyms

Cardamin, Coramine, Corazon, Kardonyl, Niamine, Nicamide, Nicorine, Nicotinoyldiaethylamidum, Percoral

Summary

Nikethamide is a central nervous system stimulant that is used in the treatment of respiratory depression.

Magnitude of Teratogenic Risk

Undetermined

Quality and Quantity of Data

None

Comment

None

No epidemiological studies of congenital anomalies among the infants of women treated with nikethamide during pregnancy have been reported.

No teratological studies of nikethamide in experimental mammals have been published.

Key References

None available.

NITRALAMINE

Synonyms

CS-12350

Summary

Nitralamine is an antifungal agent.

Magnitude of Teratogenic Risk

Undetermined

Quality and Quantity of Data

None

Comment

None

No epidemiological studies of congenital anomalies in infants born to women who used nitralamine during pregnancy have been reported.

No animal teratology studies of nitralamine have been published.

Key References

None available.

NITROFURANTOIN

Synonyms

Furadantin, Furadoninum, Furan, Macrodantin, Urantoin

Summary

Nitrofurantoin is an antimicrobial agent used frequently in prophylaxis and treatment of urinary tract infections.

Magnitude of Teratogenic Risk

None To Minimal

Quality and Quantity of Data

Poor To Fair

Comment

None

The Collaborative Perinatal Project included 83 women who took nitrofurantoin during the first trimester of pregnancy and 590 women who took the drug anytime during pregnancy. The frequency of congenital abnormalities in the children of these women was no greater than expected (Heinonen et al., 1977).

The frequency of malformations was not increased among the offspring of pregnant rats and rabbits given 2-6 times the usual human dose of nitrofurantoin (Prytherch et al., 1984). The frequency of malformations was slightly but significantly increased among the offspring of mice given nitrofurantoin during pregnancy in doses about 50 times greater than those used clinically (Nomura et al., 1976). The relevance of this finding to the risks associated with therapeutic use of nitrofurantoin in human pregnancy is unknown.

Key References

Heinonen OP, Slone D, Shapiro S: Birth Defects and Drugs in Pregnancy. Littleton, Mass.: John Wright-PSG, 1977, pp 435, 486. [E]

Nomura T, Kimura S, Isa Y, Tanaka H, et al.: Teratogenic effects of some antimicrobial agents on mouse embryo. Teratology 14:250, 1976. [A]

Prytherch JP, Sutton ML, Denine EP: General reproduction, perinatal-postnatal, and teratology studies of nitrofurantoin macrocrystals in rats and rabbits. J Toxicol Environ Health 13:811-823, 1984. [A]

NITROFURAZONE

Synonyms

Acutol, Becafurazone, Furacilinum, Furacin, Furacine, Furesol, Germex, Nitrofural, Rivafurazon

Summary

Nitrofurazone is a nitrofuran derivative with antibacterial and antiprotozoal activity. It is used topically in the prevention and treatment of infections.

Magnitude of Teratogenic Risk

None To Minimal

Quality and Quantity of Data

Poor To Fair

Comment

None

The frequencies of congenital anomalies in general, of major malformations, and of minor anomalies were not increased among the children of 234 women treated topically with nitrofurazone during the first four lunar months of pregnancy in the Collaborative Perinatal Project (Heinonen et al., 1977).

Increased frequencies of skeletal malformations were observed among the offspring of mice given injections of nitrofurazone during pregnancy in a dose of 300 mg/kg (Nomura et al., 1984). No such effect was seen among the offspring of animals treated systemically with 6-100 mg/kg/d, although a dose-dependent decrease in fetal weight was noted (Nomura et al., 1984; Price et al., 1985). The relevance of these observations to the clinical use of topical nitrofurazone in human pregnancy is uncertain.

Please see nitrofurantoin summary for information on a related agent.

Key References

Heinonen OP, Slone D, Shapiro S: Birth Defects and Drugs in Pregnancy. Littleton, Mass.: John Wright-PSG, 1977, pp 300, 302, 309, 311. [E]

Nomura T, Kimura S, Kanzaki T, Tanaka H, et al.: Induction of tumors and malformations in mice after prenatal treatment with some antibiotic drugs. Med J Osaka Univ 35:13-17, 1984. [A]

Price CJ, George JD, Marr MC: Teratologic evaluation of nitrofurazone (CAS No. 59-87-0) administered to CD-1 mice on gestational days 6 through 15. NTIS (National Technical Information Service) Report/PB86-145844, 1985. [A]

NITROGLYCERIN

Synonyms

Glyceryl Trinitrate, Nitro-Bid, Nitro-Dur, Nitroglycerol, Nitroglyn, Nitrol, Nitrolingual, Nitrostat, Transderm-Nitro, Tridil

Summary

Nitroglycerin is a smooth muscle relaxant used to treat angina pectoris and cardiac failure.

Magnitude of Teratogenic Risk

Undetermined

Quality and Quantity of Data

Poor

Comment

None

No epidemiological studies of congenital anomalies among infants born to women treated with nitroglycerin during pregnancy have been reported.

The frequency of malformations was not increased among the offspring of rats or rabbits injected with 2-50 times or 1-10 times the usual human dose of nitroglycerin during pregnancy (Oketani et al., 1981a, b). Similarly, the frequency of malformations was not increased among the offspring of pregnant rats or rabbits treated with nitroglycerin ointment in doses 2.5-1170 times those used in humans (Sato et al., 1984a, b; Miller et al., 1985; Skutt et al., 1985; Imoto et al., 1986).

Key References

Imoto S, Nakao M, Kuramoto M, et al.: Teratological test of 10% nitroglycerin (NT-1 ointment) in rabbits. J Toxicol Sci 11(Suppl 2):59-70, 1986. [A]

Miller LG, Schardein J, Matsubara Y, Ohgo T: Teratology study of nitroglycerin ointment by dermal administration in rabbits. Shin'yaku to Rinsho 34:2024-2032, 1985. [A]

Oketani Y, Mitsuzono T, Ichikawa K, Itono Y, et al.: Toxicological studies on nitroglycerin (NK-843) (6) Teratological study in rabbits. Oyo Yakuri 22:633-638, 1981b. [A]

Oketani Y, Mitsuzono T, Ichikawa K, Itono Y, et al.: Toxicological studies on nitroglycerin (NK-843) (8) Teratological study in rats. Oyo Yakuri 22:737-751, 1981a. [A]

Sato K, Taniguchi H, Himeno Y, Hoshino K, et al.: Toxicity studes of nitroglycerin. 8. Cutaneous

Sato K, Taniguchi H, Ohtsuka T, Himeno Y, et al.: Toxicity studies of nitroglycerin. 7. Cutaneous administration during organogenesis in rats. Kiso To Rinsho(Clin Rep) 18:3525-3552, 1984a. [A]

Skutt VM, Schardein J, Matsubara Y, Ohgo T: Teratology study of nitroglycerin oitment by dermal administration in rats. Shin'yaku to Rinsho 34:2009-2023, 1985. [A]

NITROUS OXIDE

Synonyms

Dinitrogen Oxide, Laughing Gas, Nitrogen Monoxide, Stickoxydul, Xenon

Summary

Nitrous oxide is a general anesthetic administered by inhalation. Occupational exposure to nitrous oxide may occur among operating room personnel, dentists, and veterinarians. The occupational exposure limit for nitrous oxide as an 8 hour time-weighted average is 50 ppm (91 mg/cu m) (Hathaway et al., 1991).

Magnitude of Teratogenic Risk

Occupational Exposure: None To Minimal

Anesthesia: None To Minimal

Quality and Quantity of Data

Occupational Exposure: Fair

Anesthesia: Fair

Comment

None

The frequency of congenital anomalies was no greater than expected among the children of 76 women who were anesthetized with nitrous oxide during the first four lunar months of pregnancy in the Collaborative Perinatal Project (Heinonen et al., 1977). The frequency of congenital anomalies was not increased among 94 children whose mothers received a brief period of inhalational anesthesia with nitrous oxide during the first 12 weeks of gestation or among 405 infants born to women who had brief inhalational anesthesia including nitrous oxide during the first two trimesters of pregnancy in another cohort study (Crawford & Lewis, 1986). Congenital anomalies did not appear to be unusually frequent among a series of children born of 175 pregnancies in which the mother received a brief nitrous oxide anesthetic (Aldridge & Tunstall, 1986). Only 3% of these exposures occurred during the first trimester of gestation; the others were in the second trimester.

The frequency of spontaneous abortion was no greater than expected among 352 pregnancies in dental assistants with occupational exposure to nitrous oxide (Heidam, 1984). No association with occupational exposure to nitrous oxide during pregnancy was observed in a case-control study of 77 women veterinarians and 85 women veterinarian assistants who had had spontaneous abortions (Johnson et al., 1987). Similarly, there was no association with occupational nitrous oxide exposure during the first trimester of pregnancy among 31 women veterinarians who had children with congenital anomalies.

A weak association with maternal nitrous oxide anesthesia during delivery was observed in a case-control study of 411 children with leukemia (OR=1.3; 95% confidence interval 1.0-1.6) (Zack et al., 1991). This observation requires independent corroboration before its clinical significance can be assessed.

A greater than expected frequency of fetal resorptions, growth retardation, and malformations has sometimes been observed among the offspring of rats exposed to anesthetic or sedative doses of nitrous oxide during pregnancy (Fink et al., 1967; Lane et al., 1980; Mazze et al., 1984, 1986, 1987, 1988; Keeling et al., 1986; Fujinaga et al., 1987, 1989, 1990). Central nervous system, ocular, vascular and skeletal anomalies are seen most often. Increased frequencies of fetal resorptions and growth retardation were also seen among the

offspring of pregnant hamsters anesthetized with nitrous oxide mixed with halothane (Bussard et al., 1974), but no consistent fetal effect was observed when pregnant hamsters were anesthetized with nitrous oxide alone (Shah et al., 1977). The frequency of malformations was not increased among the offspring of rabbits treated with subanesthetic doses or of mice treated with anesthetic or subanesthetic doses of nitrous oxide during pregnancy (Hardin et al., 1981; Mazze et al., 1982). Fetal growth retardation was sometimes seen among the offspring of exposed mice (Rodier et al., 1986).

In contrast, growth retardation and fetal loss have usually been observed among the offspring of rats treated repeatedly during pregnancy with nitrous oxide in subanesthetic doses similar to those that occur in human occupational exposure (Corbett et al., 1973; Pope et al., 1978; Vieira et al., 1980, 1983). The frequency of malformations among the offspring of rats exposed to such subanesthetic doses of nitrous oxide during pregnancy does not appear to be increased (Hardin et al., 1981; Mazze et al., 1984). No teratogenic effect was observed among the offspring of mice chronically exposed to subanesthetic doses of nitrous oxide during pregnancy (Satoh et al., 1982).

Persistent alterations of behavior have been observed among the offspring of rats and mice treated with sedative doses of nitrous oxide during pregnancy (Koeter & Roedier, 1986; Mullenix et al., 1986; Rodier, 1986; Rodier & Koeter, 1986; Tassinari et al., 1986; Rice, 1990).

An increased frequency of chromosomal aberrations was observed in bone marrow cells and spermatogonia of rats treated chronically with a mixture of nitrous oxide and halothane in doses similar to human occupational exposure (Coate et al., 1979). The clinical relevance of this observation is unknown.

Key References

Aldridge LM, Tunstall ME: Nitrous oxide and the fetus. Br J Anaesth 58:1348-1356, 1986. [R] & [S]

439

Bussard DA, Stoelting RK, Peterson C, Ishaq M: Fetal changes in hamsters anesthetized with nitrous oxide and halothane. Anesthesiology 41:275-278, 1974. [A]

Coate WB, Kapp RW, Lewis TR: Chronic exposure to low concentrations of halothane--Nitrous oxide. Reproductive and cytogenetic effects in the rat. Anesthesiology 50:310-318, 1979. [A]

Corbett TH, Cornell RG, Endres JL, Millard RI: Effects of low concentrations of nitrous oxide on rat pregnancy. Anesthesiology 39:299-301, 1973. [A]

Crawford JS, Lewis M: Nitrous oxide in early human pregnancy. Anaesthesia 41:900-905, 1986. [E]

Fink BR, Shepard TH, Blandau RJ: Teratogenic activity of nitrous oxide. Nature 214:146-148, 1967. [A]

Fujinaga M, Baden JM, Mazze RI: Susceptible period of nitrous oxide teratogenicity in Sprague-Dawley rats. Teratology 40:439-444, 1989. [A]

Fujinaga M, Baden JM, Shepard TH, Mazze RI: Nitrous oxide alters body laterality in rats. Teratology 41:131-135, 1990. [A]

Fujinaga M, Baden JM, Yhap EO, et al.: Reproductive and teratogenic effects of nitrous oxide, isoflurane, and their combination in Sprague-Dawley rats. Anesthesiology 67:960-964, 1987. [A]

Hardin BD, Bond GP, Sikov MR, Andrew FD, et al.: Testing of selected workplace chemicals for teratogenic potential. Scand J Work Environ Health 7(Suppl 4):66-75, 1981. [A]

Hathaway GJ, Proctor NH, Hughes JP, Fischman ML (Eds): Proctor and Hughes' Chemical Hazards of the Workplace, 3rd ed. New York: Van Nostrand Reinhold, 1991, pp 443-445. [O]

Heidam LZ: Spontaneous abortions among dental assistants, factory workers, painters, and gardening workers: A follow up study. J Epidemiol Comm Health 38:149-155, 1984. [E]

Heinonen OP, Slone D, Shapiro S: Birth Defects and Drugs in Pregnancy. Littleton, Mass.: John Wright-PSG, 1977, pp 358, 360. [E]

Johnson JA, Buchan RM, Reif JS: Effect of waste anesthetic gas and vapor exposure on reproductive outcome in veterinary personnel. Am Ind Hyg Assoc J 48(1):62-66, 1987. [E]

Keeling PA, Rocke DA, Nunn JF, et al.: Folinic acid protection against nitrous oxide terato-genicity in the rat. Br J Anaesth 58:528-534, 1986. [A]

Koeter HBWM, Rodier PM: Behavioral effects in mice exposed to nitrous oxide or halothane: Prenatal vs. postnatal exposure. Neurobehav Toxicol Teratol 8:189-194, 1986. [A]

Lane GA, Nahrworld ML, Tait AR, Taylor-Busch M, et al.: Anesthetics as teratogens: Nitrous oxide is fetotoxic, xenon is not. Science 210:899-901, 1980. [A]

Mazze RI, Fujinaga M, Baden JM: Halothane prevents nitrous oxide teratogenicity in Sprague-Dawley rats; folinic acid does not. Teratology 38:121-127, 1988. [A]

Mazze RI, Fujinaga M, Baden JM: Reproductive and teratogenic effects of nitrous oxide, fentanyl and their combination in Sprague-Dawley rats. Br J Anaesth 59:1291-1297, 1987. [A]

Mazze RI, Fujinaga M, Rice SA, et al.: Reproductive and teratogenic effects of nitrous oxide, halothane, isoflurane, and enflurane in Sprague-Dawley rats. Anesthesiology 64:339-344, 1986. [A]

Mazze RI, Wilson AI, Rice SA, Baden JM: Reproduction and fetal development in mice chronically exposed to nitrous oxide. Teratology 26:11-16, 1982. [A]

Mazze RI, Wilson AI, Rice SA, Baden JM: Reproduction and fetal development in rats exposed to nitrous oxide. Teratology 30:259-265, 1984. [A]

Mullenix PJ, Moore PA, Tassinari MS: Behavioral toxicity of nitrous oxide in rats following prenatal exposure. Toxicol Ind Health 2(3):273-287, 1986. [A]

Pope WDB, Halsey MJ, Lansdown ABG, Simmonds A, et al.: Fetotoxicity in rats following chronic exposure to halothane, nitrous oxide, or methoxyflurane. Anesthesiology 48:11-16, 1978. [A]

Rice SA: Effect of prenatal N2O exposure on startle reflex reactivity. Teratology 42:373-381, 1990. [A]

Rodier PM: Inhalant anesthetics as neuroteratogens. Ann NY Acad Sci 477:42-48, 1986. [R] & [A]

Rodier PM, Aschner M, Lewis LS, et al.: Cell proliferation in developing brain after brief exposure to nitrous oxide or halothane. Anesthesiology 64:680-687, 1986. [A]

Rodier PM, Koeter HBWM: General activity from weaning to maturity in mice exposed to halothane or nitrous oxide. Neurobehav Toxicol Teratol 8:195-199, 1986. [A]

Satoh T, Fuyuta M, Awata M, et al.: Effects of maternal exposure to low concentrations of nitrous oxide and halthane. Masui (J Japan Anesthesiol) 31:944-949, 1982. [A]

Shah RM, Burdett DN, Donaldson D: The effects of nitrous oxide on the developing hamster embryos. Can J Physiol Pharmacol 24:361-370, 1977. [A]

Tassinari MS, Mullenix PJ, Moore PA: The effects of nitrous oxide after exposure during middle and late gestation. Toxicol Ind Health 2(3):261-271, 1986. [A]

Vieira E, Cleaton-Jones P, Austin JC, Moyes DG, et al.: Effects of low concentrations of nitrous oxide on rat fetuses. Anesth Analg 59:175-177, 1980. [A]

Vieira E, Cleaton-Jones P, Moyes D: Effects of low intermittent concentrations of nitrous oxide on the developing rat fetus. Br J Anaesth 55:67-69, 1983. [A]

Zack M, Adami H-O, Ericson A: Maternal and perinatal risk factors for childhood leukemia. Cancer Res 51:3696-3701, 1991. [E]

NIZATIDINE

Synonyms

Axid

Summary

Nizatidine is a histamine H2 receptor antagonist administered orally in the treatment of peptic ulcers.

Magnitude of Teratogenic Risk

Undetermined

Quality and Quantity of Data

None To Poor

Comment

None

No epidemiological studies of congenital anomalies in the infants whose mothers were treated with nizatidine during pregnancy have been reported.

The frequency of malformations was not increased among the offspring of rats treated during pregnancy with 6-250 times the human dose of nizatidine (Buelke-Sam, 1989). Decreased maternal and fetal weights were seen at the highest dose.

Please see agent summary on cimetidine for information on a related agent.

Key References

Buelke-Sam JL, Hagopian GS, Probst KS, Fisher LF III: Nizatidine: Teratogenicity study in rats. Yakuri to Chiryo 17(2):547-570, 1989. [A]

NONOXYNOLS

Synonyms

Because Contraceptor, C-Film, Delfen, Double Check, Emko, Encare, Gynol II, Koromex, Ramses, Semicid

Summary

The nonoxynols are a series of nonionic surfactants of various chain lengths. Nonoxynol 9, 10, and 11 are used as vaginal spermicides. Nonoxynol 4, 15, and 30 are used as solubilizing and emulsifying agents.

Magnitude of Teratogenic Risk

None

Quality and Quantity of Data

Good

Comment

None

The frequency of malformations was no greater than expected among the infants of 1,355 women who used nonoxynol-containing contraceptives before the last menstrual period preceding their pregnancy or among the infants of 943 women who used such contraceptives after their last menstrual period (Mills et al., 1982). Similarly, no increase in the frequency of malformations was observed among the children of 342 women who used local contraceptives containing nonoxynol 9 early in pregnancy in the Collaborative Perinatal Project (Heinonen et al., 1977). Negative findings have also been reported in five large cohort studies in which data for nonoxynol were included with those for other spermicides (Huggins et al., 1982; Polednak et al., 1982; Linn et al., 1983; Harlap et al., 1985; Strobino et al., 1988).

In case/control studies, no association was observed with maternal use of spermicides containing nonoxynol around the time of conception or in the first trimester of pregnancy among infants with a variety of anomalies including 264 with Down syndrome, 396 with hypospadias, 146 with limb reduction defects, and 115 with neoplasms (Louik et al., 1987). Similarly, no association was found with maternal use of various vaginal spermicides around the time of conception in large studies involving cases with stillbirth, chromosomal abnormalities, limb reduction defects, or a variety of other congenital anomalies (Bracken & Vita, 1983; Cordero & Layde, 1983; Porter et al., 1986; Warburton et al., 1987; Adams et al., 1989).

Jick et al. (1981) reported that the frequency of a heterogenous group of anomalies (especially limb reduction defects, neoplasms, chromosomal abnormalities, and hypospadias) was greater than expected among the offspring of 763 women who had obtained a vaginal spermicide (nonoxynol 9 in about 20%) within 10 months of becoming pregnant. This study has serious methodological limitations (Cordero & Layde, 1983; Bracken, 1985; Watkins, 1986) and is not supported by the findings in other investigations (Einarson et al., 1990).

The frequency of malformations was not increased among the offspring of pregnant rats administered nonoxynol 9 vaginally in doses 2 and 20 times those used in humans (Abrutyn et al., 1982). Similarly, no teratogenic effect was observed among the offspring of pregnant rats given nonoxynol 9 orally or parenterally in a dose 25 times that used vaginally in humans (Meyer et al., 1988). Increased frequencies of skeletal variants were observed among the offspring of rats treated orally or parenterally with 125-250 times the human vaginal dose, but such doses were toxic to the mothers. Embryonic loss occurred with increased frequency among rats given 25 times the human dose of nonoxynal 9 intravaginally early in pregnancy (Tryphonas & Buttar, 1986).

Key References

Abrutyn D, McKenzie BE, Nadaskay N: Teratology study of intravaginally administered nonoxynol-9-containing contraceptive cream in rats. Fertil Steril 37:113-117, 1982. [A]

Adams MM, Mulinare J, Dooley K: Risk factors for conotruncal cardiac defects in Atlanta. J Am Coll Cardiol 14:432-442, 1989. [E]

Bracken MB: Spermicidal contraceptives and poor reproductive outcomes: The epidemiologic evidence against an association. Am J Obstet Gynecol 151(5):552-556, 1985. [R]

Bracken MB, Vita K: Frequency of non-hormonal contraception around conception and association with congenital malformations in offspring. Am J Epidemiol 117(3):281-291, 1983. [E]

Cordero JF, Layde PM: Vaginal spermicides, chromosome abnormalities and limb reduction defects. Am J Hum Genet 33:74A, 1981. [S]

Einarson TR, Koren G, Mattice D, Schechter-Tsafriri O: Maternal spermicide use and adverse reproductive outcome: A meta-analysis. Am J Obstet Gynecol 162:655-660, 1990. [O]

Harlap S, Shiono PH, Ramcharan S: Congenital abnormalities in the offspring of women who used oral and other contraceptives around the time of conception. Int J Fertil 30(2):39-47, 1985. [E]

Heinonen OP, Slone D, Shapiro S: Birth Defects and Drugs in Pregnancy. Littleton, Mass.: John Wright-PSG, 1977, p 392. [E]

Huggins G, Vessey M, Flavel R, Yeates D, et al.: Vaginal spermicides and outcome of pregnancy: Findings in a large cohort study. Contraception 25:219-230, 1982. [E]

Jick H, Walker AM, Rothman KJ, Hunter JR, et al.: Vaginal spermicides and congenital disorders. JAMA 245:1329-1332, 1981. [E]

Linn Shai, Schoenbaum SC, Monson RR, et al.: Lack of association between contraceptive usage and congenital malformations in offspring. Am J Obstet Gynecol 147:923-928, 1983. [E]

Louik C, Mitchell AA, Werler MM, et al.: Maternal exposure to spermicides in relation to certain birth defects. N Engl J Med 317:474-478, 1987. [E]

Meyer O, Andersen PH, Hansen EV, et al.: Teratogenicity and in vitro mutagenicity studies on nonoxynol-9 and -30. Pharmacol Toxicol 62:236-238, 1988. [A]

Mills JL, Harley EE, Reed GF, Berendes HW: Are spermicides teratogenic? JAMA 248:2148-2151, 1982. [E]

Polednak AP, Janerich DT, Glebatis DM: Birth weight and birth defects in relation to maternal spermicide use. Teratology 26:27-38, 1982. [E]

Porter JB, Hunter-Mitchell J, Jick H, Walker AM: Drugs and stillbirth. Am J Public Health 76(12):1428-1431, 1986. [E]

Strobino B, Kline J, Warburton D: Spermicide use and pregnancy outcome. Am J Public Health 78(3):260-263, 1988. [E]

Tryphonas L, Buttar HS: Effects of the spermicide nonoxynol-9 on the pregnant uterus and the conceptus of rat. Toxicology 39:177-186, 1986. [A]

Warburton D, Neugut RH, Lustenberger A, et al.: Lack of association between spermicide use and trisomy. N Engl J Med 317(8):478-482, 1987. [E]

Watkins RN: Vaginal spermicides and congenital disorders: The validity of a study. JAMA 256(22):3095, 1986. [O]

NORETHINDRONE

Synonyms

Aygestin, Ethinylnortestosterone, Micronor, Mini-Pill, Nor-QD, Norethisterone, Norgestin, Norlutate, Norlutin

Summary

Norethindrone is a synthetic progestin that is used as an oral contraceptive and in treatment of menstrual disorders. Norethindrone is often formulated with an estrogenic compound.

Magnitude of Teratogenic Risk

Virilization Of Female Fetus: Minimal To Small

Nongenital Congenital Anomalies: None

Quality and Quantity of Data

Virilization Of Female Fetus: Poor To Fair

Nongenital Congenital Anomalies: Fair To Good

Comment

A small risk for virilization of the genitalia in a female fetus may exist with maternal use of large doses of this agent during pregnancy. Assessment of this risk is based primarily on human studies involving use of progestational hormones at doses that are much greater than those currently employed.

The frequency of congenital anomalies was not significantly greater than expected among the children of 132 women who took norethindrone during the first four lunar months of pregnancy or of 148 women who took this drug anytime in pregnancy in the Collaborative Perinatal Project (Heinonen et al., 1977). In a case-control study, maternal use of norethindrone during pregnancy was not found significantly more often than expected among 171 children with congenital anomalies (Spira et al., 1972). Similarly, the frequency of hormonal pregnancy tests using norethindrone and ethinyl estradiol (an estrogenic agent) during the second month of pregnancy was not increased among the mothers of 194 infants with major malformations or 551 infants with minor anomalies (Kullander & Kallen, 1976).

Maternal use of norethindrone during pregnancy has been associated with the occurrence of masculinization of the external genitalia in female infants (Schardein, 1980; 1985). The genital anomalies observed include various degrees of clitoral hypertrophy with or without labioscrotal fusion (Wilkins et al., 1958; Overzier, 1963). Internal genitalia and pubertal development are not affected. Labioscrotal fusion is associated with exposure between the seventh and thirteenth week of gestation, but clitoral hypertrophy can develop with exposure at this time or later in pregnancy. The risk of pseudohermaphroditism among daughters of women who take norethindrone during pregnancy is probably on the order of a few percent (Bongiovonni & McPadden, 1960; Ishizuka et al., 1962). Masculinization of the genitalia of female offspring can be induced in several species of experimental animals by treatment of the mother with norethindrone during pregnancy (Hendrickx et al., 1983; Shardein, 1985).

No alteration in the frequency of congenital anomalies was apparent among the offspring of three species of nonhuman primates treated during pregnancy with norethindrone in combination with ethinyl estradiol (an estrogenic agent) in doses 10-100 times those used for human contraception (Hendrickx et al., 1987). Embryonic loss and genital alterations were observed at higher doses in cynomologus monkeys, but such doses were also toxic to the mothers. Pregnancy loss occurred in rhesus monkeys treated with this drug combination at 100 times the human contraceptive dose (Prahalada & Hendrickx, 1983). The frequency of malformations was no greater than expected among the offspring of mice or rabbits treated during pregnancy with norethindrone in combination with an estrogenic agent in doses respectively 50-500 and 50-150 times those used in human contraception (Takano et al., 1966). Fetal loss occurred with increased frequency in both species at the higher doses. No serious behavioral abnormalities were observed among the offspring of rhesus monkeys during pregnancy with 20-100 times the human therapeutic dose of an oral contraceptive containing norethindrone and ethinyl etradiol (Golub et al., 1983).

Key References

Bongiovanni AM, McPadden AJ: Steroids during pregnancy and possible fetal consequences. Fertil Steril 11:181-184, 1960. [R]

Golub MS, Hayes L, Prahalada S, et al.: Behavioral tests in monkey infants exposed embryonically to an oral contraceptive. Neurobehav Toxicol Teratol 5:301-304, 1983. [A]

Heinonen OP, Slone D, Shapiro S: Birth Defects and Drugs in Pregnancy. Littleton, Mass.: John Wright-PSG, 1977, pp 389-391, 443. [E]

Hendrickx AG, Binkerd PE, Rowland JM: Developmental toxicity and nonhuman primates. Issues Rev Teratol 1:149-180, 1983. [A]

Hendrickx AG, Korte R, Leuschner F, Neumann BW: Embryotoxicity of sex steroidal hormone combinations in nonhuman primates: I. Norethisterone acetate + ethinylestradiol and progesterone + estradiol benzoate (Macaca mulatta, Macaca fascicularis, and Papio cynocephalus). Teratology 35:119-127, 1987. [A]

Ishizuka N, Kawashima Y, Nakanishi T, Sugawa T, et al.: [Statistical observations on genital anomalies of newborns following the administration of progestins to their mothers.] J Jpn Obstet Gynecol Soc 9:271, 1962. [S]

Kullander S, Kallen B: A prospective study of drugs and pregnancy. 3. Hormones. Acta Obstet Gynecol Scand 55:221-224, 1976. [S]

Overzier C: Induced pseudo-hermaphroditism. In: Intersexuality. New York: Academic Press, 1963, pp 387-401. [R]

Prahalada S, Hendrickx AG: Embryotoxicity of norlestrin, a combined synthetic oral contraceptive, in rhesus macaques (Macaca mulatta). Teratology 27:215-222, 1983. [A]

Schardein JL: Chemically Induced Birth Defects. New York: Marcel Dekker, 1985, pp 275-312. [R]

Schardein JL: Congenital abnormalities and hormones during pregnancy: A clinical review. Teratology 22:251-270, 1980. [R]

Spira N, Goujard J, Huel G, Rumeau-Rouquette C: [Investigation into the teratogenic action of sex hormones first results of an epidemiologic survey involving 20,000 women]. Rev Med 41:2683-2694, 1972. [S]

Takano K, Yamamura H, Suzuki M, Nishimura H: Teratogenic effect of chlormadinone acetate in mice and rabbits. Proc Soc Exp Biol Med 121:455-457, 1966. [A]

Wilkins L, Jones HW, Holman GH, Stempfel RS: Masculinization of the female fetus associated with administration of progestins during gestation: Non adrenal female pseudo hermaphrodism. J Clin Endocrinol Metab 18:559-585, 1958. [S]

NORETHYNODREL

Synonyms

Norethinodrel

Summary

Norethynodrel is a synthetic progestin that is used in combination with an estrogenic compound as an oral contraceptive and in treatment of menstrual disorders.

Magnitude of Teratogenic Risk

None To Minimal

Quality and Quantity of Data

None To Poor

Comment

Risk is for virilization of female fetus at high doses. A minimal risk for virilization of the genitalia in a female may exist with maternal use of large doses of this agent during pregnancy. Assessment of this is based primarily on human studies involving use of progestational hormones at doses that are often much greater than those currently employed.

The frequency of congenital anomalies was no greater than expected among the infants of 154 women who took norethynodrel during the first four lunar months of pregnancy or of 180 women who took this drug anytime during pregnancy in the Collaborative Perinatal Project (Heinonen et al., 1977).

Increased frequencies of fetal loss were observed among pregnant rats treated with norethynodrel in doses 1-100 times those used in human contraception (Takano et al., 1966; Roy & Kar, 1967). Masculinization of the genitalia of female rat fetuses was demonstrated after maternal treatment with 200, but not 40, times the human contraceptive dose of norethynodrel during pregnancy (Kawashima et al., 1977). Delayed craniofacial maturation and increased resorption were found among the offspring of mice treated with 3-6 times the human contraceptive dose of norethynodrel during pregnancy (Gidley et al., 1970). Another study found behavioral alterations among male mice born to mothers that had been treated during pregnancy with norethynodrel in combination with an estrogenic agent in doses similar to those used in humans (Abbatiello & Scudder, 1970). The relevance of these observations to the clinical use of norethynodrel in human pregnancy is unknown.

Key References

Abbatiello E, Scudder CL: The effect of nore-thynodrel with mestranol treatment of pregnant mice on the isolation-induced aggression of their male offspring. Int J Fertil 15:182-189, 1970. [A]

Gidley JT, Christensen HD, Hall IH, Palmer KH, et al.: Teratogenic and other effects produced in mice by norethynodrel and its 3-hydroxyme-tabolites. Teratology 3:339-344, 1970. [A]

Heinonen OP, Slone D, Shapiro S: Birth Defects and Drugs in Pregnancy. Littleton, Mass.: John Wright-PSG, 1977, pp 389-391, 443. [E]

Kawashima K, Nakaura S, Nagao S, Tanaka S, et al.: Virilizing activities of various steroids in female rat fetuses. Endocrinol Japon 24:77-81, 1977. [A]

Roy SK, Kar AB: Foetal effect of norethyno-drel in rats. Indian J Exp Biol 5:14-16, 1967. [A]

Takano K, Yamamura H, Suzuki M, Nishimura H: Teratogenic effect of chlormadinone acetate in mice and rabbits. Proc Soc Exp Biol Med 121:455-457, 1966. [A]

NORFLOXACIN

Synonyms

Buccidal, Lexinor, Noroxin, Primoxin

Summary

Norfloxacin is a fluorinated quinolone antibiotic that is administered orally in the treatment of urinary tract infections.

Magnitude of Teratogenic Risk

Undetermined

Quality and Quantity of Data

Poor

Comment

A small risk cannot be excluded, but a high risk of congenital anomalies in the children of women treated with norfloxacin during pregnancy is unlikely.

No epidemiological studies of congenital anomalies among the infants of women treated with norfloxacin during pregnancy have been reported.

No increase in malformations was observed among the offspring of cynomolgus monkey treated during pregnancy with 3-12 times the human therapeutic dose of norfloxacin (Cukierski et al., 1989). Maternal toxicity and embryonic death were frequent at the highest dose. The rate of malformations was no greater than expected among the offspring of mice, rats, or rabbits treated during pregnancy with norfloxacin in doses respectively 8-31, 8-31, or 1.5-6 times those used in humans (Irikura et al., 1981a, b; Aruga et al., 1982; Clark et al., 1986). Fetal death and maternal toxicity occurred at the highest dose in rabbits.

Please see agent summary on nalidixic acid for information on a related agent that has been more thoroughly studied.

Key References

Aruga M, Kurata K, Miyazaki Y, Kanoh M, et al.: Teratological study of 1-Ethyl-6-fluoro-1, 4-dihydro-4-oxo-7-(1-piperazinyl)-3-quinolinecarboxylic acid in rabbits. Kiso to Rinsho 16(2):667-675, 1982. [A]

Clark RL, Robertson RT, Peter CP, Bland JA, et al.: Association between adverse maternal and embryo-fetal effects in norfloxacin-treated and food-deprived rabbits. Fundam Appl Toxicol 7:272-286, 1986. [A]

Cukierski MA, Prahalada S, Zacchei AG, et al.: Embryotoxicity studies of norfloxacin in cynomolgus monkeys: I. Teratology studies and norfloxacin plasma concentration in pregnant and nonpregnant monkeys. Teratology 39:39-52, 1989. [A]

Irikura T, Imada O, Suzuki H, Abe J: Teratological study of 1- ethyl-6-fluoro-1,4-dihydro-4-oxo-7-(1-piperazinyl)-3-quinolinecarboxilic acid (AM-715). Kiso To Rinsho 5(11):5251- 5263, 1981b. [A]

Irikura T, Suzuki H, Sugimoto T: Reproduction studies of AM-715 in mice. II. Teratological study. Chemotherapy 29:895-914, 1981a. [A]

NORFLURANE

Synonyms

R 134a

Summary

Norflurane is a general anesthetic administered by inhalation.

Magnitude of Teratogenic Risk

Undetermined

Quality and Quantity of Data

None

Comment

None

No epidemiological studies of congenital anomalies in children born to women exposed to norflurane during pregnancy have been reported.

No investigations of teratologic effects of norflurane in experimental animals have been published.

Key References

None available.

NORGESTREL

Synonyms

Dexnorgestrel, Microlut, Microluton, Microval, Norplant, Ovrette

Summary

Norgestrel is a synthetic progestin that is used alone or in combination with an estrogenic compound as an oral contraceptive and in treatment of menstrual disorders.

Magnitude of Teratogenic Risk

None To Minimal

Quality and Quantity of Data

Poor To Fair

Comment

A minimal risk for virilization of the genitalia in a female fetus may exist with maternal use of large doses of norgestrel during prenancy. This assessment is based primarily on studies involving use of progestational hormones at doses much greater than those currently employed.

No epidemiological studies of congenital anomalies in infants born to women who took norgestrel specifically during pregnancy have been reported, but many investigations of children of women who took oral contraceptives or related agents during gestation are available.

The frequency of malformations was not consistently increased among the offspring of mice treated during pregnancy with norgestrel in doses 200-20,000 times those used in human contraception (Klaus, 1983). Similarly, no alteration of the malformation frequency was seen among the offspring of rabbits treated with 100 times the human contraceptive dose of this agent during pregnancy. (Heinecke & Kohler, 1983.)

Key References

Heinecke H, Kohler D: Prenatal toxic effects of STS 557. II. Investigation in rabbits--preliminary results. Exp Clin Endocrinol 81:206-209, 1983. [A]

Klaus S: Prenatal toxic effects of STS 557. I. Investigations in mice. Exp Clin Endocrinol 81:197-205, 1983. [A]

NORTRIPTYLINE

Synonyms

Allegron, Aventyl, Demethylamitryptyline, Pamelor

Summary

Nortriptyline is a tricyclic antidepressant that is administered orally.

Magnitude of Teratogenic Risk

Undetermined

Quality and Quantity of Data

None

Comment

None

No epidemiological studies of congenital anomalies among the infants of women treated with nortriptyline during pregnancy have been reported.

No animal teratology studies of nortriptyline have been published.

Urinary retention, a recognized complication of nortriptyline therapy in adults, has been reported in the newborn infant born to a women who took this drug throughout pregnancy. (Shearer et al., 1972).

Please see agent summary on amitriptyline for information on a closely related drug that has been studied.

Key References

Shearer WT, Schreiner RL, Marshall RE: Urinary retention in a neonate secondary to maternal ingestion of nortriptyline. J Pediatr 81(3):570-572, 1972. [C]

NYLIDRIN

Synonyms

Arlidin, Buphenin, Dilatol, Nilidrine, Verina

Summary

Nylidrin is a beta-sympathomimetic agent that is used as a vasodilator in the treatment of peripheral vascular disease and abnormalities of the inner ear. Nylidrin has also been used to arrest or prevent premature labor.

Magnitude of Teratogenic Risk

Undetermined

Quality and Quantity of Data

None To Poor

Comment

None

No epidemiological studies of congenital anomalies among the infants of women treated with nylidrin during pregnancy have been reported.

The frequency of wavy ribs was increased among the offspring of rats treated with 750 times the usual human dose of nylidrin during pregnancy (Sterz et al., 1985). The relevance, if any, of this observation to the use of nylidrin in human pregnancy is unknown.

Increased fetal heart rate but no effect on blood flow in the fetal ductus arteriosus was seen after maternal tocolytic treatment with nylidrin during the second or third trimester of pregnancy (Eronen et al., 1991).

Please see agent summary on albuterol for information on a related agent that has been more thoroughly studied.

Key References

Eronen M, Pesonen E, Kurki T, et al.: The effects of indomethacin and a beta-sympathomimetic agent on the fetal ductus arteriosus during treatment of premature labor: A randomized double-blind study. Am J Obstet Gynecol 164:141-146, 1991. [E]

Sterz H, Sponer G, Neubert P, Hebold G: A postulated mechanism of beta-sympathomimetic induction of rib and limb anomalies in rat fetuses. Teratology 31:401-412, 1985. [A]

NYSTATIN

Synonyms

Korostatin, Micostatin, Mycostatin, Nilstat, Nystex, O-V Statin

Summary

Nystatin is a polyene antibiotic used in local treatment of candidiasis and other fungal infections. Nystatin is poorly absorbed from the gastrointestinal tract and is not absorbed through the skin or mucous membranes when applied topically.

Magnitude of Teratogenic Risk

None

Quality and Quantity of Data

Fair To Good

Comment

None

The frequencies of malformations in general, of major malformations, and of minor malformations were no greater than expected among infants born to 142 women treated with nystatin during the first four lunar months of pregnancy in the Collaborative Perinatal Project (Heinonen et al., 1977). Similarly, the frequency of congenital anomalies was not increased among the offspring of 230 women treated with nystatin anytime during pregnancy. In two separate cohorts of the Collaborative Drug Surveillance Program, malformations were no more frequent than expected among children born to 401 women treated with nystatin during the first trimester of gestation (Jick et al., 1981; Aselton et al., 1985).

The frequency of malformations was not increased among the offspring of rats that had been given 8-230 times the usual human oral dose of nystatin during pregnancy (Slonitskaya & Mikhailets, 1975).

Key References

Aselton P, Jick H, Milunsky A, Hunter JR, et al.: First-trimester drug use and congenital disorders. Obstet Gynecol 65:451-455, 1985. [S]

Heinonen OP, Slone D, Shapiro S: Birth Defects and Drugs in Pregnancy. Littleton, Mass.: John Wright-PSG, 1977, pp 305, 435. [E]

Jick H, Holmes LB, Hunter JR, Madsen S, et al.: First-trimester drug use and congenital disorders. JAMA 246:343-346, 1981. [S]

Rosa FW, Baum C, Shaw M: Pregnancy outcomes after first-trimester vaginitis drug therapy. Obstet Gynecol 69:751-755, 1987. [E]

Slonitskaya NM, Mikhailets GA: Study of nystatin and mycoheptin effect on intrauterine development of rat fetus. Antibiotiki 20:45-47, 1975. [A]

OCTANOIC ACID

Synonyms

Candistat, Caprylic acid, Caprystatin, Sodium Caprylate, Sodium Octanoate

Summary

Octanoic acid is used as a topical antifungal agent.

Magnitude of Teratogenic Risk

Undetermined

Quality and Quantity of Data

None To Poor

Comment

A small risk cannot be excluded, but there is no indication that the risk of congenital anomalies in the children of women treated with octanoic acid during pregnancy is likely to be great.

No epidemiological studies of congenital anomalies in infants born to women who used octanoic acid during pregnancy have been reported.

The frequency of malformations was no greater than expected among the offspring of mice treated parenterally with very large doses (600 mg/kg) of octanoic acid during pregnancy in one study (Nau et al., 1986).

Key References

Nau H, Loscher W: Pharmacologic evaluation of various metabolites and analogs of valproic acid: Teratogenic potencies in mice. Fund Appl Toxicol 6:669-676, 1986. [A]

OCTOCRYLENE

Synonyms

Agent AT 539, Octocrilene, UV Absorber-3, Uvinul N 539

Summary

Octocrylene is a substituted acrylate used topically as a sunscreen.

Magnitude of Teratogenic Risk

Undetermined

Quality and Quantity of Data

None To Poor

Comment

A small risk cannot be excluded, but a high risk of congenital anomalies in the children of women who use octocrylene topically during pregnancy is unlikely.

No epidemiological studies of congenital anomalies in infants born to mothers who used octocrylene during pregnancy have been reported.

No teratogenic effect was observed among the offspring of pregnant rats treated orally with up to 1000 mg/kg/d of octocrylene or the offspring of pregnant rabbits treated dermally with up to 300 mg/kg/d (Odio et al., 1992).

Key References

Odio MR, Azri-Meehan S, Robison SH, Kraus AL: Toxicological profile of 2-ethylhexyl-2-cyano-3,3-diphenylacrylate (Octocrylene). Toxicologist 12(1):96, 1992. [A]

OCTODRINE

Synonyms

Amidrine, Ottodrina, Vaporpac

Summary

Octodrine is a local anesthetic that has vasoconstrictor activity.

Magnitude of Teratogenic Risk

Undetermined

Quality and Quantity of Data

None

Comment

None

No epidemiological studies of congenital anomalies in children born to women exposed to octodrine during pregnancy have been reported.

No investigations of teratologic effects of octodrine in experimental animals have been published.

Please see agent summary on procaine for information on a closely related drug that has been more thoroughly studied.

Key References

None available.

OCTYL METHOXY-CINNAMATE

Synonyms

Sola Stick Broad Spectrum, Sunscreen AV, UV Sun Block, UV Sun Filter

Summary

Octyl methoxycinnamate is used topically as a sunscreen.

Magnitude of Teratogenic Risk

Undetermined

Quality and Quantity of Data

None

Comment

A small risk cnanot be excluded, but a high risk of congenital anomalies in the children of women treated with octyl methoxycinnamate during pregnancy is unlikely.

No epidemiological studies of congenital anomalies in infants born to women who used octyl methoxycinnamate during pregnancy have been reported.

No animal teratology studies of octyl methoxycinnamate have been published.

Key References

None available.

OLSALAZINE

Synonyms

Azodisalicylate, 5,5'-Azodisalicylic Acid, Disodium Azodisalicylate

Summary

Olsalazine is a salicylate that is administered orally in the treatment of ulcerative colitis. Olsalazine is metabolized to mesalamine in the colon.

Magnitude of Teratogenic Risk

Undetermined

Quality and Quantity of Data

None

Comment

A small risk cannot be excluded, but a high risk of congenital anomalies in the infants of women treated with olsalazine during pregnancy is unlikely.

No epidemiological studies of congenital anomalies among infants whose mothers were treated with olsalazine during pregnancy have been reported.

No animal teratology studies of olsalazine have been published.

Please see agent summaries on sulfasalazine and aspirin for information on two related agents that have been studied.

Key References

None available.

OMEGA-3 POLYUNSATURATES

Summary

Omega-3 polyunsaturates are fatty acids derived from fish oils. They are taken orally as a nutritional supplement.

Magnitude of Teratogenic Risk

Undetermined

Quality and Quantity of Data

None

Comment

None

No epidemiological studies of congenital anomalies in infants born to women who took supplemental omega-3 polyunsaturates during pregnancy have been reported.

No animal teratology studies of omega-3 polyunsaturates have been published.

Key References

None available.

OMEGA-6 POLYUNSATURATES

Summary

Omega-6 polyunsaturates are fatty acids derived from fish oils. They are taken orally as a nutritional supplement.

Magnitude of Teratogenic Risk

Undetermined

Quality and Quantity of Data

None

Comment

None

No epidemiological studies of congenital anomalies in infants born to women who took supplemental omega-6 polyunsaturates during pregnancy have been reported.

No animal teratology studies of omega-6 polyunsaturates have been published.

Key References

None available.

OPIUM

Synonyms

Omnopone, Pantopan, Pantopon, Papaveretum, Parapectolin Suspension, Paregoric, Tetrapon

Summary

Opium is a mixture of narcotic alkaloids obtained from the opium poppy. Its effects are due primarily to the morphine it contains. Opium is used orally as an antidiarrheal agent and parenterally as an analgesic.

Magnitude of Teratogenic Risk

None To Minimal

Quality and Quantity of Data

Poor To Fair

Comment

Chronic maternal use of opium late in pregnancy would be expected to produce neonatal withdrawal symptoms after delivery.

The frequency of congenital anomalies was no greater than expected among the children of 36 women who were treated with opium during the first four lunar months of pregnancy or of 181 women who were treated with this drug anytime during pregnancy in the Collaborative Perinatal Project (Heinonen et al., 1977).

No animal teratology studies of opium have been published.

Please see agent summary on morphine for information on this principal component of opium.

Key References

Heinonen OP, Slone D, Shapiro S: Birth Defects and Drugs in Pregnancy. Littleton, Mass.: John Wright-PSG, 1977, pp 287-288, 434, 485. [E]

ORCONAZOLE

Synonyms

Orconazole Nitrate

Summary

Orconazole is an antifungal agent.

Magnitude of Teratogenic Risk

Undetermined

Quality and Quantity of Data

None

Comment

None

No epidemiological studies of congenital anomalies in infants born to women who used orconazole during pregnancy have been reported.

No animal teratology studies of orconazole have been published.

Key References

None available.

ORGANIC MERCURY

Summary

Long chain organic mercury compounds include those of the aryl and alkyloxy-alkyl groups. They are widely used as preservatives in the paint industry and as agricultural fungicides. Long chain organic mercury compounds are absorbed through the skin or gastrointestinal tract. They are believed to be less toxic than methyl mercury compounds (Clarkson & Marsh, 1982).

Magnitude of Teratogenic Risk

Undetermined

Quality and Quantity of Data

None To Poor

Comment

Although the teratogenic risk associated with maternal exposure to this agent during pregnancy is undetermined, it may be substantial.

No epidemiological studies of congenital anomalies among infants born to women exposed to long chain organic mercury compounds during pregnancy have been reported.

Increased frequencies of embryonic death, growth retardation, and malformations, especially of the central nervous system, were observed among the offspring of mice treated with phenylmercuric acetate in a dose of about 3 mg/kg (Murakami et al., 1955).

Key References

Clarkson TW, Marsh DO: Mercury toxicity in man. In: Prasad AS (ed). Current Topics in Nutrition and Disease, Vol. 6. Clinical, Biochemical, and Nutritional Aspects of Trace Elements. New York: Alan R. Liss, 1982, pp 549-568. [R]

Murakami U, Kameyama Y, Kato T: Effects of a vaginally applied contraceptive with phenylmercuric acetate upon developing embryos and their mother animals. Res Inst Environ Med Nagoya Univ 4:88-99, 1956. [A]

ORPHENADRINE

Synonyms

Biorphen, Brocadisipal, Disipal, Mephenamine Hydrochloride, Norflex, Orpadrcx, Orphenadin Hydrochloride, Orphenate

Summary

Orphenadrine is an anticholinergic used in the treatment of parkinsonian movement disorders. It is also employed as a muscle relaxant.

Magnitude of Teratogenic Risk

Undetermined

Quality and Quantity of Data

None To Poor

Comment

None

No epidemiological studies of congenital anomalies in children born to women treated with orphenadrine during pregnancy have been reported.

No clear teratogenic effect was seen among the offspring of rats treated with 0.5-5 times the usual human dose of orphenadrine during pregnancy in one study, although a few pups with unusual abnormalities of the urinary bladder were noted (Beall, 1972). Fetal malformations and death were seen often among the offspring of rabbits treated during pregnancy with 3-6 times the usual human dose of orphenadrine in one study (McBride & Hicks, 1987), but too few animals were included to permit reliable interpretation of the data.

Key References

Beall JR: A teratogenic study of chlorpromazine, orphenadrine, perphenazine, and LSD-25 in rats. Toxicol Appl Pharmacol 21:230-236, 1972. [A]

McBride WG, Hicks LJ: Acetylcholine and choline levels in rabbit fetuses exposed to anticholinergics. Int J Devl Neuroscience 5(2):117-125, 1987. [A]

ORTHOCAINE

Synonyms

3-Amino-4-hydroxybenzoic Acid Methyl Ester, Orthoform

Summary

Orthocaine is a local anesthetic of the ester class that has been used topically.

Magnitude of Teratogenic Risk

Undetermined

Quality and Quantity of Data

None

Comment

None

No epidemiological studies of congenital anomalies in children born to women exposed to orthocaine during pregnancy have been reported.

No investigations of teratologic effects of orthocaine in experimental animals have been published.

Please see agent summary on procaine for information on a related agent that has been studied.

Key References

None available.

OUABAIN

Synonyms

Acocantherin, g-Strofantin, Strophanthin-G, Strophoperm

Summary

Ouabain is a cardiac glycoside that is administered intravenously in the acute treatment of cardiac failure and dysrhythmias.

Magnitude of Teratogenic Risk

Undetermined

Quality and Quantity of Data

None

Comment

None

No epidemiological studies of congenital anomalies in infants born to mothers treated with ouabain during pregnancy have been reported.

No animal teratology studies of ouabain have been published.

Please see agent summary on digoxin for information on a related drug that has been studied.

Key References

None available.

OX BILE EXTRACT

Synonyms

Desicol, Felkreon, Hog Bile Extract, Opobyl

Summary

Ox bile extract is given orally as a purgative and in the treatment of conditions associated with a deficiency of bile in the gastrointestinal tract.

Magnitude of Teratogenic Risk

Undetermined

Quality and Quantity of Data

None

Comment

A small risk cannot be excluded, but a high risk of congenital anomalies in children of women treated with ox bile extract during pregnancy is unlikely.

No epidemiological studies of congenital anomalies in infants born to women who used ox bile extract during pregnancy have been reported.

No animal teratology studies of ox bile extract have been published.

Key References

None available.

OXACILLIN

Synonyms

Bactocill, Bristopen, Cryptocillin, Penistafil, Penstapho, Prostaphlin, Sodium Oxacillin, Stapenor, Staphcillin V

Summary

Oxacillin is a penicillin derivative used to treat infections by penicillinase-resistant bacteria.

Magnitude of Teratogenic Risk

Undetermined

Quality and Quantity of Data

Poor

Comment

A small risk cannot be excluded, but a substantial risk of congenital anomalies in the children of women treated with oxacillin during pregnancy is unlikely.

No epidemiological studies of congenital anomalies among infants born to women treated with oxacillin during pregnancy have been reported.

Animal teratology studies of oxacillin have produced inconsistent results. One study found an increased frequency of fetal death and growth retardation after exposure of pregnant rats to oxacillin in doses similar to those used in humans (Korzhova et al., 1981). Another study found no teratogenic effect when doses 4-5 times greater were used (Persianinov & Kirjushenkov, 1976).

Please see agent summary on penicillin for information on a related drug that has been more thoroughly studied.

Key References

Korzhova VV, Lisitsyna NT, Mikhailova EG: Effect of ampicillin and oxacillin on fetal and neonatal development. Bull Exp Biol Med 91:169-171, 1981. [A]

Persianinov LS, Kirjushenkov AN: Transplacental transport of antibiotics and their influence upon embryonic and fetal development. Excerpta Med Int Congr Ser, 412:110-114, 1976. [A]

OXAMNIQUINE

Synonyms

Vansil

Summary

Oxamniquine is an oral antihelmintic agent used to treat schistosomiasis.

Magnitude of Teratogenic Risk

Undetermined

Quality and Quantity of Data

None To Poor

Comment

None

No epidemiological studies of congenital anomalies among infants born to women treated with oxamniquine during pregnancy have been reported.

No teratogenic effect was observed among the offspring of mice or rabbits treated during pregnancy with oxamniquine in doses 3-13 or 2.5-10 times those used in humans (Chvedoff et al., 1984).

Key References

Chvedoff M, Faccini MH, Gregory RM, Hull AM, et al.: The toxicology of the schistosomicidal agent oxamniquine. Drug Devel Res 4:229-235, 1984. [A]

OXANDROLONE

Synonyms

Anavar, Ossandrolone, Protivar, Provitar, Vasorome

Summary

Oxandrolone is an androgenic steroid that is administered orally as an anabolic agent. It is also used in the treatment of osteoporosis.

Magnitude of Teratogenic Risk

Virilization Of Female Fetus: Undetermined

Congenital Anomalies: Undetermined

Quality and Quantity of Data

Virilization Of Female Fetus: None

Congenital Anomalies: None

Comment

Because oxandrolone is an androgen, it would be expected to produce virilization of the external genitalia of an exposed female fetus.

No epidemiological studies of congenital anomalies in the infants of women who were treated with oxandrolone during pregnancy have been reported.

No viable offspring were delivered by pregnant rats that had been treated with oxandrolone during gestation in doses more than 500 times that used in humans (Selye et al., 1971).

Please see agent summary on testosterone for information on a related agent that has been more thoroughly studied.

Key References

Selye H, Tache Y, Szabo S: Interruption of pregnancy by various steroids. Fertil Steril 22:735-740, 1971. [A]

OXAZEPAM

Synonyms

Adumbran, Alepam, Serax , Serenal

Summary

Oxazepam is a benzodiazepine tranquilizer. It is administered orally in the treatment of anxiety, as a sedative, and as a preoperative medication.

Magnitude of Teratogenic Risk

Undetermined

Quality and Quantity of Data

None To Poor

Comment

None

No epidemiological studies of malformations in infants born to women who took oxazepam during pregnancy have been reported. The suggestion that there exists a "benzodiazepine embryofetopathy" comprised of typical facial features, neurological dysfunction, and other anomalies (Laegreid et al., 1987, 1989, 1990) is not generally accepted.

The frequency of malformations was not increased among the offspring of rabbits or rats treated during pregnancy with oxazepam in doses respectively 10-21 and 42 times those used in humans (Owen et al., 1970; Saito et al., 1984). Behavioral alterations were noted among the offspring of mice treated during pregnancy with 4-42 times the usual human dose of oxazepam (Alleva et al., 1985; Laviola et al., 1991a, b).

Oxazepam is a major metabolite of diazepam. *Please see agent summary on diazepam for information on a more thoroughly studied benzodiazepine tranquilizer.*

Key References

Alleva E, Laviola G, Tirelli E, et al.: Short-, medium-, and long-term effects of prenatal oxazepam on neurobehavioural development of mice. Psychopharmacology 87:434-441, 1985. [A]

Laegreid L, Olegard R, Conradi N, et al.: Congenital malformations and maternal consumption of benzodiazepines: A case-control study. Dev Med Child Neurol 32:432-441, 1990. [E]

Laegreid L, Olegard R, Wahlstrom J, Conradi N: Abnormalities in children exposed to benzodiazepines in utero. Lancet 1:108-109, 1987. [S]

Laegreid L, Olegard R, Walstrom J, Conradi N: Teratogenic effects of benzodiazepine use during pregnancy. J Pediatr 114:126-131, 1989. [S]

Laviola G, Bignami G, Alleva E: Interacting effects of oxazepam in late pregnancy and fostering procedure on mouse maternal behavior. Neurosci Biobehav Rev 15:501-504, 1991. [A]

Laviola G, de Acetis L, Bignami G, Alleva E: Prenatal oxazepam enhances mouse maternal aggression in the offspring, without modifying acute chlordiazepoxide effects. Neurotoxicol Teratol 13:75-81, 1991. [A]

Owen G, Smith THF, Agersborg HPK: Toxicity of some benzodiazepine compounds with CNS activity. Toxicol Appl Pharmacol 16:556-570, 1970. [A]

Saito H, Kobayashi H, Takeno S, Sakai T: Fetal toxicity of benzodiazepines in rats. Res Commun Chem Pathol Pharmacol 46:437-447, 1984. [A]

OXETHAZAINE

Synonyms

Emoren, Mucoxin, Mutesa, Oxaine, Tepilta

Summary

Oxethazaine is a local anesthetic of the amide class that is used topically.

Magnitude of Teratogenic Risk

Undetermined

Quality and Quantity of Data

None

Comment

None

No epidemiological studies of congenital anomalies in children born to women exposed to oxethazaine during pregnancy have been reported.

No investigations of teratologic effects of oxethazaine in experimental animals have been published.

Please see agent summary on lidocaine for information on a related agent that has been studied.

Key References

None available.

OXIDIZED CELLULOSE

Synonyms

Carboxycellulose, Cellulosic Acid, Oxycel, Surgicel

Summary

Oxidized cellulose is an absorbable hemostatic agent that is applied to control local bleeding during surgical procedures.

Magnitude of Teratogenic Risk

None

Quality and Quantity of Data

None

Comment

None

No epidemiological studies have been reported of congenital anomalies in infants born to women upon whom oxidized cellulose was used during pregnancy.

No animal teratology studies of oxidized cellulose have been published.

Key References

None available.

OXIFUNGIN

Summary

Oxifungin is an antifungal agent.

Magnitude of Teratogenic Risk

Undetermined

Quality and Quantity of Data

None

Comment

None

No epidemiological studies of congenital anomalies in infants born to women who used oxifungin during pregnancy have been reported.

No animal teratology studies of oxifungin have been published.

Key References

None available.

OXYBENZONE

Synonyms

Aduvex 24, Advastab 45, Cyasorb UV 9

Summary

Oxybenzone is used topically as a sunscreen.

Magnitude of Teratogenic Risk

Undetermined

Quality and Quantity of Data

None

Comment

A small risk cannot be excluded, but a high risk of congenital anomalies in the children of women treated with oxybenzone during pregnancy is unlikely.

No epidemiological studies of congenital anomalies in infants born to women who used oxybenzone during pregnancy have been reported.

No animal teratology studies of oxybenzone have been published.

Key References

None available.

OXYBUTYNIN

Synonyms

Ditropan, Dridase, Tropax

Summary

Oxybutynin is an anticholinergic tertiary amine that is used orally in the treatment of neurogenic bladder and enuresis.

Magnitude of Teratogenic Risk

Undetermined

Quality and Quantity of Data

None To Poor

Comment

A small risk cannot be excluded, but a high risk of congenital anomalies in the children of women treated with oxybutynin during pregnancy is unlikely.

No epidemiological studies of congenital anomalies among infants born to women who were treated with oxybutynin during pregnancy have been reported.

An increased frequency of ventricular septal defects and decreased postnatal growth were observed among the offspring of pregnant rats treated with 250 times the usual human dose of oxybutynin in one study (Edwards et al., 1986). Such doses also produced maternal toxicity. No teratogenic effects were seen in rats after maternal treatment with 10-50 times the human therapeutic dose or in rabbits after maternal treatment with 8-120 times the human therapeutic dose of oxybutynin during pregnancy (Edwards et al., 1986).

Please see agent summary on atropine for information on a related agent that has been more thoroughly studied.

Key References

Edwards JA, Reid YJ, Cozens DD: Reproductive toxicity studies with oxybutynin hydrochloride. Toxicology 40:31-44, 1986. [A]

OXYCHLOROSENE

Synonyms

Chlorpactin WCS-90

Summary

Oxychlorosene is a chlorine disinfectant used topically.

Magnitude of Teratogenic Risk

Undetermined

Quality and Quantity of Data

None

Comment

None

No epidemiological studies of congenital anomalies among infants whose mothers used oxychlorosene during pregnancy have been reported.

No animal teratology studies of oxychlorosene have been published.

Key References

None available.

OXYCODONE

Synonyms

Dihydrone Hydrochloride, Endone, Noroxycodone, Pancodone Retard, Pectinate, Percodan Tablets, Proladone, Roxicodone Tablets, Supeudol

Summary

Oxycodone is a narcotic analgesic.

Magnitude of Teratogenic Risk

Undetermined

Quality and Quantity of Data

Poor

Comment

1) A small risk cannot be excluded, but there is no indication that the risk of congenital anomalies in the children of women treated with oxycodone during pregnancy is likely to be great.

2) Possible effects on perinatal adaptation are discussed below.

The frequency of maternal exposure to oxycodone during the first trimester of pregnancy was not significantly greater than expected among 1370 infants with malformations in one case-control study, but only five exposed cases were included (Bracken & Holford, 1981).

Teratogenicity studies of oxycodone in experimental animals have not been published.

Neonatal withdrawal and respiratory depression following chronic exposure in late gestation have been observed with chemically related narcotics (see agent summary for codeine), but this complication has not been reported with oxycodone.

Please see agent summary on codeine for information on a related agent.

Key References

Bracken MB, Holford TR: Exposure to prescribed drugs in pregnancy and association with congenital malformations. Obstet Gynecol 58:336-344, 1981. [E]

OXYMETAZOLINE

Synonyms

Afrin, Duration, Nafrine, Oxylazine, Sinerol

Summary

Oxymetazoline is a vasoconstrictor that is used topically as a nasal decongestant.

Magnitude of Teratogenic Risk

None To Minimal

Quality and Quantity of Data

Poor To Fair

Comment

None

The frequency of congenital anomalies was no greater than expected among the infants of more than 250 women who used oxymetazoline during the first trimester of pregnancy in two cohorts of the Boston Collaborative Drug Surveillance Program (Jick et al., 1981; Aselton et al., 1985).

No animal teratology studies of oxymetazoline have been published.

Abnormal heart rate patterns were observed in the term fetus of a mother who had chronically used oxymetazoline as a nasal decongestant (Baxi et al., 1985). In contrast, no evidence of altered fetal circulation was observed among 12 fetuses whose mothers were given a single dose of oxymetazoline nasal spray in the third trimester of pregnancy (Rayburn et al., 1990).

Key References

Aselton P, Jick H, Milunsky A, Hunter JR, et al.: First-trimester drug use and congenital disorders. Obstet Gynecol 65:451-455, 1985. [S]

Baxi LV, Gindoff PR, Pregenzer GJ, Parras MK: Fetal heart rate changes following maternal administration of a nasal decongestant. Am J Obstet Gynecol 153:799-800, 1985. [C]

Jick H, Holmes LB, Hunter JR, Madsen S, et al.: First-trimester drug use and congenital disorders. JAMA 246:343-346, 1981. [S]

Rayburn WF, Anderson JC, Smith CV, et al.: Uterine and fetal doppler flow changes from a single dose of a long-acting intranasal decongestant. [S]

OXYMETHOLONE

Synonyms

Anadrol, Anapolon, Anasteron, Dynasten, Methabol, Nastenon, Ossimetolone, Oxymethenolone, Pavisoid, Synasteron

Summary

Oxymetholone is an anabolic and androgenic steroid that is used in the treatment of anemia.

Magnitude of Teratogenic Risk

Undetermined

Quality and Quantity of Data

None To Poor

Comment

Because it is an androgen, oxymetholone would be expected to have the capacity to cause virilization of the external genitalia of female fetuses.

No epidemiological studies of congenital anomalies among the infants of women treated with oxymetholone during pregnancy have been reported.

Embryonic loss frequently occurred after injection of about 4 times the usual human dose of oxymetholone to rats in early pregnancy (Naqvi & Warren, 1971).

Please see agent summary on testosterone for information on a related agent that has been more thoroughly studied.

Key References

Naqvi RH, Warren JC: Interceptives: Drugs interrupting pregnancy after implantation. Steroids 18:731-739, 1971. [A]

OXYMORPHONE

Summary

Oxymorphone is a narcotic analgesic that is administered rectally or by injection.

Magnitude of Teratogenic Risk

Undetermined

Quality and Quantity of Data

Poor

Comment

1) A small risk cannot be excluded, but a high risk of congenital anomalies in the children of women treated with oxymorphone during pregnancy is unlikely.

2) Transient neonatal respiratory depression has been observed among infants born to women treated with oxymorphone during labor (Sentnor et al., 1960; Simeckova et al., 1960).

No epidemiological studies of congenital anomalies among the infants of women treated with oxymorphone during pregnancy have been reported.

An increased frequency of various congenital anomalies was observed among the offspring of pregnant hamsters treated with a single dose of oxymorphone 5000 times that used in humans (Geber & Schramm, 1975). This treatment was often lethal to the mothers.

Please see agent summary on heroin for information on a related agent that has been more thoroughly studied.

Key References

Geber WF, Schramm LC: Congenital malformations of the central nervous system produced by narcotic analgesics in the hamster. Am J Obstet Gynecol 123:705-713, 1975. [A]

Sentnor MH, Solomons E, Kohl SG: An evaluation of oxymorphone in labor. Am J Obstet Gynecol 84:956-961, 1960. [E]

Simeckova M, Shaw W, Pool E, Nichols EE: Numorphan in labor. Obstet Gynecol 16:119-123, 1960. [S]

OXYQUINOLINE

Synonyms

Chinosol, Hydroxyquinoline Sulfate, Oxychinolin, Oxykin, Semori, Serorhinol, Superol

Summary

Oxyquinoline is an antimicrobial agent that is used topically to treat fungal and bacterial infections, as well as amebiasis. It is also used as a preservative and in cosmetics.

Magnitude of Teratogenic Risk

Undetermined

Quality and Quantity of Data

None

Comment

A small risk cannot be excluded, but a high risk of congenital anomalies in the children of women

treated with oxyquinoline during pregnancy is unlikely.

No congenital anomalies were observed among the infants of 21 women treated systemically with oxyquinoline during the first four lunar months of gestation in the Collaborative Perinatal Project (Heinonen et al., 1977).

No animal teratology studies of oxyquinoline have been published.

Key References

Heinonen OP, Slone D, Shapiro S: Birth Defects and Drugs in Pregnancy. Littleton, Mass.: John Wright-PSG, 1977, pp 299, 302. [E]

OXYTETRACYCLINE

Synonyms

Berkmycen, Imperacin, Oxycyclin, Oxymycin, Terramycin, Unimycin, Uri-Tet

Summary

Oxytetracycline is a broad spectrum antibiotic that is used in the treatment of a variety of bacterial infections.

Magnitude of Teratogenic Risk

Dental Staining: Small To Moderate

Malformations: None To Minimal

Quality and Quantity of Data

Dental Staining: Fair To Good

Malformations: Fair

Comment

Oxytetracycline causes staining of the primary dentition in fetuses exposed during the second or third trimesters of pregnancy (Toaff & Ravid, 1966; Cohlan, 1977).

The frequency of congenital anomalies was increased among the children of 119 women treated with oxytetracycline during the first four lunar months of pregnancy in the Collaborative Perinatal Project (Heinonen et al., 1977). This increase was due entirely to a higher frequency of inguinal hernias, an anomaly reported with very different frequencies by various participating centers. It is unlikely that this association is of any biological significance. The frequency of congenital anomalies was not increased among the children of 328 women in this study treated with oxytetracycline anytime during pregnancy.

The frequency of malformations was no greater than expected among the offspring of rats or mice treated orally with oxytetracycline during pregnancy in doses 15-19 or 17-26 times those used in humans despite the production of considerable maternal toxicity at such doses (Morrissey et al., 1986). Increased frequencies of skeletal and other malformations were observed among the offspring of rabbits treated with 10 times the human dose and dogs treated with twice the human dose of oxytetracycline intramuscularly during pregnancy (Savini et al., 1968; Sobkowiak & Radtke, 1977). The relevance of these observations to the clinical use of oxytetracycline in human pregnancy is unknown.

Please see agent summary on tetracycline for information on a closely related agent that has been more thoroughly studied.

Key References

Cohlan SQ: Tetracycline staining of teeth. Teratology 15:127-130, 1977. [R]

Heinonen OP, Slone D, Shapiro S: Birth Defects and Drugs in Pregnancy. Littleton, Mass.: John Wright-PSG, 1977, pp 297-298, 301, 313, 435, 472, 485. [E]

Morrissey RE, Tyl RW, Price CJ, Ledoux TA, et al.: The developmental toxicity of orally administered oxytetracycline in rats and mice. Fundam Appl Toxicol 7:434-443, 1986. [A]

Savini EC, Moulin MA, Herrou MFJ: Effets teratogenes de l'oxytetracycline. Therapie 23:1247-1260, 1968. [A]

Sobkowliak E-M, Radtke G: Teratogenic action of tetracyclines with special reference to otesolut and terramycin in animal experiments. Zahn Mund Kieferheilkd 65:163-167, 1977. [A]

Toaff R, Ravid R: Tetracyclines and the teeth. Lancet 2:281-282, 1966. [S]

OXYTOCIN

Synonyms

Orasthin, Partocon, Pitocin, Piton-S, Syntocinon, Syntometrine

Summary

Oxytocin is a peptide hormone made by the posterior pituitary. It is used to induce and maintain labor, to control postpartum hemorrhage, and to facilitate lactation.

Magnitude of Teratogenic Risk

Undetermined

Quality and Quantity of Data

None To Poor

Comment

None

No epidemiological studies of malformations in infants born to mothers treated with oxytocin early in pregnancy have been reported.

Treatment of rats with oxytocin early in pregnancy in doses thousands of times greater than those used to induce labor in humans caused fetal loss in one study (Buchanan & Smith, 1972). The relevance of this observation to the clinical use of oxytocin in humans is unknown.

Several studies have demonstrated an association between oxytocin induction or augmentation of labor in women and hyperbilirubinemia in their newborns (Beazley & Alderman, 1975; Sims & Neligan, 1975; Chalmers et al., 1976; Chew & Swan, 1977; Davis, 1984). Interpretation of this association is difficult because the women treated with oxytocin in these studies differed in a number of important ways from the untreated control mothers. No such association was seen in two of three randomized trials (Leijon et al., 1980; Lange et al., 1982; Augensen et al., 1987). Hyperbilirubinemia has been induced in the offspring of pregnant rats treated with oxytocin just prior to delivery (Hollingsworth & Oyewo, 1985), but the dose used (5000 times that employed in humans) also increased the neonatal death rate.

In another study in rats, administration of oxytocin to pregnant females for four days prior to term at a dose more than 100 times that used in humans resulted in reduced birth weights in the offspring (Boer & Kruisbrink, 1984). No effect on birth weight has been found among human infants whose mothers were treated with oxytocin before or during labor (Scanlon et al., 1978; Tylleskar et al., 1979).

Key References

Augensen K, Bergsjo P, Eikeland T, et al.: Randomised comparison of early versus late induction of labour in post-term pregnancy. Br Med J 294:1192-1195, 1987. [E]

Beazley JM, Alderman B: Neonatal hyperbilirubinaemia following the use of oxytocin in labour. Br J Obstet Gynaecol 82:265-271, 1975. [E]

Boer GJ, Kruisbrink J: Effects of continuous administration of oxytocin by an Accurel device on parturition in the rat and on development and diuresis in the offspring. J Endocrinol 101:121-129, 1984. [A]

Buchanan GD, Smith MD: Effects of estrogen and oxytocin on pregnancy in the rat. Anat Rec 172:280, 1972. [A]

Chalmers I, Campbell H, Turnbull AC: Oxytocin and neonatal jaundice. Br Med J 1:647-648, 1976. [E]

Chew WC, Swan IL: Influence of simultaneous low amniotomy and oxytocin infusion and other maternal factors on neonatal jaundice: A prospective study. Br Med J 1:72-73, 1977. [S]

Davis GH: Effects of oxytocin-induction of labor on neonatal hyperbilirubinemia. J Am Osteopath Assoc 84:365-367, 1984. [E]

Hollingsworth M, Oyewo EA: Hyperbilirubinaemia in neonatal rats after oxytocin or prostaglandin F2a treatment of pregnant rats. Biol Neonate 47:288-294, 1985. [A]

Lange AP, Secher NJ, Westergaard JG, Skovgard I: Neonatal jaundice after labour induced or stimulated by prostaglandin E2 or oxytocin. Lancet 1:991-994, 1982. [E]

Leijon I, Finnstrom O, Hedenskog S, Ryden G, et al.: Spontaneous labor and elective induction--A prospective randomized study. Acta Obstet Gynecol Scand 59:103-106, 1980. [E]

Scanlon JW, Suzuki K, Shea E, Tronick E: Clinical and neurobehavioral effects of repeated intrauterine exposure to oxytocin: A prospective study. Am J Obstet Gynecol 132:294-296, 1978. [E]

Sims DG, Neligan GA: Factors affecting the increasing incidence of severe non-hemolytic neonatal jaundice. Br J Obstet Gynaecol 82:863-867, 1975. [E]

Tylleskar J, Finnstrom O, Leijon I, Hedenskog S, et al.: Spontaneous labor and elective induction--A prospective randomized study. Acta Obstet Gynecol Scand 58:513-518, 1979. [E]

PADIMATE O

Synonyms

Chapstick, Lip-Sed Jel, Lip-Sed Stick, Octyl Dimethyl PABA, Paba-Tan, Pabafilm 5, Phiasol, Presun 4, Spectraban 4, Uvasorb DMO

Summary

Padimate O is used topically as a sunscreen.

Magnitude of Teratogenic Risk

Undetermined

Quality and Quantity of Data

None

Comment

A small risk cannot be excluded, but a high risk of congenital anomalies in the children of women treated with padimate O during pregnancy is unlikely.

No epidemiological studies of congenital anomalies in infants born to women who used padimate O during pregnancy have been reported.

No animal teratology studies of padimate O have been published.

Key References

None available.

PAMABROM

Synonyms

Odrinil, Premesyn

Summary

Pamabrom is a mild diuretic used for the relief of premenstrual edema.

Magnitude of Teratogenic Risk

Undetermined

Quality and Quantity of Data

None

Comment

None

No epidemiological studies of congenital anomalies in infants whose mothers took pamabrom during pregnancy have been reported.

No animal teratology studies of pamabrom have been published.

Key References

None available.

PANCURONIUM

Synonyms

Bromuro de Pancuronio, Mioblock, Pavulon

Summary

Pancuronium is a nondepolarizing neuromuscular blocking agent that is used as a skeletal muscle relaxant. Pancuronium is administered intravenously as an adjunct to anesthesia and mechanical ventilation.

Magnitude of Teratogenic Risk

Undetermined

Quality and Quantity of Data

None

Comment

None

No epidemiological studies of congenital anomalies in infants born to women who had been treated with pancuronium during pregnancy have been reported.

No teratogenic effect was observed among the offspring of pregnant rats or rabbits given single daily injections of pancuronium 1.6 or 0.2 times that used as the initial intravenous dose in humans (Speight & Avery, 1972).

Intravascular or intramuscular injection of pancuronium into the fetus has been used to induce paralysis for prenatal diagnostic and therapeutic procedures (Copel et al., 1988;

Pielet et al., 1988; Moise et al., 1989; Williamson et al., 1989; Weiner et al., 1991). No persistent adverse effects related to this medication have been reported.

Please see agent summary on tubocurarine for information on a related drug that has been more thoroughly studied.

Key References

Copel JA, Grannum PA, Harrison D, Hubbins JC: The use of intravenous pancuronium bromide to produce fetal paralysis during intravascular transfusion. Am J Obstet Gynecol 158:170-171, 1988. [S]

Moise KJ Jr, Deter RL, Kirshon B, et al.: Intravenous pancuronium bromide for fetal neuromuscular blockade during intrauterine transfusion for red-cell alloimmunization. Obstet Gynecol 74:905-908, 1989. [S]

Pielet BW, Socol ML, MacGregor SN, et al.: Fetal heart rate changes after fetal intravascular treatment with pancuronium bromide. Am J Obstet Gynecol 159:640-643, 1988. [E]

Speight TM, Avery GS: Pancuronium bromide: A review of its pharmacological properties and clinical application. Drugs 4:163-226, 1972. [R]

Weiner CP, Wenstrom KD, Sipes SL, Williamson RA: Risk factors for cordocentesis and fetal intravascular transfusion. Am J Obstet Gynecol 165:1020-1025, 1991. [E]

Williamson RA, Weiner CP, Yuh WTC, Abu-Yousef MM: Magnetic resonance imaging of anomalous fetuses. Obstet Gynecol 73:952-956, 1989. [S]

PANTOTHENATE

Synonyms

Calcium Pantothenate, d-Pantothenic Acid, Vitamin B3, Vitamin B5

Summary

Pantothenate is a B vitamin. A component of coenzyme A, pantothenate is essential to carbohydrate, protein, and fat metabolism. The daily requirement of pantothenate is 10 mg.

Magnitude of Teratogenic Risk

Undetermined

Quality and Quantity of Data

None

Comment

None

No epidemiological studies of congenital anomalies among infants born to women who consumed excessive amounts of pantothenate during pregnancy have been reported.

No animal teratology studies of excessive pantothenate administration have been published, but deficiency of pantothenate has been shown to be teratogenic in experimental animals. Pregnant rats maintained on a pantothenate-deficient diet had increased frequencies of fetal deaths as well as offspring with central nervous system, ocular, cardiovascular, limb and other anomalies (Lefebvres, 1954; Nelson et al., 1957; Kalter & Warkany, 1959). Abnormalities have also been observed in the offspring of swine and mice after such treatment (Ullrey, et al., 1955; Kimura & Ariyama, 1961). Isolated deficiency of pantothenate is rare in humans because it is widely distributed in foods.

Key References

Kalter H, Warkany J: Experimental production of congenital malformations in mammals by metabolic procudure. Physiol Rev 39:69-115, 1959. [A]

Kimura S, Ariyama H: Teratogenic effects of pantothenic acid antagonists on animal embryos. J Vitaminol 7:231-236, 1961. [A]

Lefebvres J: Influence d'une deficience pantothenique legere sur les resultats dc la gestation chez la ratte. C R Acad Sci 238:2123-2125, 1954. [A]

Nelson MM, Wright HV, Baird CDC, Evans HM: Teratogenic effects of pantothenic acid deficiency in the rat. J Nutr 62:395-406, 1957. [A]

Ullrey DE, Becker DE, Terrill SW, Notzold RA: Dietary levels of pantothenic acid and reproductive performance of female swine. J Nutr 57:401-414, 1955. [A]

PAPAIN

Synonyms

Benase, Carica Papaya, Carofem, Caroid, Extenzyme, Papase, Papayotin, Soflens, Summetrin, Velardon

Summary

Papain is a proteolytic enzyme or enzyme mixture obtained from papaya. Papain is used topically as a debriding agent and given orally in the treatment of malabsorption. Papain is employed as a meat tenderizer and to clarify liquids such as beer.

Magnitude of Teratogenic Risk

Undetermined

Quality and Quantity of Data

Poor

Comment

A small risk cannot be excluded, but a substantial risk of congenital anomalies in the children of women treated with papain during pregnancy is unlikely.

No epidemiological studies of congenital anomalies among infants born to women treated with papain during pregnancy have been reported.

Dose-dependent increases in the frequency of fetal death, growth retardation, and hemorrhages were observed in the offspring of rats and rabbits treated during pregnancy with 375-

1000 or 375-500 mg/kg/d of papain in one series of studies (Singh & Devi, 1978; Devi & Singh, 1979). In contrast, no teratogenic effect was observed among the offspring of mice or rats subjected to similar treatment in another investigation (Food and Drug Research Laboratories, 1974).

Key References

Devi S, Singh S: Teratogenic effect of papain in rabbit fetuses. J Anat Soc India 28:6-10, 1979. [A]

Food and Drug Research Laboratories: Teratologic evaluation of FDA 73-54, papain in mice and rats. NTIS (National Technical Information Service) Report/PB245-533, 1974. [A]

Singh S, Devi S: Teratogenic and embryotoxic effect of papain in rat. Indian J Med Res 67:499-510, 1978. [A]

PAPAVERINE

Synonyms

Cardoverina, Cerespan, Dispamil, Pavabid, Pavacap Unicelles

Summary

Papaverine is an isoquinoline smooth muscle relaxant that is used in the treatment of ischemia.

Magnitude of Teratogenic Risk

Undetermined

Quality and Quantity of Data

None To Poor

Comment

A small risk cannot be excluded, but a high risk of congenital anomalies in the children of women treated with papaverine during pregnancy is unlikely.

No epidemiological studies of congenital anomalies among infants born to women treated with papaverine during pregnancy have been reported.

No teratogenic effect was observed among the offspring of mice treated with up to 5 times the maximum dose of papaverine used in humans (Jurand, 1980).

Key References

Jurand A: Malformations of the central nervous system induced by neurotropic drugs in mouse embryos. Dev Growth Differ 22:61-78, 1980. [A]

PARALDEHYDE

Synonyms

Acetaldehyde, Trimer, Elaldehyde, Hypnotets, Paracetaldehyde, Paral, Paraldeide, Triacetaldehyde

Summary

Paraldehyde is used as a sedative, hypnotic, and anticonvulsant.

Magnitude of Teratogenic Risk

Undetermined

Quality and Quantity of Data

None To Poor

Comment

A small risk cannot be excluded, but there is no indication that the risk of congenital anomalies in the children of women treated with paraldehyde during pregnancy is likely to be great.

No epidemiological studies of congenital anomalies in children born to women treated with paraldehyde during pregnancy have been reported.

The frequency of malformations was not increased among the offspring of rats treated with 2-3 times the usual human dose of paraldehyde during pregnancy in one study (Webster et al., 1985).

Maternal treatment with paraldehyde during delivery has been associated with drowsiness in the newborn infant (Baker, 1960).

Key References

Baker, JBE: The effects of drugs on the foetus. Pharmacol Rev 12:37-90, 1960. [R]

Webster WS, Germain MA, Edwards MJ: The induction of microphthalmia, encephalocele, and other head defects following hyperthermia during the gastrulation process in the rat. Teratology 31:73-82, 1985. [A]

PARCONAZOLE

Synonyms

R 39,500

Summary

Parconazole is an antifungal agent.

Magnitude of Teratogenic Risk

Undetermined

Quality and Quantity of Data

None

Comment

None

No epidemiological studies of congenital anomalies in infants born to women who used parconazole during pregnancy have been reported.

No animal teratology studies of parconazole have been published.

Key References

None available.

PARGYLINE

Synonyms

Eutonyl, Eutron, Pargilina, Pargylamine

Summary

Pargyline is a monoamine oxidase inhibitor used as an oral antihypertensive agent.

Magnitude of Teratogenic Risk

Undetermined

Quality and Quantity of Data

None To Poor

Comment

A small risk cannot be excluded, but a high risk of congenital anomalies in the children of women treated with pargyline during pregnancy is unlikely.

No epidemiological studies of congenital anomalies among the infants of women treated with pargyline during pregnancy have been reported.

Increased frequencies of fetal death were observed among pregnant mice treated with about 50 times the human dose of pargyline (Poulson & Robson, 1963) and among pregnant mice given intra-amniotic injections of pargyline (Koren et al., 1965). The frequency of cleft palate was not increased among the offspring of rats treated with 80 times the human therapeutic dose of pargyline during pregnancy (King et al., 1972).

Key References

King CTG, Horigan E, Wilk AL: Fetal outcome from prolonged versus acute drug administration in the pregnant rat. Adv Exp Med Biol 27:61-75, 1972. [A]

Koren Z, Pfeifer Y, Sulman FG: Deleterious effect of the monoamine oxidase inhibitor pargyline on pregnant rats. Fertil Steril 16:393-400, 1965. [A]

Poulson E, Robson JM: The effect of amine oxidase inhibitors on pregnancy. J Endocrinol 27:147-152, 1963. [A]

PAROMOMYCIN

Synonyms

Aminosidine Sulfate, Catenulin, Crestomycin Sulfate, Estomycin, Gabbromycin, Gabroral, Humagel, Humatin, Hydroxymycin, Sinosid

Summary

Paromomycin is an aminoglycoside antibiotic that is poorly absorbed from the gastrointestinal tract after oral administration. It is used in the treatment of intestinal parasitic infections and to suppress the growth of gastrointestinal bacteria.

Magnitude of Teratogenic Risk

Undetermined

Quality and Quantity of Data

None

Comment

None

No epidemiological studies of congenital anomalies among the children of women treated with paromomycin during pregnancy have been reported.

No animal teratology studies of paromomycin have been published.

Please see agent summary on neomycin for information on a related agent.

Key References

None available.

PARTRICIN

Synonyms

Ayfactin, SPA-S132

Summary

Partricin is an antifungal and antiprotozoal agent.

Magnitude of Teratogenic Risk

Undetermined

Quality and Quantity of Data

None

Comment

None

No epidemiological studies of congenital anomalies in infants born to women who used partricin during pregnancy have been reported.

No animal teratology studies of partricin have been published.

Key References

None available.

PARVOVIRUS B19

Synonyms

Erythema Infectiosum, Fifth Disease, Protein VP 1, Protein VP 2

Summary

Parvoviruses are small single-stranded DNA viruses that cause fifth disease (erythema infectiosum) in children (Anonymous, 1989; Rotbart, 1990; Shmoys & Kaplan, 1990). Parvovirus infections in adults may be asymptomatic or may produce a rash that is often associated with athralgia.

Magnitude of Teratogenic Risk

Hydrops/Fetal Death: Moderate

Malformations: Minimal

Quality and Quantity of Data

Hydrops/Fetal Death: Good

Malformations: Fair

Comment

Risk assessment is for parvovirus B19 and not for infections with other parvoviruses, such as canine parvovirus.

Fetal infection with parvovirus B19 can cause severe anemia, hydrops, and death (Brown et al., 1984; Bond et al., 1986; Gray et al., 1986; Anonymous, 1989; Brown, 1989; Mead, 1989; Shmoys & Kaplan, 1990). Most infected fetuses that develop hydrops die, but survival after intrauterine transfusion has been reported (Enders & Biber, 1990; Peters & Nicolaides, 1990). Resolution of hydrops in parvovirus-infected fetuses also occurs without treatment in some cases (Torok, 1990; Morey et al., 1991).

In a prospective series of pregnant women with proven parvovirus B19 infection during pregnancy, there was a fetal loss rate of 17% (28/166) with maternal infection before 20 weeks and 6% (1/17) with maternal infection later in gestation (Public Health Laboratory Service Working Party on Fifth Disease, 1990). Many of these miscarriages would have been expected even if the women had not been infected by parvovirus B19. The rate of miscarriage among these women attributable to fetal parvovirus infection is probably less than 10% (Public Health Laboratory Service Working Party on Fifth Disease, 1990; Torok, 1990). In another series of 114 pregnant women with documented parvovirus B19 infection, hydrops fetalis occurred in 8.7% (Enders & Biber, 1990). Thirty-six of these 114 women were infected in the first trimester, 62 in the second trimester, and 16 in the third.

The rate of congenital anomalies among liveborn infants of women who were infected with parvovirus B19 during pregnancy does not appear to be greatly increased. Malformations were not unusually common among 156 liveborn infants of women with documented parvovirus B19 infection during pregnancy in one series (Public Health Laboratory Service Working Party on Fifth Disease, 1990). Ninety-six of these women were infected in the first 12 weeks of gestation. In another series, all 51 infants of mothers who had documented parvovirus B19 infection during pregnancy were said to be "healthy at birth" (Enders & Biber, 1990). In a case-control study conducted after an outbreak of parvovirus B19, none of 47 infants with congenital anomalies had serologic evidence of parvovirus infection (Kinney et al., 1988). However, a therapeutically-aborted fetus was found to have ocular malformations and generalized myocarditis and myositis in association with documented first-trimester parvovirus infection (Weiland et al., 1987; Hartwig et al., 1989).

The single most useful diagnostic study in evaluation of a pregnant woman exposed to parvovirus is testing for specific IgM antibody in her serum (Rodis et al., 1988; Torok, 1990; Plotkin et al., 1990). Many exposed women will be found to have pre-existing antibody and therefore not be susceptible to infection; only a few percent of exposed women are likely to have evidence of primary infection (Enders & Biber, 1990; Cartter et al., 1991).

Prenatal diagnosis of affected fetuses is often possible by ultrasonography and maternal serum alpha-fetoprotein screening (Carrington et al., 1987; Bernstein & Capeless, 1989). Measurement of IgM in amniotic fluid or fetal blood is not a sensitive indicator of fetal infection, but detection of viral DNA in such specimens may be useful (Torok, 1990; Peters & Nicolaides, 1990; Morey et al., 1991).

Various parvoviruses have been shown to cause transplacental infection and fetal death in rats, hamsters, and swine (Kilham & Margolis, 1975; Mengeling, 1979; Mengeling & Paul, 1981). Ataxia associated with cerebellar hypoplasia has been observed among the offspring of cats, ferrets, rats, and hamsters infected with parvovirus during pregnancy (Kilham & Margolis, 1975; Catalano & Sever, 1973). A variety of central nervous system, facial, and other anomalies have been produced in the offspring of hamsters infected with parvovirus during pregnancy (Kilham & Margolis, 1975).

Key References

Anonymous: Risks associated with human parvovirus B19 infection. MMWR 38(6):81-88, 93-97, 1989. [R]

Bernstein IM, Capeless EL: Elevated maternal serum alpha-fetoprotein and hydrops fetalis in association with fetal parvovirus B-19 infection. Obstet Gynecol 74(3):456-7, 1989. [C]

Bond PR, Caul EO, Usher J, Cohen BJ, et al.: Intrauterine infection with human parvovirus. Lancet 1:448-449, 1986. [C]

Brown KE: What threat is human parvovirus B19 to the fetus? A review. Br J Obstet Gynaecol 96(7):764-767, 1989. [R]

Brown T, Anand A, Ritchie LD, Clewley JP, et al.: Intrauterine parvovirus infection associated with hydrops fetalis. Lancet 2:1033-1034, 1984. [C]

Carrington D, Gilmore DH, Whittle MJ, Aitken D, et al.: Maternal serum alpha-fetoprotein--A marker of fetal aplastic crisis during intrauterine human parvovirus infection. Lancet 1:433-435, 1987. [C]

Cartter ML, Farley TA, Rosengren S, et al.: Occupational risk factors for infection with parvovirus B19 among pregnant women. J Infect Dis 163:282-285, 1991. [S]

Catalano LW, Sever JL: The role of viruses as causes of congenital defects. Annu Rev Microbiol 25:255-282, 1971. [A]

Enders G, Biber M: Parvovirus B19 infections in pregnancy. Behring Inst Mitt 85:74-78, 1990. [S]

Gray ES, Anand A, Brown T: Parvovirus infections in pregnancy. Lancet 1:208, 1986. [C]

Hartwig NG, Vermeij-Keers C, van Elsacker-Niele AMW, Fleuren GJ: Embryonic malformations in a case of intrauterine parvovirus B19 infection. Teratology 39:295-302, 1989. [C]

Kilham L, Margolis G: Problems of human concern arising from animal models of intrauterine and neonatal infections due to viruses: A review. Progr Med Virol 20:113-143, 1975. [A]

Kinney JS, Anderson LJ, Farrar J, et al.: Risk of adverse outcomes of pregnancy after human parvovirus B19 infection. J Infect Dis 157(4):663-667, 1988. [E]

Mead PB: Parvovirus B19 infection and pregnancy. Contemp Ob Gyn 34:56-70, 1989. [R]

Mengeling WL: Prenatal infection following maternal exposure to porcine parvovirus on either the seventh or fourteenth day of gestation. Can J Comp Med 43:106-109, 1979. [A]

Mengeling WL, Paul PS: Reproductive performance of gilts exposed to porcine parvovirus at 56 or 70 days of gestation. Am J Vet Res 42:2074-2076, 1981. [A]

Morey AL, Nicolini U, Welch CR, et al.: Parvovirus B19 infection and transient fetal hydrops. Lancet 337:496, 1991. [C]

Peters MT, Nicolaides KH: Cordocentesis for the diagnosis and treatment of human fetal parvovirus infection. Obstet Gynecol 75(3):501-504, 1990. [C]

Plotkin SA, Halsey NA, Lepow ML, et al.: Parvovirus, erythema infectiosum, and pregnancy. Pediatrics 85(1):131-133, 1990. [R]

Public Health Laboratory Service Working Party on Fifth Disease: Prospective study of human parvovirus (B19) infection in pregnancy. BMJ 300:1166-1170, 1990. [E]

Rodis JF, Hovick TJ, Quinn DL, et al.: Human parvovirus infection in pregnancy. Obstet Gynecol 72(5):733-738, 1988. [S] & [R]

Rotbart HA: Human parvovirus infections. Annu Rev Med 41:25-34, 1990. [R]

Shmoys S, Kaplan C: Parvovirus and pregnancy. Clin Obstet Gynecol 33(2):268-275, 1990. [R]

Torok TJ: Human parvovirus B19 infections in pregnancy. Pediatr Infect Dis J 9(10):772-776, 1990. [R]

Weiland HT, Vermeij-Keers C, Salimans MM, Fleuren GJ, et al.: Parvovirus B19 associated with fetal abnormality. Lancet 1:682-683, 1987. [C]

PECTIN

Synonyms

Amforol, Methoxypectin, Methyl Pectinate, Parelixir

Summary

Pectin is a methoxylated derivative of galacturonic acids extracted from the rind of citrus fruits. It is used as a gelling agent and as a protectant and suspending agent in pharmaceutical preparations.

Magnitude of Teratogenic Risk

Undetermined

Quality and Quantity of Data

None

Comment

A small risk cannot be excluded, but a high risk of congenital anomalies in the children of women treated with pectin during pregnancy is unlikely.

No epidemiological studies of congenital anomalies in infants whose mothers were exposed to pectin during pregnancy have been reported.

No animal teratology studies of pectin have been published.

Key References

None available.

PELRINONE

Synonyms

Myotrope

Summary

Pelrinone is a cardiotonic drug.

Magnitude of Teratogenic Risk

Undetermined

Quality and Quantity of Data

None

Comment

None

No epidemiological studies of congenital anomalies in infants born to women who were treated with pelrinone during pregnancy have been reported.

No animal teratology studies of pelrinone have been published.

Key References

None available.

PEMOLINE

Synonyms

Cylert, Deltamine, Dinergil, Dynalert, Kethamed, Phenylisohydantoin, Phenylpseudohydantoin, Tamilan, Volital

Summary

Pemoline, an oxazolidine, is a central nervous system stimulant that is administered orally in the treatment of attention deficit disorders.

Magnitude of Teratogenic Risk

Undetermined

Quality and Quantity of Data

None

Comment

None

No epidemiological studies of congenital anomalies among infants born to women treated with pemoline during pregnancy have been reported.

No animal teratology studies of pemoline have been published.

Key References

None available.

PEMPIDINE

Synonyms

Perolysen, Pyrilene, Tenormal

Summary

Pempidine is a tertiary amine ganglionic-blocking agent used as an oral antihypertensive agent.

Magnitude of Teratogenic Risk

Undetermined

Quality and Quantity of Data

None

Comment

None

No epidemiological studies of congenital anomalies in infants whose mothers were treated with pempidine during pregnancy have been reported.

No animal teratology studies of pempidine have been published.

Key References

None available.

PENICILLAMINE

Synonyms

Cuprimine, D-3-Mercaptovaline, Depen, Dimethylcysteine, Distamine, Pendramine

Summary

Penicillamine is administered orally as a chelating agent and in the treatment of rheumatoid arthritis and cystinuria.

Magnitude of Teratogenic Risk

Small To Moderate

Quality and Quantity of Data

Fair To Good

Comment

None

Five infants with connective tissue abnormalities resembling cutis laxa whose mothers were treated with penicillamine during most or all of pregnancy have been reported (Mjolnerod et al., 1971; Solomon et al., 1977; Linares et al., 1979; Beck et al., 1981; Harpey et al., 1983). In addition to lax skin, some of these infants had inguinal hernias, loose joints, flat facies, small jaw, or vascular or tissue fragility. Three of the children died in infancy; one also had features of DiGeorge anomaly. The appearance of the skin in the two infants who survived improved markedly within a few months. The striking and unusual connective tissue abnormalities in these infants who were born to women who all received the same unusual therapy during pregnancy is consistent with a causal relationship. Nevertheless, connective tissue abnormalities appear to be uncommon among infants born to women who are treated with penicillamine during pregnancy (Endres, 1981; Gregory & Mansell, 1983; Rosa, 1986). In a series of 93 infants born to women treated with penicillamine during pregnancy and reported in the medical literature, only four with congenital anomalies were observed (Roubenoff et al., 1988). These four abnormal infants were all among those described above with connective tissue abnormalities.

Increased frequencies of cutis laxa and abdominal herniation were observed among the offspring of pregnant rats fed diets containing penicillamine in doses similar to those used therapeutically in humans (Keen et al., 1982). Conventional teratogenic malformations have been reported among the offspring of experimental animals treated with larger doses of penicillamine during pregnancy. Fetal death and congenital anomalies such as cleft palate have been observed with increased frequency among the offspring of mice and rats treated with penicillamine during pregnancy in doses 67-130 or about 50 times greater than those used in humans (Steffek et al., 1972; Kilburn & Hess, 1982; Myint, 1984; Rousseaux & MacNabb, 1992). Increased frequencies of neural tube and skeletal defects were noted among the offspring of pregnant hamsters treated with 110-160 times the usual human dose of penicillamine (Wiley & Joneja, 1978). The teratogenic effect in mice and rats can be prevented by dietary copper supplementation (Irino et al., 1982; Mark-Savage et al., 1983).

Key References

Beck RB, Rosenbaum KN, Byers PH, Holbrook KA, Perry LW: Ultrastructural findings in fetal penicillamine syndrome. Presentation and abstract. March of Dimes 14th Annual Birth Defects Conference, San Diego, Calif.: June 16, 1981. [C]

Endres W: D-penicillamine in pregnancy--to ban or not to ban? Klin Wochenschr 59:535-537, 1981. [R]

Gregory MC, Mansell MA: Pregnancy and cystinuria. Lancet 2:1158- 160, 1983. [S]

Harpey J-P, Jaudon M-C, Clavel J-P, et al.: Cutix laxa and low serum zinc after antenatal exposure to penicillamine. Lancet 2:858, 1983. [C]

Irino M, Sanada H, Tashiro S-I, et al.: D-penicillamine toxicity in mice. III. Pathological study of offspring of penicillamine-fed pregnant and lactating mice. Toxicol Appl Pharmacol 65:273-285, 1982. [A]

Keen CL, Marks-Savage P, Loneeerdal B, Hurley LS: Teratogenesis and low copper status resulting form D-penicillamine in rats. Teratology 26:163-165, 1982. [A]

Kilburn KH, Hess RA: Neonatal deaths and pulmonary dysplasia du to D-penicillamine in the rat. Teratology 26:1-9, 1982. [A]

Linares A, Zarranz JJ, Rodriguez-Alarcon J, Diaz-Perez JL: Reversible cutix laxa due to maternal D-penicillamine treatment. Lancet 2:43, 1979. [C]

Mark-Savage P, Keen CL, Hurley LS: Reduction by copper supplementation of teratogenic effects of D-penicillamine. J Nutr 113:501-510, 1983. [A]

Mjolnerod OK, Rasmussen K, Dommerud SA, Gjeruldsen ST: Congenital connective-tissue defect probably due to D-penicillamine treatment in pregnancy. Lancet 1:673-675, 1971. [C]

Myint BA: D-penicillamine-induced cleft palate in mice. Teratology 30:333-340, 1984. [A]

Rosa FW: Teratogen update: Penicillamine. Teratology 33:127-131, 1986. [R]

Roubenoff R, Hoyt J, Petri M, et al.: Effects of antiinflammatory and immunosuppressive drugs on pregnancy and fertility. Semin Arthritis Rheum 18(2):88-110, 1988. [R]

Rousseaux CG, MacNabb LG: Oral administration of d-penicillamine causes neonatal mortality without morphological defects in CD-1 mice. J Appl Toxicol 12(1):35-38, 1992. [A]

Solomon L, Abrams G, Dinner M, Berman L: Neonatal abnormalities associated with D-penicillamine treatment during pregnancy. N Engl J Med 296:54-55, 1977. [C]

Steffek AJ, Verrusio AC, Watkins CA: Cleft palate in rodents after maternal treatment with various lathyrogenic agents. Teratology 5:33-38, 1972. [A]

Wiley MJ, Joneja MG: Neural tube lesions in the offspring of hamsters given single oral doses of lathyrogens early in gestation. Acat Anat 100:347-353, 1978. [A]

PENICILLIN

Synonyms

Benzathine Penicillin, Benzylpenicillin Sodium, Bicillin L-A, Crystalline Penicillin G, Pentids 400 & 800, Permapen Isoject, Pfizerpen for Injection

Summary

Penicillin is a very widely used antibiotic.

Magnitude of Teratogenic Risk

None

Quality and Quantity of Data

Good

Comment

Available data deal with the use of penicillin in usual therapeutic doses. No information is available on the effects of exposure to exceptionally large doses as may be used to treat bacterial endocarditis.

The Collaborative Perinatal Project included 3546 infants born to women who had been treated with penicillin or its derivatives during the first four lunar months of pregnancy and 7171 pregnancies so treated anytime during gestation. The frequencies of congenital anomalies in general and of major classes of malformations were no greater than expected among the children born of these pregnancies (Heinonen et al., 1977). Similarly, the frequency of congenital anomalies was no greater than expected among the infants of 646 women who had been treated with penicillin during the first trimester of pregnancy in two cohorts of the Boston Collaborative Drug Surveillance

Program (Jick et al., 1981; Aselton et al., 1985). In a case-control study of 194 infants with major malformations, the frequency of first-trimester penicillin use was no greater among the cases than among the controls (Kullander & Kallen, 1976).

No teratogenic effect was observed among the offspring of rabbits treated during pregnancy with pencillin in doses similar to those used in humans (Brown et al., 1968).

Key References

Aselton P, Jick H, Milunsky A, Hunter JR, Stergachis A: First-trimester drug use and congenital disorders. Obstet Gynecol 65(4): 451-455, 1985. [S]

Brown DM, Harper KH, Palmer AK, Tesh SA: Effect of antibiotics upon pregnancy in the rabbit. Toxicol Appl Pharmacol 12:295, 1968. [A]

Heinonen OP, Slone D, Shapiro S: Birth Defects and Drugs in Pregnancy. Littleton, Mass.: John Wright-PSG, 1977, pp 312, 435. [E]

Jick H, Holmes LB, Hunter JR, Madsen S, et al.: First-trimester drug use and congenital disorders. JAMA 246:343-346, 1981. [S]

Kullander S, Kallen B: A prospective study of drugs and pregnancy. Acta Obstet Gynecol Scand 55:287-295, 1976. [S]

PENTACHLOROPHENOL

Synonyms

Chlorophen, Penchlorol, Penta, Santobrite, Santophen

Summary

Pentachlorophenol is widely used as a pesticide and as a preservative in wood, textiles, starch and glues. It acts as an uncoupler of oxidative phosphorylation and can produce considerable toxicity in adults (Choudhury et al., 1986). Pentachlorophenol is absorbed through the skin, lungs, and gastrointestinal tract. The 1991 ACGIH Threshold Limit Value for occupational exposure to pentachlorophenol is

0.5 mg/cu m of air as an 8-hour time-weighted average (Hathaway et al., 1991).

Magnitude of Teratogenic Risk

Undetermined

Quality and Quantity of Data

None To Poor

Comment

1) The abbreviation "PCP", which is sometimes used to refer to pentachlorophenol, has also been used as a name for phencyclidine, an hallucinogenic drug of abuse.

2) A small risk cannot be excluded, but a high risk of congenital anomalies in the children of women exposed to pentachlorophenol during pregnancy is unlikely.

No epidemiological studies of congenital anomalies among infants born to women exposed to pentachlorophenol during pregnancy have been reported.

Increased frequencies of fetal death, growth retardation, subcutaneous edema and skeletal anomalies were observed among the offspring of rats treated during pregnancy with both maternally toxic (30-50 mg/kg/d) and subtoxic (13-15 mg/kg/d) doses of pentachlorophenol (Schwetz et al., 1974; Welsh et al., 1987).

Key References

Choudhury H, Coleman J, De Rosa CT, Stara JF: Pentachlorophenol: Health and environmental effects profile. Toxicol Ind Health 2(4):483-571, 1986. [R]

Hathaway GJ, Proctor NH, Hughes JP, Fischman ML (eds): Proctor and Hughes' Chemical Hazards of the Workplace, 3rd edition. New York: Van Nostrand Reinhold, 1991, p 460. [R]

Schwetz BA, Keeler PA, Gehring PJ: The effect of purified and commercial grade pentachlorophenol on rat embryonal and fetal development. Toxicol Appl Pharmacol 28:151-161, 1974. [A]

Welsh JJ, Collins TFX, Black TN, et al.: Teratogenic potential of purified pentachlorophenol and pentachloroanisole in subchronically exposed Sprague-Dawley rats. Food Chem Toxicol 25(2):163-172, 1987. [A]

PENTAERYTHRITOL TETRANITRATE

Synonyms

Cardiacap, Duotrate, Mycardol, Pentanitrine, Peritrate, Tetrahydroxymethylmethane, Tetramethylolmethane

Summary

Pentaerythritol tetranitrate is an oral nitrate vasodilator used in the treatment of angina pectoris.

Magnitude of Teratogenic Risk

Undetermined

Quality and Quantity of Data

None

Comment

None

No epidemiological studies of congenital anomalies among infants born to women treated with pentaerythritol tetranitrate during pregnancy have been reported.

No animal teratology studies of pentaerythritol tetranitrate have been published.

Please see agent summary on nitroglycerin for information on a related agent that has been studied.

Key References

None available.

PENTAGASTRIN

Synonyms

Gastrodiagnost, Peptavlon, Petavlon, Petogasrin

Summary

Pentagastrin is a synthetic polypeptide hormone that stimulates gastric and pancreatic secretion. Pentagastrin is administered parenterally as a diagnostic test.

Magnitude of Teratogenic Risk

Undetermined

Quality and Quantity of Data

None To Poor

Comment

None

No epidemiological studies of congenital anomalies among infants born to women who had been given pentagastrin during pregnancy have been reported.

No animal teratology studies of pentagastrin have been published. Increased frequencies of pyloric hypertrophy and peptic ulceration have been observed among the offspring of dogs treated repeatedly during late pregnancy with 17-250 times the human diagnostic dose of pentagastrin (Dodge & Karim, 1976). The clinical relevance of this observation is uncertain.

Fasting plasma gastrin levels were not increased among 15 human infants with pyloric stenosis (Rogers et al., 1975).

Key References

Dodge JA, Karim AA: Induction of pyloric hypertrophy by pentagastrin. Gut 17:280-284, 1976. [A]

Rogers IM, Drainer IK, Moore MR, Buchanan KD: Plasma gastrin in congenital hypertrophic pyloric stenosis. Arch Dis Child 50:467, 1975. [E]

PENTAMIDINE

Synonyms

Diamidine, Lomidine, M & B-800, Pentacarinat, Pentam

Summary

Pentamidine is an antibiotic that is administered parenterally in the treatment of serious parasitic infestations such as pneumocystis pneumonia, trypanosomiasis, and leishmaniasis. Pentamidine has also been given for prophylaxis against trypanosomiasis.

Magnitude of Teratogenic Risk

Undetermined

Quality and Quantity of Data

None

Comment

None

No epidemiological studies of congenital anomalies among the children of women treated with pentamidine during pregnancy have been reported.

The frequency of malformations was not increased among the offspring of rats treated during pregnancy with 1-5 times the human therapeutic dose of pentamidine in one study (Harstad et al., 1990).

Key References

Harstad TW, Little BB, Bawdon RE, et al.: Embryofetal effects of pentamidine isethionate administered to pregnant Sprague-Dawley rats. Am J Obstet Gynecol 163:912-916, 1990. [A]

PENTAZOCINE

Synonyms

Algopent, Fortral, Pentafen, Talwin

Summary

Pentazocine is a narcotic analgesic that is used for the relief of moderate to severe pain. Pentazocine is also used as a "recreational" drug, often in combination with other drugs.

Magnitude of Teratogenic Risk

Minimal

Quality and Quantity of Data

Poor To Fair

Comment

Withdrawal symptoms have been observed in newborn infants of women who used pentazocine during pregnancy. These symptoms resemble those seen in infants of heroin and morphine addicts (see below).

No congenital anomalies were observed among the infants of 51 female drug abusers who used a pentazocine and tripelennamine combination ("Ts and Blues") during pregnancy (von Almen & Miller, 1986). In another series of 23 infants born to women who abused pentazocine and tripelennamine during pregnancy, the frequency of cardiac anomalies was increased, but the abnormalities observed seem unlikely to be attributable to the mothers' use of this medication (Little et al., 1990). Lower than expected birth weight, length, and head circumference have been noted among infants born to women who abused pentazocine and tripelennamine during pregnancy (Dunn & Reynolds, 1982; Chasnoff et al., 1983; von Almen & Miller, 1986; Little et al., 1990), but it is difficult to determine whether this is an effect of the drug or of factors associated with the lifestyle of these women.

An increased frequency of cranial neural tube defects was observed among the offspring of hamsters treated at a critical point in pregnancy with single doses of pentazocine 30 or more times greater than those used clinically (Geber & Schramm, 1975). No teratogenic effect was noted after administration of 15 times the usual human therapeutic dose. Long-term behavioral alterations have been observed among the offspring of rats treated with 2-4 times the human dose of pentazocine and tripelennamine during pregnancy (Driscoll et al., 1986).

Transient neonatal withdrawal symptoms occur in infants born to women who take pentazocine chronically late in pregnancy (Goetz & Bain, 1974; Scanlon, 1974; Kopelman, 1975; Dunn & Reynolds, 1982; Chasnoff et al., 1983; von Almen & Miller, 1986). The infants' symptoms resemble those seen in neonatal withdrawal from other narcotics: irritability, hyperactivity, vomitting, and high-pitched cry.

Please see agent summary on morphine for information on a closely related drug that has been more thoroughly studied.

Key References

Chasnoff IJ, Hatcher R, Burns WJ, et al.: Pentazocine and tripelennamine ('T's and Blue's'): Effects on the fetus and neonate. Dev Pharmacol Ther 6:162-169, 1983. [E]

Driscoll CD, Meyer LS, Riley EP: Behavioral and developmental effects of prenatal exposure to pentazocine and tripelennamine combinations. Neurobehav Toxicol Teratol 8(6):605-613, 1986. [A]

Dunn DW, Reynolds J: Neonatal withdrawal symptoms associated with 'T's and Blues' (pentazocine and tripelennamine). Am J Dis Child 136:644-645, 1982. [S]

Geber WF, Schramm LC: Congenital malformations of the central nervous system produced by narcotic analgesics in the hamster. Am J Obstet Gynecol 123:705-713, 1975. [A]

Goetz RL, Bain RV: Neonatal withdrawal symptoms associated with maternal use of pentazocine. J Pediatr 84:887-888, 1974. [C]

Kopelman AE: Fetal addiction to pentazocine. Pediatrics 55:888-889, 1975. [C]

Little BB, Snell LM, Breckenridge JD, Knoll KA, et al.: Effects of T's and Blues abuse on pregnancy outcome and infant health status. Am J Perinatol 7(4):359-362, 1990. [E]

Scanlon JW: Pentazocine and neonatal withdrawal symptoms. J Pediatr 85:735-736, 1974. [C]

von Almen WF, Miller JM: "Ts and Blues" in pregnancy. J Reprod Med 31:236-239, 1986. [E]

PENTOBARBITAL

Synonyms

Embutal, Ethaminal Sodium, Insom Rapido, Mebubarbital Sodium, Mebumal Sodium, Nembutal, Nova-Rectal

Summary

Pentobarbital is a short-acting barbiturate that is used as a sedative and hypnotic.

Magnitude of Teratogenic Risk

None To Minimal

Quality and Quantity of Data

Fair To Good

Comment

None

The frequencies of congenital anomalies in general, of major malformations, and of minor anomalies were no greater than expected among the children of 250 women who took pentobarbital during the first four lunar months of pregnancy in the Collaborative Perinatal Project (Heinonen et al., 1977). The frequency of congenital anomalies was not increased among the infants of 1523 women who used pentobarbital anytime during pregnancy in this study. No increase in the frequency of congenital anomalies was seen among the children of more than 50 women who took pentobarbital during the first trimester of pregnancy

in the Boston Collaborative Drug Surveillance Program (Jick et al., 1981).

Increased frequencies of skeletal and craniofacial anomalies as well as of fetal death were observed among the offspring of mice treated during pregnancy with about 25 times the usual human sedative dose of pentobarbital (Setala & Nyyssonen, 1964). No increase in malformations but increased frequencies of fetal growth retardation and death were observed among the offspring of golden hamsters treated during pregnancy with 16 times the usual human sedative dose of pentobarbital (Hilbelink, 1982). No fetal effect was seen at 4-12 times the usual human sedative dose. Similarly, no increase in malformations but an increased frequency of fetal death were observed among the offspring of pregnant rabbits treated with 20 times the usual human sedative dose of pentobarbital (Johnson, 1971). Long-lasting alterations of behavior and decreased brain/body weight ratios were observed among the offspring of rats treated with 20-40 times the usual human sedative dose of pentobarbital during pregnancy (Martin, et al., 1985). The relevance of these observations to the clinical use of pentobarbital in human pregnancy is unknown.

Key References

Heinonen OP, Slone D, Shapiro S: Birth Defects and Drugs in Pregnancy. Littleton, Mass.: John Wright-PSG, 1977, pp 336-337, 341, 438, 476, 490. [E]

Hilbelink DR: Effects of prolonged sodium pentobarbital anesthesia on the embryonic development of the golden hamster. Teratology 25:48A, 1982. [A]

Jick H, Holmes LB, Hunter JR, Madsen S, et al.: First-trimester drug use and congenital disorders. JAMA 246:343-346, 1981. [S]

Johnson WE: Fetal loss from anesthesia and surgical trauma in the rabbit. Toxicol Appl Pharmacol 18:773-779, 1971. [A]

Martin JC, Martin DC, Mackler B, Grace R, et al.: Maternal barbiturate administration and offspring response to shock. Psychopharmacology 85:214-220, 1985. [A]

Setala K, Nyyssonen O: Hypnotic sodium pentobarbital as a teratogen for mice. Naturwissenschaften 51:413, 1964. [A]

PENTOXIFYLLINE

Synonyms

Azutrentat, Dimethyloxohexylxanthine, Durapental, Hemovas, Oxpentifylline, Pento-Puren, Rentylin, Torental, Trental

Summary

Pentoxifylline is a methylxanthine derivative that is administered orally in the treatment of peripheral vascular disease.

Magnitude of Teratogenic Risk

Undetermined

Quality and Quantity of Data

Poor

Comment

A small risk cannot be excluded, but a high risk of congenital anomalies in the children of women treated with pentoxyfylline during pregnancy is unlikely.

No epidemiological studies of congenital anomalies among infants born to women treated with pentoxifylline during pregnancy have been reported.

No teratogenic effect was observed among the offspring of rabbits treated with 0.25-1 times the usual human dose of pentoxifylline during pregnancy (Sugisaki et al., 1981). The frequency of malformations is said to have been no greater than expected among the offspring of pregnant rats or rabbits respectively treated with up to 25 or up to 10 times the usual human dose of pentoxifylline, but these studies have not been published in sufficient detail to permit independent evaluation (Aviado & Porter, 1984).

Key References

Aviado DM, Porter JM: Pentoxifylline: A new drug for the treatment of intermittent claudication. Pharmacotherapy 4:297-307, 1984. [R]

Sugisaki T, Hayashi S, Miyamoto M: Teratological study of pentoxifylline in rabbits by the intravenous route. Oyo Yakuri 22:451-458, 1981. [A]

PEPSIN

Synonyms

Lactated Pepsin

Summary

Pepsin is a proteolytic enzyme found in the gastric juice of animals. It is administered orally as an aid to digestion.

Magnitude of Teratogenic Risk

Undetermined

Quality and Quantity of Data

None

Comment

A small risk cannot be excluded, but a high risk of congenital anomalies in the children of women treated with pepsin during pregnancy is unlikely.

No epidemiological studies of congenital anomalies among infants born to women treated with pepsin during pregnancy have been reported.

No animal teratology studies of pepsin have been published.

Key References

None available.

PERMETHRIN

Synonyms

Ambush, Corsair, Dragnet, Ectiban, Nix, Pounce, Pynosect, Ridect Pour-On

Summary

Permethrin is a pyrethroid insecticide used topically to treat lice infestations. Skin absorption after topical application is less than 2%. Permethrin is also used as an agricultural and garden insecticide.

Magnitude of Teratogenic Risk

Undetermined

Quality and Quantity of Data

None To Poor

Comment

A small risk cannot be excluded, but there is no indication that the risk of congenital anomalies in the children of women treated topically with permethrin during pregnancy is likely to be great.

No epidemiological studies of congenital anomalies in infants whose mothers were exposed to permethrin during pregnancy have been reported.

No teratogenic effects were observed among the offspring of mice fed 15-150 mg/kg/d of permethrin during pregnancy (Miyamoto, 1976; WHO, 1990). Similarly, the frequency of malformations was not increased among the offspring of rats or rabbits fed permethrin during pregnancy in doses of 4-225 mg/kg/d or 600-1800 mg/kg/d, respectively (WHO, 1990).

Key References

Miyamoto J: Degradation, metabolism and toxicity of synthetic pyrethroids. Environ Health Persp 14:15-28, 1976. [A]

WHO (World Health Organization): Environmental health criteria 94: Permethrin. Environ Health Criter 94:1-125, 1990. [R]

PERPHENAZINE

Synonyms

Trilafon

Summary

Perphenazine is a phenothiazine tranquilizer used in the treatment of psychoses. It is also used to control nausea and vomiting.

Magnitude of Teratogenic Risk

None To Minimal

Quality and Quantity of Data

Poor To Fair

Comment

None

The frequency of congenital anomalies was not increased among the children of 63 women treated with perphenazine during the first four lunar months of pregnancy or of 166 women treated with the drug anytime during pregnancy in the Collaborative Perinatal Project (Heinonen et al., 1977).

Increased frequencies of cleft palate and micromelia were observed among the offspring of rats treated with 40-300 times the usual human dose of perphenazine during pregnancy, but no teratogenic effect was observed in the offspring of rats treated with 1.5-14 times the usual human dose (Beall, 1972; Druga, 1976).

Fetal loss was increased throughout the entire dose-range studied. An increased frequency of cleft palate was also found among the offspring of mice treated during pregnancy with 30-100 times the usual therapeutic dose of perphenazine, but this effect was shown to be due largely to suppression of eating in the mothers (Szabo & Brent, 1974, 1975). The relevance of these observations to the risks associated with therapeutic use of perphenazine in human pregnancy is unknown.

An increased frequency of chromosome breaks and rearrangements has been reported in peripheral blood lymphocytes of patients taking perphenazine (Nielen et al., 1969). No studies of the gametes or offspring of these patients have been reported; the clinical significance of these findings is unknown.

Please see agent summary on chlorpromazine for information on a related agent that has been more thoroughly studied.

Key References

Beall JR: A teratogenic study of chlorpromazine, orphenadrine, perphenazine, and LSD-25 in rats. Toxicol Appl Pharmacol 21:230-236, 1972. [A]

Druga A: The effect of perphenazine treatment during the organogenesis in rats. Acta Biol Acad Sci Hung 27:15-23, 1976. [A]

Heinonen OP, Slone D, Shapiro S: Birth Defects and Drugs in Pregnancy. Littleton, Mass.: John Wright-PSG, 1977, pp 323-324, 437. [E]

Nielen J, Friedrich U, Tsuboi T: Chromosome abnormalities in patients treated with chlorpromazine, perphenazine, and lysergide. Br Med J 3:634-636, 1969. [E]

Szabo KT, Brent RL: Reduction of drug-induced cleft palate in mice. Lancet 1:1296-1297, 1975. [A]

Szabo KT, Brent RL: Species differences in experimental teratogenesis by tranquillising agents. Lancet 1:565, 1974. [A]

PERUVIAN BALSAM

Synonyms

Balsam Peru Oil, Branolind, Dera, Linitul, Oil Balsam Peru

Summary

Peruvian balsam is a plant resin that has mild antiseptic properties. It is used topically to treat bedsores, chronic ulcers, eczema, and pruritis. It is an ingredient in some rectal suppositories used for symptomatic treatment of hemorrhoids.

Magnitude of Teratogenic Risk

Undetermined

Quality and Quantity of Data

None

Comment

None

No epidemiological studies of congenital anomalies in infants whose mothers used peruvian balsam during pregnancy have been reported.

No animal teratology studies of peruvian balsam have been published.

Key References

None available.

PETROLATUM

Synonyms

Fonoline White, Fonoline Yellow, Jelonet, Mineral Jelly, Ocu-Lube, Paraffin Jelly, Petro-Phylic, Petroleum Jelly, Soft Paraffin, Vaseline, White Petrolatum, Yellow Petroleum Jelly

Summary

Petrolatum is a purified semi-solid mixture of hydrocarbons. It is used topically as an ointment base and protectant. Petrolatum is poorly absorbed through the skin.

Magnitude of Teratogenic Risk

None

Quality and Quantity of Data

None

Comment

None

No epidemiological studies of congenital anomalies in the infants of women who used petrolatum during pregnancy have been reported.

No animal teratology studies of petrolatum have been published.

Key References

None available.

PHENACAINE

Synonyms

Holocaine

Summary

Phenacaine is a local anesthetic that has been used in ophthalmology.

Magnitude of Teratogenic Risk

Undetermined

Quality and Quantity of Data

None

Comment

None

No epidemiological studies of congenital anomalies in children born to women exposed to phenacaine during pregnancy have been reported.

No investigations of teratologic effects of phenacaine in experimental animals have been published.

Please see agent summary on procaine for information on a related agent that has been studied.

Key References

None available.

PHENACETIN

Synonyms

Acetophenetidin

Summary

Phenacetin is an analgesic and antipyretic agent that is used orally, usually in combination with other agents of this class. Acetaminophen is a metabolic product of phenacetin.

Magnitude of Teratogenic Risk

None

Quality and Quantity of Data

Good

Comment

This risk is for use at conventional therapeutic doses.

The frequencies of congenital anomalies in general, major malformations, minor anomalies, and principal classes of congenital anomalies were not increased among the children of 5546 women who took phenacetin during the first four lunar months of pregnancy in the Collaborative Perinatal Project (Heinonen et al., 1977). Similarly, no increase in the frequency of malformations was observed among more than 100 infants whose mothers took phenacetin in combination with aspirin, caffeine, and codeine during the first trimester of pregnancy in the Boston Collaborative Drug Surveillance Program (Jick et al., 1981). The frequency of congenital anomalies was no greater than expected among the children of 13,031 women who took phenacetin anytime during pregnancy in the Collaborative Perinatal Project (Heinonen et al., 1977).

No malformations were observed among the infants of four women who took large overdoses of phenacetin and other medications at various times during pregnancy (Czeizel et al., 1984).

The frequency of malformations was not increased among the offspring of rats treated with 2-17 times the maximum human therapeutic dose of phenacetin during pregnancy (Baethke & Muller, 1965). Maternal toxicity and reduced fetal weight occurred at the highest doses.

Please see agent summary on acetaminophen for information on a related agent.

Key References

Baethke R, Muller B: Investigation of the chronic toxicity of phenacetin in rat embryos. Klin Wochenschr 43:364-368, 1965. [A]

Czeizel A, Szentesi, Szekeres I, et al.: Pregnancy outcome and health conditions of offspring of self-poisoned pregnant women. Acta Paaediatr Hung 25(3):209-236, 1984. [S]

Heinonen OP, Slone D, Shapiro S: Birth Defects and Drugs in Pregnancy. Littleton, Mass.: John Wright-PSG, 1977, pp 11, 287, 289, 291, 294-295, 370, 434, 471, 483. [E]

Jick H, Holmes LB, Hunter JR, Madsen S, et al.: First-trimester drug use and congenital disorders. JAMA 246:343-346, 1981. [S]

PHENAZOPYRIDINE

Synonyms

Azo Gantrisin, Giracid, Phenazo, Pyridacil, Pyridium, Uropyrine

Summary

Phenazopyridine is used to relieve urinary tract pain and irritability in cystitis, urethritis, and prostatitis.

Magnitude of Teratogenic Risk

None

Quality and Quantity of Data

Fair To Good

Comment

None

The frequency of malformations in general, of major malformations, and of minor malformations was no greater than expected among the offspring of 219 women who used phenazopyridine during the first four lunar months of pregnancy in the Collaborative Perinatal Project (Heinonen et al., 1977). Similarly, in the Boston Collaborative Drug Surveillance program, the frequency of malformations in infants born to more than 300 women who used phenazopyridine during the first trimester of pregnancy was no greater than expected (Jick et al., 1981; Aselton et al., 1985). No association between congenital anomalies in the infants and maternal use of phenazopyridine anytime during pregnancy was observed among 1109 exposed women in the Collaborative Perinatal Project (Heinonen et al., 1977).

No animal teratology studies of phenazopyridine have been published.

Key References

Aselton P, Jick H, Milunsky A, et al.: First-trimester drug use and congenital disorders. Obstet Gynecol 65:451-455, 1985. [S]

Heinonen OP, Slone D, Shapiro S: Birth Defects and Drugs in Pregnancy. Littleton, Mass.: John Wright-PSG, 1977, pp 308, 486. [E]

Jick H, Holmes LB, Hunter JR, et al.: First-trimester drug use and congenital disorders. JAMA 246:343-346, 1981. [S]

PHENCYCLIDINE

Synonyms

Angel Dust, Cyclone, Mist, Peace Pills, Super Weed, Surfer

Summary

Phencyclidine is widely used as a "recreational" drug (Harry & Howard, 1992). It was formerly employed as a human and veterinary anesthetic.

Magnitude of Teratogenic Risk

Minimal

Quality and Quantity of Data

Poor To Fair

Comment

Neurobehavioral alterations have been observed in infants of women who abused phencyclidine during pregnancy (see below), but it is not known if persistent drug-related effects occur.

No malformations were noted in series of 94 and 37 infants of women who abused phencyclidine at some time during pregnancy (Golden et al., 1987; Tabor et al., 1990). In another series of 57 infants whose mothers abused phencyclidine during pregnancy, two of the children looked "morphologically unusual," but no consistent pattern of congenital anomalies was found (Wachsman et al., 1989). One of the children in this series exhibited severe developmental delay. The cause of these abnormalities is unknown, and no direct relationship to the maternal use of phencyclidine has been established.

Alterations of neonatal neurological function and behavior have frequently been observed among the children of women who abused phencyclidine during pregnancy (Golden et al., 1980, 1987; Strauss et al., 1981; Chasnoff et al., 1983; Wachsman et al., 1989; Tabor et al., 1990; Harry & Howard, 1992). The abnormalities seen include symptoms resembling narcotic withdrawal (jitteriness, abnormal suck, irritability) as well as alterations of tone, abnormal eye movements, sudden outbursts of agitation, and rapid changes in the level of consciousness. Lower than expected weight, length, and head circumference have also been noted among these infants (Wachsman et al., 1989). Various mild behavioral and developmental abnormalities have been found among preschool children whose mothers abused phencyclidine during pregnancy (Harry & Howard, 1992). It is difficult to know if these findings are due to an effect of the phencyclidine or to other socioeconomic or biological factors associated with children of women who abuse phencyclidine.

An increased frequency of limb and cranial defects occurred in the offspring of pregnant rats given phencyclidine in doses 25-30 times those used in humans (Jordan et al., 1978). Teratogenic effects were observed in mice at doses of phencyclidine that were toxic to the mothers (120 times the usual human dose) but not at lower doses (5-100 times the usual human dose) (Goodwin et al., 1980; Marks et al., 1980; Nicholas & Schreiber, 1983). Behavioral abnormalities occur among the offspring of mice and rats treated with phencyclidine during pregnancy in doses 10-20 times those used by humans (Goodwin et al., 1980; Nicholas & Schreiber, 1983; Nabeshima et al., 1987, 1988; Yanai et al., 1992).

Key References

Chasnoff IJ, Burns WJ, Hatcher RP, et al.: Phencyclidine: Effects on the fetus and neonate. Dev Pharmacol Ther 6:404-408, 1983. [E]

Golden NL, Kuhnert BR, Sokol RJ, et al.: Neonatal manifestations of maternal phencyclidine exposure. J Perinat Med 15:185-191, 1987. [E]

Golden NL, Sokol RJ, Rubin IL: Angel dust: Possible effects on the fetus. Pediatrics 65(1):18-20, 1980. [C]

Goodwin PJ, Perez VJ, Eatwell JC, Palet JL, et al.: Phencyclidine: Effects of chronic administration in the female mouse on gestation, maternal behavior, and the neonates. Psychopharmacology 69:63-67, 1980. [A]

Harry GJ, Howard J: Phencyclidine: Experimental studies in animals and long-term developmental effects on humans. In: Sonderegger TB (ed). Perinatal Substance Abuse: Research Findings and Clinical Implications. Baltimore: The Johns Hopkins University Press, 1992, pp 254-278. [R]

Jordan RL, young TR, Harry GJ: Teratology of phencyclidine in rats: Preliminary studies. Teratology 17:40A, 1978. [A]

Marks TA, Worthy WC, Staples RE: Teratogenic potential of phencyclidine in the mouse. Teratology 21:241-246, 1980. [A]

Nabeshima T, Hiramatsu M, Yamaguchi K, et al.: Effects of prenatal administration of phencyclidine on the learning and memory processes of rat offspring. J Pharmacobio-Dyn 11:816-823, 1988. [A]

Nabeshima T, Yamaguchi K, Hiramatsu M, et al.: Effects of prenatal and perinatal administration of phencyclidine on the behavioral development of rat offspring. Pharmacol Biochem Behav 28:411-418, 1987. [A]

Nicholas JM, Schreiber EC: Phencyclidine exposure and the developing mouse: Behavioral teratological implications. Teratology 28:319-326, 1983. [A]

Strauss AA, Modanlou HD, Bosu SK: Neonatal manifestations of maternal phencyclidine (PCP) abuse. Pediatrics 68:550-552, 1981. [C]

Tabor BL, Smith-Wallace T, Yonckura ML: Perinatal outcome associated with PCP versus cocaine use. Am J Drug Alcohol Abuse 16(3,4):337-348, 1990. [E]

Wachsman L, Schuetz S, Chan LS, et al.: What happens to babies exposed to phencyclidine (PCP) in utero? Am J Drug Alcohol Abuse 15(10):31-39, 1989. [E]

Yanai J, Avraham Y, Levy S, Maslaton J, et al.: Alterations in septohippocampal cholinergic innervations and related behaviors after early exposure to heroin and phencyclidine. Dev Brain Res 69(2):207-214, 1992. [A]

PHENDIMETRAZINE

Synonyms

Adipost, Anorex, Bacarate, Prelu-2, Sprx, Statobex, Trimtabs, Wehless

Summary

Phendimetrazine is a sympathomimetic agent that is taken orally as an appetite suppressant.

Magnitude of Teratogenic Risk

Undetermined

Quality and Quantity of Data

None

Comment

None

No adequate epidemiological studies of congenital anomalies in infants born to women who took phendimetrazine during pregnancy have been reported.

No animal teratology studies of phendimetrazine have been published.

Please see agent summary on dextroamphetamine for information on a related agent that has been studied.

Key References

None available.

PHENELZINE

Synonyms

Estinerval, Fenelzin, Kalgan, Nardelzine, Nardil, Phenethylhydrazine, Stinerval

Summary

Phenelzine is a monoamine oxidase inhibitor that is used orally as an antidepressant.

Magnitude of Teratogenic Risk

Undetermined

Quality and Quantity of Data

None To Poor

Comment

None

No epidemiological studies of congenital anomalies among infants born to women treated with phenelzine during pregnancy have been reported.

Increased frequencies of embryonic loss and fetal death were observed among pregnant mice and rats treated with 7-14 times the usual human dose of phenelzine (Poulson & Robson, 1964; Samojlik, 1965; Robson et al., 1971).

Key References

Poulson E, Robson JM: Effect of phenelzine and some related compounds on pregnancy and on sexual development. J Endocrinol 30:205-215, 1964. [A]

Robson JM, Sullivan FM, Wilson C: The maintenance of pregnancy during the pre-implantation period in mice treated with phenelzine derivatives. J Endocrinol 49:635-648, 1971. [A]

Samojlik E: Studies of the effect of monoaminooxidase inhibitors on the fertility, fetuses and reproductive organs of rats. 1. The effect of monoaminooxidase inhibitors on the fertility, fetuses and on the sexual cycle. Pol Endocrinol 16(1-2):21-29, 1965. [A]

PHENINDAMINE

Synonyms

Nolahist, Thephorin

Summary

Phenindamine is used orally as an antihistamine.

Magnitude of Teratogenic Risk

Undetermined

Quality and Quantity of Data

None

Comment

A small risk cannot be excluded, but a high risk of congenital anomalies in the children of women treated with phenindamine during pregnancy is unlikely.

No adequate epidemiological studies of congenital anomalies among infants born to women treated with phenindamine during pregnancy have been reported.

No animal teratology studies of phenindamine have been published.

Please see agent summary on chlorpheniramine for information on a related agent that has been studied.

Key References

None available.

PHENIRAMINE

Synonyms

Acovil, Avil, Avilettes, Daneral SA, Fenamine, Inhiston, Prophenpyridamine Maleate, Rynabond, Verstat

Summary

Pheniramine is an alkylamine derivative used to treat allergic symptoms.

Magnitude of Teratogenic Risk

None To Minimal

Quality and Quantity of Data

Fair

Comment

None

The frequencies of congenital anomalies in general, major malformations, minor anomalies, and major classes of anomalies were not significantly increased among the children of 831 women who used pheniramine during the first four lunar months of pregnancy in the Collaborative Perinatal Project (Heinonen et al., 1977). Similarly, the frequency of congenital anomalies was no greater than expected among the children of 2442 women who used this drug anytime during pregnancy.

No animal teratology studies of pheniramine have been published.

Please see the agent summary on chlorpheniramine for information on a closely related agent that has been more thoroughly studied.

Key References

Heinonen OP, Slone D, Shapiro S: Birth Defects and Drugs in Pregnancy. Littleton, Mass.: John Wright-PSG, 1977, pp 323-324, 329, 437, 475, 488. [E]

PHENMETRAZINE

Synonyms

Fenmetrazina, Mefolin, Oxazimedrine, Preludin, Probese-P

Summary

Phenmetrazine is a sympathomimetic agent that is administered orally as an appetite suppressant.

Magnitude of Teratogenic Risk

None To Minimal

Quality and Quantity of Data

Poor To Fair

Comment

None

The frequency of congenital anomalies was no greater than expected among the children of 58 women who used phenmetrazine during the first four lunar months of pregnancy or among the children of 257 women who used this drug anytime during pregnancy in the Collaborative Perinatal Project (Heinonen et al., 1977). Similarly, the frequency of severe congenital anomalies was not significantly increased among the children of 55 women who took phenmetrazine during the first 84 days of pregnancy or among the children of 406 women who took this medication anytime during pregnancy in another large cohort study (Milkovich & van den Berg, 1977). Phenmetrazine was used relatively often in pregnancy in the 1950s and 1960s (e.g., in 3.75% of the pregnancies reported by Milkovich and van den Berg, 1977). In light of this fact and the epidemiological studies cited above, anecdotal case reports from this era of congenital anomalies among infants born to women who took phenmetrazine during pregnancy probably represent chance occurrences (Powell & Johnstone, 1962; Moss, 1962; Lenz, 1962; Fogh-Anderson, 1967).

No teratological studies of phenmetrazine in experimental animals have been published.

Key References

Fogh-Andersen P: Genetic and non-genetic factors in the etiology of facial clefts. Scand J Plast Reconstr Surg 1:22-29, 1967. [R]

Heinonen OP, Slone D, Shapiro S: Birth Defects and Drugs in Pregnancy. Littleton, Mass.: John Wright-PSG, 1977, pp 346-347, 439. [E]

Lenz W: Drugs and congenital abnormalities. (Letters to the Editor.) Lancet 2:1332-1333, 1962. [C]

Milkovich L, van den Berg BJ: Effects of antenatal exposure to anorectic drugs. Am J Obstet Gynecol 129:637-642, 1977. [E]

Moss PD: Phenmetrazine and foetal abnormalities. (Correspondence) Br Med J 2:1610, 1962. [C]

Powell PD, Johnstone JM: Phenmetrazine and foetal abnormalities. (Correspondence) Br Med J 2:1327, 1962. [C]

PHENOBARBITAL

Synonyms

Blues, Fenobarbital, Gardenal, Luminal, Phenobarbitone, Phenylethylmalonylurea, Sedofen, Solfoton, Yellow Jackets

Summary

Phenobarbital is a barbiturate used as a hypnotic, sedative, and anticonvulsant.

Magnitude of Teratogenic Risk

Minimal To Small

Quality and Quantity of Data

Fair To Good

Comment

This assessment is for chronic treatment with phenobarbital in usual therapeutic doses. The risk of teratogenic effects may be greater with a toxic overdose of phenobarbital in pregnancy.

The frequencies of congenital anomalies in general, of major malformations, of minor anomalies, and of anatomic classes of congenital anomalies were no greater than expected among the children of 1415 women treated with phenobarbital during the first four lunar months of pregnancy in the Collaborative Perinatal Project (Heinonen et al., 1977). Similarly, there was no increase in the frequency of congenital anomalies among the children of 8037 women treated with phenobarbital anytime during pregnancy in this study.

The frequency of congenital anomalies appears to be somewhat increased among the children of women who take phenobarbital for treatment of a seizure disorder during pregnancy (Shapiro et al., 1976). Several epidemiological studies in which phenobarbital was taken for maternal epilepsy have demonstrated a higher-than-expected frequency of malformations, especially facial clefts and congenital heart disease, among the children when compared with children of untreated women (Greenberg et al., 1977; Rothman et al., 1979; Nakane et al., 1980; Robert et al., 1986; Dansky & Finnell, 1991). One interpretation of the data is that the increased risk of malformations seen in some studies may be due to teratogenic effects of factors associated with the mother's seizure disorder rather than to a specific effect of phenobarbital (Kelly, 1984).

The frequency of congenital anomalies among 250 infants born to epileptic women treated with phenobarbital monotherapy was no greater than that in infants of epileptic women treated with other anticonvulsant monotherapy in a multinational European collaborative study (Bertollini et al., 1987). The risk of congenital anomalies appears to be greater among infants whose mothers were treated with phenobarbital and phenytoin (and/or other anticonvulsants) during pregnancy than among infants of mothers treated with phenobarbital alone (Nakane et al., 1980; Dansky & Finnell, 1991; Dravet et al., 1992; Lindhout et al., 1992; Tanganelli & Regesta, 1992).

A characteristic pattern of minor dysmorphic features has been observed in children born to women treated with anticonvulsant drugs during pregnancy. The features of this "fetal anticonvulsant syndrome" include nail hypoplasia and typical facial appearance produced by midface hypoplasia, depressed nasal bridge, epicanthal folds, and ocular hypertelorism *(See phenytoin agent summary for further discussion)*. A similar pattern of minor anomalies has been reported in children of epileptic women who were treated only with phenobarbital during pregnancy (Seip, 1976; Robert et al., 1986; Rating et al., 1987; Thakker et al., 1991; Koch et al., 1992; Jones et al, 1992).

A small but statistically significant decrease in the birthweight and head circumference was observed among 55 infants born to epileptic women treated with phenobarbital when compared with the infants of nonepileptic women in one study, but a similar effect on head circumference was observed among the infants of epileptic women who were untreated (Mastroiacovo et al., 1988). Smaller than expected head circumferences were seen among six to 13 year-old children whose mothers had been treated during pregnancy with phenobarbital for a seizure disorder in another study (van der Pol et al., 1991).

The adjusted intelligence quotient at age four years was no different in children exposed to phenobarbital during gestation than in unexposed children in the Collaborative Perinatal Project (Shapiro et al., 1976). Poor performance in arithmetic and spelling and short attention span were seen more frequently than expected among six to 13 year-old children whose mothers had been treated with phenobarbital during pregnancy for a seizure disorder in another study (van der Pol et al., 1991). The relative contribution of anticonvulsant drug exposure, maternal seizures during pregnancy, genetic factors, and psychosocial influences on developmental differences that have been observed in children

of women treated with anticonvulsants during pregnancy is uncertain (Gaily et al., 1990; Fisher & Vorhees, 1992).

In a follow-up study of children born to women who had participated in a controlled trial of third-trimester phenobarbital therapy for prevention of neonatal jaundice, boys born to women in the treatment group were taller, had smaller testicular volumes, and scored higher on standardized intelligence tests as adolescents (Yaffe & Dorn, 1990). It is not clear whether the associations observed are due to the treatment or to other differences between the treated and untreated groups.

None of three children whose mothers took phenobarbital overdoses in the first trimester of pregnancy had congenital anomalies (Czeizel et al., 1984, 1988). Four of 18 children born to women who had taken overdoses of phenobarbital during the second or third trimester of pregnancy had congenital anomalies (Czeizel et al., 1984, 1988). The problems differed among the affected children and may not be attributable to the phenobarbital.

In animal studies, increased frequencies of cleft palate, cardiovascular malformations, and other congenital anomalies have been observed among the offspring of pregnant mice or rats treated with many times the usual human dose of phenobarbital (Fritz et al., 1976; Sullivan & McElhatton, 1977; Nishimura et al., 1979; Vorhees, 1983; Finnell & Dansky, 1991). A dose-dependent increase in the frequency of congenital anomalies was observed among the offpring of mice treated chronically with 8-33 times the human dose of phenobarbital in one study; although the doses used in this investigation were large, they produced blood levels that were near or within the human therapeutic range (Finnell et al., 1987a, b). Some of the affected mice had facial features reminiscent of the "fetal anticonvulsant syndrome" seen among the children of epileptic women treated with phenobarbital during pregnancy.

Behavioral alterations and abnormalities of central nervous system structure and function have been reported among the offspring of rodents treated during pregnancy with phenobarbital in doses many times those used in humans (Bergman et al., 1980; Middaugh et al., 1981; Vorhees, 1983, 1985; Takagi et al., 1986;

Yanai et al., 1989; Ransom & Elmore, 1991; Livezey et al., 1992; Rogel-Fuchs et al., 1992). Alterations in reproductive and endocrine function have also been observed in such offspring (Yaffe & Gupta, 1981; Gupta et al., 1982; Sonawane & Yaffe, 1983).

Chronic maternal use of phenobarbital late in pregnancy has been associated with transient neonatal sedation or withdrawal symptoms in the infants (Desmond et al., 1972; Koch et al., 1985). Features include hyperactivity, irritability, and tremors.

Maternal treatment with phenobarbital shortly before delivery has been used to prevent intraventricular hemorrhage in premature infants (Morales & Koerten, 1986; Shankaran et al., 1986; De Carolis et al., 1988; Kaempf et al., 1990; Paneth & Pinto-Martin, 1991).

Key References

Bergman A, Rosselli-Austin L, Yedwab G, Yanai J: Neuronal deficits in mice following phenobarbital exposure during various periods in fetal development. Acta Anat 108:370-373, 1980. [A]

Bertollini R, Kallen B, Mastroiacovo P, et al.: Anticonvulsant drugs in monotherapy. Effect on the fetus. Eur J Epidemiol 3(2):164-171, 1987. [E]

Czeizel A, Szentesi I, Szekeres I, Glauber A, et al.: Pregnancy outcome and health conditions of offspring of self-poisoned pregnant women. Acta Paediatr Hung 25(3):209-236, 1984. [S]

Czeizel A, Szentesi I, Szekeres I, Molnar G, et al.: A study of adverse effects on the progeny after intoxication during pregnancy. Arch Toxicol 62:1-7, 1988. [S]

Dansky LV, Finnell RH: Parental epilepsy, anticonvulsant drugs, and reproductive outcome: Epidemiologic and experimental findings spanning three decades. 2: Human studies. Reprod Toxicol 5(4):301-335, 1991. [R]

De Carolis S, De Carolis MP, Caruso A, Oliva GC, et al.: Antenatal phenobarbital in preventing intraventricular hemorrhage in premature newborns. Fetal Ther 3:224-229, 1988. [E]

Desmond MM, Schwanecke RP, Wilson GS, Yasunaga S, et al.: Maternal barbiturate utilization and neonatal withdrawal symptomatology. J Pediatr 80:190-197, 1972. [S]

Dravet C, Julian C, Legras C, Magaudda A, et al.: Epilepsy, antiepileptic drugs, and malformations in children of women with epilepsy: A French prospective cohort study. Neurology 42(Suppl 5):75-82, 1992. [E]

Finnell RH, Dansky LV: Parental epilepsy, anticonvulsant drugs, and reproductive outcome: Epidemiologic and experimental findings spanning three decades. 1: Animal studies. Reprod Toxicol 5:281-299, 1991. [R]

Finnell RH, Shields HE, Chernoff GF: Variable patterns in anticonvulsant drug-induced malformations in mice: Comparisons of phenytoin and phenobarbital. Teratog Carcinog Mutagen 7:541-549, 1987b. [A]

Finnell RH, Shields HE, Taylor SM, et al.: Strain differences in phenobarbital-induced teratogenesis in mice. Teratology 35:177-185, 1987a. [A]

Fisher JE, Vorhees CV: Developmental toxicity of antiepileptic drugs: Relationship to postnatal dysfunction. Pharmacol Res 26(3):207-221, 1992. [R]

Fritz H, Muller D, Hess R: Comparative study of the teratogenicity of phenobarbitone, diphenylhydantoin and carbamazepine in mice. Toxicology 6:323-330, 1976. [A]

Gaily E, Kantola-Sorsa E, Granstrom M-L: Specific cognitive dysfunction in children with epileptic mothers. Dev Med Child Neurol 32:403-414, 1990. [E]

Greenberg G, Inman WHW, Weatherall JAC, Adelstein AM, et al.: Maternal drug histories and congenital abnormalities. Br Med J 2:853-856, 1977. [E]

Gupta C, Yaffe SJ, Shapiro BH: Prenatal exposure to phenobarbital permanently decreases testosterone and causes reproductive dysfunction. Science 216:640-642, 1982. [A]

Heinonen OP, Slone D, Shapiro S: Birth Defects and Drugs in Pregnancy. Littleton, Mass.: John Wright-PSG, 1977, p 343. [E]

Jones KL, Johnson KA, Chamber CC: Pregnancy outcome in women treated with phenobarbital monotherapy. Teratology 45:452-453, 1992. [S]

Kaempf JW, Porreco R, Molina R, Hale K, et al.: Antenatal phenobarbital for the prevention of periventricular and intraventricular hemorrhage: A double-blind, randomized, placebo-controlled, multihospital trial. J Pediatr 117:933-938, 1990. [E]

Kelly TE: Teratogenicity of anticonvulsant drugs. I: Review of the literature. Am J Med Genet 19:413-434, 1984. [R]

Koch S, Goepfert-Geyer I, Haeuser I, et al.: Neonatal behaviour disturbances in infants of epileptic women treated during pregnancy. In: Prevent of Phys and Mental Congen Defects, Part B: Epidemiol, Early Detect and Therapy, and Environ Factors. Prog Clin Biol Res 163B:453-461, 1985. [E]

Koch S, Losche G, Jager-Roman E, Jakob S, et al.: Major and minor birth malformations and antiepileptic drugs. Neurology 42(Suppl 5):83-88, 1992. [E]

Lindhout D, Meinardi H, Meijer JWA, Nau H: Antiepileptic drugs and teratogenesis in two consecutive cohorts: Changes in prescription policy paralleled by changes in pattern of malformations. Neurology 42(Suppl 5):94-110, 1992. [E]

Livezey GT, Rayburn WF, Smith CV: Prenatal exposure to phenobarbital and quantifiable alterations in the electroencephalogram of adult rat offspring. Am J Obstet Gynecol 167:1611-1615, 1992. [A]

Mastroiacovo P, Bertollini R, Licata D, et al.: Fetal growth in the offspring of epileptic women: Results of an Italian multicentric cohort study. Acta Neurol Scand 78:110-114, 1988. [E]

Middaugh LD, Thomas TN, Simpson LW, Zemp JW: Effects of prenatal maternal injections of phenobarbital on brain neurotransmitters and behavior of young C57 mice. Neurobehav Toxicol Teratol 3(3):271-275, 1981. [A]

Morales WJ, Koerten J: Prevention of intraventricular hemorrhage in very low birth weight infants by maternally administered phenobarbital. Obstet Gynecol 68(3):295-299, 1986. [E]

Nakane Y, Okuma T, Takahashi R, Sato Y, et al.: Multi-institutional study on the teratogenicity and fetal toxicity of antiepileptic drugs: A report of a collaborative study group in Japan. Epilepsia 21:663-680, 1980. [E]

Nishimura KY, Terada Y, Mukumoto K, Syoji K, et al.: Teratogenic effects of phenobarbital in fetal rats. Teratology 20:156-157, 1979. [A]

Paneth N, Pinto-Martin J: The epidemiology of germinal matrix/intraventricular hemorrhage. In: Kiely M (ed). Reproductive and Perinatal Epidemiology. Boca Raton, Fla.: CRC Press, 1991, pp 371-399. [R]

Ransom BR, Elmore JG: Effects of antiepileptic drugs on the developing central nervous system. Adv Neurol 55:225-237, 1991. [R]

Rating D, Jager-Roman E, Koch S, Deichl A, et al.: Major malformations and minor anomalies in the offspring of epileptic parents: The role of antiepileptic drugs. Pharmacokinet Teratog Vol 1. Interspecies Compar Maternal/Embryonic-Fetal Drug Transfer 1:205-223, 1987. [E]

Robert E, Lofkvist E, Mauguiere F, et al.: Evaluation of drug therapy and teratogenic risk in a Rhone-Alpes District population of pregnant epileptic women. Eur Neurol 25:436-443, 1986. [E]

Rogel-Fuchs Y, Newman ME, Trombka D, Zahalka EA, et al.: Hippocampal cholinergic alterations and related behavioral deficits after early exposure to phenobarbital. Brain Res Bull 29(1):1-6, 1992. [A]

Rothman KJ, Fyler DC, Goldblatt A, Kreidberg MB: Exogenous hormones and other drug exposures of children with congenital heart disease. Am J Epidemiol 109:433-439, 1979. [E]

Seip ML: Growth retardation, dysmorphic facies and minor malformations following massive exposure to phenobarbitone in utero. Acta Paediatr Scand 65:617-621, 1976. [R]

Shankaran S, Cepeda EE, Hagan N, et al.: Antenatal phenobarbital for the prevention of neonatal intracerebral hemorrhage. Am J Obstet Gynecol 154(1):53-57, 1986. [E]

Shapiro S, Hartz SC, Siskind V, Mitchell AA, et al.: Anticonvulsants and parental epilepsy in the development of birth defects. Lancet 1:272-275, 1976. [S]

Sonawane BR, Yaffe SJ: Delayed effects of drug exposure during pregnancy: Reproductive function. Biol Res Pregnancy 4(2):48-55, 1983. [R]

Sullivan FM, McElhatton PR: A comparison of the teratogenic activity of the antiepileptic drugs carbamazepine, clonazepam, ethosuximide, phenobarbital, phenytoin, and primidone in mice. Toxicol Appl Pharmacol 40:365-378, 1977. [A]

Takagi S, Alleva FR, Seth PK, et al.: Delayed development of reproductive functions and alteration of dopamine receptor binding in hypothalamus of rats exposed prenatally to phenytoin and phenobarbital. Toxicol Lett 34:107-113, 1986. [A]

Tanganelli P, Regesta G: Epilepsy, pregnancy, and major birth anomalies: An Italian prospective, controlled study. Neurology 42(Suppl 5):89-93, 1992. [E]

Thakker JC, Kothari SS, Deshmukh CT, Deshpande PG: Hypoplasia of nails and phalanges: A teratogenic manifestation of phenobarbitone. Indian Pediatr 28(1):73-75, 1991. [C]

van der Pol MC, Hadders-Algra M, Huisjes HJ, Touwen BCL: Antiepileptic medication in pregnancy: Late effects on the children's central nervous system development. Am J Obstet Gynecol 164:121-128, 1991. [E]

Vorhees CV: Fetal anticonvulsant syndrome in rats: Dose- and period-response relationships of prenatal diphenylhydantoin, trimethadione and phenobarbital exposure on the structural and functional development of the offspring. J Pharmacol Exp Ther 227:274-287, 1983. [A]

Vorhees CV: Fetal anticonvulsant syndrome in rats: Effects on postnatal behavior and brain amino acid content. Neurobehav Toxicol Teratol 7:471-482, 1985. [A]

Yaffe SJ, Dorn LD: Effects of prenatal treatment with phenobarbital. Dev Pharmacol Ther 15:215-223, 1990. [E]

Yaffe SJ, Gupta C: Prenatal administration of phenobarbital and reproductive dysfunction in the offspring. In: Semm K, Mettler L (eds). Human Reproduction. Amsterdam: Excerpta Medica, 1981, pp 250-258. [A]

Yanai J, Fares F, Gavish M, Greenfeld Z, et al.: Neural and behavioral alterations after early exposure to phenobarbital. Neurotoxicology 10:543-554, 1989. [A]

PHENOL

Synonyms

Carbolic Acid, Cepastat, Chloraseptic, Fenol, Hydroxybenzene, Phenyl Hydrate

Summary

Phenol, a hydroxylated derivative of benzene, is an acidic hydrocarbon. It is used as a disinfectant, a local anesthetic (in weak solutions), and in the manufacture of resins, dyes, and other chemicals. It is readily absorbed after oral, inhalation, or dermal exposure. The threshold limit value for industrial exposure is 5 ppm; the short-term exposure limit is 10 ppm (38 mg/cubic meter) (Bruce et al., 1987). Acute toxicity produces gastrointestinal irritation (including nausea and vomiting), cardiorespiratory symptoms or collapse, muscle weakness, seizures, and coma.

Magnitude of Teratogenic Risk

Undetermined

Quality and Quantity of Data

None To Poor

Comment

None

No epidemiological studies of congenital anomalies among infants born to women exposed to phenol during pregnancy have been reported.

The frequency of malformations was not increased among the offspring of mice or rats given phenol in doses of 70-140 mg/kg/d or 20-200 mg/kg/d, respectively (Minor & Bechard, 1971; Jones-Price et al., 1983a, b; Price et al., 1986). Dose-related fetal growth retardation was seen in the treated rats.

Key References

Bruce RM, Santodonato J, Neal MW: Summary review of the health effects associated with phenol. Toxicol Ind Health 3:535-568, 1987. [R]

Jones-Price C, Ledoux TA, Reel JR, Fisher PW, et al.: Teratologic evaluation of phenol (CAS No. 108-95-2) in CD rats. NTIS (National Technical Information Service) Report/PB83-247726, 1983b. [A]

Jones-Price C, Ledoux TA, Reel JR, Langhoff-Paschke L, et al.: Teratologic evaluation of phenol (CAS No. 108-95-2) in CD-1 mice. NTIS (National Technical Information Service) Report/PB85-104461, 1983a. [A]

Minor JL, Becker BA: A comparison of the teratogenic properties of sodium salicylate, sodium benzoate, and phenol. Toxicol Appl Pharmacol, 19:373, 1971. [A]

Price CJ, Ledoux TA, Reel JR, Fisher PW, et al.: Teratologic evaluation of phenol in rats and mice. Teratology 33:92c-93c, 1986. [A]

PHENOLPHTHALEIN

Synonyms

Alophen Pill, Dihydroxyphthalophenone, Evac-Q-Kwik, Ex-Lax Pills, Feen-A-Mint Gum, Fenolftaleina, Phenolax, Prulet

Summary

Phenolphthalein is used as a purgative.

Magnitude of Teratogenic Risk

None

Quality and Quantity of Data

Fair

Comment

None

The frequencies of congenital anomalies in general, of major malformations, and of minor anomalies were no greater than expected among the children of 236 women who took phenolphthalein during the first four lunar months of pregnancy in the Collaborative Perinatal Project. The frequency of congenital anomalies was also not increased among the children of 806 women who took this drug anytime during pregnancy (Heinonen et al., 1977).

No animal teratology studies of phenolphthalein have been published.

Key References

Heinonen OP, Slone D, Shapiro S: Birth Defects and Drugs in Pregnancy. Littleton, Mass.: John Wright-PSG, 1977, pp 385-387, 442, 497. [E]

PHENSUXIMIDE

Synonyms

Milontin

Summary

Phensuximide is a succinimide anticonvulsant used in the treatment of petit mal epilepsy.

Magnitude of Teratogenic Risk

Undetermined

Quality and Quantity of Data

Poor

Comment

None

No epidemiological studies of congenital anomalies in the infants of women treated with phensuximide during pregnancy have been reported.

The frequency of malformations, especially of the heart and skeleton, was increased among the offspring of mice treated with phensuximide in doses nine or more times greater than those used in humans (Kao et al., 1979; Fabro et al., 1982). The relevance of this observation in human pregnancy is unknown.

Key References

Fabro S, Shull G, Brown NA: The relative teratogenic index and teratogenic potency: Proposed components of developmental toxicity risk assessment. Teratogenesis Carcinog Mutagen 2:61-76, 1982. [A]

Kao J, Brown NA, Shull G, Fabro S: Chemical structure and teratogenicity of anticonvulsants. Fed Proc 38:438, 1979. [A]

PHENTERMINE

Synonyms

Adipex-P, Duromine, Fastin, Ionamin, Phentermyl

Summary

Phentermine is a sympathomimetic agent used as an anorectic in the treatment of obesity.

Magnitude of Teratogenic Risk

Undetermined

Quality and Quantity of Data

None

Comment

None

No human epidemiological studies of malformations in infants born to women who took phentermine during embryogenesis have been reported.

No animal teratology studies of phentermine have been published.

Key References

None available.

PHENYLBUTAZONE

Synonyms

Azolid, Butazolidin

Summary

Phenylbutazone is a nonsteroidal anti-inflammatory with analgesic and antipyretic action. It is used to treat gout and rheumatic diseases.

Magnitude of Teratogenic Risk

Undetermined

Quality and Quantity of Data

Poor

Comment

None

No epidemiological studies of congenital anomalies in infants born to women who took phenylbutazone during pregnancy have been reported.

The frequency of malformations was no greater than expected among the offspring of rats or rabbits treated with phenylbutazone in doses 5-15 times those used in humans (Schardein et al., 1969; Kato et al., 1979a, b).

Please see agent summary on indomethacin for information on a related agent that has been more thoroughly studied.

Key References

Kato M, Matsuzawa K, Enjo H, Makita T, Hashimoto Y: [Reproduction studies of feprazone. II. Teratogenicity study in rats and rabbits.] Iyakuhin Kenkyu 10:149-162, 1979a. [A]

Kato M, Matsuzawa K, Enjo H, Makita T, Hashimoto Y: [Reproduction studies of feprazone. III. Perinatal and postnatal studies in rats.] Iyakuhin Kenkyu 10:164-175, 1979b. [A]

Schardein JL, Blatz AT, Woosley ET, Kaump DH: Reproduction studies on sodium meclofenamate in comparison to aspirin and phenylbutazone. Toxicol Appl Pharmacol 15:46-55, 1969. [A]

PHENYLEPHRINE

Synonyms

Fenilefrina Cloridrato, Mesatonum, Metaoxedrini Chloridum, Mydfrin, Neophryn, Neosyn, Nostril, Prefrin, Sinarest Nasal, Sinex Decongestant Nasal

Summary

Phenylephrine is a sympathomimetic agent used as a nasal decongestant and for temporary relief of glaucoma. It is also used as a vasoconstrictor to treat hypotensive states.

Magnitude of Teratogenic Risk

None To Minimal

Quality and Quantity of Data

Fair To Good

Comment

None

Epidemiological studies of congenital anomalies among infants born to women treated with phenylephrine during pregnancy have produced inconsistent results. The Collaborative Perinatal Project included 1249 pregnancies exposed to phenylephrine during the first four lunar months and 4194 exposed anytime during gestation (Heinonen et al., 1977). A weak but statistically significant association was observed between maternal exposure to phenylephrine during the first four lunar months and the occurrence of congenital anomalies in the infants. This association primarily involved minor anomalies, although "malformations of the eye and ear" as a group occurred more often than expected among the children of exposed pregnancies. In contrast, the frequency of malformations was no greater than expected among more than 225 infants born to women treated with phenylephrine during the first trimester in the Boston Collaborative Drug Surveillance Project (Jick et al., 1981; Aselton et al., 1985). In a case-control study of 390 children with congenital heart disease, Rothman et al. (1979) observed a slightly higher rate of exposure to phenylephrine early in pregnancy in the cases than in the controls. This observation was confirmed in a later and more rigorous study by the same investigators of 298 children with congenital heart disease (Zierler & Rothman, 1985). No association between first-trimester maternal use of phenylephrine and congenital heart disease in the offspring was seen in a large cohort study (Heinonen et al., 1977). Interpretation of these studies is complicated by the fact that phenylephrine is usually used as part of a multi-drug combination in treatment of viral illnesses. The possibility exists that the weak associations observed with maternal phenylephrine use, if real, might be due to another drug or the underlying illness.

Increased frequencies of fetal growth retardation and premature delivery have been reported in the offspring of rabbits treated chronically during gestation with phenylephrine in doses equivalent to those used in humans (Shabanah et al., 1969a, b). Similar doses of phenylephrine, when administered to sheep late in pregnancy, produced acidosis and hypoxemia in the fetuses (Cottle et al., 1982). These effects have not been studied in human pregnancies.

Key References

Aselton P, Jick H, Milunsky A, Hunter JR, et al.: First-trimester drug use and congenital disorders. Obstet Gynecol 65:451-455, 1985. [S]

Cottle MKW, van Petten GR, van Muyden P: Effects of phenylephrine and sodium salicylate on maternal and fetal cardiovascular indices and blood oxygenation in sheep. Am J Obstet Gynecol 143:170-176, 1982. [A]

Heinonen OP, Slone D, Shapiro S: Birth Defects and Drugs in Pregnancy. Littleton, Mass.: John Wright-PSG, 1977, pp 345-347, 439. [E]

Jick H, Holmes LB, Hunter JR, Madsen S, et al.: First-trimester drug use and congenital disorders. JAMA 246:343-346, 1983. [S]

Rothman KJ, Fyler DC, Goldblatt A, Kreidberg MB: Exogenous hormones and other drug exposures of children with congenital heart disease. Am J Epidemiol 109:433-439, 1979. [E]

Shabanah EH, Tricomi V, Suarez JR: Effect of epinephrine on fetal growth and the length of gestation. Surg Gynecol Obstet 129:341-343, 1969a. [A]

Shabanah EH, Tricomi V, Suarez JR: Fetal environment and its influence on fetal development. Surg Gynecol Obstet 129:556-564, 1969b. [A]

Zierler S, Rothman KJ: Congenital heart disease in relation to maternal use of Bendectin and other drugs in early pregnancy. N Engl J Med 313:347-352, 1985. [E]

PHENYLPROPANOL-AMINE

Synonyms

Acutrim, Dexatrim, Mydriatin, Oxyfedrine, Poly-Histine D Capsules, Prolamine, Propagest, Rhindecon, Triaminic Chewables, Tuss-Ornade Liquid

Summary

Phenylpropanolamine is a sympathomimetic agent usually given for relief of nasal congestion. It has also been used for urinary incontinence and as an anorectic.

Magnitude of Teratogenic Risk

None To Minimal

Quality and Quantity of Data

Fair To Good

Comment

None

The frequency of major malformations was not increased among the children of 726 women who took phenlypropanolamine during the first four lunar months of pregnancy in the Collaborative Perinatal Project, but increased frequencies of minor anomalies (RR=1.67, 95% confidence interval 1.01-2.59) and of eye and ear defects (RR=4.04, 95% confidence interval 1.63-8.29) were observed (Heinonen et al., 1977). The frequency of congenital anomalies was no greater than expected among the infants of 2489 women who took phenylpropanolamine anytime during pregnancy. The frequency of malformations was not increased among more than 350 infants born to women who took phenylpropanolamine during the first trimester of pregnancy in two cohorts of the Boston Collaborative Drug Surveillance Project (Jick et al., 1981; Aselton et al., 1985). No significant association was observed with maternal phenylpropanolamine use during the first trimester of pregnancy in a case-control study of 76 children with gastroschisis (Werler et al., 1992).

No animal studies of the phenylpropanolamine exposure during embryogenesis have been published.

Key References

Aselton P, Jick H, Milunsky A, Hunter JR, et al.: First-trimester drug use and congenital disorders. Obstet Gynecol 65:451-455, 1985. [S]

Heinonen OP, Slone D, Shapiro S: Birth Defects and Drugs in Pregnancy. Littleton, Mass.: John Wright-PSG, 1977, pp 346-347, 439. [E]

Jick H, Holmes LB, Hunter JR, Madsen S, et al.: First-trimester drug use and congenital disorders. JAMA 246:343-346, 1981. [S]

Werler MM, Mitchell AA, Shapiro S: First trimester maternal medication use in relation to gastroschisis. Teratology 45:361-367, 1992. [E]

PHENYLTOLOXAMINE

Synonyms

C 5581

Summary

Phenyltoloxamine is an antihistamine of the ethanolamine class used to treat allergic symptoms.

Magnitude of Teratogenic Risk

None

498

Comment

None

The frequency of congenital anomalies was not significantly increased among the children of 45 women who took phenyltoloxamine during the first four lunar months of pregnancy or the children of 142 women who took this drug anytime during pregnancy in the Collaborative Perinatal Project (Heinonen et al., 1977).

No animal teratology studies of phenyltoloxamine have been published.

Please see agent summary on diphenhydramine for information on a closely related agent that has been more thoroughly studied.

Key References

Heinonen OP, Slone D, Shapiro S: Birth Defects and Drugs in Pregnancy. Littleton, Mass.: John Wright-PSG, 1977, p 437. [E]

PHENYTOIN

Synonyms

Dilantin, Diphenin, Diphenylan, Diphenylhydantoin, DPH, Epanutin, Epilantin, Fenitoina

Summary

Phenytoin is an anticonvulsant used in the treatment of seizure disorders.

Magnitude of Teratogenic Risk

Small To Moderate

Quality and Quantity of Data

Fair To Good

Comment

This assessment is based on data for continuous gestational exposure to phenytoin in treatment of maternal seizure disorders. No data are available on the effects of acute exposure.

A "fetal hydantoin syndrome," which consists of an unusual and characteristic pattern of anomalies, has been described in about 10% of infants born to epileptic women who took phenytoin during pregnancy (Speidel & Meadow, 1972; Hanson et al., 1976; Kelly, 1984; Kelly et al., 1984a; Hanson, 1986). Typical features of this syndrome include apparent ocular hypertelorism, flat nasal bridge, and distal digital hypoplasia with nail hypoplasia. None of these features is of great clinical importance, but some authors believe that cleft palate, congenital heart disease, microcephaly, developmental delay, and prenatal and postnatal growth retardation also occur as occasional manifestations of fetal hydantoin syndrome (Speidel & Meadow, 1972; Hanson et al., 1976; Bracken, 1986; Hanson, 1986; Friis, 1989; Adams et al., 1990). This conclusion is controversial, however. Other authorities believe that most of the anomalies which occur more frequently among the children of epileptic women taking phenytoin during pregnancy than among the children of normal untreated women are due to underlying familial factors or effects of maternal epilepsy per se rather than to the teratogenic action of phenytoin (Shapiro et al., 1976; Dieterich et al., 1980; Kelly, 1984; Kelly et al., 1984a, b; Gaily et al., 1988a, b, 1990; Gaily & Granstrom, 1989; Kaneko et al., 1991). Distal digital hypoplasia is one feature in the children that does appear to be due to maternal phenytoin treatment during pregnancy (Kelly et al., 1984a; Gaily, 1990; D'Souza et al., 1990).

Although many large epidemiologic studies of the offspring of epileptic women have been published, currently available data are incapable of resolving this controversy because assessment of the effects of phenytoin exposure is confounded by many other factors (Kelly, 1984; Schardein, 1985; Hanson, 1986).

Among these confounders are the facts that most women with seizures are treated with some anticonvulsant drug, that many women are treated with more than one anticonvulsant at a time, that women who are not treated or are treated with a single agent probably have milder disease, and that phenytoin exposure rarely occurs in women without seizures.

This much seems clear: The frequency of major malformations among the children of epileptic women treated with phenytoin during pregnancy is about twice as great as the frequency of such anomalies in the general population (Kelly, 1984). The risk of malformations in the offspring is probably even greater if the mother requires treatment with other anticonvulsants in addition to phenytoin during pregnancy (Fedrick, 1973; Lindhout et al., 1984; Kaneko et al., 1988) or if the mother has previously had a child with features of fetal hydantoin syndrome (Van Dyke et al., 1988). Genetic factors in the fetus may be important in determining whether or not congenital anomalies occur when a pregnant epileptic woman is treated with phenytoin (Phelan et al., 1982; Buehler et al., 1990).

Prenatal diagnosis by means of ultrasound examination has been advocated for pregnant epileptic women who are being treated with anticonvulsant medication, but such screening does not appear to be very sensitive for the kinds of anomalies most often seen in the children of these women (Wladimiroff et al., 1988).

Phenytoin, in doses producing therapeutic blood levels or in greater doses, is teratogenic in mice, rats, and rabbits (McClain & Langhoff, 1980; Finnell, 1981; Finnell & Chernoff, 1984; Finnell et al., 1989; Zengel et al., 1989; Collins et al., 1990; Rowland et al., 1990). Cleft palate, cardiac defects, and skeletal anomalies are the malformations most frequently observed. A typical dose-response relationship has been demonstrated for the induction of malformations by phenytoin in the mouse (Finnell, 1981; McDevitt et al., 1981; Finnell et al., 1989). Frequent embryonic death but no increase in fetal malformations was observed among pregnant rhesus monkeys treated with phenytoin in doses that produced blood levels 1-2 times those considered to be therapeutic in humans; considerable maternal toxicity was seen with these doses in the monkeys (Hendrie et al., 1990). Behavioral alterations have been demonstrated among the offspring of rats and rhesus monkeys treated during pregnancy with phenytoin in doses that produce blood levels similar to those used therapeutically in humans (Elmazar & Sullivan, 1981; Mullenix et al., 1983; Phillips & Lockard, 1985; Vorhees, 1987; Vorhees & Minck, 1989; Weisenburger et al., 1990; Adams et al., 1990).

Exposure to phenytoin during embryogenesis has also been associated with an increased risk of tumor development in humans; neuroblastoma and other neoplasms have been reported in such children with surprisingly high frequency (Lipson & Bale, 1985; Koren et al., 1989). Malignancy in childhood is rare, however, and the risk of neoplasia in a given child who was exposed to phenytoin during gestation is probably small.

Perinatal and neonatal hemorrhage associated with deficiency of vitamin K-dependent clotting factors has been observed in infants of women treated with phenytoin during pregnancy (Mountain et al., 1970; Solomon et al., 1972; Gimovsky & Petrie, 1986). Administration of vitamin K to these infants appears to be useful both prophylactically and therapeutically.

Key References

Adams J, Vorhees CV, Middaugh LD: Developmental neurotoxicity of anticonvulsants: Human and animal evidence on phenytoin. Neurotoxicol Teratol 12:203-214, 1990. [R]

Bracken MB: Drug use in pregnancy and congenital heart disease in offspring. N Engl J Med 314:1120, 1986. [E]

Buehler BA, Delimont D, van Waes M, Finnell RH: Prenatal prediction of risk of the fetal hydantoin syndrome. N Engl J Med 322:1567-1572, 1990. [S]

Collins MD, Fradkin R, Scott WJ: Induction of postaxial forelimb ectrodactyly with anticonvulsant agents in A/J mice. Teratology 41:61-70, 1990. [A]

Dieterich E, Steveling A, Lukas A, Seyfeddinipur N, et al.: Congenital anomalies in children of epileptic mothers and fathers. Neuropediatrics 11:274-283, 1980. [E]

D'Souza SW, Robertson IG, Donnai D, Mawer G: Fetal phenytoin exposure, hypoplastic nails, and jitteriness. Arch Dis Child 65:320-324, 1990. [E]

Elmazar MMA, Sullivan FM: Effect of phenytoin administration on postnatal development of the rat: A behavioral teratology study. Teratology 24:115-124, 1981. [A]

Fedrick J: Epilepsy and pregnancy: A report from the Oxford record linkage study. Br Med J 2:442-448, 1973. [E]

Finnell RH: Phenytoin-induced teratogenesis: A mouse model. Science 211:483-484, 1981. [A]

Finnell RH, Abbott LC, Taylor SM: The fetal hydantoin syndrome: Answers from a mouse model. Reprod Toxicol 3:127-133, 1989. [A]

Finnell RH, Chernoff GF: Variable patterns of malformation in the mouse fetal hydantoin syndrome. Am J Med Genet 19:463-471, 1984. [A]

Friis ML: Facial clefts and congenital heart defects in children of parents with epilepsy: Genetic and environmental etiologic factors. Acta Neurol Scand 79:433-459, 1989. [R]

Gaily E: Distal phalangeal hypoplasia in children with prenatal phenytoin exposure: Results of a controlled anthropometric study. Am J Med Genet 35:574-578, 1990. [E]

Gaily E, Granstrom M-L: A transient retardation of early postnatal growth in drug-exposed children of epileptic mothers. Epilepsy Res 4:147-155, 1989. [E]

Gaily E, Granstrom M-L, Hiilesmaa V, Bardy A: Minor anomalies in offspring of epileptic mothers. J Pediatr 112:520-529, 1988a. [E]

Gaily E, Granstrom M-L, Hiilesmaa VK, Bardy AH: Head circumference in children of epileptic mothers: Contributions of drug exposure and genetic background. Epilepsy Res 5:217-222, 1990. [E]

Gaily E, Kantola-Sorsa E, Granstrom M-L: Intelligence of children of epileptic mothers. J Pediatr 113:677-684, 1988b. [E]

Gimovsky ML, Petrie R: Maternal anticonvulsants and fetal hemorrhage. A report of two cases. J Reprod Med 31:61-62, 1986. [C]

Hanson JW: Teratogen update: Fetal hydantoin effects. Teratology 33:349-353, 1986. [R]

Hanson JW, Myrianthopoulos NC, Harvey MAS, Smith DW: Risks to the offspring of women treated with hydantoin anticonvulsants, with emphasis on the fetal hydantoin syndrome. J Pediatr 89:662-668, 1976. [E]

Hendrie TA, Rowland JR, Binkerd PE, Hendrickx AG: Developmental toxicity and pharmacokinetics of phenytoin in the rhesus macaque: An interspecies comparison. Reprod Toxicol 4:257-266, 1990. [A]

Kaneko S: Antiepileptic drug therapy and reproductive consequences: Functional and morphologic effects. Reprod Toxicol 5:179-198, 1991. [R]

Kaneko S, Otani K, Fukushima Y, et al.: Teratogenicity of antiepileptic drugs: Analysis of possible risk factors. Epilepsia 29(4):459-467, 1988. [E]

Kelly TE: Teratogenicity of anticonvulsant drugs. I: Review of the literature. Am J Med Genet 19:413-434, 1984. [R]

Kelly TE, Edwards P, Rein M, Miller JQ, et al.: Teratogenicity of anticonvulsant drugs. II: A prospective study. Am J Med Genet 19:435-443, 1984a. [S]

Kelly TE, Rein M, Edwards P: Teratogenicity of anticonvulsant drugs. IV: The association of clefting and epilepsy. Am J Med Genet 19:451-458, 1984b. [S]

Koren G, Deitrakoudis D, Weksberg R, Rieder M, et al.: Neuroblastoma after prenatal exposure to phenytoin: Cause and effect? Teratology 40:157-162, 1989. [S]

Lindhout D, Hoppener RJEA, Meinardi H: Teratogenicity of antiepileptic drug combinations with special emphasis on epoxidation (of carbamazepine). Epilepsia 25:77-83, 1984. [E]

Lipson A, Bale P: Ependymoblastoma associated with prenatal exposure to diphenylhydantoin and methylphenobarbitone. Cancer 55:1859-1862, 1985. [C]

McClain RM, Langhoff L: Teratogenicity of diphenylhydantoin in the New Zealand white rabbit. Teratology 21:371-379, 1980. [A]

McDevitt JM, Gautieri RF, Mann DE: Comparative teratogenicity of cortisone and phenytoin in mice. J Pharm Sci 70:631-634, 1981. [A]

Mountain KR, Hirsh J, Gallus AS: Neonatal coagulation defect due to anticonvulsant drug treatment in pregnancy. Lancet 1:265-268, 1970. [S]

Mullenix P, Tassinari S, Keith DA: Behavioral outcome after prenatal exposure to phenytoin in rats. Teratology 27:149-157, 1983. [A]

Phelan MC, Pellock JM, Nance WE: Discordant expression of fetal hydantoin syndrome in heteropaternal dizygotic twins. N Engl J Med 307(2):99-101, 1982. [C]

Phillips NK, Lockard JS: A gestational monkey model: Effects of phenytoin versus seizures on neonatal outcome. Epilepsia 26(6):697-703, 1985. [A]

Rowland JF, Binkerd PE, Hendrickx AG: Developmental toxicity and pharmacokinetics of oral and intravenous phenytoin in the rat. Reprod Toxicol 4:191-202, 1990. [A]

Schardein JL: Chemically Induced Birth Defects. New York: Marcel Dekker, 1985, pp 142-189. [R]

Shapiro S, Hartz SC, Siskind V, Mitchell AA, et al.: Anti-convulsants and parental epilepsy in the development of birth defects. Lancet 1:272-275, 1976. [E]

Solomon GE, Hilgartner MW, Kutt H: Coagulation defects caused by diphenylhydantoin. Neurology 22:1165-1171, 1972. [C] & [A]

Speidel BD, Meadow SR: Maternal epilepsy and abnormalities of the fetus and newborn. Lancet 2:839-843, 1972. [E]

Van Dyke DC, Hodge SE, Heide F, Hill LR: Family studies in fetal phenytoin exposure. J Pediatr 113:301-306, 1988. [S]

Vorhees CV: Fetal hydantoin syndrome in rats: Dose-effect relationships of prenatal phenytoin on postnatal development and behavior. Teratology 35:287-303, 1987. [A]

Vorhees CV, Minck DR: Long-term effects of prenatal phenytoin exposure on offspring behavior in rats. Neurotoxicol Teratology 11:295-305, 1989. [A]

Weisenburger WP, Minck DR, Acuff KD, Vorhees CV: Dose-response effects of prenatal phenytoin exposure in rats: Effects on early locomotion, maze learning, and memory as a function of phenytoin- induced circling behavior. Neurotoxicol Teratol 12:145-152, 1990. [A]

Wladimiroff JW, Stewart PA, Reuss A, et al.: The role of ultrasound in the early diagnosis of fetal structural defects following maternal anticonvulsant therapy. Ultrasound Med Biol 14(8):657-660, 1988. [S]

Zengel AE, Keith DA, Tassinari MS: Prenatal exposure to phenytoin and its effect on postnatal growth and craniofacial proportion in the rat. J Craniofac Genet Dev Biol 9:147-160, 1989. [A]

PILOCARPINE

Synonyms

Adsorbocarpine, Akarpine, Alcon Opulets Pilocarpine, Isopto Carpine, Minims Pilocarpine, Ocu-Carpine, Ocusert Pilo, Pilocar, Pilopine

Summary

Pilocarpine is a muscarinic parasympathomimetic agent. Ophthalmic preparations are used to induce pupillary contraction and to decrease intraocular pressure in glaucoma and retinal detachment. Pilocarpine is sometimes given orally to counteract side effects of ganglion-blocking agents.

Magnitude of Teratogenic Risk

Undetermined

Quality and Quantity of Data

None

Comment

None

No epidemiological studies of congenital anomalies in infants born after maternal use of pilocarpine during pregnancy have been reported.

Behavioral alterations were observed among the offspring of pregnant rats treated parenterally with 5 mg/kg/d of pilocarpine (Watanabe et al., 1985). The relevance of this observation to the clinical use of pilocarpine in human pregnancy is unknown.

Key References

Watanabe T, Matsuhashi K, Takayama S: Study on the postnatal neurobehavioral development in rats treated prenatally with drugs acting on the autonomic nervous systems. Folia Pharmacol Japon 85:79-90, 1985. [A]

PIMOZIDE

Synonyms

Orap

Summary

Pimozide is a major tranquilizer of the diphenylbutylpiperadine class. Pimozide is used orally in the treatment of Tourette syndrome and psychoses.

Magnitude of Teratogenic Risk

Undetermined

Quality and Quantity of Data

None To Poor

Comment

A small risk cannot be excluded, but a high risk of congenital anomalies in the children of women treated with pimozide during pregnancy is unlikely.

No epidemiological studies of congenital anomalies among infants born to women treated with pimozide during pregnancy have been published.

No teratogenic effect was reportedly observed among the offspring of rats or rabbits treated with pimozide during pregnancy in doses <1-8 times the maximum human therapeutic dose (Pinder et al., 1976; Baldwin & Ridings, 1986).

Please see agent summary on haloperidol for information on a related agent that has been more thoroughly studied.

Key References

Baldwin J, Ridings J: Teratogenicity in rats of two dopaminergic agonists. Toxicology 42:291-302, 1986. [A]

Pinder RM, Brogden RN, Sawyer PR, Speight TM, et al.: Pimozide: A review of its pharmacological properties and therapeutic uses in psychiatry. Drugs 12:1-40, 1976. [R]

PINDOLOL

Synonyms

Visken

Summary

Pindolol is a beta-adrenergic blocking agent that is given orally in the treatment of hypertension and angina pectoris.

Magnitude of Teratogenic Risk

None To Minimal

Quality and Quantity of Data

Poor To Fair

Comment

None

No epidemiological studies of congenital anomalies among infants born to women treated with pindolol during pregnancy have been reported. No adverse effects related to maternal treatment with pindolol for hypertension during pregnancy have been noted in several clinical series which include 16 to 38 newborn infants each (Dubois et al., 1982; Sukerman-Voldman, 1982; Ellenbogen et al., 1986; Tuimala & Hartikainen-Sorri, 1988; Montan et al., 1992).

The frequency of malformations was not increased among the offspring of rats treated during pregnancy with 83-167 times the maximal human dose of pindolol (Koga et al., 1985). Fetal skeletal anomalies and growth retardation were more frequent at the higher dose, which was maternally toxic.

Please see agent summary on propranolol for information on a related agent.

Key References

Dubois D, Petitcolas J, Temperville B, Klepper A, et al.: Treatment of hypertension in pregnancy with beta-adrenoceptor antagonists. Br J Clin Pharmac 13:375S-378S, 1982. [S]

Ellenbogen A, Jaschevatzky O, Davidson A, Anderman S, et al.: Management of pregnancy-induced hypertension with pindolol--Comparative study with methyldopa. Int J Gynaecol Obstet 24:3-7, 1986. [S]

Koga T, Ohta T, Aoki Y, Sugasawa M, et al.: Teratological study of nipradilol (K-351) in rats and rabbits. Oral administration during the period of fetal organogenesis. Oyo Yakuri 29:747-759, 1985. [A]

Montan S, Ingemarsson I, Marsal K, Sjoberg N-O: Randomised controlled trial of atenolol and pindolol in human pregnancy: Effects on fetal haemodynamics. Br Med J 304:946-949, 1992. [E]

Sukerman-Voldman E: Pindolol therapy in pregnant hypertensive patients. Br J Clin Pharm 13:379S, 1982. [S]

Tuimala R, Hartikainen-Sorri A-L: Randomized comparison of atenolol and pindolol for treatment of hypertension in pregnancy. Curr Ther Res 44:579-584, 1988. [E]

PIPERACILLIN

Synonyms

Avocin, Ivacin, Pentcillin, Pipracil, Pipril, Sodium Piperacillin

Summary

Piperacillin is a broad spectrum semisynthetic penicillin that is administered parenterally to treat serious infections.

Magnitude of Teratogenic Risk

Undetermined

Quality and Quantity of Data

None To Poor

Comment

A small risk cannot be excluded, but a high risk of congenital anomalies in the children of women treated with piperacillin during pregnancy is unlikely.

No epidemiological studies of congenital anomalies among infants born to women treated with piperacillin during pregnancy have been reported.

The frequency of malformations was not increased among the offspring of mice or rats treated during pregnancy with 1-4 or <1-4 times the maximum human therapeutic dose of piperacillin (Takai et al., 1977a, b; Lochry et al., 1991).

Please see agent summary on ampicillin for information on a related agent that has been more thoroughly studied.

Key References

Lochry EA, Hoberman AM, Filler R, et al.: Embryo-fetal toxicity and teratogenic potential of tazobactam alone and in combination with piperacillin rats. Teratology 43(5):453, 1991. [A]

Takai A, Yoneda T, Nakada H, Nakamura S, et al.: Toxicity tests of T-1220 (VI): Reproduction study in mice. Chemotherapy 25:915-927, 1977a. [A]

Takai A, Yoneda T, Nakada H, Nakamura S, et al.: Toxicity tests of T-1220 (VII): Teratological study in rats. Chemotherapy 25:928-988, 1977b. [A]

PIPERAZINE

Synonyms

Antepar, Ascalix, Diethylenediamine, Ectodyne, Hitepar, Piperasol, Rotape Worm, Uvilon, Vermizine

Summary

Piperazine is an anthelmintic used orally to treat intestinal parasite infestations.

Magnitude of Teratogenic Risk

Undetermined

Quality and Quantity of Data

None To Poor

Comment

A small risk cannot be excluded, but a high risk of congenital anomalies in the children of women treated with piperazine during pregnancy is unlikely.

No adequate epidemiological studies of congenital anomalies among infants born to women treated with piperazine during pregnancy have been reported.

No malformations were observed among rat fetuses subjected to direct intrauterine application of piperazine in a dose of 50 mcg/fetus (Wilk, 1969).

Key References

Wilk AL: Relation between teratogenic activity and cartilage-binding affinity of norchlorcyclizine analogues. Teratology 2:272, 1969. [A]

PIPEROCAINE

Synonyms

Metycaine, Neothesin

Summary

Piperocaine is a local anesthetic of the ester class.

Magnitude of Teratogenic Risk

Undetermined

Quality and Quantity of Data

None

Comment

A small risk cannot be excluded, but there is no indication that the risk of congenital anomalies in the children of women treated with piperocaine during pregnancy is likely to be great.

No epidemiological studies of congenital anomalies in children born to women exposed to piperocaine during pregnancy have been reported.

No investigations of teratologic effects of piperocaine in experimental animals have been published.

Please see agent summary on procaine for information on a related agent that has been studied.

Key References

None available.

PIPERONYL BUTOXIDE

Synonyms

Butacide, Butocide, Butoxide

Summary

Piperonyl butoxide is a glycol ether that is used as an insecticide synergist, especially with pyrethrum and rotenone. Piperonyl butoxide is contained in a variety of insecticide preparations, including some that are used topically in the treatment of lice.

Magnitude of Teratogenic Risk

Undetermined

Quality and Quantity of Data

None

Comment

A small risk cannot be excluded, but a high risk of congenital anomalies in the children of women treated with piperonyl butoxide during pregnancy is unlikely.

No epidemiological studies of congenital anomalies among infants born to women exposed to piperonyl butoxide during pregnancy have been reported.

Increased frequencies of microphthalmia and other congenital anomalies were observed among the offspring of one strain of mice treated during pregnancy with 1000 mg/kg/d of piperonyl butoxide (Anonymous, 1968), a dose that also produced maternal toxicity. No teratogenic effect was seen in another strain of mice at the same dose or in a third strain treated with 300 mg/kg/d (Anonymous, 1968; Schwetz et al., 1976). Decreased body weight was noted among the offspring of mice fed diets containing 0.15-0.6% piperonyl butoxide throughout pregnancy (Tanaka, 1992). No teratogenic effect was noted among the offspring of pregnant rats treated with 62.5-1000 mg/kg/d of piperonyl butoxide (Kennedy et al., 1977; Khera et al., 1979). An increased frequency of malformations was seen in the offspring of rabbits treated during pregnancy with 100 mg/kg/d of piperonyl butoxide (Schwetz et al., 1976).

Key References

Anonymous: Evaluation of carcinogenic, teratogenic, and mutagenic activities of selected pesticides and industrial chemicals. Volume II. Teratogenic study in mice and rats. NTIS (National Technical Information Service) Report/PB-223 160, 1968. [A]

Kennedy GL, Smith SH, Kinoshita FK, Keplinger ML, et al.: Teratogenic evaluation of piperonyl butoxide in the rat. Food Cosmet Toxicol 15:337-339, 1977. [A]

Khera KS, Whalen C, Angers G, Trivett G: Assessment of the teratogenic potential of piperonyl butoxide, biphenyl, and phosalone in the rat. Toxicol Appl Pharmacol 47:353-358, 1979. [A]

Schwetz BA, Murray FJ, Staples RE: Teratology studies on the metabolic inhibitors SKF-525A and piperonyl butoxide in mice and rabbits. Toxicol Appl Pharmacol 37:150-151, 1976. [A]

Tanaka T: Effects of piperonyl butoxide on F1 generation mice. Toxicol Lett 60:83-90, 1992. [A]

PIROXICAM

Synonyms

Felden, Feldene, Larapam, Novopirocam, Reudene

Summary

Piroxicam is a nonsteroidal anti-inflammatory agent with antipyretic action. It is used in the treatment of arthritis and other musculoskeletal disorders.

Magnitude of Teratogenic Risk

Undetermined

Quality and Quantity of Data

Poor

Comment

Maternal treatment with piroxicam late in pregnancy may be associated with premature closure of the fetal ductus arteriosus.

No epidemiological studies of infants born to women treated with piroxicam during pregnancy have been reported.

No increase in the frequency of malformations was observed among the offspring of rats or rabbits treated with piroxicam during pregnancy in doses 5 to 25 times the usual human dose (Sakai et al., 1980; Perraud et al., 1984), but fetal growth retardation was noted in rats at the highest dose level (Sakai et al., 1980). The relevance of these results to human exposure during pregnancy is unknown.

In rats, piroxicam administered in late pregnancy was found to delay parturition (Powell & Cochrane, 1982). The effect of piroxicam on human parturition has not been studied, but other nonsteroidal anti-inflammatory agents may delay parturition in humans (Grella & Zanor, 1978).

Constriction or closure of the ductus arteriosus was observed in fetal rats exposed to 1-10 times the human therapeutic dose of piroxicam late in pregnancy (Momma et al., 1984). Treatment of women late in pregnancy with chemically related nonsteroidal anti-inflammatory agents has been associated with premature closure of the ductus arteriosus in utero and postnatal pulmonary hypertension. *Please consult the agent summary on indomethacin for more information on this point.*

Key References

Grella P, Zanor P: Premature labor and indomethacin. Prostaglandins 16:1007-1017, 1978. [S]

Momma K, Hagiwara H, Konishi T: Constriction of fetal ductus arteriosus by non-steroidal anti-inflammatory drugs: Study of additional 34 drugs. Prostaglandins 28:527-536, 1984. [A]

Perraud J, Stadler J, Kessedjlan MJ, Monro AM: Reproductive studies with the anti-inflammatory agent, piroxicam: Modification of classical protocols. Toxicology 30:59-63, 1984. [A]

Powell JG, Cochrane RL: The effects of a number of non-steroidal anti-inflammatory compounds on parturition in the rat. Prostaglandins 23:469-488, 1982. [A]

Sakai T, Ohtsuki I, Noguchi Y: Reproduction studies of piroxicam. Effects of piroxicam on fertility. Yakuri to Chiryo 8:4655-4671, 1980. [A]

PIROXIMONE

Synonyms

MDL 19205

Summary

Piroximone is a cardiotonic drug.

Magnitude of Teratogenic Risk

Undetermined

Quality and Quantity of Data

None

Comment

None

No epidemiological studies of congenital anomalies in infants born to women who were treated with piroximone during pregnancy have been reported.

No animal teratology studies of piroximone have been published.

Key References

None available.

PITCHER PLANT DISTILLATE

Summary

Pitcher plant (Sarracenia purpurea) distillate is administered parenterally for the relief of neuromuscular and neuralgic pain.

Magnitude of Teratogenic Risk

Undetermined

Quality and Quantity of Data

None

Comment

None

No epidemiological studies of congenital anomalies in infants whose mothers were treated with pitcher plant distillate during pregnancy have been reported.

No animal teratology studies of pitcher plant distillate have been published.

Key References

None available.

PLAGUE VACCINE

Summary

Plague vaccine is a preparation of killed bacteria that is administered intramuscularly for immunization against plague.

Magnitude of Teratogenic Risk

Undetermined

Quality and Quantity of Data

None

Comment

A small risk cannot be excluded, but a high risk of congenital anomalies in the children of women treated with plague vaccine during pregnancy is unlikely.

No epidemiological studies of congenital anomalies in infants whose mothers were immunized with plague vaccine during pregnancy have been reported.

No animal teratology studies of plague vaccine have been published.

Key References

None available.

PLASMA PROTEIN FRACTION

Synonyms

Plasmanate, Plasma-Plex, Plasmatein, Protemate

Summary

Plasma protein fraction contains human serum albumin and globulins obtained from fractionated human plasma. Plasma protein fraction is administered intravenously in the treatment of hypovolemic shock.

Magnitude of Teratogenic Risk

Undetermined

Quality and Quantity of Data

None

Comment

A small risk cannot be excluded, but a high risk of congenital anomalies in the children of women treated with plasma protein fraction during pregnancy is unlikely.

No epidemiological studies of congenital anomalies among infants born to women treated with plasma protein fraction during pregnancy have been reported.

No animal teratology studies of plasma protein fraction have been published.

Key References

None available.

PLICAMYCIN

Synonyms

Aureolic acid, Mithracin, Mithramycin

Summary

Plicamycin is a toxic antibiotic that is administered intravenously as an antineoplastic agent and in the treatment of hypercalcemia associated with malignancies.

Magnitude of Teratogenic Risk

Undetermined

Quality and Quantity of Data

None To Poor

Comment

Although the risk of plicamycin is unknown, it may be substantial because it is an antineoplastic agent.

No epidemiological studies of congenital anomalies among infants born to women treated with plicamycin during pregnancy have been reported.

Increased frequencies of fetal death were observed among the offspring of rats treated with 33-100 times the usual human dose of plicamycin during pregnancy (Chaube & Murphy, 1968; Thiersch, 1971). The relevance of this finding to the clinical use of plicamycin in human pregnancy is unknown.

Key References

Chaube S, Murphy ML: The teratogenic effects of the recent drugs active in cancer chemotherapy. Adv Teratol 3:181-237, 1968. [R]

Thiersch JB: Investigations into the differential effect of compounds on rat litter and mother. Malform Congenitales Mammiferes :95-113, 1971. [A]

PNEUMOCOCCAL VACCINE

Synonyms

Pneumovax 23

Summary

Pneumococcal vaccine is a sterile mixture of purified capsular polysaccharides. It is administered parenterally for immunization against pneumococcal infections.

Magnitude of Teratogenic Risk

Undetermined

Quality and Quantity of Data

None

Comment

A small risk cannot be excluded, but a high risk of congenital anomalies in the children of women treated with pneumococcal vaccine during pregnancy is unlikely.

No epidemiological studies of congenital anomalies in infants whose mothers were immunized with pneumococcal vaccine during pregnancy have been reported.

No animal teratology studies of pneumococcal vaccine have been published.

Key References

None available.

POLIOVIRUS VACCINE, INACTIVATED

Synonyms

Inactivated Poliovirus Vaccine, IPV, Poliomyelitis Vaccine (Salk), Salk Vaccine

Summary

Inactivated poliovirus vaccine is a killed virus preparation that is given parenterally to induce immunization against poliomyelitis.

Magnitude of Teratogenic Risk

None

Quality and Quantity of Data

Fair To Good

Comment

None

The frequencies of congenital anomalies in general, of major malformations, of minor anomalies, and of principal classes of malformations were no greater than expected among the children of 6774 women who had been given inactivated poliovirus vaccine during the first four lunar months of pregnancy in the Collaborative Perinatal Project (Heinonen et al., 1977). Similarly, the frequency of congenital anomalies was not increased among the children of 18,219 women who had been given inactivated poliovirus vaccine anytime during pregnancy in this study. A possible association between maternal immunization with inactivated poliovirus vaccine during pregnancy and subsequent development of malignant neoplasms has been suggested on the basis of the occurrence of 14 malignancies in these children (Heinonen et al., 1973). If such an association does in fact exist, it may be attributable to contamination of early batches of the vaccine with SV-40, a potentially oncogenic virus. Current vaccines no longer contain the SV-40 virus.

No animal teratology studies of inactivated poliovirus vaccine have been published.

Key References

Heinonen OP, Shapiro S, Monson R, Hartz SC, et al.: Immunization during pregnancy against poliomyelitis and influenza in relation to childhood malignancy. Int J Epidemiol 2:229, 1973. [E]

Heinonen OP, Slone D, Shapiro S: Birth Defects and Drugs in Pregnancy. Littleton, Mass.: John Wright-PSG, 1977, pp 276-277, 317-318, 436, 445, 473, 486. [E]

POLIOVIRUS VACCINE, LIVE

Synonyms

OPV, Orimune, Sabin Vaccine, TOPV

Summary

Live poliovirus vaccine is a living attenuated virus preparation that is given orally to induce immunization against poliomyelitis.

Magnitude of Teratogenic Risk

None

Quality and Quantity of Data

Fair To Good

Comment

None

The frequencies of congenital anomalies in general, of major malformations, of minor anomalies, and of principal classes of malformations were no greater than expected among the children of 1628 women who had been given live poliovirus vaccine during the first four lunar months of pregnancy in the Collaborative Perinatal Project (Heinonen et al., 1977). Similarly, the frequency of congenital anomalies was not increased among the children of 3059 women who had been given live poliovirus vaccine anytime during pregnancy in this study. The frequencies of congenital anomalies, of central nervous system malformations, and of orofacial clefts were no greater than expected among approximately 15,000 children who were born to women who had been vaccinated in early pregnancy during a Finnish immunization campaign that provided live poliovirus vaccine to 94% of adults (Harjulehto et al., 1989). No difference in the number of spontaneous abortions was recorded in a four-month period following an Israeli immunization campaign that provided live poliovirus vaccine to 90% of the population in comparison to the same period in the previous year (Ornoy et al., 1990).

No animal teratology studies of live poliovirus vaccine have been published.

Key References

Harjulehto T, Aro T, Hovi T, Saxen L: Congenital malformations and oral poliovirus vaccination during pregnancy. Lancet 1:771-772, 1989. [E]

Heinonen OP, Slone D, Shapiro S: Birth Defects and Drugs in Pregnancy. Littleton, Mass.: John Wright-PSG, 1977, pp 314-319, 436, 445, 474, 487. [E]

Ornoy A, Arnon J, Feingold M, Ben Ishai P: Spontaneous abortions following oral poliovirus vaccination in first trimester. Lancet 335:800, 1990. [E]

POLYESTRADIOL PHOSPHATE

Synonyms

Estradurin

Summary

Polyestradiol phosphate is administered intramuscularly in the treatment of prostatic carcinoma. The large polyestradiol phosphate molecules slowly release estradiol, an estrogenic compound, into the circulation.

Magnitude of Teratogenic Risk

Undetermined

Quality and Quantity of Data

None

Comment

Polyestradiol phosphate is used therapeutically in men only. The risk assessment therefore pertains to potential occupational exposures in women.

No epidemiological studies of congenital anomalies among infants born to women exposed to polyestradiol phosphate have been published.

No animal teratology studies of polyestradiol phosphate have been published.

Please see agent summary on ethinyl estradiol for information on a related agent that has been studied.

Key References

None available.

POLYETHYLENE GLYCOL

Synonyms

Blink-N-Clean, Carbowax, Lutrol, Macrogols, Polyhydroxyethylene, Polyoxyethylene Glycols

Summary

Polyethylene glycols are polymeric dihydroxy derivatives of paraffins. They are named according to their average molecular weight. (For example, polyethylene glycol 200 is a mixture of polymers of molecular weight around 200). High molecular weight polyethylene glycol and electrolyte mixtures are given orally to induce osmotic diarrhea. Polyethylene glycols are widely employed as bases for ointments and suppositories; as industrial lubricants, plasticizers, and binders; in paints, polishes, and paper coatings; in cosmetics and hair preparations; and as food additives.

Magnitude of Teratogenic Risk

Undetermined

Quality and Quantity of Data

None

Comment

A small risk cannot be excluded, but a high risk of congenital anomalies in the children of women exposed to polyethylene glycol during pregnancy is unlikely.

No epidemiological studies of congenital anomalies among infants born to women treated with polyethylene glycol during pregnancy have been reported.

No animal teratology studies of polyethylene glycol have been published.

Key References

None available.

POLYMYXIN B

Synonyms

Aerosporin Powder

Summary

Polymyxin B is a polypeptide antibiotic. It is used parenterally, topically, and in ophthalmic and dermatologic preparations.

Magnitude of Teratogenic Risk

Undetermined

Quality and Quantity of Data

None

Comment

None

No epidemiological studies of infants born after maternal polymyxin B use during pregnancy have been reported.

No adequate teratology studies of polymyxin B in experimental animals have been published.

Key References

None available.

POLYTHIAZIDE

Synonyms

Drenusil, Nephril, Politiazida, Renese

Summary

Polythiazide is a thiazide diuretic that is administered orally in the treatment of hypertension and edema.

Magnitude of Teratogenic Risk

Undetermined

Quality and Quantity of Data

Poor

Comment

A small risk cannot be excluded, but a high risk of congenital anomalies in the children of women treated with polythiazide during pregnancy is unlikely.

The frequency of congenital anomalies was no greater than expected among the children of 505 women treated with polythiazide during pregnancy in the Collaborative Perinatal Project (Heinonen et al., 1977). Only 10 of these women received polythiazide therapy during the first four lunar months of gestation.

No animal teratology studies of polythiazide have been published.

Please see agent summary on chlorothiazide for information on a related agent that has been more thoroughly studied.

Key References

Heinonen OP, Slone D, Shapiro S: Birth Defects and Drugs in Pregnancy. Littleton, Mass.: John Wright-PSG, 1977, pp 372, 436, 441. [E]

POTASSIUM CHLORIDE

Synonyms

K-Lor, K-Lyte/Cl, K-Tab, Kaochlor, Kaon Cl, Kato, Kay-Cee-L, Klor-Con, Klotrix, Micro-K, Rum-K, Slow-K

Summary

Potassium is an essential element, the concentration of which is closely regulated in body fluids. Potassium chloride is used for replenishment of depletion due to factors such as malnutrition, dehydration, or diuretic therapy. It is also used as a dietary substitute for table salt.

Magnitude of Teratogenic Risk

None

Quality and Quantity of Data

Poor

Comment

This assessment is for maternal treatment with potassium chloride.

No epidemiological studies of congenital anomalies in children of women who took large amounts of potassium chloride during pregnancy have been reported.

The frequency of malformations among the offspring of mice treated with 0.6-60 times the usual human dose of potassium chloride during pregnancy was no greater than expected (Food & Drug Research Labs, 1975).

Direct injection of potassium chloride into the fetal thorax, pericardium, or heart has been used for selective fetocide in multifetal pregnancies (Evans et al., 1990; Wapner et al., 1990).

Key References

Evans MI, May M, Drugan A, et al.: Selective termination: Clinical experience and residual risks. Am J Obstet Gynecol 162(6):1568-1575, 1990. [S]

Food and Drug Research Labs.: Teratologic evaluation of FDA 73-78, Potassium Chloride, in mice and rats. NTIS (National Technical Information Service) Report/PB-245 528, 1975. [O]

Wapner RJ, Davis GH, Johnson A, et al.: Selective reduction of multifetal pregnancies. Lancet 335:90-93, 1990. [S]

POVIDONE

Synonyms

Betadine Skin Cleanser, Efodine Ointment, Iodex-P, Plasdone, Polyvidone, Polyvinylpyrrolidone, PVP

Summary

Povidone is a polyvinylpyrrolidone polymer used as a suspending, dispersing, and coating agent in pharmaceutical preparations.

Magnitude of Teratogenic Risk

Undetermined

Quality and Quantity of Data

None To Poor

Comment

None

No epidemiological studies of congenital anomalies in infants born to women who took povidone during pregnancy have been reported.

The frequency of malformations was not increased among rabbits that had povidone injected directly into their yolk sacs during embryonic development (Claussen & Breuer, 1975).

Key References

Claussen U, Breuer HW: The teratogenic effects in rabbits of doxycycline, dissolved in polyvinylpyrrolidone, injected into the yolk sac. Teratology 12:297-302, 1975. [A]

PRAMOXINE

Synonyms

Fleet Relief, Prame Gel, Pramocaine Hydrochloride, Prax, Proctofoam, Tronolane Cream, Tronothane, Zone-A-Cream 1%

Summary

Pramoxine is a local anesthetic that is used topically.

Magnitude of Teratogenic Risk

Undetermined

Quality and Quantity of Data

None

Comment

None

No epidemiological studies of congenital anomalies in children born to women exposed to pramoxine during pregnancy have been reported.

No investigations of teratologic effects of pramoxine in experimental animals have been published.

Key References

None available.

PRAZEPAM

Synonyms

Centrax, Demetrin, Equipaz, Lysanxia, Prazene, Reapam, Verstran

Summary

Prazepam is a benzodiazepine minor tranquilizer used to treat anxiety.

Magnitude of Teratogenic Risk

Undetermined

Quality and Quantity of Data

Poor

Comment

None

No epidemiological studies of malformations in the offspring of women who took prazepam during pregnancy have been published.

In one study, the frequency of malformations (mostly hydrops fetalis and short tail) was increased among the offspring of rats treated with prazepam during pregnancy in doses 1700-3300 times those used clinically, but such doses were toxic to the mothers (Kuriyama et al., 1978). The frequency of congenital anomalies was not increased in the offspring of rats treated during pregnancy with 40-400 times the usual human dose. Similarly, the frequency of malformations was not increased among the offspring of rabbits treated with 8-80 times the usual human dose of prazepam during pregnancy (Ota et al., 1979).

Please see agent summary on diazepam for information on a closely related drug that has been more thoroughly studied.

Key References

Kuriyama T, Nishigaki K, Ota T, Koga T, et al.: [Safety studies of prazepam (K-373). VI. Teratological study in rats]. Oyo Yakuri (Pharmacometrics) 15:797-811, 1978. [A]

Ota T, Okubo M, Kuriyama T, Koga T, et al.: [Safety studies of prazepam (K-373). VIII. Teratological study in rabbits]. Oyo Yakuri (Pharmacometrics) 17:673-681, 1979. [A]

PRAZIQUANTEL

Synonyms

Biltricide, Cesol, Droncit, Embay 8440, Livera, Pontel, Prazi, Prazite, Pyquiton

Summary

Praziquantel is an oral anthelmintic agent used to treat fluke and tapeworm infestations.

Magnitude of Teratogenic Risk

Undetermined

Quality and Quantity of Data

None To Poor

Comment

None

No epidemiological studies of congenital anomalies among infants born to women treated with praziquantel during pregnancy have been reported.

No teratogenic effect was observed among the offspring of rats or rabbits treated with 0.5-7.5 or 0.5-5 times the usual human dose of praziquantel during pregnancy (Muermann et al., 1976; Ni et al., 1982).

Key References

Muermann P, Von Eberstein M, Frohberg H: Notes on the tolerance of DroncitR. Summary of trial results. Vet Med Rev 2:142-165, 1976. [A]

Ni Y-C, Shao B-R, Zhan C-Q, Xu Y-Q, et al.: Mutagenic and teratogenic effects of anti-schistosomal praziquantel. Chin Med J 95:494-498, 1982. [A]

PRAZOSIN

Synonyms

Furazosin Hydrochloride, Hypovase, Minipres, Minizide Capsules, Peripres, Sinetens

Summary

Prazosin is an oral antihypertensive agent.

Magnitude of Teratogenic Risk

Undetermined

Quality and Quantity of Data

Poor

Comment

None

No epidemiological studies of congenital anomalies among infants born to women treated with prazosin during pregnancy have been reported.

The frequency of malformations was not increased in the offspring of either rats or rabbits treated during pregnancy with prazosin in doses hundreds to thousands of times greater than those used in humans (Noguchi & Oh-waki, 1979).

Key References

Noguchi Y, Ohwaki Y: Prazosin hydrochloride. Reproductive and teratologic studies with prazosin hydrochloride in rats and rabbits. Oyo Yakuri 17:57-62, 1979. [A]

PREDNISONE/ PREDNISOLONE

Synonyms

Ak-Tate, Cortisolone, Deltacortisone, Deltadehydrocortisone, Econopred, Hydeltrasol, Hydeltra TBA, Inflamase, Metacortandralone, Meticorten, Pediapred, Predalone T.B.A., Predate, Prednicen-M, Prelone, Sterapred

Summary

Prednisolone and prednisone are synthetic glucocorticoids. Prednisone is biologically inert; it is converted to prednisolone, a biologically active compound, in the liver. Prednisone and prednisolone are used to treat a variety of allergic and inflammatory conditions.

Magnitude of Teratogenic Risk

None To Minimal

Quality and Quantity of Data

Poor To Fair

Comment

None

The frequency of malformations was not increased among the children of 43 women who had been treated with prednisone during the first four lunar months of pregnancy in the Collaborative Perinatal Project (Heinonen et al., 1977). Similarly, malformations do not appear to be unusually frequent among the infants of women treated with prednisone during pregnancy in uncontrolled series of 20-40 livebirths (Nielsen et al., 1984; O'Donnell et al., 1985).

Congenital immunodeficiency and lymphopenia have been reported in two infants born to women who had been treated with prednisone and azathioprine during pregnancy (Cote et al., 1974; DeWitte et al., 1984). It is uncertain whether or not the maternal immunosuppressive therapy played a role in development of this disease in the infants.

A high frequency of perinatal death has been observed in some series of women treated throughout gestation with prednisolone or prednisone (Walsh & Clark, 1967; Warrell & Taylor, 1968; Brown et al., 1991), but the perinatal death cannot be attributed to maternal steroid therapy because these women had serious illnesses requiring treatment, often with several drugs. Fetal growth retardation is also seen in some series of women treated during pregnancy with prednisone or prednisolone (Reinisch et al., 1978; Pirson et al., 1985), but the same confounding factors affect interpretation of the studies.

Dose-related fetal growth retardation occurs with increased frequency among the offspring of mice and rats treated in pregnancy with prednisone or prednisolone in doses within or above the human therapeutic range (Reinisch et al., 1978; Gandelman & Rosenthal, 1981; Gandelman & Guerriero, 1982; Neumann et al., 1986). Dose-dependent constriction of the ductus arteriosus was observed among the offspring of pregnant rats injected with prednisolone near term in doses 10-1000 times those used in humans (Momma et al., 1981).

Prednisolone, like other corticosteroids, produces a dose-dependent increase in the frequency of cleft palate in the offspring of mice treated with 1-40 times the human therapeutic dose during pregnancy (Pinsky & DiGeorge, 1965; Ballard et al., 1977). Increased frequencies of cleft palate are also observed among the offspring of pregnant rabbits and hamsters treated during pregnancy with prednisolone in doses respectively <1-2 and 80-240 times that used in humans (Walker, 1967; Shah & Kilistoff, 1976). A dose-dependent increase in the frequency of genital anomalies has been observed among the offspring of mice treated with 2-10 times the human therapeutic dose of prednisolone during pregnancy (Ballard et al., 1977; Gandelman & Rosenthal, 1981). Developmental and other behavioral alterations have been noted in mice born to mothers treated during pregnancy with prednisolone in doses 1-4 times those used in humans (Reinisch et al., 1980; Gandelman & Rosenthal, 1981; Gandelman & Guerriero, 1982).

Key References

Ballard PD, Hearney EF, Smith MB: Comparative teratogenicity of selected glucocorticoids applied ocularly in mice. Teratology 16:175-180, 1977. [A]

Brown JH, Maxwell AP, McGeown MG: Outcome of pregnancy following renal transplantation. Ir J Med Sci 160:255-256, 1991. [S]

Cote CJ, Hilaire MD, Meuwissen JH, et al.: Effects on the neonate of prednisone and azathioprine administered to the mother during pregnancy. J Pediatr 85(3):324-328, 1974. [C]

DeWitte DB, Buick MK, Cyran SE, et al.: Neonatal pancytopenia and severe combined immunodeficiency associated with antenatal administration of azathioprine and prednisone. J Pediatr 105(4):625-628, 1984. [C]

Gandelman R, Guerriero LA: Brief prenatal exposure to prednisolone adversely affects behavioral development and body weight. Neurobehav Toxicol Teratol 4:289-292, 1982. [A]

Gandelman R, Rosenthal C: Deleterious effects of prenatal prednisolone exposure upon morphological and behavioral development of mice. Teratology 24:293-301, 1981. [A]

Heinonen OP, Slone D, Shapiro S: Birth Defects and Drugs in Pregnancy. Littleton, Mass.: John Wright-PSG, 1977, pp 389, 391. [E]

Momma K, Nishihara S, Ota Y: Constriction of the fetal ductus arteriosus by glucocorticoid hormones. Pediatr Res 15:19-21, 1981. [A]

Neumann H-J, Garling H, Towe J: Zur wirkung von prednisolonbisuccinat auf die pranatale entwicklung der Wistar-ratte. Arzneimittelforsch 36:216-219, 1986. [A]

Nielsen OH, Andreasson B, Bondesen S, et al.: Pregnancy in ulcerative colitis. Scand J Gastroenterol 19:724-732, 1984. [S]

O'Donnell D, Sevitz H, Seggie JL, et al.: Pregnancy after renal transplantation. Aust NZ J Med 15:320-325, 1985. [S]

Pinsky L, DiGeorge AM: Cleft palate in the mouse: A teratogenic index of glucocorticoid potency. Science 147:402-403, 1965. [A]

Pirson Y, van Lierde M, Ghysen J, et al.: Retardation of fetal growth in patients receiving immunosuppressive therapy. N Engl J Med 313:328, 1985. [E]

Reinisch JM, Simon NG, Gandelman R: Prenatal exposure to prednisone permanently alters fighting behavior of female mice. Pharmacol Biochem Behav 12:213-216, 1980. [A]

Reinisch JM, Simon NG, Karow WG, Gandelman RG: Prenatal exposure to prednisone in humans and animals retards intrauterine growth. Science 202:436-438, 1978. [A]

Shah RM, Kilistoff A: Cleft palate induction in hamster fetuses glucocorticoid hormones and their synthetic analogues. J Embryol Exp Morphol 36:101-108, 1976. [A]

Walker BE: Induction of cleft palate in rabbits by several glucocorticoids. Proc Soc Exp Biol Med 125:1281-1284, 1967. [A]

Walsh SD, Clark FR: Pregnancy in patients on long-term corticosteroid therapy. Scot Med J 12:302-306, 1967. [S]

Warrell DW, Taylor R: Outcome for the foetus of mothers receiving prednisolone during pregnancy. Lancet 1:117-118, 1968. [E]

PRILOCAINE

Synonyms

Citanest, Xylonest

Summary

Prilocaine is a local anesthetic of the amide class.

Magnitude of Teratogenic Risk

Undetermined

Quality and Quantity of Data

None

Comment

A small risk cannot be excluded, but there is no indication that the risk of congenital anomalies in the children of women treated with prilocaine during pregnancy is likely to be great.

No epidemiological studies of congenital anomalies in children born to women exposed to prilocaine during pregnancy have been reported.

No investigations of teratologic effects of prilocaine in experimental animals have been published.

Maternal epidural analgesia with prilocaine during labor has been associated with the occurrence of methemoglobinemia in newborn children (Climie et al., 1967).

Please see agent summary on lidocaine for information on a related agent that has been studied.

Key References

Climie CR, McLean S, Starmer GA, Thomas J: Methaemoglobinaemia in mother and fetus following continuous analgesia with prilocaine. Br J Anaesth 39:155-160, 1967. [A]

PRIMIDOLOL

Synonyms

UK 11-443

Summary

Primidolol is a beta-adrenoreceptor blocking agent used to treat hypertension.

Magnitude of Teratogenic Risk

Undetermined

Quality and Quantity of Data

None

Comment

A small risk cannot be excluded, but there is no indication that the risk of congenital anomalies in the children of women treated with primidolol during pregnancy is likely to be great.

No epidemiological studies of malformations in infants born to mothers who used primidolol during pregnancy have been reported.

No animal teratology studies of primidolol have been published.

Please see agent summary on propranolol for information on a more thoroughly studied drug with similar action.

Key References

None available.

PRIMIDONE

Synonyms

Desoxyphenobarbitone, Hexamidinum, Midone, Mysoline, Neurosyn, Primaclone, Sertan

Summary

Primidone is an anticonvulsant used to treat grand mal, psychomotor, and focal motor seizures. It is partially metabolized to phenobarbital.

Magnitude of Teratogenic Risk

Small To Moderate

Quality and Quantity of Data

Fair To Good

Comment

None

In a study of children of epileptic women, the frequency of congenital anomalies, especially cleft lip and palate, was greater among the infants of 146 women who were treated with primidone during the first trimester of pregnancy than among the infants of women not treated with this drug (Nakane et al., 1980). Similarly, the frequency of congenital anomalies was greater than expected among the infants of 24 epileptic women treated with primidone during the first trimester of pregnancy in another cohort study (Fedrick, 1973). The rate of major and/or minor congenital anomalies among 92 infants born to women treated with primidone in one study was 17%, but this was not significantly different from the outcome in women treated with other anticonvulsants (Kaneko et al., 1988). Most of the women in these investigations were treated with more than one drug, and it is unclear whether the associations observed were due to the severity of the maternal epilepsy, enhancement of the teratogenic action of another agent, a primary teratogenic effect of primidone, or some other factor (Janz, 1982). The risk of congenital anomalies among infants born to epileptic women treated with multiple drugs appears to be greater than the risk among infants born to women treated with a single anticonvulsant (Kaneko et al., 1988; Lander & Eadie, 1990).

A pattern of minor dysmorphic features has been observed among a few children born to women treated with primidone for epilepsy during pregnancy (Rudd & Freedom, 1979; Myhre & Williams, 1981; Rating et al., 1982; Hoyme et al., 1990). This pattern may represent a "fetal primidone syndrome," but the phenotype has not been completely delineated. Poor growth, especially of the head, seems unusually frequent among the infants of epileptic women treated with primidone during preg-

nancy (Rating et al., 1982; Neri et al., 1983; Majewski and Steger, 1984).

A greater-than-expected frequency of cleft palate has been reported among the offspring of mice given primidone in doses 1-80 times those used in humans, but the effect did not increase with increasing dose (Sullivan & McElhatton, 1975; McElhatton et al., 1977).

Please see agent summary on phenobarbital, a metabolic product of primidone, that has been more thoroughly studied.

Key References

Fedrick J: Epilepsy and pregnancy: A report from the Oxford Record Linkage Study. Br Med J 2:442-448, 1973. [E]

Hoyme HE: Teratogenically induced fetal anomalies. Clin Perinatol 17(3):547-567, 1990. [R]

Janz D: On major malformations and minor anomalies in the offspring of parents with epilepsy: Review of the literature. In: Janz D et al. (eds). Epilepsy, Pregnancy and the Child. New York: Raven Press, 1982, pp 211-222. [R]

Kaneko S, Otani K, Fukushima Y, et al.: Teratogenicity of antiepileptic drugs: Analysis of possible risk factors. Epilepsia 29(4):459-467, 1988. [E]

Lander CM, Eadie MJ: Antiepileptic drug intake during pregnancy and malformed offspring. Epilepsy Res 7:77-82, 1990. [E]

Majewski F, Steger M: Fetal head growth retardation associated with maternal phenobarbitone/primidone and/or phenytoin therapy. Eur J Pediatr 141:188-189, 1984. [E]

McElhatton PR, Sullivan FM, Toseland PA: Teratogenic activity and metabolism of primidone in the mouse. Epilepsia 18:1-11, 1977. [A]

Myhre SA, Williams R: Teratogenic effects associated with maternal primidone therapy. J Pediatr 99:160-162, 1981. [C]

Nakane Y, Okuma T, Takahashi R, Sato Y, et al.: Multi-institutional study on the teratogenicity and fetal toxicity of antiepileptic drugs: A report of a collaborative study group in Japan. Epilepsia 21:663-680, 1980. [E]

Neri A, Heifetz L, Nitke S, et al.: Neonatal outcome in infants of epileptic mothers. Eur J Obstet Gynecol Reprod Biol 16:263-268, 1983. [E]

Rating D, Nau H, Jager-Roman E, et al.: Teratogenic and pharmacokinetic studies of primidone during pregnancy and in the offspring of epileptic women. Acta Paediatr Scand 71:301-311, 1982. [E]

Rudd NL, Freedom RM: A possible primidone embryopathy. J Pediatr 94:835-837, 1979. [C]

Sullivan FM, McElhatton PR: Teratogenic activity of the antiepileptic drugs phenobarbital, phenytoin, and primidone in mice. Toxicol Appl Pharmacol 34:271-282, 1975. [A]

PROBENECID

Synonyms

Benemid, Benuryl, Ethamide

Summary

Probenecid is a uricosuric agent that is administered orally to treat gout and hyperuricemia of other causes.

Magnitude of Teratogenic Risk

Undetermined

Quality and Quantity of Data

None

Comment

None

No epidemiological studies of congenital anomalies among the infants of women treated with probenecid during pregnancy have been reported.

No animal teratology studies of probenecid have been published.

Key References

None available.

PROBUCOL

Synonyms

Bifenabid, Biphenabid, Lesterol, Lorelco, Lurselle, Panesclerina, Superlid

Summary

Probucol is an antioxidant that is given orally to treat hyperlipidemia. The drug is stored in adipose tissue and persists in the body for several months after discontinuation of therapy.

Magnitude of Teratogenic Risk

Undetermined

Quality and Quantity of Data

None To Poor

Comment

None

No epidemiological studies of congenital anomalies among infants born to women treated with probucol during pregnancy have been reported.

No increase in malformations was observed among the offspring of rats or rabbits treated during pregnancy with up to 50 times the human dose of probucol (Molello et al., 1980).

Key References

Molello JA, Thompson DJ, Stephenson MF, Gerbig CG, et al.: Eight-year toxicity study in monkeys and reproduction studies in rats and rabbits treated with probucol. J Toxicol Environ Health 6:529-545, 1980. [A]

PROCAINAMIDE

Synonyms

Procamide, Procan SR, Procapan, Pronestyl

Summary

Procainamide is used to treat cardiac arrhythmias.

Magnitude of Teratogenic Risk

Undetermined

Quality and Quantity of Data

None

Comment

A small risk cannot be excluded, but there is no indication that the risk of congenital anomalies in the children of women treated with procainamide during pregnancy is likely to be great.

No epidemiological studies of congenital anomalies in the children of women treated with procainamide during pregnancy have been reported.

No animal teratology studies of procainamide have been published.

Procainamide has been used successfully in the treatment of fetal cardiac arrhythmia in the third trimester of pregnancy (Dumesic et al., 1982; Given et al., 1984).

Key References

Dumesic DA, Silverman NH, Tobias S, Golbus MS: Transplacental cardioversion of fetal supraventricular tachycardia with procainamide. N Engl J Med 307:1128-1131, 1982. [C]

Given BD, Phillippe M, Sanders SP, et al.: Procainamide cardioversion of fetal supraventricular tachyarrhythmia. Am J Cardiol 53:1460-1461, 1984. [C]

PROCAINE

Synonyms

Allocaine, Ethocaine, Novocain, Syncaine

Summary

Procaine is an injectable local anesthetic of the ester class.

Magnitude of Teratogenic Risk

None

Quality and Quantity of Data

Poor To Fair

Comment

None

The frequencies of malformations in general, of major malformations, of minor malformations, and of major classes of congenital anomalies were not increased among the children of 1340 women who had been treated with procaine during the first four lunar months of pregnancy in the Collaborative Perinatal Project (Heinonen et al., 1977). In the same study, the frequency of congenital anomalies was no greater than expected among the children born to 3395 women treated with procaine anytime during pregnancy. In a case-control study of 266 infants with congenital anomalies, the frequency of maternal treatment with procaine during the first trimester was no greater than expected (Mellin, 1964).

No teratologic studies of procaine in experimental animals have been published.

Key References

Heinonen OP, Slone D, Shapiro S: Birth Defects and Drugs in Pregnancy. Littleton, Mass.: John Wright-PSG, 1977, pp 358, 360, 362, 440, 477, 493. [E]

Mellin GW: Drugs in the first trimester of pregnancy and the fetal life of Homo sapiens. Am J Obstet Gynecol 90:1169-1180, 1964. [E]

PROCHLORPERAZINE

Synonyms

Compazine, Nibromin-A, Prochlorpemazine, Stemetil, Vertigon Spansule

Summary

Prochlorperazine is a phenothiazine tranquilizer used in treatment of psychosis and as an antiemetic.

Magnitude of Teratogenic Risk

None

Quality and Quantity of Data

Good To Excellent

Comment

None

The frequencies of congenital anomalies in general, of major malformations, of minor anomalies, and of principle classes of anomalies were no greater than expected among the children of 877 women who took prochlorperazine during the first four lunar months of pregnancy in the Collaboarative Perinatal Project (Heinonen et al., 1977). There was also no increase in the frequency of congenital anomalies among the children of 2023 women who took this medication anytime during pregnancy. Similarly, no association between first-trimester maternal use of prochlorperazine and malformations in the infants was observed in three other cohort studies that included, respectively, 433, 91, and more than 50 exposed pregnancies (Milkovich & van den Berg, 1976; Kullander & Kallen, 1976; Jick et al., 1981).

An increased frequency of cleft palate was observed among the offspring of mice and rats treated during pregnancy with prochlorperazine in doses 17 or more and 3-23 times those used in humans (Roux, 1959; Szabo & Brent, 1974). The relevance of these observations to the therapeutic use of prochlorperazine in human pregnancy is unknown.

Key References

Heinonen OP, Slone D, Shapiro S: Birth Defects and Drugs in Pregnancy. Littleton, Mass.: John Wright-PSG, 1977, pp 323-324, 437. [E]

Jick H, Holmes LB, Hunter JR, Madsen S, et al.: First-trimester drug use and congenital disorders. JAMA 246:343-346, 1981. [E]

Kullander S, Kallen B: A prospective study of drugs and pregnancy: II. Anti-emetic drugs. Acta Obstet Gynecol Scand 55:105-111, 1976. [E]

Milkovich L, van den Berg BJ: An evaluation of the teratogenicity of certain antinauseant drugs. Am J Obstet Gynecol 125:244-248, 1976. [E]

Roux CH: Teratogenic action of prochlorperazine. Arch Fr Pediatr 16:968-971, 1959. [A]

Szabo KT, Brent RL: Species differences in experimental teratogenesis by tranquillising agents. Lancet 1:565, 1974. [A]

PROCLONOL

Synonyms

Kilacar

Summary

Proclonol is an antihelmintic and antifungal agent.

Magnitude of Teratogenic Risk

Undetermined

Quality and Quantity of Data

None

Comment

None

No epidemiological studies of congenital anomalies in infants born to women treated with proclonol during pregnancy have been reported.

No animal teratology studies of proclonol have been published.

Key References

None available.

PROCYCLIDINE

Synonyms

Arpicolin Syrup, Elorine, Kemadrin, Lergine, Prociclidina, Tricoloid, Tricyclamol, Vagosin

Summary

Procyclidine is an anticholinergic agent that is administered orally in the symptomatic treatment of parkinsonism and drug-induced extrapyramidal syndromes.

Magnitude of Teratogenic Risk

Undetermined

Quality and Quantity of Data

None

Comment

None

No adequate epidemiological studies of congenital anomalies in infants born to mothers who were treated with procyclidine during pregnancy have been reported.

No animal teratology studies of procyclidine have been published.

Please see agent summary on atropine for information on a related agent that has been studied.

Key References

None available.

PROMETHAZINE

Synonyms

BayMeth, Ganphen, Histantil, Phencen, Phenergan, Promet, Prothazine, Remsed, V-Gan

Summary

Promethazine is a phenothiazine with antihistaminic, antiemetic, and sedative actions. It is used to treat allergic disorders, as a preoperative medication, and in the management of parkinsonian symptoms.

Magnitude of Teratogenic Risk

None

Quality and Quantity of Data

Good To Excellent

Comment

This rating is for usual therapeutic doses of promethazine; the risk associated with toxic overdoses of this drug is unknown but may be greater.

The frequency of congenital anomalies was no greater than expected among the children of 63, 55, 114, and 529 women who were treated with promethazine during the first trimester of pregnancy in four cohort studies (Farkas & Farkas, 1971; Heinonen et al., 1977; Rumeau-Rouquette et al., 1977; Aselton et al., 1985). In one of these investigations, the frequency of congenital anomalies was no greater than expected among 746 children born to women who took promethazine anytime during pregnancy (Heinonen et al., 1977). No association with maternal use of promethazine during the first trimester of pregnancy was seen in case-control studies of 175 and 836 children with congenital anomalies (Nelson & Forfar, 1971; Greenberg et al., 1977).

Among 19 pregnancies that were continued after the mother had taken a toxic overdose of promethazine, usually in combination with other drugs, there were two fetal deaths (one thought to be unrelated to the overdose), two children with mental retardation (who were siblings), and one child with borderline intellectual function (Czeizel et al., 1984; Czeizel et al., 1988). Three children had multiple naevi and one had strabismus; no malformations were noted. Most of the overdoses occurred in the second or third trimester; only two were in the first trimester of pregnancy.

The frequency of malformations was no greater than expected among the offspring of pregnant rats treated with 50-250 times the usual human dose of promethazine (King et al., 1965).

Maternal promethazine treatment during pregnancy has been used for Rh hemolytic disease (Gusdon, 1981). Altered immunological function has been demonstrated in the newborn infants of such treated women (Rubinstein et al., 1976; Eidelman et al., 1977).

Abnormal in vitro tests of platelet function have been observed in infants born to women treated with promethazine during labor (Corby & Schulman, 1971). The clinical relevance of this observation is unknown.

Key References

Aselton P, Jick H, Milunsky A, Hunter JR, et al.: First-trimester drug use and congenital disorders. Obstet Gynecol 65:451-455, 1985. [S]

Corby DG, Schulman I: The effects of antenatal drug administration on aggregation of platelets of newborn infants. J Pediatr 79:307-313, 1971. [E]

Czeizel A, Szentesi I, Szekeres I, et al.: Pregnancy outcome and health conditions of offspring of self-poisoned pregnant women. Acta Paediatr Hung 25(3):209-236, 1984. [S]

Czeizel A, Szentesi I, Szekeres I, et al.: A study of adverse effects on the progeny after intoxication during pregnancy. Arch Toxicol 62:1-7, 1988. [S]

Eidelman AI, Rubinstein A, Melamed J, et al.: More on the effect of maternal promethazine (P-HCl) on neonatal immunologic functions. J Pediatr 90(2):332-333, 1977. [O]

Farkas VG, Farkas G: Teratogenic action of hyperemesis in pregnancy and of medication used to treat it. Zentralbl Gynaekol 93:325-330, 1971. [S]

Greenberg G, Inman WHW, Weatherall JAC, Adelstein AM, et al.: Maternal drug histories and congenital abnormalities. Br Med J 2:853-856, 1977. [E]

Gusdon JP: The treatment of erythroblastosis with promethazine hydrochloride. J Reprod Med 26(9):454-458, 1981. [E]

Heinonen OP, Slone D, Shapiro S: Birth Defects and Drugs in Pregnancy. Littleton, Mass.: John Wright-PSG, 1977, pp 323, 437. [E]

King CTG, Weaver SA, Narrod SA: Antihistamines and teratogenicity in the rat. J Pharmacol Exp Ther 147:391-398, 1965. [A]

Nelson MM, Forfar JO: Associations between drugs administered during pregnancy and congenital abnormalities of the fetus. Br Med J 1:523-527, 1971. [E]

Rubinstein A, Eidelman AI, Melamed J, et al.: Possible effect of maternal promethazine therapy on neonatal immunologic functions. J Ped 89(1):136-138, 1976. [S]

Rumeau-Rouquette C, Goujard J, Huel G: Possible teratogenic effect of phenothiazines in human beings. Teratology 15:57-64, 1977. [S]

PROPANIDID

Synonyms

Epontol, Fabantol

Summary

Propanidid is a short-acting nonbarbiturate intravenous general anesthetic.

Magnitude of Teratogenic Risk

Undetermined

Quality and Quantity of Data

None To Poor

Comment

None

No epidemiological studies of congenital anomalies in children born to women exposed to propanidid during pregnancy have been reported.

No teratogenic effect was noted among the offspring of rats anesthetized briefly with propanidid during pregnancy (Giovanelli et al., 1979). The frequency of fetal loss was apparently increased among the offspring of dogs treated every other day during early pregnancy with propanidid in doses about 6 times those used in humans (Lear et al., 1964). The relevance of this observation to the clinical use of propanidid in human pregnancy is unknown.

Key References

Giovanelli L, Brandolin P, Zanozi A, Fregnan L, Savorelli M: Fetal abnormalities induced by anesthetic drugs in the early stages of pregnancy. Riv Ital Ginecol 53:770-777, 1969. [A]

Lear E, Tangoren G, Chiron AE, Pallin IM, et al.: New phenoxyacetamide systemic anaesthetic. Toxicity and clinical studies. NY State J Med 64:2177-2184, 1964. [A]

PROPANOCAINE

Synonyms

467D3

Summary

Propanocaine is a local anesthetic that has been used topically.

Magnitude of Teratogenic Risk

Undetermined

Quality and Quantity of Data

None

Comment

None

No epidemiological studies of congenital anomalies in children born to women exposed to propanocaine during pregnancy have been reported.

No investigations of teratologic effects of propanocaine in experimental animals have been published.

Please see agent summary on procaine for information on a related agent that has been studied.

Key References

None available.

PROPARACAINE

Synonyms

AK-Taine, Alcaine, I-Paracaine, Kainair, Ocu-Caine, Ophthaine, Ophthetic, Proxymetacaine

Summary

Proparacaine is a surface anesthetic of the ester class used in ophthalmology.

Magnitude of Teratogenic Risk

Undetermined

Quality and Quantity of Data

None

Comment

A small risk cannot be excluded, but there is no indication that the risk of congenital anomalies in

the children of women treated with proparacaine during pregnancy is likely to be great.

No epidemiological studies of congenital anomalies in children born to women exposed to proparacaine during pregnancy have been reported.

No investigations of teratologic effects of proparacaine in experimental animals have been published.

Please see agent summary on procaine for information on a related agent that has been studied.

Key References

None available.

PROPIONATE

Synonyms

Propionic Acid, Sodium Propionate

Summary

Propionate is an antifungal agent that is used topically. It is also used as a mold inhibitor in food and pharmaceutical agents.

Magnitude of Teratogenic Risk

Undetermined

Quality and Quantity of Data

None

Comment

A small risk cannot be excluded, but a high risk of congenital anomalies in the children of women treated with propionate during pregnancy is unlikely.

No epidemiological studies of congenital anomalies in infants whose mothers were treated with propionate during pregnancy have been reported.

No animal teratology studies of propionate have been published.

Key References

None available.

PROPOFOL

Synonyms

Diprivan

Summary

Propofol is a general anesthetic that is administered intravenously.

Magnitude of Teratogenic Risk

Undetermined

Quality and Quantity of Data

None

Comment

None

No epidemiological studies of congenital anomalies in children born to women treated with propofol during pregnancy have been reported.

No studies of teratologic effects of propofol in experimental animals have been published.

Alterations of neonatal behavior have been noted among the infants of women anesthetized with propofol during cesarean delivery (Celleno et al., 1989).

Key References

Celleno D, Capogna G, Tomassetti M, et al.: Neurobehavioural effects of propofol on the neonate following elective Caesarean section. Br J Anaesth 62:649-654, 1989. [E]

PROPOXYCAINE

Summary

Propoxycaine is an injectable local anesthetic of the ester class.

Magnitude of Teratogenic Risk

Undetermined

Quality and Quantity of Data

None To Poor

Comment

A small risk cannot be excluded, but there is no indication that the risk of congenital anomalies in the children of women treated with propoxycaine during pregnancy is likely to be great.

The frequency of congenital anomalies was not significantly greater than expected among the children of 41 women treated with propoxycaine during the first four lunar months of pregnancy or among the children of 90 women treated anytime in pregnancy in the Collaborative Perinatal Project (Heinonen et al., 1977).

No investigations of teratologic effects of propoxycaine in experimental animals have been published.

Please see agent summary on procaine for information on a related agent that has been more thoroughly studied.

Key References

Heinonen OP, Slone D, Shapiro S: Birth Defects and Drugs in Pregnancy. Littleton, Mass.: John Wright-PSG, 1977, pp 358-360, 440. [E]

PROPOXYPHENE

Synonyms

Darvon, Dolene, Doloxene, Novopropoxyn, Proxagesic, SK-65

Summary

Propoxyphene is a widely prescribed oral analgesic agent.

Magnitude of Teratogenic Risk

None

Quality and Quantity of Data

Good

Comment

Available data concern use of propoxyphene in usual therapeutic doses.

The frequencies of congenital anomalies in general, major malformations, minor anomalies, and major classes of congenital anomalies were no greater than expected among the children of 686 women who took propoxyphene during the first four lunar months of pregnancy in the Collaborative Perinatal Project (Heinonen et al., 1977). Similar findings were reported by Jick et al. (1981) in another cohort study involving more than 100 pregnancies exposed to propoxyphene during the first trimester. The frequency of congenital anomalies was no greater than expected among the infants of 2914 women who took propoxyphene anytime during pregnancy in the Collaborative Perinatal Project (Heinonen et al., 1977). A few anecdotal cases of malformations in infants born after maternal exposure to propoxyphene during pregnancy have been reported (Boelter, 1980; Golden et al., 1982; Williams et al., 1983), but no recurrent pattern of anomalies is apparent and a causal relationship of the maternal exposure to the infants' malformations seems unlikely.

No teratogenic effect was observed in rats, rabbits, or hamsters after treatment with propoxyphene in doses as large as 10-40 times those used clinically (Emmerson et al., 1971; Geber & Schramm, 1975; Buttar & Moffatt, 1983). An increased frequency of malformations was observed among the offspring of hamsters treated during pregnancy with 40-95 times the usual human dose, but substantial maternal mortality occurred in the upper part of this range (Geber & Schramm, 1975). Long-lasting behavioral alterations have been noted among the offspring of rats treated during pregnancy with 6-10 times the human dose of propoxyphene (Vorhees et al., 1979; Sallenfait & Vannier, 1988).

Transient neonatal withdrawal symptoms have been reported in infants born to mothers who took propoxyphene chronically during pregnancy (Tyson, 1974; Klein et al., 1975; Quillian & Dunn, 1976; Ente & Mehra, 1978). Irritability, hyperactivity, tremors, and high-pitched cry are the usual clinical features.

Key References

Boelter W: Proposed fetal propoxyphene (DarvonR) syndrome. Clin Res 28:115A, 1980. [C]

Buttar HS, Moffatt JH: Pre- and postnatal development of rats following concomitant intrauterine exposure to propoxyphene and chlordiazepoxide. Neurobehav Toxicol Teratol 5:549-556, 1983. [A]

Emmerson JL, Owen NV, Koenig GR, Markham JK, et al.: Reproduction and teratology studies on propoxyphene napsylate. Toxicol Appl Pharmacol 19:471-479, 1971. [A]

Ente G, Mehra MC: Neonatal withdrawal from propoxyphene hydrochloride. NY State J Med 78:2084-2085, 1978. [C]

Geber WF, Schramm LC: Congenital malformations of the central nervous system produced by narcotic analgesics in the hamster. Am J Obstet Gynecol 123:705-713, 1975. [A]

Golden NL, King KC, Sokol RJ: Propoxyphene and acetaminophen. Possible effects on the fetus. Clin Pediatr 21:752-754, 1982. [C]

Heinonen OP, Slone D, Shapiro S: Birth Defects and Drugs in Pregnancy. Littleton, Mass.: John Wright-PSG, 1977, pp 287-288, 294, 434, 471, 484. [E]

Jick H, Holmes LB, Hunter JR, Madsen S, et al.: First-trimester drug use and congenital disorders. JAMA 246:343-346, 1981. [E]

Klein RB, Blatman S, Little GA: Probable neonatal propoxyphene withdrawal: A case report. Pediatrics 55:882-884, 1975. [C]

Quillian WW, Dunn CA: Neonatal drug withdrawal from propoxyphene. JAMA 235:2128, 1976. [C]

Saillenfait AM, Vannier B: Methodological proposal in behavioural teratogenicity testing: Assessment of propoxyphene, chlorpromazine, and vitamin A as positive controls. Teratology 37:185-199, 1988. [A]

Tyson HK: Neonatal withdrawal symptoms associated with maternal use of propoxyphene hydrochloride (Darvon). J Pediatr 85:684-685, 1974. [C]

Vorhees CV, Brunner RL, Butcher RE: Psychotropic drugs as behavioral teratogens. Science 205:1220-1225, 1979. [A]

Williams DA, Weiss T, Wade E, Dignan P: Prune perineum syndrome: Report of a second case. Teratology 28:145-148, 1983. [C]

PROPRANOLOL

Synonyms

Angilol, Apsolol, Berkolol, Inderal, Novopranol

Summary

Propranolol is a widely used beta-adrenergic receptor blocking agent. It is employed in the treatment of hypertension, cardiac arrhythmias, hypertrophic subaortic stenosis, hyperthyroidism, and migraine headaches.

Magnitude of Teratogenic Risk

Undetermined

Quality and Quantity of Data

Poor

Comment

A small risk cannot be excluded, but there is no indication that the risk of malformations in the children of women treated with propranolol during pregnancy is likely to be great. Possible effects on fetal growth and perinatal adaptation are discussed below.

No adequate study of congenital anomalies in the infants of women treated with propranolol during pregnancy has been published.

The frequency of malformations was not increased among the offspring of rats or mice treated with propranolol during pregnancy in doses respectively 2-4 and 2-10 times those usually employed in humans (Fuji & Nishimura, 1974; Speiser et al., 1983; Kang & Manson, 1987).

Chronic propranolol treatment of pregnant women in late pregnancy has been associated with intrauterine growth retardation of the fetus (Eliahou et al., 1978; Lieberman et al., 1978; Oakley et al., 1979; Pruyn et al., 1979; Redmond, 1982). However, it is difficult in most studies to separate an action of the drug from an effect of the disease for which it has been given, and not all investigations show this association (Rubin, 1981). Fetal weight appears to be most consistently affected; head circumference may also be involved (Pruyn et al., 1979), but this measurement is not recorded in most studies. There are no data available in humans regarding whether or not the growth retardation associated with maternal propranolol use persists into childhood. The possibility that head (and presumably also brain) growth is deficient in offspring of mothers treated with propranolol is of concern, but no studies of neurological or intellectual function in these children have been reported.

Studies in rodents employing doses several times larger than those used in humans have shown decreased fetal weight after chronic maternal propranolol treatment late in pregnancy (Schoenfeld et al., 1978; Harmon et al., 1986). Rats exposed prenatally to propranolol in doses slightly larger than those used in humans have been reported to exhibit long-lasting alterations of behavior (Speiser et al., 1983).

The occurrence of difficulties in perinatal adaptation including neonatal apnea, respiratory distress, bradycardia, and hypoglycemia has been associated with maternal treatment with propranolol, especially if the drug is administered in a high dose and/or shortly before delivery (Tunstall, 1969; Habib & McCarthy, 1977; Oakley et al., 1979; Pruyn et al., 1979; Rubin, 1981; Buechler & Palmer, 1982). Such effects are compatible with the known pharmacological actions of propranolol (Ayromlooi, 1983). The magnitude of these risks is uncertain.

Key References

Ayromlooi J: Effect of propranolol on the acid base balance and hemodynamics of 'chronically instrumented' pregnant sheep. Dev Pharmacol Ther 6:207-216, 1983. [A]

Buechler AA, Palmer SK: Intrapartum fetal death associated with propranolol; case report and review of physiology. Wis Med J 81:23-25, 1982. [C] & [R]

Eliahou HE, Silverberg DS, Reisin E, Romem I, et al.: Propranolol for the treatment of hypertension in pregnancy. Br J Obstet Gynaecol 85:431-436, 1978. [S]

Fuji T, Nishimura H: Reduction in frequency of fetopathic effects of caffeine in mice by pretreatment with propranolol. Teratology 10:149-152, 1974. [A]

Habib A, McCarthy JS: Effects on the neonate of propranolol administered during pregnancy. J Pediatr 91:808-811, 1977. [C]

Harmon JR, Delongchamp RR, Kimmel GL, et al.: Effect of prenatal propranolol exposure on development of the postnatal rat heart. Teratogenesis Carcinog Mutagen 6:139-150, 1986. [A]

Kang YJ, Manson JM: Effect of prenatal propranolol-nitrofen exposure on pregnant rats. Teratology 35(2):58A, 1987. [A]

Lieberman BA, Stirrat GM, Cohen SL, Beard RW, et al.: The possible adverse effect of propranolol on the fetus in pregnancies complicated by severe hypertension. Br J Obstet Gynaecol 85:678-683, 1978. [S]

Oakley GG, McGarry K, Limb DG, Oakley CM: Management of pregnancy in patients with hypertrophic cardiomyopathy. Br Med J 1:1749-1750, 1979. [S]

Pruyn SC, Phelan JP, Buchanan GC: Long-term propranolol therapy in pregnancy: Maternal and fetal outcome. Am J Obstet Gynecol 135:485-489, 1979. [S]

Redmond GP: Propranolol and fetal growth retardation. Semin Perinatol 6(2):142-147, 1982. [R]

Rubin PC: Beta-blockers in pregnancy. N Engl J Med 305:1323-1326, 1981. [R]

Schoenfeld N, Epstein O, Nemesh L, Rosen M, et al.: Effects of propranolol during pregnancy and development of rats. I. Adverse effects during pregnancy. Pediatr Res 12:747-750, 1978. [A]

Speiser Z, Shved A, Gitter S: Effect of propranolol treatment in pregnant rats on motor activity and avoidance learning of the offspring. Psychopharmacology 79:148-154, 1983. [A]

Tunstall ME: The effect of propranolol on the onset of breathing at birth. Br J Anaesth 41:792, 1969. [S]

PROPYLPARABEN

Synonyms

Nipasol, Nipazol, Paseptol, Propyl-p-Hydroxybenzoate, Propylparasept

Summary

Propylparaben is a propyl ester of hydroxybenzoic acid. It is used as a preservative in foods and pharmaceuticals.

Magnitude of Teratogenic Risk

Undetermined

Quality and Quantity of Data

None

Comment

None

No epidemiological studies of congenital anomalies among infants born to women exposed to large amounts of propylparaben during pregnancy have been reported.

No animal teratology studies of propylparaben have been published.

Key References

None available.

PROPYLTHIOURACIL

Synonyms

Propycil, Propyl-Thyracil, PTU, Thyreostat II, Tiotil

Summary

Propylthiouracil is a thioamide derivative that is administered orally to treat hyperthyroidism.

Magnitude of Teratogenic Risk

Malformations: None

Goiter: Small To Moderate

Quality and Quantity of Data

Malformations: Poor To Fair

Goiter: Good

Comment

None

Propylthiouracil, when given to a pregnant woman, crosses the placenta and can cause suppression of fetal thyroid function. Since maternal thyroid hormones do not readily cross the placenta, fetal thyroid hyperplasia and goiter may develop as the fetus attempts to compensate for its hypothyroidism (Burrow, 1978; Solomon, 1981). It has been estimated that 1-5% of infants born to women treated with propylthiouracil during pregnancy develop significant transient neonatal hypothyroidism (Davis et al., 1989; Becks & Burrow, 1991), although clinically inapparent mild hypothyroxinemia is much more common (Cheron et al., 1981). Neonatal goiter is also seen in a few percent of infants born to women treated with propylthiouracil during pregnancy but is rarely large enough to cause respiratory compromise (Davis et al., 1989; Becks & Burrow, 1991). Large goiters are much more common in infants of women treated with both propylthiouracil and iodides during pregnancy (Seligman & Pescovitz, 1950; Burrow, 1965; Mujtaba & Burrow, 1975). Since either hypothyroidism or hyperthyroidism may occur among infants of women who have Graves' disease treated with propylthiouracil during pregnancy, thyroid function should be assessed in these children at the time of birth (Hayek & Brooks, 1975; Burrow, 1985).

The frequency of malformations was not significantly increased among the children of 65 women with Graves' disease who were treated with propylthiouracil during pregnancy when compared to the children of untreated Graves' disease patients in one study (Momotani & Ito, 1991). Interpretation of this investigation is difficult because it appears to lack epidemiological rigor. The frequency of congenital anomalies not related to the thyroid gland does not appear unusual in clinical series of infants born to mothers treated with propylthiouracil during pregnancy (Burrow, 1965; Talbert et al., 1970; Goluboff et al., 1974). No difference in intelligence test scores were found among 28 children born of propylthiouracil-treated pregnancies and 32 of their siblings who were born of pregnancies without such exposure (Burrow et al., 1978).

Maternal antithyroid treatment with imidazole derivatives during pregnancy has been associated with congenital scalp defects (cutis aplasia) in the infants (Milham, 1985). No such defects were observed in 20 infants born to women treated with propylthiouracil late in pregnancy (Mujtaba & Burrow, 1975).

Maternal treatment with propylthiouracil has been used to provide transplacental therapy to fetuses with hyperthyroidism (Serup & Petersen, 1977; Serup, 1978; Bruinse et al., 1988).

Thyroid enlargement but no malformations were observed among the offspring of rabbits treated during pregnancy with propylthiouracil in a dose slightly greater than that used in humans (Krementz et al., 1957).

Key References

Becks GP, Burrow GN: Thyroid disease and pregnancy. Med Clin North Am 75(1):121-150, 1991. [R]

Bruinse HW, Vermeulen-Meiners C, Wit JM: Fetal treatment for thyrotoxicosis in non-thyrotoxic pregnant women. Fetal Ther 3:152-157, 1988. [C] & [R]

Burrow GN: Hyperthyroidism during pregnancy. N Engl J Med 298(3):150-153, 1978. [R]

Burrow GN: The management of thyrotoxicosis in pregnancy. N Engl J Med 313(9):562-565, 1985. [R]

Burrow GN: Neonatal goiter after maternal propylthiouracil therapy. J Clin Endocrinol Metab 25:403-408, 1965. [S]

Burrow GN, Klatskin EH, Genel M: Intellectual development in children whose mothers received propylthiouracil during pregnancy. Yale J Biol Med 51:151-156, 1978. [E]

Cheron RG, Kaplan MM, Larsen PR, et al.: Neonatal thyroid function after propylthiouracil therapy for maternal Graves' disease. N Engl J Med 304(9):525-528, 1981. [S]

Davis LE, Lucas MJ, Hankins GDV, et al.: Thyrotoxicosis complicating pregnancy. Am J Obstet Gynecol 160(1):63-70, 1989. [E]

Goluboff LG, Sisson JC, Hamburger JI: Hyperthyroidism associated with pregnancy. Obstet Gynecol 44(1):107-116, 1974. [S]

Hayek A, Brooks M: Neonatal hyperthyroidism following intrauterine hypothyroidism. J Pediatr 87(3):446-448, 1975. [C]

Krementz ET, Hooper RG, Kempson RL: The effect on the rabbit fetus of the maternal administration of propylthiouracil. Surgery 41(4):619-631, 1957. [A]

Milham, Jr S: Scalp defects in infants of mothers treated for hyperthyroidism with methimazole and carbimazole during pregnancy. Teratology 32:321, 1985. [O]

Momotani N, Ito K: Treatment of pregnant patients with Basedow's Disease. Exp Clin Endocrinol 97(2/3):268-274, 1991. [E]

Mujtaba Q, Burrow GN: Treatment of hyperthyroidism in pregnancy with propylthiouracil and methimazole. Obstet Gynecol 46:282-286, 1975. [S]

Seligman B, Pescovitz H: Suffocative goiter in newborn infant. NY State J Med 50:1845-1847, 1950. [C]

Serup J: Maternal propylthiouracil to manage fetal hyperthyroidism. Lancet 2:896, 1978. [C]

Serup J, Petersen S: Hyperthyroidism during pregnancy treated with propylthiouracil. Acta Obstet Gynecol Scand 56:463-466, 1977. [C]

Solomon DH: Pregnancy and PTU. N Engl J Med 304(9):538-539, 1981. [O]

Talbert LM, Thomas Jr CG, Holt WA, Rankin P: Hyperthyroidism during pregnancy. Obstet Gynecol 36(5):779-785, 1970. [S]

PROSCILLARIDIN

Synonyms

Caradrin, Proscillan, Stellarid

Summary

Proscillaridin is a cardiac glycoside. It is used to treat heart failure.

Magnitude of Teratogenic Risk

Undetermined

Quality and Quantity of Data

None

Comment

None

No epidemiological studies of congenital anomalies in infants whose mothers took proscillaridin during pregnancy have been reported.

No animal teratology studies of proscillaridin have been published.

Please see agent summary on digoxin for information on a related agent that has been studied.

Key References

None available.

PROTIRELIN

Synonyms

Antepan, Lopremone, Relefact TRH, Thypinone, Thyrefact, TRH-Roche

Summary

Protirelin is the hypothalamic tripeptide hormone that promotes release of thyroid-stimulating hormone from the anterior pituitary. Protirelin is administered intravenously as a diagnostic test of pituitary and thyroid function. Maternal treatment with protirelin in combination with glucocorticoids has been used in early premature labor to reduce morbidity associated with neonatal respiratory distress syndrome (Ballard et al., 1992).

Magnitude of Teratogenic Risk

Undetermined

Quality and Quantity of Data

None To Poor

Comment

A small risk cannot be excluded, but a high risk of congenital anomalies in the children of women tested or treated with protirelin during pregnancy is unlikely.

No epidemiological studies of congenital anomalies among infants born to women who had been given protirelin during pregnancy have been reported.

The frequency of malformations was no greater than expected among the offspring of mice or rats treated repeatedly during pregnancy with protirelin in doses 30-3000 or 20-2000 times those used in humans (Asano et al., 1974).

Transient alterations of somatosensory evoked potentials have been observed among premature infants born to mothers who had been treated before delivery with betamethasone and protirelin to induce fetal pulmonary maturation (de Zegher et al., 1992). Increased activity of the fetal pituitary-thyroid axis and alterations of fetal heart rate have been noted in pregnant women treated with protirelin in the second or third trimester (Moya et al., 1991; Thorpe-Beeston et al., 1991; Gyselaers et al., 1992).

Key References

Asano Y, Fumio A, Higaki K: The effects of administration of synthetic thyrotropin-releasing-hormone (TRH) on mouse and rat fetuses. Oyo Yakuri 8:807-816, 1974. [A]

Ballard RA, Ballard PL, Creasy RK, et al.: Respiratory disease in very-low-birthweight infants after prenatal thyrotropin-releasing hormone and glucocorticoid. Lancet 339:510-515, 1992. [E]

de Zegher F, de Vries L, Pierrat V, et al.: Effect of prenatal betamethasone/thyrotropin releasing hormone treatment on somatosensory evoked potentials in preterm newborns. Pediatr Res 32:212-214, 1992. [E]

Gyselaers W, Spitz B, de Zegher F, et al.: Effects of thyrotropin-releasing hormone on fetal heart rate. Lancet 339:1417, 1992. [E]

Moya F, Mena P, Foradori A, et al.: Effect of maternal administration of thyrotropin releasing hormone on the preterm fetal pituitary-thyroid axis. J Pediatr 119:966-971, 1991. [E]

Thorpe-Beeston JG, Nicolaides KH, Snijders RJM, et al.: Fetal thyroid-stimulating hormone response to maternal administration of thyrotropin-releasing hormone. Am J Obstet Gynecol 164:1244-1245, 1991. [E]

PROTRIPTYLINE

Synonyms

Amimetilina, Concordin, Maximed, Triptil, Vivactil

Summary

Protriptyline is a tricyclic antidepressant that is administered orally.

Magnitude of Teratogenic Risk

Undetermined

Quality and Quantity of Data

None

Comment

A small risk cannot be excluded, but a high risk of congenital anomalies in the children of women treated with protriptyline during pregnancy is unlikely.

No epidemiological studies of congenital anomalies among the infants of women treated with protriptyline during pregnancy have been reported.

No teratological studies of protriptyline in experimental animals have been published.

Please see agent summary on amitriptyline for information on a related agent that has been studied.

Key References

None available.

PSEUDOEPHEDRINE

Synonyms

Afrinol, Dorcol Decongestant, Novafed, Pediacare, Robidrine, Sudafed

Summary

Pseudoephedrine is a sympathomimetic agent which is widely used as a nasal and bronchial decongestant, often in combination with other drugs.

Magnitude of Teratogenic Risk

None To Minimal

Quality and Quantity of Data

Fair

Comment

None

The frequency of malformations was no higher than expected among the offspring of 902 women who took pseudoephedrine during the first trimester of pregnancy in two cohorts of the Boston Collaborative Drug Surveillance Program (Jick et al., 1981; Aselton et al., 1985). Similarly, the risk of congenital anomalies was not increased among children born to 39 women who took pseudoephedrine during the first trimester of gestation or to 194 women who took the drug anytime during pregnancy in the Collaborative Perinatal Project (Heinonen et al., 1977). An association with maternal use of pseudoephedrine during the first trimester of pregnancy (RR=3.2, 95% confidence interval = 1.3-7.7) was observed in a case-control study of 76 children with gastroschisis (Werler et al., 1992b). No association was seen with such exposure in 416 infants with other congenital anomalies of possible vascular etiology. The authors concluded that the positive association of gastroschisis with maternal use of pseudoephedrine should be considered tentative until independent confirmation is obtained. The prevalence of gastroschisis in the general population is rare, affecting 1/10,000 live-births (Werler et al., 1992a).

No animal teratology studies of pseudoephedrine have been published.

Key References

Aselton P, Jick H, Milunsky A, Hunter JR, et al.: First-trimester drug use and congenital disorders. Obstet Gynecol 65:451-455, 1985. [S]

Heinonen OP, Slone D, Shapiro S: Birth Defects and Drugs in Pregnancy. Littleton, Mass.: John Wright-PSG, 1977, pp 346-347, 439. [E]

Jick H, Holmes LB, Hunter JR, Madsen S, et al.: First-trimester drug use and congenital disorders. JAMA 246:343-346, 1981. [S]

Werler MM, Mitchell AA, Shapiro S: Demographic, reproductive, medical, and environmental factors in relation to gastroschisis. Teratology 45:353-360, 1992a. [E]

Werler MM, Mitchell AA, Shapiro S: First trimester maternal medication use in relation to gastroschisis. Teratology 45:361-367, 1992b. [E]

PSILOCYBINE

Synonyms

Agaricacceae, Conocybe, Magic Mushrooms

Summary

Psilocybine is a naturally occurring hallucinogenic alkaloid found in several species of mushrooms. Psilocybine is used as a "recreational drug."

Magnitude of Teratogenic Risk

Undetermined

Quality and Quantity of Data

None

Comment

None

No epidemiological studies of malformations in infants born to mothers who used psilocybine during pregnancy have been reported.

No animal teratology studies of psilocybine have been published.

Key References

None available.

PSYLLIUM

Synonyms

Effersyllium, Fiberall, Hydrocil Instant, Indian Plantago Seed, Konsyl, Metamucil, Modane Bulk, Naturacil, Perdiem Plain Granules, Plantago Seed, Siblin, Syllact

Summary

Psyllium is a dietary fiber obtained from the husks of Plantago seeds. It is used as a bulk laxative.

Magnitude of Teratogenic Risk

None

Quality and Quantity of Data

Poor To Fair

Comment

None

The Boston Collaborative Drug Surveillance Program included more than 100 women who took psyllium during the first trimester of pregnancy (Jick et al., 1981). The frequency of malformations among the infants born to these women was no greater than expected.

No animal teratology studies of psyllium have been published.

Key References

Jick H, Holmes LB, Hunter JR, Madsen S, et al.: First-trimester drug use and congenital disorders. JAMA 246:343-346, 1981. [S]

PYRANTEL

Synonyms

Anthel, Antiminth, Combantrin, Nemocid, Pirantel, Vermisan

Summary

Pyrantel is an antihelmintic that is given orally to treat intestinal nematodes. Pyrantel is poorly absorbed from the gastrointestinal tract.

Magnitude of Teratogenic Risk

Undetermined

Quality and Quantity of Data

None To Poor

Comment

A small risk cannot be excluded, but a substantial risk of congenital anomalies in the children of women treated with pyrantel during pregnancy is unlikely.

No epidemiological studies of congenital anomalies among infants born to women treated with pyrantel during pregnancy have been reported.

The frequency of congenital anomalies was no greater than expected among the offspring of rabbits treated during pregnancy with 5-50 times the maximum human therapeutic dose of pyrantel (Owaki et al., 1971). No teratogenic effect was observed among the offspring of dogs treated during pregnancy with pyrantel in a dose similar to that used in humans (Clark et al., 1992).

Key References

Clark JN, Pulliam JD, Daurio CP: Safety study of a beef-based chewable tablet formulation of ivermectin and pyrantel pamoate in growing dogs, pups, and breeding adult dogs. Am J Vet Res 53(4):608-612, 1992. [A]

Owaki Y, Sakai T, Momiyama H: Teratological studies on pyrantel pamoate in rabbits. Oyo Yakuri 5:33-39, 1971. [A]

PYRAZINAMIDE

Synonyms

Isopas, Pyrazine Carboxylamide, Pyrazinoic Acid Amide, Rozide, Tebrazid, Zinamide

Summary

Pyrazinamide is used orally to treat tuberculosis.

Magnitude of Teratogenic Risk

Undetermined

Quality and Quantity of Data

None

Comment

None

No epidemiological studies of congenital anomalies among infants born to women treated with pyrazinamide during pregnancy have been reported.

No animal teratology studies of pyrazinamide have been published.

Key References

None available.

PYRETHRINS

Synonyms

Insect Powder, Pyrethrum

Summary

Pyrethrins are a group of insecticidal esters obtained from flowers of the genus Chrysanthemum. Pyrethrins are widely used in domestic and agricultural insecticide sprays and dusting powders. Pyrethrins have also been used topically in the treatment of pediculosis. The Threshold Limit Value for occupational exposure as a time-weighted average is 5 mg/cu m of air (ACGIH, 1990).

Magnitude of Teratogenic Risk

Undetermined

Quality and Quantity of Data

None To Poor

Comment

None

No epidemiological studies of congenital anomalies among the children of women exposed to pyrethrins during pregnancy have been reported.

Dose-related increases in the frequencies of fetal resorptions and skeletal anomalies were observed among pregnant rats fed 50-150 mg/kg/d of pyrethrins (Khera et al., 1982). The relevance of this observation to the risks associated with human exposure to pyrethrins during pregnancy is unknown.

Key References

ACGIH: 1990-1991 Threshold Limit Values For Chemical Substances and Physical Agents and Biological Exposure Indices. Cincinnati, Ohio: Am Conference Govt Ind Hyg, 1990. [O]

Khera KS, Whalen C, Angers G: Teratogenicity study on pyrethrum and rotenone (natural origin) and ronnel in pregnant rats. J Toxicol Environ Health 10:111-119, 1982. [A]

PYRIDOSTIGMINE

Synonyms

Mestinon, Regonol

Summary

Pyridostigmine is a cholinesterase inhibitor used to treat myasthenia gravis, paralytic ileus, and post-operative urinary retention.

Magnitude of Teratogenic Risk

Undetermined

Quality and Quantity of Data

None To Poor

Comment

None

No epidemiological studies of congenital anomalies in infants born to women who took pyridostigmine during pregnancy have been reported.

The frequency of malformations was not increased among the offspring of rats treated during pregnancy with various doses of pyridostigmine in a range similar to that used in humans (Levine and Parker, 1991). At the highest dose, which produced maternal toxicity, increased rates of embryonic death and delayed fetal skeletal ossification were seen.

Key References

Levine BS, Parker RM: Reproductive and developmental toxicity studies of pyridostigmine bromide in rats. Toxicology 69:291-300, 1991. [A]

PYRIDOXINE

Synonyms

Adermine Hydrochloride, Beesix, Benadon, Hexa-Betalin, Hexabione Hydrochloride, Paxadon, Piridossina Cloridrato, Pyridoxinium Chloride, Rodex, Vitamin B_6

Summary

Pyridoxine, vitamin B_6, is an essential nutrient which serves as an enzyme co-factor in intermediary metabolism. The dietary requirement for pyridoxine appears to be greater in pregnant women than in non-pregnant individuals (Schuster et al., 1984). The U.S. Recommended Dietary Allowance of pyridoxine in pregnancy is 2.2 mg/d.

Magnitude of Teratogenic Risk

None

Quality and Quantity of Data

Fair

Comment

This assessment refers to very high doses (hundreds of milligrams per day) of pyridoxine. Pyridoxine in small doses is a necessary dietary component.

No epidemiological studies of congenital anomalies among children born to women who used large ("megavitamin") doses of pyridoxine during pregnancy have been reported.

The frequency of malformations was not increased among the offspring of rats treated during pregnancy with pyridoxine in doses of 20-800 mg/kg/d (up to 100 times larger than those used in human megavitamin therapy) (Khera, 1975; Marathe & Thomas, 1986).

Please see agent summary for bendectin, an agent which contains pyridoxine in combination with other drugs.

Key References

Khera KS: Teratogenicity study in rats given high doses of pyridoxine (vitamin B6) during organogenesis. Experientia 31:469-470, 1975. [A]

Marathe MR, Thomas GP: Absence of teratogenicity of pyridoxine in Wistar rats. Indian J Physiol Pharmacol 30:264-266, 1986. [A]

Schuster K, Bailey LB, Mahan CS: Effect of maternal pyridoxine HCL supplementation on the vitamin B-6 status of mother and infant and on pregnancy outcome. J Nutr 114:977-988, 1984. [S]

PYRILAMINE

Synonyms

Allergon, Anthisan, Fluidasa, Mepyramine, Pymal

Summary

Pyrilamine is an antihistamine of the ethylenediamine class. It is used to treat allergic symptoms and as an antinauseant.

Magnitude of Teratogenic Risk

None

Quality and Quantity of Data

Poor To Fair

Comment

None

The frequency of congenital anomalies was no greater than expected among the children of 121 women treated with pyrilamine during the first four lunar months of pregnancy or the children of 392 women treated with the drug anytime during pregnancy in the Collaborative Perinatal Project (Heinonen et al., 1977).

An increased frequency of embryonic, fetal, or perinatal death was observed among the offspring of mice and rats treated with pyrilamine, during pregnancy, in doses 10-20 times those used in humans (Naranjo & de Naranjo, 1968; Bovet-Nitti et al., 1963). In mice, no such effect was seen after maternal treatment with 1-2 times the usual human dose.

Key References

Bovet-Nitti, Mignami G, Bovet D: Antihistamine drugs on rat pregnancy: Effects of pyrilamine and meclizine. Life Sci 5:303-310, 1963. [A]

Heinonen OP, Slone D, Shapiro S: Birth Defects and Drugs in Pregnancy. Littleton, Mass.: John Wright-PSG, 1977, pp 437, 489. [E]

Naranjo P, de Naranjo E: Embryotoxic effects of antihistamines. Arzneimittelforsch 18:188-195, 1968. [A]

PYRIMETHAMINE

Synonyms

Chloridin, Daraprim, Erbaprelina, Ethylpyrimidine, Fansidar Injection, Fansimef, Maloprim Tablets, Pirimetamina, Tindurin

Summary

Pyrimethamine is a folic acid antagonist used to treat malaria and toxoplasmosis.

Magnitude of Teratogenic Risk

Minimal

Quality and Quantity of Data

Poor To Fair

Comment

Two other folic acid antagonists (methotrexate and aminopterin) are recognized human teratogens. Please see summaries on these agents for more information.

No controlled epidemiological studies of congenital anomalies in children born to women treated with pyrimethamine during pregnancy have been reported. The frequency of malformations did not appear to be unusually great among 64 infants born to women treated with pyrimethamine in the first trimester of pregnancy in one clinical series (Hengst, 1972).

The frequency of congenital anomalies was increased among the offspring of rats treated with 1-25 times the usual human dose of pyrimethamine during pregnancy (Dyban et al., 1965; Sullivan & Takacs, 1971; Horvath et al., 1989; Hayama et al., 1991). Cleft palate, other craniofacial defects, limb anomalies, and neural tube defects were seen most often. Increased frequencies of malformations have also been observed among the offspring of mice, rabbits, and minipigs treated with pyrimethamine during pregnancy in doses, respectively, 9, 20, and 2 times those used clinically (Schvartsman, 1979; Hayama & Kokue, 1985). No teratogenic effect was seen in minipigs with smaller doses or in hamsters with doses 80 times those used in humans (Sullivan & Takacs, 1971). The relevance of these observations to the therapeutic use of pyrimethamine in human pregnancy is unknown.

Key References

Dyban AP, Akimova IM, Svetlova VA: Effect of 2,4-diamino-5-chlorophenyl-6-ethylpyrimidine on the embryonic development of rats. Doklady Biological Sciences (English Translation) 163:455-458, 1965. [A]

Hayama T, Kokue E: Use of the Goettingen Miniature Pig for studying pyrimethamine teratogenesis. CRC Crit Rev Toxicol 14:403-421, 1985. [A]

Hayama T, Tsunematsu K, Shimoda M, Kokue E: Oral folic acid potentiates pyrimethamine teratogenesis in rat. Acta Vet Scand Suppl 87:340-341, 1991. [A]

Hengst VP: [Investigations of the teratogenicity of daraprim (pyrimethamine) in humans.] Zentralbl Gynakol 94:551-555, 1972. [S]

Horvath C, Tangapregassom AM, Tangapregassom MJ, et al.: Pathogenesis of limb and facial malformations induced by pyrimethamine in the rat. Acta Morphol Hung 36(1-2):53-61, 1989. [A]

Schvartsman S: Teratogenicity of pyrimethamine. Toxicol Appl Pharmacol 48:A123, 1979. [A]

Sullivan GE, Takacs E: Comparative teratogenicity of pyrimethamine in rats and hamsters. Teratology 4:205-209, 1971. [A]

PYRITHIONE

Synonyms

Zincon Shampoo

Summary

Pyrithione is an antifungal and antibacterial agent used in antidandruff shampoos. It is poorly absorbed from the skin.

Magnitude of Teratogenic Risk

None

Quality and Quantity of Data

Poor

Comment

None

No epidemiological studies of congenital anomalies in infants born to women who used pyrithione during pregnancy have been reported.

No teratogenic effect was observed among the offspring of pigs, rats, and rabbits treated topically during pregnancy with pyrithione in doses several to hundreds of times greater than the usual human exposure during shampooing (Wedig et al., 1976; Nolen & Dierkman, 1979; Nolen, 1984). Maternal toxicity and fetal growth retardation occurred after oral administration of this agent to rats or rabbits during pregnancy in doses 2-5 or 1.5-3 times those used in shampooing in humans (Nolen & Dierkman, 1979).

Key References

Nolen GA: Reproduction and teratology studies of topically applied materials: Zinc pyrithione. In: Drill VA, Lazar P (ed)s. Cutaneous Toxicity. New York: Raven Press, 1984, pp 109-125. [A]

Nolen GA, Dierckman TA: Reproduction and teratology studies of zinc pyrithione administered orally or topically to rats and rabbits. Fd Cosmet Toxicol 17:639-649, 1979. [A]

Wedig JH, Kennedy GL, Jenkins DH, Henderson R, et al.: Teratologic evaluation of dermally applied zinc pyrithione on swine. Toxicol Appl Pharmacol 36:255-259, 1976. [A]

PYRROCAINE

Synonyms

EN 1010

Summary

Pyrrocaine is an injectable local anesthetic of the amide class that has been used in dentistry.

Magnitude of Teratogenic Risk

Undetermined

Quality and Quantity of Data

None

Comment

None

No epidemiological studies of congenital anomalies in children born to women exposed to pyrrocaine during pregnancy have been reported.

No investigations of teratologic effects of pyrrocaine in experimental animals have been published.

Please see agent summary on lidocaine for information on a related agent that has been studied.

Key References

None available.

PYRROLNITRIN

Synonyms

Micutrin, Pirrolnitrina, Pyroace

Summary

Pyrrolnitrin is an antifungal antibiotic. It is used in topical preparations from which it is poorly absorbed.

Magnitude of Teratogenic Risk

Undetermined

Quality and Quantity of Data

None To Poor

Comment

A small risk cannot be excluded, but a high risk of congenital anomalies in the children of women treated with pyrrolnitrin during pregnancy is unlikely.

No epidemiological studies of congenital anomalies among infants born to women treated with pyrrolnitrin during pregnancy have been reported.

No teratogenic effect was observed among the offspring of mice or rats given 3-30 mg/kg/d of pyrrolnitrin subcutaneously during pregnancy (Nishida et al., 1965). Although this dose is many times that used in humans, absorption from the subcutaneous site seemed to be poor.

Key References

Nishida M, Matsubara T, Watanabe N: Pyrrolnitrin, a new antifungal antibiotic. J Antiobiotics 18:211-219, 1965. [A]

QUAZEPAM

Synonyms

Doral

Summary

Quazepam is a benzodiazepine used orally as a hypnotic agent.

Magnitude of Teratogenic Risk

Undetermined

Quality and Quantity of Data

None To Poor

Comment

A small risk cannot be excluded, but a high risk of congenital anomalies in the children of women treated with quazepam during pregnancy is unlikely.

No epidemiological studies of congenital anomalies among infants born to women treated with quazepam during pregnancy have been reported.

The frequency of malformations was not increased among the offspring of mice or rabbits treated during pregnancy with quazepam in doses respectively 10-400 or 33-133 times those used in humans (Black et al., 1987). Fetal growth retardation was seen in the rabbits and delayed skeletal maturation in the mice at the higher doses.

Please see agent summary on diazepam for information on a related agent that has been more thoroughly studied.

Key References

Black HE, Szot RJ, Arthaud LE, et al.: Preclinical safety evaluation of the benzodiazepine quazepam. Arzneimittelforsch 37(8):906-913, 1987. [A]

QUAZINONE

Summary

Quazinone is a cardiotonic agent.

Magnitude of Teratogenic Risk

Undetermined

Quality and Quantity of Data

None

Comment

None

No epidemiological studies of congenital anomalies in infants born to women who used quazinone during pregnancy have been reported.

No animal teratology studies of quazinone have been published.

Key References

None available.

QUAZODINE

Summary

Quazodine is a bronchodilator and cardiotonic agent.

Magnitude of Teratogenic Risk

Undetermined

Quality and Quantity of Data

None

Comment

None

No epidemiological studies of congenital anomalies in infants born to women who used quazodine during pregnancy have been reported.

No animal teratology studies of quazodine have been published.

Key References

None available.

QUINACRINE

Synonyms

Acrichinum, Acrinamine, Antimalarinae Chlorhydras, Atabrine Hydrochloride, Chinacrina, Mepacrine, Mepacrini Hydrochloridum

Summary

Quinacrine is an anthelmintic and antiprotozoal agent.

Magnitude of Teratogenic Risk

Undetermined

Quality and Quantity of Data

None To Poor

Comment

None

No epidemiological studies of congenital anomalies among infants born to women treated with quinacrine during pregnancy have been reported.

Fetal deaths were increased but no malformations were observed among the offspring of rats treated during pregnancy with about 7 times the usual human dose of quinacrine (Rothschild & Levy, 1950). A dose-dependent increase in fetal death but no increase in the frequency of fetal malformations was observed after intrauterine instillation of 0.4-4.0 mg of quinacrine during pregnancy in the rat (Blake et al., 1983). Fetal death was also observed after intrauterine instillation of 3 mg of quinacrine in three pregnant cynomolgus monkeys (Blake et al., 1983).

Please see agent summary on chloroquine for information on a related agent that has been more thoroughly studied.

Key References

Blake DA, Dubin NH, DiBlasi MC, et al.: Teratologic and mutagenic studies with intrauterine quinacrine hydrochloride. In: Female Transcervical Steril Proc Int Workshop Non-Surg Methods Female Occlusion, 1983, 71-88. [A]

Rothschild B, Levy G: Action de la quinacrine sur la gestation chez le rat. C R Soc Biol 144:1350-1352, 1950. [A]

QUINESTROL

Synonyms

Estrovis, Estrovister, Plestrovis

Summary

Quinestrol is an estrogen that is administered orally to treat atrophic vaginitis or vulvar dystrophy, ovariectomy, primary ovarian failure, and menopausal symptoms.

Magnitude of Teratogenic Risk

Undetermined

Quality and Quantity of Data

None

Comment

Although the risk of this agent is undetermined, it may be substantial because it is an estrogen.

No epidemiological studies of congenital anomalies in infants whose mothers were treated with quinestrol during pregnancy have been reported.

No animal teratology studies of quinestrol have been published.

Please see agent summary on diethylstilbestrol for information on a related agent that has been more thoroughly studied.

Key References

None available.

QUINETHAZONE

Synonyms

Aquamox, Chinetazone, Chinethazone, Hydromox, Idrokin, Quinetazona

Summary

Quinethazone is a diuretic that is administered orally in the treatment of edema and hypertension.

Magnitude of Teratogenic Risk

Undetermined

Quality and Quantity of Data

None To Poor

Comment

None

No congenital anomalies were observed in the infants of eight mothers who were treated with quinethazone during the first four lunar months of pregnancy in the Collaborative Perinatal Project (Heinonen et al., 1977).

No animal teratology studies of quinethazone have been published.

Key References

Heinonen OP, Slone D, Shapiro S: Birth Defects and Drugs in Pregnancy. Littleton, Mass.: John Wright-PSG, 1977, p 372. [E]

QUINIDINE

Synonyms

Cardioquin, Cin-Quin, Duraquin, Quinaglute, Quinate, Quinidex, Quinora

Summary

Quinidine is a drug used to prevent and treat cardiac arrhythmias.

Magnitude of Teratogenic Risk

Undetermined

Quality and Quantity of Data

None

Comment

None

No epidemiological studies of congenital anomalies in infants born to women who used quinidine during pregnancy have been reported.

No animal teratology studies of quinidine have been published.

Administration of quinine to the mother has been used successfully to treat fetal supraventricular tachycardia in the late second and third trimesters of pregnancy (Spinnato et al., 1984; Guntheroth et al., 1985).

Key References

Guntheroth WG, Cyr DR, Mack LA, et al.: Hydrops from reciprocating atrioventricular tachycardia in a 27-week fetus requiring quinidine for conversion. Obstet Gynecol 66:29S-33S, 1985. [C]

Spinnato JA, Shaver DC, Flinn GS, Sibai BM, et al.: Fetal supraventricular tachycardia: In utero therapy with digoxin and quinidine. Obstet Gynecol 64:730-735, 1984. [C]

QUININE

Synonyms

Legatrin, Quin-Amino, Quinaminoph, Quindan, Quine, Quiphile

Summary

Quinine is a cinchona alkaloid that is administered in small doses (300-500 mg per day) to treat night leg cramps and in large doses (about 2000 mg per day) to treat malaria. Quinine has sometimes been taken illicitly in large doses to induce abortion. The drug is used as a cold remedy, to "cut" narcotics, and, in very small amounts, as a flavoring agent. It is also contained in some shampoos and hair lotions.

Magnitude of Teratogenic Risk

Large Doses Taken To Induce Abortion: Moderate

Low Therapeutic Doses: Minimal

Quality and Quantity of Data

Large Doses Taken To Induce Abortion: Fair To Good

Low Therapeutic Doses: Poor

Comment

The magnitude of risk with large doses of quinine is primarily for deafness

The frequency of congenital anomalies was not increased among the infants of 104 women who took quinine during the first four lunar months of pregnancy in the Collaborative Perinatal Project (Heinonen et al., 1977). Although this study does not provide information regarding the dosage used, it is likely to be less than that employed in the treatment of malaria or in attempted induction of abortion. This distinction is important because the risk is probably greater with higher doses.

Dannenberg et al. (1983) have summarized 70 published cases in which quinine was taken by pregnant women in an attempt to induce abortion. Maternal toxicity occurred in many of these instances, and at least 11 women died. More than 40 of the infants had congenital anomalies. Ascertainment of these patients is clearly biased, and it is likely that some of these anomalies were not due to the maternal ingestion of quinine. However, 18 of the children had deafness, and ototoxicity is a known complication of quinine therapy in adults. Taylor (1937) reported four deaf children whose mothers had taken large doses of quinine at various times during pregnancy and who had themselves developed deafness during treatment. These observations suggest that fetal ototoxicity may occur with high-dose maternal quinine ingestion during pregnancy, although the frequency of this complication is unknown.

Major malformations reported anecdotally among infants born to women who took large doses of quinine during the first trimester of pregnancy, often in an attempt to induce abortion, include central nervous system anomalies (especially hydrocephalus), limb defects, cardiac defects, and gastrointestinal tract anomalies (Nishimura & Tanimura, 1976). No characteristic pattern of anomalies has been identified, and the relationship of these malformations to the maternal quinine therapy remains uncertain.

Hemolysis in G6PD deficient males and thrombocytopenic purpura are rare complications of quinine therapy in adults. Similar effects in neonates have been attributed to placental transmission of quinine after maternal treatment late in pregnancy (Mauer et al., 1957; Glass et al., 1973).

Although teratology studies of quinine have been reported in several animal species, most of these investigations were not conducted according to currently accepted standards (Tanimura, 1972). Fetal death has been observed in pregnant rabbits, chinchillas, and mice treated with quinine in doses well above those used therapeutically in humans. The frequency of malformations was not increased among the offspring of pregnant rats treated with 1-5 times the human antimalarial dose of quinine despite the occurrence of maternal toxicity at the highest dose (Colley et al., 1989). Central nervous system malformations have been observed among the offspring of rabbits and chinchillas treated with very large doses of quinine during pregnancy (Belkina, 1958; Klosovskii, 1963), and auditory nerve and cochlear abnormalities have been reported in fetal rabbits and guinea pigs after similar treatment (Covell, 1936; West, 1938; Mosher, 1938). No malformations were found in a series of six macaque fetuses after maternal treatment with quinine in doses equivalent to 0.5-5 times the dose used to treat malaria in humans (Tanimura, 1972).

Key References

Belkina AP: Effect of quinine administered to pregnant rabbits on the development of the fetal brain. Arkh Patol 20:64-69, 1958. [A]

Colley JC, Edwards JA, Heywood R, Purser D: Toxicity studies with quinine hydrochloride. Toxicology 54:219-226, 1989. [A]

Covell WP: A cytological study of the effects of drugs on the cochlea. Arch Otolaryngol 23:633-641, 1936. [A]

Dannenberg AL, Dorfman SF, Johnson J: Use of quinine for self-induced abortion. Southern Medical J 76:846-849, 1983. [C]

Glass L, Rajegowda BK, Bowen E; Evans H.: Exposure to quinine and jaundice in a glucose-6-phosphate dehydrogenase-deficient newborn infant. J Pediatr 82:734-735, 1973. [C]

Heinonen OP, Slone D, Shapiro: Birth Defects and Drugs in Pregnancy. Littleton: Mass.: John Wright-PSG, 1977, pp 229, 302, 333. [E]

Klosovskii BN: The Development of the Brain and Its Disturbance by Harmful Factors. New York: Macmillan Co., 1963. [A]

Mauer AM, DeVaux W, Lahey ME: Neonatal and maternal thrombocytopenic purpura due to quinine. Pediatrics 19:84-87, 1957. [C]

Mosher HP: Does animal experimentation show similar changes in the ear of mother and fetus after the ingestion of quinine by the mother? Laryngoscope 48:361-395, 1938. [A]

Nishimura H, Tanimura T: Clinical Aspects of the Teratogenicity of Drugs. New York: Excerpta Medica, American Elsevier Publishing Co., pp 140-143, 1976. [C]

Tanimura T: Effects on macaque embryos of drugs reported or suspected to be teratogenic to humans. Acta Endocrinol 71(Suppl 166):293-308, 1972. [A]

Taylor HM: Prenatal medication and its relation to the fetal ear. Surg Gynecol Obstet 64:542-546, 1937. [C]

West RA: Effect of quinine upon auditory nerve. Am J Obstet Gynecol 36:241-248, 1938. [A]

RABIES ANTISERUM

Summary

Rabies antiserum contains antibodies to rabies obtained from the blood of an animal immunized with rabies vaccine. Rabies antiserum is administered parenterally in conjunction with vaccine to prevent rabies in exposed persons.

Magnitude of Teratogenic Risk

Undetermined

Quality and Quantity of Data

None

Comment

None

No epidemiological studies of congenital anomalies in infants whose mothers were given rabies antiserum during pregnancy have been reported.

No animal teratology studies of rabies antiserum have been published.

Key References

None available.

RABIES IMMUNE GLOBULIN

Synonyms

Hyperab, Imogam, RIG

Summary

Rabies immune globulin is a passive immunizing agent derived from the blood of human donors hyperimmunized with rabies vaccine. It is administered intramuscularly, in conjunction with rabies vaccine, to prevent the development of rabies in exposed individuals.

Magnitude of Teratogenic Risk

Undetermined

Quality and Quantity of Data

None

Comment

A small risk cannot be excluded, but a high risk of congenital anomalies in the children of women treated with rabies immune globulin during pregnancy is unlikely.

No epidemiological studies of congenital anomalies in infants whose mothers were immunized with rabies immune globulin during pregnancy have been reported.

No animal teratology studies of rabies immune globulin have been published.

Key References

None available.

RADON

Summary

Radon is a chemically inert but radioactive gas that is often found in uranium mines and caves. Radon contributes substantially to natural (background) radiation.

Magnitude of Teratogenic Risk

Undetermined

Quality and Quantity of Data

None

Comment

1)   A small risk cannot be excluded, but a substantial risk of congenital anomalies in the children of women with usual exposures to radon during pregnancy is unlikely.

2)   Natural levels of radiation produced by usual exposures to radon, even on a protracted basis, are far below those associated with a measurably increased risk of teratogenic or genetic damage.

3)   Because radon is chemically inert, any teratogenic effects related to this gas would be expected to be related to the radiation that it produces.

No epidemiological studies of congenital anomalies among infants born to women exposed to high concentrations of radon during pregnancy have been reported.

No animal teratology studies of radon have been published.

Key References

None available.

RANITIDINE

Synonyms

Zantac

Summary

Ranitidine is a histamine H2-receptor antagonist used to reduce gastric acidity.

Magnitude of Teratogenic Risk

Undetermined

Quality and Quantity of Data

Poor

Comment

None

No epidemiological studies of congenital anomalies in infants born to women treated with ranitidine during pregnancy have been published.

The frequency of malformations was not increased among the offspring of pregnant rats or rabbits treated with ranitidine in doses, respectively, 8-130 or 4-70 times those used clinically (Higashida et al., 1983; Tamura et al., 1983).

Key References

Higashida N, Kamada S, Sakanoue M, Takeuchi M, et al.: Teratogenicity study on ranitidine hydrochloride in rats. J Toxicol Sci 8(Suppl I):101-122, 1983. [A]

Tamura J, Sato N, Ezaki H, Yokoyama S: Teratological study on ranitidine hydrochloride in rabbits. J Toxicol Sci 8:141-150, 1983. [A]

RESCINNAMINE

Synonyms

Anaprel, Cartric, Moderil

Summary

Rescinnamine is an alkaloid related to reserpine. Rescinnamine is given orally in the treatment of hypertension.

Magnitude of Teratogenic Risk

Undetermined

Quality and Quantity of Data

None

Comment

None

No epidemiological studies of congenital anomalies in infants born to women who were treated with rescinnamine during pregnancy have been reported.

No animal teratology studies of rescinnamine have been published.

Key References

None available.

RESERPINE

Synonyms

Serpalan, Serpasil

Summary

Reserpine is a Rauwolfia alkaloid with central nervous system depressant action. It is used as an antihypertensive agent.

Magnitude of Teratogenic Risk

None To Minimal

Quality and Quantity of Data

Fair

Comment

Transient neonatal respiratory distress may occur in infants born to women treated with reserpine late in pregnancy.

The frequency of maternal reserpine use during pregnancy was no greater than expected among 6227 infants with various congenital anomalies in the Hungarian Case-Control Surveillance System (Czeizel, 1988). There was no association with maternal use of reserpine during pregnancy among the infants in 11 malformation subgroups in this study. No information was provided regarding when in pregnancy the maternal exposures occurred, but it seems likely that most were late in gestation.

The frequency of congenital anomalies was not significantly greater than expected among the children of 48 women treated with reserpine or Rauwolfia alkaloids during the first four lunar months of pregnancy or among 475 women treated with these agents anytime during pregnancy in the Collaborative Perinatal Project (Heinonen et al., 1977). The frequency of hydronephrosis and hydroureter appeared high among the children of women treated with reserpine or Rauwolfia alkaloids anytime in pregnancy, but the statistical and clinical significance of this observation is uncertain. If maternal reserpine therapy during pregnancy does increase the risk of congenital anomalies in the offspring, the magnitude of the increase appears to be small in comparison to the background risk that accompanies every pregnancy.

Increased frequencies of anophthalmia and other malformations were observed among the offspring of rats treated with reserpine in doses 80-200 times that used in humans (Goldman & Yakovac, 1965; Moriyama et al.,1978). Such doses were toxic to the mothers, and no teratogenic effect was observed at a nontoxic dose 10 times that used in human therapy.

Fetal death often occurs in pregnant rats treated with reserpine in doses 50 or more times greater than those used in humans (West, 1962; Buelke-Sam et al., 1984). In guinea pigs, fetal death occurred with increased frequency when pregnant animals were treated with reserpine in doses 0.5-10 or more times those used therapeutically in humans (Towell & Hyman, 1966; Deanesly, 1966). An increased frequency of death in early postnatal life has been observed among the offspring of rats treated with 10-150 times the usual human dose of reserpine during pregnancy (Werboff et al., 1961; Buelke-Sam et al., 1984; Harmon et al., 1987).

Some studies, but not others, have demonstrated long-lasting behavioral alterations among the offspring of rats treated with 10 or more times the usual human dose of reserpine during pregnancy (Werboff et al., 1961, Hoffeld & Webster 1965; Jewett & Norton, 1966; Murai, 1966; Hoffeld et al., 1967, 1968; Buelke-Sam et al., 1989). The relevance of these findings to the clinical use of reserpine in humans is unknown.

Maternal treatement with reserpine near term can produce transient nasal congestion, respiratory distress, and lethargy in newborn children (Budnick et al., 1955).

Key References

Budnick IS, Leikin S, Hoeck LE: Effect in the newborn infant of reserpine administered ante partum. Am J Dis Child 90:286-289, 1955. [C]

Buelke-Sam J, Ali SF, Kimmel GL, et al.: Postnatal function following prenatal reserpine exposure in rats: Neurobehavioral toxicity. Neurotoxicol Teratol 11:515-522, 1989. [A]

Buelke-Sam J, Kimmel GL, Webb PJ, et al.: Postnatal toxicity following prenatal reserpine exposure in rats: Effects of dose and dosing schedule. Fundam Appl Toxicol 4:983-991, 1984. [A]

Czeizel A: Reserpine is not a human teratogen. J Med Genet 25:787, 1988. [E]

Deanesly R: The effects of reserpine on ovulation and on the corpus luteum of the guinea-pig. J Reprod Fert 11:429-438, 1966. [A]

Goldman AS, Yakovac WC: Teratogenic action in rats of reserpine alone and in combination with salicylate and immobilization. Proc Soc Exp Biol Med 118:857-862, 1965. [A]

Harmon JR, Kimmel GL, Webb PJ, Delongchamp RR: Effect of prenatal reserpine exposure on development of the postnatal rat heart. Teratogenesis Carcinog Mutagen 7:347-355, 1987. [A]

Heinonen OP, Slone D, Shapiro S: Birth Defects and Drugs in Pregnancy. Littleton, Mass.: John Wright-PSG, 1977, pp 372-373, 441, 495. [E]

Hoffeld DR, McNew J, Webster RL: Effect of tranquillizing drugs during pregnancy on activity of offspring. Nature 218:357-358, 1968. [A]

Hoffeld DR, Webster RL: Effect of injection of tranquillizing drugs during pregnancy on offspring. Nature 205:1070-1072, 1965. [A]

Hoffeld DR, Webster RL, McNew J: Adverse effects on offspring of tranquillizing drugs during pregnancy. Nature 215:182-183, 1967. [A]

Jewett RE, Norton S: Effect of tranquilizing drugs on postnatal behavior. Exp Neurol 14:33-43, 1966. [A]

Moriyama I, Kanoh S: Effect of reserpine on the pregnant rat. Acta Obstet Gynaecol Jpn 30(2):161-166, 1978. [A]

Murai N: Effect of maternal medication during pregnancy upon behavioral development of offspring. Tohoku J Exp Med 89:265-272, 1966. [A]

Towell ME, Hyman AI: Catecholamine depletion in pregnancy. J Obstet Gynaecol Br Commonw 73:431-438, 1966. [A]

Werboff J, Gottlieb JS, Havlena J, Word TJ: Behavioral effects of prenatal drug administration in the white rat. Pediatrics 27:318-324, 1961. [A]

West GB: Drugs and rat pregnancy. J Pharm Pharmacol 14:828-830, 1962. [A]

RESORCINOL

Synonyms

M-Dihydroxybenzene, Resorcin

Summary

Resorcinol is an aromatic alcohol that is used topically in the treatment of dermatologic conditions such as acne, seborrhea, eczema, and psoriasis. Industrial uses of resorcinol occur in the manufacture of rubber products, dyes, explosives, adhesives and cosmetics. Resorcinol may be absorbed through the skin or lungs. The threshold limit value for occupational exposure is 10 ppm in air as a time-weighted average; the short-term exposure limit is 20 ppm (Hathaway et al., 1991).

Magnitude of Teratogenic Risk

None

Quality and Quantity of Data

Poor To Fair

Comment

None

The frequency of congenital anomalies was no greater than expected among the children of 118 women treated with resorcinol anytime during pregnancy in the Collaborative Perinatal Project (Heinonen et al., 1977). Only 18 of these patients were treated in the first four lunar months of gestation.

No teratogenic effect was observed among the offspring of pregnant rats or rabbits fed 40-500 or 25-100 mg/kg/d of resorcinol, respectively (DiNardo et al., 1985; Spengler et al., 1986).

Key References

DiNardo JC, Picciano JC, Schnetzinger RW, Morris WE, et al.: Teratological assessment of five oxidative hair dyes in the rat. Toxicol Appl Pharmacol 78:163-166, 1985. [A]

Hathaway GJ, Proctor NH, Hughes JP, Fischman ML (eds): Proctor and Hughes' Chemical Hazards of the Workplace, 3rd ed. New York: Van Nostrand Reinhold, 1991, pp 501-502. [R]

Heinonen OP, Slone D, Shapiro S: Birth Defects and Drugs in Pregnancy. Littleton, Mass.: John Wright-PSG, 1977, pp 410-411, 444, 499. [E]

Spengler J, Osterburg I, Korte R: Teratogenic evaluation of p-toluenediamine sulphate, resorcinol and p-aminophenol in rats and rabbits. Teratology 33:31A, 1986. [A]

RHO(D) IMMUNE GLOBULIN

Synonyms

Gamulin Rh, HypRho-D, MICRhoGAM, Mini-Gamulin, RhoGAM

Summary

Rho(D) immune globulin is a preparation of human immunoglobulin containing antibody to the major rhesus blood group antigen. Rho(D) immune globulin is administered by intramuscular injection to prevent the development of Rh isoimmunization.

Magnitude of Teratogenic Risk

Undetermined

Quality and Quantity of Data

None

Comment

A small risk cannot be excluded, but a high risk of congenital anomalies in the children of women treated with rho(d) immune globulin during pregnancy is unlikely.

No epidemiological studies of congenital anomalies among the infants of women treated with Rho(D) immune globulin during pregnancy have been reported. The frequency of Rh sensitization is reduced among Rh negative women treated with Rho(D) immune globulin during pregnancy (Thornton, 1989; Trolle, 1989; Bowman, 1991). The frequencies of fetal death, low birth weight, and prematurity do not appear to be substantially altered in treated pregnancies (Crane et al., 1984; Thornton et al., 1989)

No animal teratology studies of Rho(D) immune globulin have been published.

Key References

Bowman JM: Antenatal suppression of Rh alloimmunization. Clin Obstet Gynecol 34(2):296-303, 1991. [R]

Bowman JM, Chown B, Lewis M, Pollock JM: Rh isoimmunisation during pregnancy; antenatal prophylaxis. Can Med Ass J 118:623-626, 1978. [S]

Crane JP, Rohland B, Larson D: Rh immune globulin after genetic amniocentesis: Impact on pregnancy outcome. Am J Med Genet 19:763-768, 1984. [E]

McMaster Conference on prevention of Rh immunisation. Vox Sang 36:50-64, 1979. [S]

Thornton JG, Page C, Foote G, et al.: Efficacy and long term effects of antenatal prophylaxis with anti-D immunoglobulin. Br Med J 298:1671-1673, 1989. [E]

Trolle B: Prenatal Rh-immune prophylaxis with 300 micrograms immune globulin anti-D in the 28th week of pregnancy. Acta Obstet Gynecol Scand 68:45-47, 1989. [E]

RHUS EXTRACTS

Summary

Rhus extracts are administered intramuscularly for the prophylaxis and treatment of contact dermatitis associated with the poison ivy, poison oak, and related species.

Magnitude of Teratogenic Risk

Undetermined

Quality and Quantity of Data

None

Comment

None

No epidemiological studies of congenital anomalies in infants whose mothers were given Rhus extracts during pregnancy have been reported.

No animal teratology studies of Rhus extracts have been published.

Key References

None available.

RIBAVIRIN

Synonyms

Tribavirin, Virazid, Virazole

Summary

Ribavirin is a nucleoside analog used to treat viral infections. It is administered orally or by aerosol inhalation. Exposure of health care workers to ribavirin aerosols under usual occupational conditions appears to be associated with minimal absorption of the drug (Anonymous, 1991; Gladu & Ecobichon, 1989; Harrison, 1990).

Magnitude of Teratogenic Risk

Undetermined

Quality and Quantity of Data

None To Poor

Comment

1) Although a risk of teratogenicity has not been demonstrated for this agent, animal studies and its pharmacologic action raise concern that such a risk may exist.

2) The risk of teratogenicity from maternal occupational exposures is not likely to be great since occupational exposures are less than therapeutic exposures.

No epidemiological studies of congenital anomalies among infants born to women treated with ribavirin during pregnancy have been reported.

No teratogenic effect was observed among the fetuses of seven baboons treated during pregnancy with 3-6 times the human oral dose of ribavirin (Johnson, 1990). In contrast, treatment of pregnant rats and hamsters with ribavirin in doses within or below the human therapeutic range increased the frequency of central nervous system, eye, and skeletal anomalies in the offspring (Kilham & Ferm, 1977; Ferm et al., 1978; Johnson, 1990). Similarly, the frequency of skeletal malformations was increased among the offspring of mice treated with ribavirin during pregnancy in doses of 1-10 times those used in humans (Kochhar et al., 1980). In all three species, typical dose- and time-dependence of the teratogenic effect was demonstrated (Ferm et al., 1978; Kochhar et al., 1980; Johnson, 1990). Because of the consistency of these findings in lower mammals, the low dosages at which they occurred, and the pharmacological nature of this agent, it must be assumed that ribavirin may be potentially teratogenic in humans.

Key References

Anonymous: Ribavirin: Is there a risk to hospital personnel? Infectious Diseases and Immunization Committee, Canadian Paediatric Society. Can Med Assoc J 144(3):285-286, 1991. [R]

Ferm VH, Willhite C, Kilham L: Teratogenic effects of ribavirin on hamster and rat embryos. Teratology 17:93-102, 1978. [A]

Gladu J-M, Ecobichon DJ: Evaluation of exposure of health care personnel to ribavirin. J Toxicol Environ Health 28:1-12, 1989. [S]

Harrison R: Reproductive risk assessment with occupational exposure to ribavirin aerosol. Pediatr Infect Dis J 9:S102-S105, 1990. [S]

Johnson EM: The effects of ribavirin on development and reproduction: A critical review of published and unpublished studies in experimental animals. J Am Coll Toxicol 9(5):551-561, 1990. [R]

Kilham L, Ferm VH: Congenital anomalies induced in hamster embryos with ribavirin. Science 195:413-414, 1977. [A]

Kochhar DM, Penner JD, Knudsen TB: Embryotoxic, teratogenic and metabolic effects of ribavirin in mice. Toxicol Appl Pharmacol 52:99-112, 1980. [A]

RIBOFLAVIN

Synonyms

B$_2$-Elite-10, Beflavin, Beflavina, Beflavit, Fladd, Flavitan, Riboflavine, Vitamin B$_2$ Phosphate, Vitamin G

Summary

Riboflavin (vitamin B$_2$) is a necessary dietary component. It functions as a coenzyme in intermediary metabolism. The U.S. Recommended Dietary Allowance of riboflavin for pregnant women is 1.6 mg/d (NRC, 1989).

Magnitude of Teratogenic Risk

Undetermined

Quality and Quantity of Data

None To Poor

Comment

A small risk cannot be excluded, but there is no indication that the risk of congenital anomalies in children of women who take large amounts of riboflavin during pregnancy is likely to be great.

No epidemiological studies of congenital anomalies in infants born to mothers who took unusually large amounts of riboflavin during pregnancy have been reported.

The frequency of malformations was not increased among the offspring of rats treated with 625 times the human recommended daily allowance of riboflavin during pregnancy (Chaube, 1973). In contrast, a variety of congenital anomalies including cleft palate, skeletal malformations, and brain abnormalities, can be induced in the offspring of rats and mice made severely riboflavin deficient during pregnancy (Kalter & Warkany, 1959; Record & Dreosti, 1988; Kalter, 1990).

Key References

Chaube S: Protective effects of thymidine, 5-aminoimidazolecarboxamide, and riboflavin against fetal abnormalities produced in rats by 5-(3,3-dimethyl-1-triazeno) imidazole-4-carboxamide. Cancer Res 33:2231-2239, 1973. [A]

Kalter H: Analysis of the syndrome of congenital malformations induced in genetically defined mice by acute riboflavin deficiency. Teratogenesis Carcinog Mutagen 10(5):385-397, 1990. [A]

Kalter H, Warkany J: Experimental production of congenital malformations in mammals by metabolic procedure. Physiol Rev 39:69-115, 1959. [A]

NRC (National Research Council): Recommended Dietary Allowances, 10th ed. Report of the Subcommittee on the Tenth Edition of the RDAs, Food and Nutrition Board, Commission on Life Sciences. Washington, D.C.: National Academy Press, 1989. [O]

Record IR, Dreosti IE: Zinc and riboflavin interactions with salicylate in pregnant rats. Nutr Rep Int 38(5):1041-1046, 1988. [A]

RICINOLEIC ACID

Synonyms

Ricinic acid, Ricinolic acid

Summary

Ricinoleic acid is a mixture of hydroxylated fatty acids obtained from castor oil. Ricinoleic acid is used in vaginal preparations as a topical antimicrobial agent and as a spermicide.

Magnitude of Teratogenic Risk

None To Minimal

Quality and Quantity of Data

Poor To Fair

Comment

None

The frequency of congenital anomalies was not increased among the infants of 110 women who used ricinoleic acid during the first four lunar months of pregnancy in the Collaborative Perinatal Project (Heinonen et al., 1977).

No animal teratology studies of ricinoleic acid have been published.

Key References

Heinonen OP, Slone D, Shapiro S: Birth Defects and Drugs in Pregnancy. Littleton, Mass.: John Wright-PSG, 1977, pp 300, 302. [E]

RIFAMPIN

Synonyms

Rifadin, Rifaldazine, Rifampicin, Rifamycin, Rimactane, Rofact

Summary

Rifampin is an antibiotic used in the treatment of tuberculosis. It is also used to treat leprosy and meningococcal carriers.

Magnitude of Teratogenic Risk

None To Minimal

Quality and Quantity of Data

Poor To Fair

Comment

None

No adequate epidemiological studies of congenital anomalies among the infants of women treated with rifampin during pregnancy have been published. The frequency of malformations did not appear unusually high among the children of 442 women reported in various studies to have been treated during pregnancy with rifampin, usually in combination with other drugs (Snider et al., 1980). In 109 of these pregnancies, treatment with rifampin occurred during the first trimester.

The frequency of congenital anomalies was not increased among the offspring of mice or rats treated with 2.5-10 times the usual human dose of rifampin during pregnancy (Stratford, 1966), but an increased frequency of cleft palate was observed among the offspring of mice and spina bifida among the offspring of rats treated with more than 15 times the human dose of rifampin (Steen & Stainton-Ellis, 1977; Anonymous, 1971). Congenital anomalies were not increased among the offspring of pregnant rabbits treated with similar doses (Stratford, 1966; Steen & Stainton-Ellis, 1977; Anonymous, 1971).

Key References

Anonymous: Evaluations on new drugs. Drugs 1:354-398, 1971. [R]

Snider DE, Layde PM, Johnson MW, Lyle MA: Treatment of tuberculosis during pregnancy. Amer Rev Resp Disease 122:65-79, 1980. [S]

Steen JSM, Stainton-Ellis DM: Rifampicin in pregnancy. Lancet 2:604-605, 1977. [O]

Stratford BF: Observations on laboratory rodents treated with "Rifamide" during pregnancy. Med J Australia 1:10-12, 1966. [A]

RISOCAINE

Synonyms

Propaesin, Propazyl, Propesin, Raythesin

Summary

Risocaine is a local anesthetic agent.

Magnitude of Teratogenic Risk

Undetermined

Quality and Quantity of Data

None

Comment

None

No epidemiological studies of congenital anomalies in children born to women exposed to risocaine during pregnancy have been reported.

No investigations of teratologic effects of risocaine in experimental animals have been published.

Key References

None available.

RODOCAINE

Summary

Rodocaine is a local anesthetic agent.

Magnitude of Teratogenic Risk

Undetermined

Quality and Quantity of Data

None

Comment

None

No epidemiological studies of congenital anomalies in children born to women exposed to rodocaine during pregnancy have been reported.

No investigations of teratologic effects of rodocaine in experimental animals have been published.

Key References

None available.

ROFLURANE

Synonyms

DA-893

Summary

Roflurane is a general anesthetic that is administered by inhalation.

Magnitude of Teratogenic Risk

Undetermined

Quality and Quantity of Data

None

Comment

None

No epidemiological studies of congenital anomalies in children born to women exposed to roflurane during pregnancy have been reported.

No investigations of teratologic effects of roflurane in experimental animals have been published.

Key References

None available.

RUBELLA VACCINE

Synonyms

Almevax, Ervevax, German Measles Vaccine, Measles Vaccine, German, Meruvax II, Rubella Vaccine, Live

Summary

Rubella vaccine is a live attenuated virus vaccine used for the prevention of German measles.

Magnitude of Teratogenic Risk

None To Minimal

Quality and Quantity of Data

Good

Comment

None

Features of congenital rubella syndrome are uncommon among children born to women vaccinated for rubella during or just before pregnancy. No abnormalities characteristic of the congenital rubella syndrome were found among the infants of 210 susceptible women immunized with RA27/3 strain vaccine, or among the infants of 94 susceptible women immunized with Cendehill or HPV-77 strain vaccine in the three months immediately pre-

ceding or following conception (Preblud et al., 1981; Preblud, 1985; Anonymous, 1989). This study included 73 women who were immunized with RA27/3 vaccine from one week before to four weeks after conception, the period of presumed highest risk for fetal malformations (Anonymous, 1989). Similarly, no cases of congenital rubella syndrome were observed in two other studies among 98 or 21 infants born to mothers who were susceptible to rubella and had been immunized with rubella vaccine during pregnancy (Enders, 1982; Sheppard et al., 1986). All strains of rubella vaccine virus studied are capable of causing infection of the embryo or fetus after maternal immunization (Bolognese et al., 1973; Fleet et al., 1974; Hayden et al., 1980; Banatvala et al., 1981; Preblud, 1985; Anonymous, 1989). One case of cataract in a fetus with documented rubella vaccine virus infection has been observed after maternal immunization (Fleet et al., 1974).

Fetal infection, but no increase in the frequency of malformations, was found among the offspring of rabbits injected with rubella vaccine virus during pregnancy (Cohen et al., 1971).

Please see agent summary on rubella for information on the teratogenic effects of natural rubella virus infection.

Key References

Anonymous. Rubella vaccination during pregnancy--United States, 1971-1988. MMWR 38(17):289-293, 1989. [S]

Banatvala JE, O'Shea S, Best JM, Nicholls MWN, et al.: Transmission of RA27/3 rubella vaccine strain to products of conception. Lancet 1:392, 1981. [C]

Bolognese RJ, Corson SL, Fuccillo DA, Sever JL, et al.: Evaluation of possible transplacental infection with rubella vaccination during pregnancy. Am J Obstet Gynecol 117:939-941, 1973. [C]

Cohen SM, Collins DN, Ward G, Deibel R: Transplacental transmission of rubella virus infection in rabbits. Appl Microbiol 21:76-78, 1971. [A]

Enders G: Rubella antibody titers in vaccinated and nonvaccinated women and results of vaccination during pregnancy. Rev Infect Dis 7(Suppl 1):S103-S107, 1985. [E]

Fleet WF, Benz EW, Karzon DT, Lefkowitz LB, et al.: Fetal consequences of maternal rubella immunization. JAMA 227:621-627, 1974. [C]

Hayden GF, Herrmann KL, Buimovici-Klein E, Weiss KE, et al.: Subclinical congenital rubella infection associated with maternal rubella vaccination in early pregnancy. J Pediatr 96:869-872, 1980. [C]

Preblud SR, Stetler HC, Frank JA, Greaves WL, et al.: Fetal risk associated with rubella vaccine. JAMA 246:1413-1417, 1981. [S]

Preblud SR: Some current issues relating to rubella vaccine. JAMA 254:253-256, 1985. [R]

Sheppard S, Smithells RW, Dickson A, et al.: Rubella vaccination and pregnancy: Preliminary report of a national survey. Br Med J (Clin Res) 292:727, 1986. [S]

RUBELLA VIRUS

Synonyms

German Measles, Rubeola Notha, Third Disease, Three-Day Measles

Summary

Rubella virus is the causative agent of German measles.

Magnitude of Teratogenic Risk

High

Quality and Quantity of Data

Excellent

Comment

None

Rubella virus infection of the embryo or fetus can produce a variety of structural and functional abnormalities, growth retardation, and death. Features of the so-called congenital rubella syndrome include growth retardation, cardiovascular disease (most often peripheral pulmonic stenosis or patent ductus arteriosis), cataracts, retinopathy, glaucoma, and deafness (Korones, 1976; Rosenberg et al., 1981; Munro et al., 1987; Preblud & Alford, 1990). In infancy, thrombocytopenic purpura, hepatosplenomegaly, and obstructive jaundice are common. Mental retardation, neurological deficits, and behavioral abnormalities are often observed in older individuals with congenital rubella syndrome (Chess et al., 1978; Desmond et al., 1978; Preblud & Alford, 1990). The infection tends to be chronic, and deterioration of hearing or mental functioning may occur in children who are initially unaffected. Endocrinopathies, especially diabetes mellitus, and progressive rubella panencephalitis occasionally develop in older individuals with intrauterine rubella infection (South & Sever, 1985; Sever et al., 1985; Ginsberg-Fellner et al., 1985).

Although several prospective studies of children born to pregnant women with clinically diagnosed rubella are available (Peckham & Marshall, 1979), investigations in which the maternal disease was diagnosed serologically are more reliable. A total of 128 pregnancies in women with documented clinical rubella were followed in the Collaborative Perinatal Project (Sever et al., 1965, 1969). Seventy percent of infants whose mothers had rubella in the first month of pregnancy had one or more anomalies characteristic of the fetal rubella syndrome. This figure dropped to about 40% with maternal rubella in the fourth month of gestation, and no rubella-associated abnormalities were seen in infants born after third-trimester exposure. In a British cohort study of 307 children born to mothers with serological evidence of rubella with or without symptoms during pregnancy (Miller et al., 1982), 80% of children who had been exposed during the first trimester of gestation also had serological evidence of rubella infection. This rate fell to 25% among infants whose mothers had had rubella at the end of the second trimester, but increased again to very high levels with maternal rubella just before term. The frequency of defects associated with the congenital rubella syndrome was 85% among children born after maternal rubella during the

556

first 12 weeks of pregnancy and 25% among children born after maternal rubella between 13 and 18 weeks of pregnancy. None of 53 children born to mothers who had rubella after the eighteenth week of pregnancy were clinically affected. In a Danish cohort of 520 infants born to women who had serologically confirmed rubella during pregnancy, only seven infants were found to have anomalies characteristic of congenital rubella syndrome in the neonatal period (Bitsch, 1987). All of these children were born to women who had developed rubella before the twelfth week of pregnancy. Among these 14 pregnancies, the rate of congenital rubella syndrome apparent at birth was 50%.

When congenital rubella syndrome occurs, it is almost always after primary maternal exposure during pregnancy, although rare cases of congenital rubella syndrome after maternal exposure several weeks prior to conception or after secondary maternal exposure during gestation have been reported (South & Sever, 1985; Best et al., 1989; Das et al., 1989; Miller, 1990).

In utero diagnosis of fetal rubella infection has been performed by measuring rubella-specific antibody in fetal blood late in the second trimester (Daffos et al., 1984).

Fetal demise, growth retardation, and ocular malformations similar to those produced in humans were observed in the offspring of rhesus monkeys injected with rubella virus during pregnancy (Delahunt & Reiser, 1967). Similar findings, as well as characteristic cardiac and skeletal anomalies, have also been noted in the offspring of rats infected with rubella virus during pregnancy (Cotlier et al., 1968).

Key References

Best JM, Banatvala JE, Morgan-Capner P, Miller E: Fetal infection after maternal reinfection with rubella: Criteria for defining reinfection. Br Med J 299:773-775, 1989. [S]

Bitsch M: Rubella in pregnant Danish women 1975-1984. Dan Med Bull 34:46-49, 1987. [S]

Chess S, Fernandez P, Korn S: Behavioral consequences of congenital rubella. J Pediatr 93:699-703, 1978. [S]

Cotlier E, Fox J, Bohigian G, Beaty C, et al.: Pathogenic effects of rubella virus on embryos and newborn rats. Nature 217:38-40, 1968. [A]

Daffos F, Forestier F, Grangeot-Keros L, Capella-Pavlovsky M, et al.: Prenatal diagnosis of congenital rubella. Lancet 2:1-3, 1984. [S]

Das BD, Lakhani P, Kurtz JB, et al.: Congenital rubella after previous maternal immunity. Arch Dis Child 65:545-546, 1990. [C]

Delahunt CS, Reiser N: Rubella-induced embryopathies in monkeys. Am J Obstet Gynecol 99:580-588, 1967. [A]

Desmond MM, Fisher ES, Vorderman AL, Schaffer HG, et al.: The longitudinal course of congenital rubella encephalitis in nonretarded children. J Pediatr 93:584-591, 1978. [S]

Ginsberg-Fellner F, Witt ME, Fedun B, et al.: Diabetes mellitus and autoimmunity in patients with the congenital rubella syndrome. Rev Infect Dis 7(Suppl 1):S170-S176, 1985. [S]

Korones SB: Congenital rubella--An encapsulated review. Teratology 14:111-114, 1976. [R]

Miller E: Rubella reinfection. Arch Dis Child 65(8):820-821, 1990. [R]

Miller E, Cradock-Watson JE, Pollock TM: Consequences of confirmed maternal rubella at successive stages of pregnancy. Lancet 2:781-784, 1982. [S]

Peckham C, Marshall WC: Rubella and other virus infections in pregnancy. J Antimicrob Chemother 5(Suppl A):71-80, 1979. [R]

Preblud SR, Alford CA: Rubella. In: Remington JS, Klein JO (eds). Infectious Diseases of the Fetus and Newborn Infant. Philadelphia: W.B. Saunders Co., 1990, pp 196-240. [O]

Rosenberg HS, Oppenheimer EH, Esterly JR: Congenital rubella syndrome: The late effects and their relation to early lesions. Perspect Pediatr Pathol 6:183-202, 1981. [R]

Sever JL, Hardy JB, Nelson KB, Gilkeson MR: Rubella in the collaborative perinatal research study II. Clinical and laboratory findings in children through 3 years of age. Am J Dis Child 118:123-132, 1969. [S]

Sever JL, Nelson KB, Gilkeson MR: Rubella epidemic, 1964: Effect on 6,000 pregnancies. Am J Dis Child 110:395-407, 1965. [S]

South MA, Sever JL: Teratogen update: The congenital rubella syndrome. Teratology 31:297-307, 1985. [R]

RUTAMYCIN

Synonyms

Oligomycin D

Summary

Rutamycin is an antifungal agent.

Magnitude of Teratogenic Risk

Undetermined

Quality and Quantity of Data

None

Comment

None

No epidemiological studies of congenital anomalies in infants born to women who used rutamycin during pregnancy have been reported.

No animal teratology studies of rutamycin have been published.

Key References

None available.

SACCHARIN

Synonyms

Gluside

Summary

Saccharin is a nonnutritive sweetener used as a sugar substitute in beverages and foods. The 1984 FAO/WHO acceptable daily intake of saccharin is 2.5 mg/kg (FAO/WHO, 1984).

Magnitude of Teratogenic Risk

None To Minimal

Quality and Quantity of Data

Poor To Fair

Comment

A small risk cannot be excluded, but there is no indication that the risk of congenital anomalies in children of women who used saccharin during pregnancy is likely to be great.

No epidemiological studies of congenital anomalies among infants born to women who used saccharin during pregnancy have been reported. Maternal use of sugar substitutes (largely or exclusively saccharin) during pregnancy was no more frequent than expected in a case-control study of 545 spontaneous abortions (Kline et al., 1978).

The frequency of malformations was not increased among the offspring of pregnant mice given 2-800 times the human maximum recommended daily intake of saccharin (Lorke, 1969; Dropkin et al., 1985; Tanaka et al., 1973). Similarly, the frequency of malformations was not increased among the offspring of pregnant rats or rabbits treated respectively with 2-1500 or 2-10 times the human maximum recommended daily intake of saccharin (Fritz & Hess, 1968; Klotzsche, 1969; Tanaka et al., 1973). A variety of ocular malformations were observed among the offspring of rats treated during pregnancy with saccharin containing organic impurities in doses 12-2000 times the human maximum recommended daily intake (Colson et al., 1984). In contrast, no increase in eye anomalies was found among the offspring of pregnant rats treated with saccharin purified to commercial standards in doses 6-200 times the human maximum recommended daily intake (Luckhaus & Machemer, 1978; Colson et al., 1984).

A slightly increased incidence of bladder tumors has been observed in some studies of rats exposed daily throughout prenatal and postnatal life to hundreds or thousands of times the recommended human intake of saccharin. Other studies do not show this effect, and prenatal exposure alone does not appear to increase the risk of bladder tumors (Kroes et al., 1977; Taylor et al., 1980; Arnold et al., 1983; Schoenig et al., 1985).

Administration of saccharin to pregnant mice in doses of 400-1600 times the human maximum daily recommended intake did not alter the frequency of fetal somatic cell chromosomal aberrations (Dropkin et al., 1985). No effect on the frequency of germ cell chromosomal abnormalities was seen among male mice treated with saccharin in doses 80-200 times the human maximum recommended daily intake (Pecevski et al., 1983).

Key References

Arnold DL, Krewski D, Munro IC: Saccharin: A toxicological and historical perspective. Toxicology 27:179-256, 1983. [R]

Colson A, Lederer J, Michiels J: Ocular lesions produced on the embryo eyes of rats by saccharin and pollutants. J Fr Ophtalmol 7:399-410, 1984. [A]

Dropkin RH, Salo DF, Tucci SM, Kaye GI: Effects on mouse embryos of in utero exposure to saccharin: Teratogenic and chromosome effects. Arch Toxicol 56:283-287, 1985. [A]

FAO/WHO: Twenty-eighth report of the Joint FAO/WHO Expert Committee on Food Additives. Tech Rep Ser Wld Hlth Org No. 710, 1984. [O]

Fritz H, Hess R: Prenatal development in the rat following administration of cyclamate, saccharin and sucrose. Experientia 24:1140-1141, 1968. [A]

Kline J, Stein ZA, Susser M, et al.: Spontaneous abortion and the use of sugar substitutes (saccharin). Am J Obstet Gynecol 130(6):708-711, 1978. [E]

Klotzsche VC: [Teratogenic and embryotoxic effects of cyclamate, saccharine, and saccharose]. Arzneimittelforsch 119:925-928, 1969. [A]

Kroes R, Peters PWJ, Berkvens JM, et al.: Long term toxicity and reproduction study (including a teratogenicity study) with cyclamate, saccharin and cyclohexylamine. Toxicology 8:285-300, 1977. [A]

Lorke VD: [Investigations into the embryotoxic and teratogenic action of cyclamate and saccharin in the mouse]. Arzneimittelforsch 19:920-922, 1969. [A]

Luckhaus G, Machemer L: Histological examination of perinatal eye development in the rat after ingestion of sodium cyclamate and sodium saccharin during pregnancy. Food Cosmet Toxicol 16:7-11, 1978. [A]

Pecevski J, Vuksanovic L, Savkovic N, Alavantic D, et al.: Effect of saccharin on the induction of chromosomal translocations in male mice and their F1 offspring. Toxicol Lett 19:267-271, 1983. [A]

Schoenig GP, Goldenthal EI, Geil RG, Frith CH, et al.: Evaluation of the dose response and in utero exposure to saccharin in the rat. Food Chem Toxicol 23:475-490, 1985. [A]

Tanaka S, Kawashima K, Nakaura S, Nagao S, et al.: Studies on the teratogenicity of food additives (1). Effects of saccharin sodium on the development of rats and mice. J Food Hyg Soc Jpn (Shokuhin Eiseigaku Zassi) 14:371-379, 1973. [A]

Taylor JM, Weinberger MA, Friedman L: Chronic toxicity and carcinogenicity to the urinary bladder of sodium saccharin in the in utero-exposed rat. Toxicol Appl Pharmacol 54:57-75, 1980. [A]

SALICYL ALCOHOL

Summary

Salicyl alcohol has been used as a local anesthetic.

Magnitude of Teratogenic Risk

Undetermined

Quality and Quantity of Data

None To Poor

Comment

A small risk cannot be excluded, but there is no indication that the risk of congenital anomalies in the children of women treated with salicyl alcohol during pregnancy is likely to be great.

No epidemiological studies of congenital anomalies in children born to mothers treated with salicyl alcohol during pregnancy have been reported.

An increased frequency of embryonic loss and of minor tail anomalies was observed in the offspring of rats treated with very large parental doses of salicyl alcohol during pregnancy (Saito et al., 1982). The relevance of this observation to the therapeutic local use of salicyl alcohol in human pregnancy is unknown.

Please see agent summary on aspirin for information on a closely related agent that has been more thoroughly studied.

Key References

Saito H, Yokoyama A, Takeno S, et al.: Fetal toxicity and hypocalcemia induced by acetylsalicylic acid analogues. Res Commun Chem Pathol Pharmacol 38:209-220, 1982. [A]

SALICYLAMIDE

Synonyms

Amid-Sal, 2-Hydroxybenzamide, Salamide, Salimed

Summary

Salicylamide is a salicylate with analgesic, antipyretic, and anti-inflammatory actions.

Magnitude of Teratogenic Risk

None

Quality and Quantity of Data

Fair

Comment

None

The frequencies of congenital anomalies in general, of major malformations, of minor anomalies, and of major classes of congenital anomalies were no greater than expected among the children of 744 women who took salicylamide during the first four lunar months of pregnancy in the Collaborative Perinatal Project (Heinonen et al., 1977). The frequency of congenital anomalies was not increased among the infants of 1623 women who took salicylamide anytime during pregnancy in this study.

The frequencies of fetal loss and anomalies were increased among hamsters treated with 3-4 times the usual human dose of salicylamide during pregnancy (Lapointe & Harvey, 1964). In rats, fetal loss and skeletal malformations were found with increased frequency among the offspring of animals given several times the usual human dose of salicylamide during pregnancy (Knight & Roe, 1978).

Please see agent summary on aspirin for information on a related agent that has been more thoroughly studied.

Key References

Heinonen OP, Slone D, Shapiro S: Birth Defects and Drugs in Pregnancy. Littleton, Mass.: John Wright-PSG, 1977, pp 291, 471, 484. [E]

Knight E, Roe DA: Effects of salicylamide and protein restriction on the skeletal development of the rat fetus. Teratology 18:17-22, 1978. [A]

Lapointe R, Harvey EB: Salicylamide-induced anomalies in hamster embryos. J Exp Zool 156:197-200, 1964. [A]

SALSALATE

Synonyms

Argesic-SA, Artha-G, Disalcid, Disalicyclic Acid, Mono-Gesic, Salflex, Salgesic, Salsitab

Summary

Salsalate is a salicylate that is used orally in the treatment of rheumatic diseases.

Magnitude of Teratogenic Risk

Undetermined

Quality and Quantity of Data

None To Poor

Comment

None

No epidemiological studies of congenital anomalies among infants born to women treated with salsalate during pregnancy have been reported.

An increased incidence of fetal death was found among the offspring of rats treated late in pregnancy with salsalate in a single dose 8 or 10 times that used therapeutically in humans (Eriksson, 1971).

Salsalate is an inhibitor of prostaglandin synthesis. This class of drugs has been used therapeutically to produce closure of the ductus arteriosus and consequent changes in cardio-vascular and pulmonary function in newborns with patent ductus arteriosus. Salsalate administration to near-term pregnant rats in doses similar to those used in humans has been shown to cause premature (in utero) closure of the ductus arteriosus in the fetuses (Momma et al., 1984). The risk of a similar occurrence in humans after maternal exposure to salsalate late in pregnancy is unknown.

Please see agent summary on aspirin for information on a related agent that has been more thoroughly studied.

Key References

Eriksson M: Salicylate-induced foetal damage during late pregnancy in mice: A comparison between sodium salicylate, acetylsalicylic acid and salicylsalicylic acid. Acta Pharmacol Toxicol 29:250-255, 1971. [A]

Momma K, Hagiwara H, Konishi T: Constriction of fetal ductus arteriosus by non-steroidal anti-inflammatory drugs: Study of additional 34 drugs. Prostaglandins 28:527-536, 1984. [A]

SCOPAFUNGIN

Synonyms

NSC-107041

Summary

Scopafungin is an antifungal and antibacterial agent.

Magnitude of Teratogenic Risk

Undetermined

Quality and Quantity of Data

None

Comment

None

No epidemiological studies of congenital anomalies in infants born to women who used scopafungin during pregnancy have been reported.

No animal teratology studies of scopafungin have been published.

Key References

None available.

SCOPOLAMINE

Synonyms

Hyoscine, Isopto Hyoscine, Transderm Scop

Summary

Scopolamine is an anticholinergic agent. It produces central nervous system depression and is frequently used as a preoperative medication. Scopolamine is also employed in the treatment of motion sickness, mania, and delirium. It is used in ophthalmic preparations to produce mydriasis and cycloplegia.

Magnitude of Teratogenic Risk

None To Minimal

Quality and Quantity of Data

Poor To Fair

Comment

None

The Collaborative Perinatal Project included 388 infants born to women treated with scopolamine during the first four lunar months of pregnancy and 1053 infants born to women treated anytime during pregnancy (Heinonen et al., 1977). The frequency of congenital anomalies was no greater than expected in either group.

No teratogenic effect was observed among the offspring of mice treated during pregnancy with 200-18,000 times the maximum human dose of scopolamine (George et al., 1987a). An increased frequency of eye and skeletal anomalies was observed in a much smaller study in mice treated during pregnancy with 92-1180 times the maximum human dose of scopolamine (Yu et al., 1988). Studies in rats showed no teratogenic effect at 200 times the maximum human dose of scopolamine, but marginal, non-dose-related effects on fetal weight and anomalies were seen in association with maternal toxicity at higher doses (George et al., 1987b). Eye anomalies were found in all 38 fetuses born to rabbits given scopolamine in their drinking water during pregnancy in one study (McBride, 1983); the doses ingested were several times the maximum used in humans. Malformations appeared to be unexpectedly frequent among the offspring of two rabbits treated with twice the human dose of scopolamine during pregnancy in another study reported from the same laboratory (McBride & Hicks, 1987). Long-lasting alterations of behavior were observed among mice born to mothers treated with scopolamine during pregnancy in doses 50 times greater than those used clinically (Richardson et al., 1972).

When given to a pregnant woman just prior to delivery, scopolamine may alter fetal cardiac rate and activity (Ayromlooi et al., 1980). The clinical significance of this observation is unclear.

Key References

Ayromlooi J, Tobias M, Berg P: The effects of scopolamine and ancillary analgesics upon the fetal heart rate recording. J Reprod Med 25:323-326, 1980. [E]

George JD, Price CJ, Marr MC: Teratologic evaluation of scopolamine hydrobromide (CAS No. 114-49-8) administered to CD rats on gestational days 6 through 15. NTIS (National Technical Information Service) Report/PB87-235412, 1987. [A]

George JD: Teratologic evaluation of scopolamine hydrobromide (CAS No. 114-49-8) administered to CD-1 mice on gestational days 6 through 15. NTIS (National Technical Information Service) Report/PB87-209516, 1987. [A]

Heinonen OP, Slone D, Shapiro S: Birth Defects and Drugs in Pregnancy. Littleton, Mass.: John Wright-PSG, 1977, pp 346, 439. [E]

McBride WG: Note on the paper 'Effects of scopolamine hydrobromide on the development of the chick and rabbit embryo' by W. G. McBride, P. H. Vardy and J. French. Aust J Biol Sci 36:171-172, 1983. [A]

McBride WG, Hicks LJ: Acetylcholine and choline levels in rabbit fetuses exposed to anticholinergics. Int J Dev Neurosci 5(2):117-125, 1987. [A]

Richardson DL, Karczmar AG, Scudder CL: Effects of pre-natal cholinergic drug treatment on post-natal behavior and brain chemistry in mice. Fed Proc Fed Am Soc Exp Biol 31:596, 1972. [A]

Yu JF, Yang YS, Wang WY, et al.: Mutagenicity and teratogenicity of chlorpromazine and scopolamine. Chin Med J [Engl] 101(5):339-345, 1988. [A]

SEBACIC ACID

Synonyms

Decanedioic Acid, Domol

Summary

Sebacic acid is a fatty acid used topically as an emollient.

Magnitude of Teratogenic Risk

Undetermined

Quality and Quantity of Data

None To Poor

Comment

A small risk cannot be excluded, but a high risk of congenital anomalies in the children of women who use sebacic acid topically during pregnancy is unlikely.

No epidemiological studies of congenital anomalies in infants whose mothers used sebacic acid during pregnancy have been reported.

No teratogenic effect was observed among the offspring of pregnant rats or rabbits fed 500 mg/kg/d or 1000 mg/kg/d of the sodium salt of sebacic acid, respectively (Greco et al., 1990).

Key References

Greco AV, Mingrone G, Mastromattei EA, et al.: Toxicity of disodium sebacate. Drugs Exp Clin Res 16(10):531-536, 1990. [A]

SECOBARBITAL

Synonyms

Quinalbarbitone Sodium, Seconal

Summary

Secobarbital is a barbiturate that is used as a sedative and hypnotic.

Magnitude of Teratogenic Risk

None

Quality and Quantity of Data

Poor To Fair

Comment

Neonatal withdrawal symptoms have been found with chronic use of secobarbital (see below).

The frequencies of congenital anomalies in general, of major malformations, of minor anomalies, and of principal classes of malformations were no greater than expected among the children of 378 women who took secobarbital during the first four lunar months of pregnancy in the Collaborative Perinatal Project (Heinonen et al., 1977). Similarly, the frequency of congenital anomalies was not increased among the children of 4248 women who took secobarbital anytime during pregnancy in this study (Heinonen et al., 1977).

No animal teratology studies of secobarbital have been published.

Hyperirritability and seizures, thought to represent neonatal withdrawal symptoms, have been reported in the infant of a woman who took very large doses of secobarbital throughout pregnancy (Bleyer & Marshall, 1972).

Key References

Bleyer WA, Marshall RE: Barbiturate withdrawal syndrome in a passively addicted infant. J Am Med Assoc 221:185-186, 1972. [C]

Heinonen OP, Slone D, Shapiro S: Birth Defects and Drugs in Pregnancy. Littleton, Mass.:

John Wright-PSG, 1977, pp 336-40, 344, 438, 476, 490. [E]

SELENIUM SULFIDE

Synonyms

Excel, Selsun, Selsun Blue

Summary

Selenium sulfide is used in topical preparations for the treatment of dandruff and fungal infections of the skin and scalp.

Magnitude of Teratogenic Risk

Undetermined

Quality and Quantity of Data

None

Comment

A small risk cannot be excluded, but a high risk of congenital anomalies in the children of women treated with selenium sulfide during pregnancy is unlikely.

No epidemiological studies of congenital anomalies among infants born to women who used preparations containing selenium sulfide during pregnancy have been reported.

No animal teratology studies of selenium sulfide have been published.

Key References

None available.

SENNA

Synonyms

Black Draught, Gentle Nature, Nytilax, Senna-Gen, Senolax, X-Prep Liquid

Summary

Senna is an anthraquinone obtained from plants of the genus Cassia. It is taken by mouth or rectum as a contact laxative. Senna is not appreciably absorbed when taken in small doses.

Magnitude of Teratogenic Risk

Undetermined

Quality and Quantity of Data

None To Poor

Comment

A small risk cannot be excluded, but a high risk of congenital anomalies in the children of women treated with senna during pregnancy is unlikely.

No epidemiological studies of congenital anomalies among infants born to women who took senna during pregnancy have been reported.

No teratogenic effect was observed among the offspring of rats or rabbits treated during pregnancy with senna in doses 2-100 or 2-20 times those used in humans (Mengs, 1986).

Key References

Mengs U: Reproductive toxicological investigations with sennosides. Arzneimittelforsch 36:1355-1358, 1986. [A]

SERTRALINE

Synonyms

Zoloft

Summary

Sertraline is an inhibitor of presynaptic sero-tonin reuptake. It is administered orally to treat depressive illnesses.

Magnitude of Teratogenic Risk

Undetermined

Quality and Quantity of Data

None

Comment

None

No epidemiological studies of congenital anomalies among the children of women who were treated with sertraline during pregnancy have been reported.

No animal teratology studies of sertraline have been published.

Key References

None available.

SEVOFLURANE

Synonyms

BAX-3084

Summary

Sevoflurane is a general anesthetic administered by inhalation.

Magnitude of Teratogenic Risk

Undetermined

Quality and Quantity of Data

None To Poor

Comment

None

No epidemiological studies of congenital anomalies in children born to women anesthe-tized with sevoflurane during pregnancy have been reported.

The frequency of cleft palate was increased among the offspring of a susceptible strain of mice exposed to sevoflurane during pregnancy (Natsume et al., 1990). This study has only been published as an abstract, and it is unclear whether the exposure was to an anesthetic or subanesthetic dose.

Key References

Natsume N, Miura S, Sugimoto S, et al.: Tera-togenicity caused by halothane, enflurane, and sevoflurane, and changes depending on O2 concen-tration. Teratology 42(6):30A, 1990. [A]

SHARK LIVER OIL

Summary

Shark liver oil is used as a topical protectant and as a source of vitamin A.

Magnitude of Teratogenic Risk

Oral: Undetermined

Topical: Undetermined

Quality and Quantity of Data

Oral: None

Topical: None

Comment

Although the risk of this agent is undetermined, it may be substantial at doses greater than 25,000 international units (IU).

No epidemiological studies of congenital anomalies among infants whose mothers used shark liver oil during pregnancy have been reported.

No animal teratology studies of shark liver oil have been published.

Although the teratogenicity of shark liver oil has not been established in humans, there is reason to suspect that the risk of congenital anomalies may be increased among the children of women who take large amounts of this substance early in pregnancy. Large doses of vitamin A are teratogenic in many species of experimental animals, and retinoic acid, a closely related compound, has been shown to be a human teratogen. Thus it seems likely that large doses of shark liver oil may also be teratogenic in humans.

Please see agent summary on vitamin A for more information on a closely related compound.

Key References

None available.

SIMETHICONE

Synonyms

Infacol, Mylicon, Silain, Windcheaters

Summary

Simethicone is a silicone-containing surfactant that is taken orally for the treatment of flatulence. Simethicone is not absorbed from the gastrointestinal tract.

Magnitude of Teratogenic Risk

Undetermined

Quality and Quantity of Data

None

Comment

A small risk cannot be excluded, but a high risk of congenital anomalies in the children of women treated with simethicone during pregnancy is unlikely.

No epidemiological studies of congenital anomalies among infants born to women who took simethicone during pregnancy have been reported.

No animal teratology studies of simethicone have been published.

Key References

None available.

SINEFUNGIN

Synonyms

Antibiotic A 9145, Compound 57926

Summary

Sinefungin is an antifungal agent.

Magnitude of Teratogenic Risk

Undetermined

Quality and Quantity of Data

None

Comment

None

No epidemiological studies of congenital anomalies in infants born to women who used sinefungin during pregnancy have been reported.

No animal teratology studies of sinefungin have been published.

Key References

None available.

SKIN TEST ANTIGENS

Synonyms

Multitest CMI

Summary

Skin test antigens are sterile solutions containing antigens that are used as a diagnostic aid in determining cellular hypersensitivity to specific antigens.

Magnitude of Teratogenic Risk

Undetermined

Quality and Quantity of Data

None

Comment

A small risk cannot be excluded, but a high risk of congenital anomalies in the children of women treated with skin test antigens during pregnancy is unlikely.

No epidemiological studies of congenital anomalies in infants whose mothers were tested with skin test antigens have been reported.

No animal teratology studies of skin test antigens have been published.

Key References

None available.

SODIUM BICARBONATE

Synonyms

Baking Soda, Monosodium Carbonate, Neut, Soda Mint

Summary

Sodium bicarbonate is an alkalinizing agent that is used as an antacid and in the treatment of metabolic acidosis. Both sodium and bicarbonate ions are major components of body fluids, and their concentrations are normally regulated within narrow limits.

Magnitude of Teratogenic Risk

Undetermined

Quality and Quantity of Data

None To Poor

Comment

A small risk cannot be excluded, but a substantial risk of congenital anomalies in the children of women who took sodium bicarbonate during pregnancy is unlikely.

No epidemiological studies of congenital anomalies among infants born to women treated with sodium bicarbonate during pregnancy have been reported.

No teratogenic effect was noted among the offspring of rats given 100 to more than 4000 mg/kg/d of sodium bicarbonate during pregnancy (Mayura et al., 1982; Khera, 1991). Similarly, no teratogenic effect was seen among the offspring of mice given 500 mg/kg/d of sodium bicarbonate during pregnancy (Reddy et al., 1981).

Key References

Khera KS: Chemically induced alterations in maternal homeostasis and histology of conceptus: Their etiologic significance in rat fetal anomalies. Teratology 44:259-297, 1991. [A]

Mayura K, Hayes AW, Berndt WO: Teratogenicity of secalonic acid d in rats. Toxicology 25:311-322, 1982. [A]

Reddy CS, Reddy RV, Hayes AW: Teratogenicity of secalonic acid d in mice. J Toxicol Environ Health 7:445-455, 1981. [A]

SODIUM CHLORIDE

Synonyms

Adsorbonac, Minims Sodium Chloride, Muro-128, NaSal, Ocean Mist, Saline, Salt

Summary

Sodium chloride is ordinary table salt. It is an essential component of all body fluids. Excessive ingestion of sodium chloride (or dehydration that produces relative excess of salt in body fluids) can produce toxic symptoms.

Magnitude of Teratogenic Risk

Undetermined

Quality and Quantity of Data

None To Poor

Comment

A small risk cannot be excluded, but a substantial risk of congenital anomalies in the children of women who ingest nontoxic amounts of sodium chloride during pregnancy is unlikely.

No epidemiological studies of congenital anomalies among infants born to women who experienced toxic exposures to sodium chloride during pregnancy have been reported. Infusion of physiologic saline solution into the amniotic sac has been used to treat oligohydramnios (Owen et al., 1990; Strong, 1992). Intra-amniotic injection of hypertonic saline has been used to induce termination of pregnancy in the second trimester (Binkin et al., 1983; Fuchs et al., 1984).

Increased frequencies of skeletal anomalies were observed among the offspring of mice treated during pregnancy with 1900-2500 mg/kg of sodium chloride (Nishimura & Miyamoto, 1969). Physiological sodium chloride solutions are often used as negative controls in teratology experiments (e.g., Blakley & Scott, 1984; Svoboda & O'Shea, 1984; Slott & Hales, 1985; Beck, 1989).

Key References

Beck SL: Prenatal ossification as an indicator of exposure to toxic agents. Teratology 40:365-374, 1989. [A]

Binkin NJ, Schulz KF, Grimes DA, Cates W: Urea-prostaglandin versus hypertonic saline for instillation abortion. Am J Obstet Gynecol 146:947-952, 1983. [E]

Blakley PM, Scott WJ: Determination of the proximate teratogen of the mouse fetal alcohol syndrome. 1. Teratogenicity of ethanol and acetaldehyde. Toxicol Appl Pharmacol 72:355-363, 1984. [E]

Fuchs A-R, Rasmussen AB, Rehnstrom J, Toth M: Prostaglandin F2alpha, oxytocin, and uterine activation in hypertonic saline-induced abortions. Am J Obstet Gynecol 150:27-32, 1984. [E]

Nishimura H, Miyamoto S: Teratogenic effects of sodium chloride in mice. Acta Anat Nippon 74:121-124, 1969. [A]

Owen J, Henson BV, Hauth JC: A prospective randomized study of saline solution amnioinfusion. Am J Obstet Gynecol 162:1146-1149, 1990. [E]

Slott V, Hales BF: Teratogenicity and embryolethality of acrolein and structurally related compounds in rats. Teratology 32:65-72, 1985. [A]

Strong TH Jr: Amnioinfusion with preterm, premature rupture of membranes. Clin Perinatol 19(2):399-409, 1992. [R]

Svoboda KK, O'Shea KS: Optic vesicle defects induced by vincristine sulfate: An in vivo and in vitro study in the mouse embryo. Teratology 29:223-239, 1984. [A]

SODIUM CITRATE

Synonyms

Citravescent, Citrosodina, Urade

Summary

Sodium citrate is an organic salt. Citrate is a critical intermediate in the metabolism of carbohydrates. Sodium citrate is used in medicine to alkalinize the urine and as an anticoagulant in stored blood.

Magnitude of Teratogenic Risk

Undetermined

Quality and Quantity of Data

None To Poor

Comment

A small risk cannot be excluded, but there is no indication that the risk of congenital anomalies in the children of women treated with sodium citrate during pregnancy is likely to be great.

No epidemiological studies of congenital anomalies in the children of women who had taken large doses of sodium citrate during pregnancy have been reported.

The frequency of malformations was no greater than expected among the offspring of rats treated during pregnancy with sodium citrate in doses smaller than those sometimes given therapeutically to humans (Nolen et al., 1972).

Key References

Nolen GA, Bohne RL, Buehler EV: Effects of trisodium nitrilotriacetate, trisodium citrate and a trisodium nitrilotriacetate-ferric chloride mixture on cadmium and methyl mercury toxicity and teratogenesis in rats. Toxicol Appl Pharmacol 23:238-250, 1972. [A]

SODIUM LAURYL SULFATE

Synonyms

Cycloryl 580, Empicol LPZ, Maprofix LK

Summary

Sodium lauryl sulfate is an anionic surfactant and emulsifying agent that is used in detergents, shampoos, and dermatological preparations.

Magnitude of Teratogenic Risk

Undetermined

Quality and Quantity of Data

None

Comment

A small risk cannot be excluded, but a high risk of congenital anomalies in the children of women treated with sodium lauryl sulfate during pregnancy is unlikely.

No epidemiological studies of congenital anomalies in infants born to women who used sodium lauryl sulfate during pregnancy have been reported.

No animal teratology studies of sodium lauryl sulfate have been published.

Key References

None available.

SODIUM OXYBATE

Synonyms

Gamma OH, Somsanit

Summary

Sodium oxybate is a general anesthetic that is administered intravenously.

Magnitude of Teratogenic Risk

Undetermined

Quality and Quantity of Data

None

Comment

None

No epidemiological studies of congenital anomalies in children born to women treated with sodium oxybate during pregnancy have been reported.

No studies of teratologic effects of sodium oxybate in experimental animals have been published.

Key References

None available.

SODIUM PHOSPHATES

Synonyms

Sodium Biphosphate, Trisodium Orthophosphate

Summary

Sodium phosphates are administered orally or rectally as cathartic agents. They are also administered orally or intravenously to correct electrolyte disorders and to lower the urinary pH. Sodium phosphates are poorly absorbed from the gastrointestinal tract.

Magnitude of Teratogenic Risk

Undetermined

Quality and Quantity of Data

None

Comment

A small risk cannot be excluded, but a high risk of congenital anomalies in the children of women treated with sodium phosphates during pregnancy is unlikely.

No epidemiological studies of congenital anomalies in infants whose mothers were given sodium phosphates during pregnancy have been reported.

No animal teratology studies of sodium phosphates have been published.

Key References

None available.

SODIUM POLYSTYRENE SULFONATE

Synonyms

Kayexalate, SPS

Summary

Sodium polystyrene sulfonate is a cation-exchange resin that is administered orally or rectally to lower potassium concentrations in the blood. The resin is not absorbed from the gastrointestinal tract.

Magnitude of Teratogenic Risk

Undetermined

Quality and Quantity of Data

None

Comment

A small risk cannot be excluded, but a high risk of congenital anomalies in the children of women

treated with sodium polystyrene sulfonate during pregnancy is unlikely.

No epidemiological studies of congenital anomalies in infants whose mothers were treated with sodium polystyrene sulfonate during pregnancy have been recorded.

No animal teratology studies of sodium polystyrene sulfonate have been published.

Key References

None available.

SODIUM SALICYLATE

Synonyms

Ancosal, Bidocyl, Ensalate, Enterosalicyl, Idocyl, Kerasalicyl, Rhumax, S-60, Saliglutin, Salisod

Summary

Sodium salicylate is used orally in the treatment of rheumatic disorders. The antipyretic, analgesic, and anti-inflammatory properties of sodium salicylate are similar to those of aspirin.

Magnitude of Teratogenic Risk

None To Minimal

Quality and Quantity of Data

Poor To Fair

Comment

1) Risk assessment is for occasional use during pregnancy and may be greater with chronic high-dose use.

2) Potential risks of prolonged labor, maternal antenatal hemorrhage, fetal or neonatal hemorrhage, and premature closure of the fetal ductus arteriosus may exist with maternal use of sodium

salicylate during the last trimester of pregnancy (see aspirin summary).

The frequency of congenital anomalies was not increased among the children of 54 women treated with sodium salicylate during the first four lunar months of pregnancy in the Collaborative Perinatal Project (Heinonen et al., 1977).

Increased frequencies of fetal death and growth retardation occur among the offspring of pregnant rats treated with sodium salicylate in doses similar to or greater than those used clinically (Warkany & Takacs, 1959; Beck & Gulamhusein, 1980; Skowronski et al., 1985; Fritz & Giese, 1990; Bergman et al., 1990). Malformations of the central nervous system, eye, skeleton, and heart were observed with doses two or more times those used clinically. Similar results have been observed in other species. Treatment of pregnant mice with sodium salicylate in doses 2.5 times those used clinically produced fetal death and treatment with doses five times that used in humans caused increased frequencies of central nervous system, skeletal, and other congenital anomalies (Larsson & Eriksson, 1966; Eriksson & Larsson, 1982). Treatment of pregnant ferrets with a dose similar to that used in humans produced an increased frequency of fetal death while treatment with doses two or more times as great produced a variety of malformations in the offspring (Beck & Gulamhusein, 1980).

Please see agent summary on aspirin for information on a closely related agent that has been more thoroughly studied.

Key References

Beck F, Gulamhusein AP: The effect of sodium salicylate on limb development. Teratol Limbs Symp Prenatal Dev 4th 1980:393-401, 1981. [A]

Bergman K, Cekan E, Slanina P, et al.: Effects of dietary sodium selenite supplementation on salicylate-induced embryo- and fetotoxicity in the rat. Toxicology 61(2):135-146, 1990. [A]

Eriksson M, Larsson KS: Influence of a low protein diet on salicylate-induced damage in mice. Biol Neonate 41:138-142, 1982. [A]

Fritz H, Fiese K: Evaluation of the teratogenic potential of chemicals in the rat. Pharmacology 40(suppl 1):1-27, 1990. [A]

Heinonen OP, Slone D, Shapiro S: Birth Defects and Drugs in Pregnancy. Littleton, Mass.: John Wright-PSG, 1977, pp 287-288. [E]

Larsson KS, Eriksson M: Salicylate-induced fetal death and malformations in two mouse strains. Acta Paediatr Scand 55:569-576, 1966. [A]

Skowronski GA, Abdel-Rahman MS, Gerges SE, Klein KM: Teratologic evaluation of Alcide liquid in rats and mice. I JAT J Appl Toxicol 5:97-103, 1985. [A]

Warkany J, Takacs E: Experimental production of congenital malformations in rats by salicylate poisoning. Am J Pathol 35:315-331, 1959. [A]

SODIUM SULFATE

Synonyms

Liquisulf

Summary

Sodium sulfate is given orally as a saline laxative; the salt is poorly absorbed from the gastrointestinal tract. Sodium sulfate may also be administered intravenously in the treatment of hypercalcemia.

Magnitude of Teratogenic Risk

Undetermined

Quality and Quantity of Data

None To Poor

Comment

A small risk cannot be excluded, but a high risk of congenital anomalies in the children of women treated with sodium sulfate during pregnancy is unlikely.

No epidemiological studies of congenital anomalies among infants born to women treated with sodium sulfate during pregnancy have been reported.

The frequency of malformations was not increased among the offspring of mice injected with 60 mg/kg of sodium sulfate during pregnancy (Arcuri & Gautieri, 1973).

Key References

Arcuri PA, Gautieri RF: Morphine-induced fetal malformations III: Possible mechanisms of action. J Pharm Sci 62:1626-1634, 1973. [A]

SODIUM TETRADECYL SULFATE

Synonyms

Sotradecol, STD, Trombovar

Summary

Sodium tetradecyl sulfate is an anionic surfactant. It is given by injection as a sclerosant to treat varicose veins. It is also used as a surfactant in disinfectants.

Magnitude of Teratogenic Risk

As A Sclerosant: Small

As A Disinfectant: Undetermined

Quality and Quantity of Data

As A Sclerosant: Poor

As A Disinfectant: None

Comment

A small risk cannot be excluded, but a high risk of congenital anomalies in the children of women who used sodium tetradecyl sulfate as a disinfectant during pregnancy is unlikely.

Congenital anomalies were observed twice as frequently as expected among the infants of 95 women who were treated with sodium tetradecyl sulfate for varicose veins during the first four lunar months of pregnancy in the Collaborative Perinatal Project (Heinonen et al., 1977). No significant increase in congenital anomalies was found among the infants of 606 women who were treated with this agent anytime during pregnancy.

No animal teratology studies of sodium tetradecyl sulfate have been published.

Key References

Heinonen OP, Slone D, Shapiro S: Birth Defects and Drugs in Pregnancy. Littleton, Mass.: John Wright-PSG, 1977, pp 410-411, 415, 444. [E]

SODIUM THIOSULFATE

Synonyms

Oligosol, S-Hydril, Soufre Oligosol

Summary

Sodium thiosulfate is used in dermatological preparations for the treatment of acne and fungal infections. Sodium thiosulfate is also administered intravenously in the treatment of cyanide poisoning.

Magnitude of Teratogenic Risk

Undetermined

Quality and Quantity of Data

Poor

Comment

A small risk cannot be excluded, but a high risk of congenital anomalies in the children of women treated with sodium thiosulfate during pregnancy is unlikely.

No epidemiological studies of congenital anomalies among infants born to women treated with sodium thiosulfate during pregnancy have been reported.

No teratogenic effect was observed among the offspring of hamsters treated repeatedly during pregnancy with sodium thiosulfate in doses similar to those given intravenously to treat cyanide poisoning in humans (Willhite, 1983). This treatment was found to ameliorate the teratogenic effects of maternal cyanide poisoning in the hamsters (Doherty et al., 1982; Willhite, 1983).

Key References

Doherty PA, Ferm VH, Smith RP: Congenital malformations induced by infusion of sodium cyanide in the golden hamster. Toxicol Appl Pharmacol 64:456-464, 1982. [A]

Willhite CC: Developmental toxicology of acetonitrile in the Syrian golden hamster. Teratology 27:313-325, 1983. [A]

SOMATREM

Synonyms

Met-HGH, Methionyl Human Growth Hormone

Summary

Somatrem is a highly purified human growth hormone produced by recombinant DNA technology. It is administered intramuscularly in the treatment of growth failure.

Magnitude of Teratogenic Risk

Undetermined

Quality and Quantity of Data

None

Comment

A small risk cannot be excluded, but a high risk of congenital anomalies in the children of women treated with somatrem during pregnancy is unlikely.

No epidemiological studies of congenital anomalies in infants whose mothers were treated with somatrem during pregnancy have been reported.

No animal teratology studies of somatrem have been published.

Key References

None available.

SOMATROPIN

Synonyms

Asellacrin, HGH, Human Growth Hormone, Humatrope, Protropin, Somatonorm, Soma-totrophin

Summary

Somatropin is human pituitary growth hormone. It is prepared by recombinant DNA technology and administered parenterally in the treatment of pituitary dwarfism.

Magnitude of Teratogenic Risk

Undetermined

Quality and Quantity of Data

None To Poor

Comment

A small risk cannot be excluded, but a high risk of congenital anomalies in the children of women treated with somatropin during pregnancy is unlikely.

No epidemiological studies of congenital anomalies among infants born to women treated with somatropin during pregnancy have been reported.

Prolonged gestation, increased birth weight, and increased brain weight have been found among the offspring of rats treated with very large doses of heterospecific pituitary growth hormone preparations during pregnancy in some experiments but not others (Hultquist & Engfeldt, 1949; Zamenof et al., 1971; Croskerry & Smith, 1975; Hendrich et al., 1984).

Please see agent summary on somatrem for information on a related agent that has been studied.

Key References

Croskerry PG, Smith GK: Prolongation of gestation by growth hormone: A confounding factor in the assessment of its prenatal action. Science 189:648-650, 1975. [A]

Hendrich CE, Jackson WJ, Porterfield SP: Behavioral testing of progenies of Tx (hypothyroid) and growth hormone-treated Tx rats: An animal model for mental retardation. Neuroendocrinology 38:429-437, 1984. [A]

Hultquist GT, Engfeldt B: Giant growth of rat fetuses produced experimentally by means of administration of hormones to the mother during pregnancy. Acta Endocrinol 3:365-376, 1949. [A]

Zamenof S, van Marthens E, Grauel L: Prenatal cerebral development: Effect of restricted diet, reversal by growth hormone. Science 174:954-955, 1971. [A]

SORBITOL

Synonyms

Cinecolex R-X, D-Glucitol, Howsorb 1, Howsorb 2, Sorbilande, Sorbostyl

Summary

Sorbitol is a simple sugar alcohol that is widely used as a sweetener in pharmaceutical preparations and some foods. It is also employed as a moistening agent in creams and as an ingredient in toothpastes. Sorbitol is used as a carbohydrate energy source in parenteral solutions and as an osmotic diuretic in the treatment of cerebral edema and increased intraocular pressure. Large doses may be given by mouth as a laxative.

Magnitude of Teratogenic Risk

Undetermined

Quality and Quantity of Data

Poor

Comment

A small risk cannot be excluded, but there is no indication that the risk of congenital anomalies in the children of women treated with sorbitol during pregnancy is likely to be great.

No epidemiological studies of congenital anomalies in children of women treated with sorbitol during pregnancy have been reported.

The frequency of congenital anomalies was not increased among the offspring of pregnant rats given diets containing 2.5-10% sorbitol or among the offspring of rats or mice treated with 16-1600 times the usual human dose of sorbitol during pregnancy (MacKenzie et al., 1968; Food & Drug Research Labs, 1972). Similarly, no teratogenic effect was observed among the offspring of hamsters treated with 4 to 1,200 times the usual human dose of sorbitol during pregnancy (Food and Drug Research Labs, 1972; Gill et al., 1981).

Key References

Food & Drug Research Labs: Teratologic evaluation of FDA 71-31 (Sorbitol). NTIS (National Technical Information Service) Report/PB-221 806, 1972. [A]

Gill TS, Guram MS, Geber WF: Comparative study of the teratogenic effects of chlordiazepoxide and diazepam in the fetal hamster. Life Sciences 29:2141-2147, 1981. [A]

MacKenzie KM, Hauck WN, Wheeler AG, Roe FJC: Three-generation reproduction study of rats ingesting up to 10% sorbitol in the diet--And a brief review of the toxicological status of sorbitol. Food Chem Toxicol 24:191-200, 1986. [A]

SPECTINOMYCIN

Synonyms

Actinospectacin, Delspectin, Kempi, Spectam, Togamycin, Trobicin

Summary

Spectinomycin is an aminocyclitol antibiotic that is given parenterally to treat gonorrhea.

Magnitude of Teratogenic Risk

Undetermined

Quality and Quantity of Data

None

Comment

None

No epidemiological studies of congenital anomalies among infants born to women treated with spectinomycin during pregnancy have been reported.

No animal teratology studies of spectinomycin have been published.

Key References

None available.

SPIRONOLACTONE

Synonyms

Aldactone, Diatensec, Espironolactona, Laractone, Spiretic, Spiroctan, Spirolactone, Spirolone

Summary

Spironolactone is a steroid that acts as a competitive inhibitor of aldosterone. It is used as a diuretic and as an antihypertensive agent.

Magnitude of Teratogenic Risk

Undetermined

Quality and Quantity of Data

None To Poor

Comment

None

No epidemiological studies of congenital anomalies in the offspring of women who used spironolactone during pregnancy have been reported.

No increase in the frequency of malformations was observed among the offspring of pregnant rats or mice treated with spironolactone in doses 2.5-10 times those used in humans (Miyakubo et al., 1977). Feminization of the genitalia was seen in the male offspring of rats treated with spironolactone during late pregnancy in doses 5 times greater than those used in humans in one study (Hecker et al., 1980). In another study, hypoprolactinemia and reduced weights of accessory sex organs were seen in adult male rats and increased ovarian and uterine weights in adult female rats born to dams that had been treated during pregnancy with spironolactone in doses 2.5 times those used in humans (Jaussan et al., 1985). The relevance of these observations to the clinical use of spironolactone in human pregnancy is unknown.

Key References

Hecker A, Hasan SH, Neumann F: Disturbances in sexual differentiation of rat foetuses following spironolactone treatment. Acta Endocrinol 95:540-545, 1980. [A]

Jaussan V, Lemarchand-Beraud T, Gomez F: Modifications of the gonadal function in the adult rat after fetal exposure to spironolactone. Biol Reprod 32:1051-1061, 1985. [A]

Miyakubo H, Saito S, Tokunaga Y, Ando H, et al.: Toxicological studies of SC-14266. 5. Teratological study of SC-14266 in rats and mice. Nichidai Igaku Zasshi 36:261-282, 1977. [A]

STANOZOLOL

Synonyms

Anasyth, Androstanazole, Methylstanazole, Stromba, Strombaject, Winstrol

Summary

Stanozolol is an anabolic androgenic steroid that is usually administered orally. It is used in the prophylaxis and treatment of hereditary angioneurotic edema.

Magnitude of Teratogenic Risk

Undetermined

Quality and Quantity of Data

None

Comment

Although the risk of congenital anomalies among infants born to women treated with stanozolol during pregnancy is unknown, it is likely that the maternal use of stanozolol can produce virilization of the external genitalia of a female fetus.

No epidemiological studies of congenital anomalies among infants born to women

treated with stanozolol during pregnancy have been reported.

No animal teratology studies of stanozolol have been published.

Please see agent summary on testosterone for information on a related agent that has been studied.

Key References

None available.

STAPHYLOCOCCUS VACCINE

Synonyms

Staphylococcus Phage Lysate

Summary

Staphylococcus vaccine is a killed bacterial lysate used to induce immunity to staphylococci.

Magnitude of Teratogenic Risk

Undetermined

Quality and Quantity of Data

None To Poor

Comment

A small risk cannot be excluded, but a high risk of congenital anomalies in the children of women treated with staphylococcus vaccine during pregnancy is unlikely.

No epidemiological studies of congenital anomalies among infants born to women immunized with staphylococcus vaccine during pregnancy have been reported.

No teratogenic effect was observed among the offspring of rats or rabbits given repeated subcutaneous injections of staphylococcus

vaccine during pregnancy (Hirayama et al., 1980a, b).

Key References

Hirayama H, Kimura T, Wada S, Enokuya Y: Reproductive evaluation of staphylococcal phage lysate (SPL). (2) Embryotoxic and teratogenic study in rats and rabbits. Oyo Yakuri 20:575-581, 1980a. [A]

Hirayama H, Wada S, Kimura T, Enokiya Y: Reproductive evaluation of staphylococcal phage lysate (SPL). (3) Peri- and postnatal study in rats. Oyo Yakuri 20:595-608, 1980b. [A]

STREPTOKINASE

Synonyms

Kabikinase, Streptase

Summary

Streptokinase is a nonenzymatic protein produced by certain streptococcal bacteria that activates plasminogen in human plasma to plasmin, a fibrinolytic enzyme. Streptokinase is administered intravenously or intra-arterially to dissolve blood clots in conditions such as pulmonary thromboembolism, deep vein thrombosis, and coronary artery thrombosis.

Magnitude of Teratogenic Risk

Undetermined

Quality and Quantity of Data

None

Comment

None

No epidemiological studies of congenital anomalies among infants born to women treated with streptokinase during pregnancy have been reported.

No animal teratology studies of streptokinase have been published.

Key References

None available.

STREPTOMYCIN

Synonyms

Hydroxystreptomycin, Orastrep, Servistrep

Summary

Streptomycin is an aminoglycoside antibiotic used parenterally in the treatment of tuberculosis and other bacterial infections.

Magnitude of Teratogenic Risk

Deafness: Small

Malformations: None

Quality and Quantity of Data

Deafness: Fair To Good

Malformations: Fair To Good

Comment

None

The frequency of congenital anomalies was no greater than expected among the children of 135 women who took streptomycin in the first four lunar months of pregnancy or among the children of 335 women who took the drug anytime in pregnancy in the Collaborative Perinatal Project (Heinonen et al., 1977). Deafness was not included among the anomalies studied in this investigation. A number of case reports of sensorineural deafness, sometimes with accompanying vestibular dysfunction, in children born to women treated with streptomycin for tuberculosis during pregnancy have been published (Warkany, 1979; Snider et al., 1980; Donald & Sellars, 1981). No relationship to drug dosage or stage of pregnancy during which exposure occurred is apparent in these reports, but since auditory nerve damage is a well-known toxic effect of streptomycin in children and adults, it seems likely that similar toxicity could occur antenatally. Although asymptomatic abnormalities of auditory or vestibular function have been observed in up to 10% of children born to women treated with streptomycin during pregnancy, symptomatic disturbances of eighth cranial nerve function appear to be much less common (Varpela et al., 1969; Warkany, 1979; Donald & Sellars, 1981).

No increase in the frequency of malformations was observed among the offspring of mice treated during pregnancy with streptomycin in doses 5-6 times those used in humans (Ericson-Strandvik & Gyllensten, 1963; Nomura et al., 1984). No abnormality of auditory response was observed in the offspring of pregnant rats and mice treated, respectively, with 2.5-7.5 and 2-10 times the usual human dose of streptomycin (Suzuki & Takeuchi, 1961), but histological evidence of inner ear damage was apparent among the offspring of pregnant mice treated with three times the human dose of streptomycin (Nakamoto et al., 1985). No functional or histological abnormality of the auditory or vestibular system was seen among the offspring of guinea pigs treated during pregnancy with streptomycin in doses similar to those used in humans (Riskaer et al., 1952).

Key References

Donald PR, Sellars SL: Streptomycin ototoxicity in the unborn child. S Afr Med J 60:316-318, 1981. [S]

Ericson-Strandvik B, Gyllensten L: The central nervous system of foetal mice after administration of streptomycin. Acta Pathol Microbiol Scand 59:292-300, 1963. [A]

Heinonen OP, Slone D, Shapiro S: Birth Defects and Drugs in Pregnancy. Littleton, Mass.: John Wright-PSG, 1977, pp 297, 435. [E]

Nakamoto Y, Otani H, Tanaka O: Effects of aminoglycosides administered to pregnant mice on postnatal development of inner ear in their offspring. Teratology 32(3):34B, 1985. [A]

Nomura T, Kimura S, Kanzaki T, et al.: Induction of tumors and malformations in mice after prenatal treatment with some antibiotic drugs. Med J Osaka Univ 35(1-2):13-17, 1984. [A]

Riskaer N, Christensen E, Hertz H: The toxic effects of streptomycin and dihydrostreptomycin in pregnancy, illustrated experimentally. Acta Tuber Pneumol Scand 27:211-216, 1952. [A]

Snider DE, Layde PM, Johnson MW, Lyle MA: Treatment of tuberculosis during pregnancy. Am Rev Respir Dis 122:65-79, 1980. [S]

Suzuki Y, Takeuchi S: Experimental studies on effects of streptomycin on the auditory mechanism of the fetus after administration of various doses to the pregnant mother. Keio J Med 10:31-41, 1961. [A]

Varpela E, Hietalahti J, Aro MJT: Streptomycin and dihydrostreptomycin medication during pregnancy and their effect on the child's inner ear. Scand J Respir Dis 50:101-109, 1969. [S]

Warkany J: Antituberculous drugs. Teratology 20:133-138, 1979. [R]

SUCRALFATE

Synonyms

Andapsin, Antepsin, Carafate, Duracralfat, Keal, Sucramal, Sugast

Summary

Sucralfate is an aluminated salt of a sulfated disaccharide. It is administered orally in the treatment of peptic ulcers. Sucralfate is poorly absorbed from the gastrointestinal tract.

Magnitude of Teratogenic Risk

Undetermined

Quality and Quantity of Data

None

Comment

A small risk cannot be excluded, but a high risk of congenital anomalies in the children of women treated with sucralfate during pregnancy is unlikely.

No epidemiological studies of congenital anomalies in infants whose mothers were treated with sucralfate during pregnancy have been reported.

No animal teratology studies of sucralfate have been published.

Key References

None available.

SULBACTAM

Synonyms

CP-45889-2

Summary

Sulbactam is a sulfone derivative of penicillin that has antibiotic activity and is a beta-lactamase inhibitor. Sulbactam is administered parenterally, often in combination with a beta-lactam antibiotic, in the treatment of infections.

Magnitude of Teratogenic Risk

Undetermined

Quality and Quantity of Data

None To Poor

Comment

A small risk cannot be excluded, but a high risk of congenital anomalies in the children of women treated with sulbactam during pregnancy is unlikely.

No epidemiological studies of congenital anomalies among infants born to women

treated with sulbactam during pregnancy have been reported.

No teratogenic effect was observed among the offspring of rats treated with 0.6-6 times the human dose of sulbactam during pregnancy (Horimoto et al., 1984).

Key References

Horimoto M, Sakai T, Ohtsuki I, Noguchi Y: Reproduction studies with sulbactam and combinations of sulbactam and cefoperazone in rats. Chemotherapy 32:115, 1984. [A]

SULCONAZOLE

Synonyms

Exelderm, Sulcosyn

Summary

Sulconazole is an imidazole antifungal agent that is used topically.

Magnitude of Teratogenic Risk

Undetermined

Quality and Quantity of Data

None To Poor

Comment

A small risk cannot be excluded, but a high risk of congenital anomalies in the children of women treated with sulconazole during pregnancy is unlikely.

No epidemiological studies of congenital anomalies in infants born to women treated with sulconazole during pregnancy have been reported.

The frequency of malformations was not increased among the offspring of pregnant rats or rabbits given subcutaneous injections of 0.3-

60 or 0.3-30 mg/kg/d of sulconazole (Kobayashi et al., 1985).

Please see agent summary on metronidazole for information on a related agent that has been studied.

Key References

Kobayashi T, Ariyuki F, Higaki K, et al.: Reproduction studies in rats and rabbits given sulconazole nitrate (RS 44872). Oyo Yakuri (Pharmacometrics) 30:451-465, 1985. [A]

SULFABENZAMIDE

Synonyms

Sulfabenzid, Sulfabenzoylamide, Vagilia

Summary

Sulfabenzamide is a sulfonamide that is used as a topical antibacterial agent in the treatment of vaginitis.

Magnitude of Teratogenic Risk

None To Minimal

Quality and Quantity of Data

Poor To Fair

Comment

None

The frequency of congenital anomalies was not increased among the infants of 88 women who were treated with sulfabenzamide during the first four lunar months of pregnancy in the Collaborative Perinatal Project (Heinonen et al., 1977).

No animal teratology studies of sulfabenzamide have been published.

Key References

Heinonen OP, Slone D, Shapiro S: Birth Defects and Drugs in Pregnancy. Littleton, Mass.: John Wright-PSG, 1977, pp 298, 301. [E]

SULFACETAMIDE

Synonyms

Acetosulfaminum, Ak-Sulf, Bleph-10, Cetamide, N-Sulphanilylacetamide, Sodium Sulamyd, Sulfair

Summary

Sulfacetamide is a sulfonamide that is used as an antibacterial agent in ophthalmic and vaginal preparations. Systemic absorption of topical sulfacetamide may occur.

Magnitude of Teratogenic Risk

None

Quality and Quantity of Data

Poor To Fair

Comment

None

The frequency of congenital anomalies was no greater than expected among the children of 93 women who were treated with sulfacetamide during the first trimester of pregnancy in the Collaborative Perinatal Project (Heinonen et al., 1977).

No animal teratology studies of sulfacetamide have been published.

Please see agent summary on sulfamethoxazole for information on a related agent that has been more thoroughly studied.

Key References

Heinonen OP, Slone D, Shapiro S: Birth Defects and Drugs in Pregnancy. Littleton, Mass.: John Wright-PSG, 1977, pp 298, 301. [E]

SULFADOXINE

Synonyms

Fanasil, Fanzil, Sulformethoxine, Sulforthomidine

Summary

Sulfadoxine is a sulfonamide that is taken orally. It is used in combination with pyrimethamine in the treatment and prophylaxis of malaria. Sulfadoxine persists in the body for a prolonged period afer administration. The half-life for elimination ranges from four to ten days.

Magnitude of Teratogenic Risk

None To Minimal

Quality and Quantity of Data

Poor To Fair

Comment

None

No congenital anomalies attributed to this drug were noted among the infants of 67 women in one series or of 33 women in another series treated during the first trimester of pregnancy with sulfadoxine in combination with pyrimethamine (Anonymous, 1983). Unfortunately, the details of these studies have not been published. No drug-related effects were noted in series of 34 and six children whose mothers had been treated with sulfadoxine and pyrimethamine in the second or third trimester of pregnancy for toxoplasmosis (Barbosa & Perreira, 1978; Daffos et al., 1988).

No teratological studies of sulfadoxine in experimental animals have been published.

Please see agent summary on sulfisoxazole for information on a related agent that has been more thoroughly studied.

Key References

Anonymous: Pyrimethamine combinations in pregnancy. Lancet 2:1005-1007, 1983. [R]

Barbosa JC, Ferreira I: Sulfadoxine-pyrimethamine (Fansidar) in pregnant women with Toxoplasma antibody titres. In: Siegenthaler W & Luthy R (eds). Current Chemotherapy (Proc X Int Congr Chemother vol 1). Washington, D.C.: Amer Soc for Microbiol, 1978, pp 134-135. [S]

Daffos F: Prenatal management of 746 pregnancies at risk for congenital toxoplasmosis. N Engl J Med 318:271-275, 1988. [S]

SULFAMETHOXAZOLE

Synonyms

Gantanol, Sulfamethylisoxazole

Summary

Sulfamethoxazole is a sulfonamide used primarily in the treatment of urinary tract infections.

Magnitude of Teratogenic Risk

None To Minimal

Quality and Quantity of Data

Poor To Fair

Comment

None

The frequency of congenital anomalies was no greater than expected among the offspring of 46 women treated with sulfamethoxazole in the first four lunar months of pregnancy or among the children of 210 women exposed to this drug anytime in pregnancy in the Collaborative Perinatal Project (Heinonen et al., 1977). Similarly, the frequency of congenital anomalies was no higher among the children of 120 women treated with sulfamethoxazole and trimethoprim in combination than among the children of 66 women treated with placebo in one controlled trial of therapy for bacteriuria of pregnancy (Williams et al., 1969). Only 10 of these women were treated with the active drugs during the first trimester.

An increased frequency of cleft palate was observed in the offspring of rats administered 15 times the usual human dose of sulfamethoxazole during pregnancy (Udall, 1969). The relevance of this observation to the therapeutic use of sulfamethoxazole in human pregnancy is unknown.

Key References

Heinonen OP, Slone D, Shapiro S: Birth Defects and Drugs in Pregnancy. Littleton, Mass.: John Wright-PSG, 1977, pp 298, 301, 435. [E]

Udall V: Toxicology of sulphonamide-trimethoprim combinations. Postgrad Med J 45(Suppl 5):42-45, 1969. [A]

Williams JD, Condie AP, Brumfitt W, Reeves DS: The treatment of bacteriuria in pregnant women with sulphamethoxazole and trimethoprim. A microbiological, clinical and toxicological study. Postgrad Med J 45(Suppl 6):71-76, 1969. [E]

SULFAPYRIDINE

Synonyms

Dagenan, M & B 693, Sulphapyridine

Summary

Sulfapyridine is a sulfonamide used orally to treat dermatitis herpetiformis and other dermatoses.

Magnitude of Teratogenic Risk

Undetermined

Quality and Quantity of Data

None

Comment

None

No epidemiological studies of congenital anomalies among infants born to women treated with sulfapyridine during pregnancy have been reported.

No animal teratology studies of sulfapyridine have been published.

Because this agent is a sulfonamide, it is capable of interfering with bilirubin binding to albumin in neonates born to women treated late in pregnancy.

For additional information on related agents, please see agent summaries on sulfasalazine, which is broken down to sulfapyridine in the bowel, and sulfisoxazole, which has been more thoroughly studied.

Key References

None available.

SULFASALAZINE

Synonyms

Azulfidine, Colo-Pleon, Salazopyridin, Salazopyrine, Salazosulfapyridine, Salicylazosulfapyridine, Salisulf

Summary

Sulfasalazine is given orally or rectally in the treatment of inflammatory bowel disease. The drug is composed of two moieties, one a sulfonamide (sulfapyridine) and the other a salicylate (mesalamine), into which sulfasalazine is

Magnitude of Teratogenic Risk

None To Minimal

Quality and Quantity of Data

Fair

Comment

None

The frequency of congenital anomalies was no greater than expected among the children of women with inflammatory bowel disease treated during pregnancy with sulfasalazine with or without steroids in studies which included 60, 100, and 186 pregnancies, respectively (Willoughby & Truelove, 1980; Mogadam et al., 1981; Nielsen et al., 1983). Interpretation of these studies is confounded by the fact that the treatment occurred at various times and for various durations during the pregnancies and underascertainment of congenital anomalies appears to have occurred, at least in the largest study. Instances of congenital anomalies among infants born to women who had been treated with sulfasalazine during pregnancy have been reported (Craxi & Pagliarello, 1980; Haxton & Bell, 1983; Newman & Correy, 1983; Hoo et al., 1988), but no consistent pattern of malformations has been noted. A causal relationship between maternal sulfasalazine therapy during pregnancy and the congenital anomalies cannot be inferred from these anecdotal observations.

No animal teratology studies of sulfasalazine have been published.

No increase in the frequency of serious neonatal jaundice was observed among the infants of women with inflammatory bowel disease treated with sulfasalazine during pregnancy in the studies cited above (Willoughby & Truelove, 1980; Mogadam et al., 1981; Nielsen et al., 1983). Although there is a theoretical risk of kernicterus among infants of women treated with sulfonamides late in pregnancy because of displacement of bilirubin from albumin in the baby's blood, this problem appears to be of little practical concern (Jarnerot et al., 1981; Esbjorner et al., 1987).

Key References

Craxi A, Pagliarello F: Possible embryotoxicity of sulfasalazine. Arch Intern Med 140:1674, 1980. [C]

Esbjorner E, Jarnerot G, Wranne L: Sulphasalazine and sulphapyridine serum levels in children to mothers treated with sulphasalazine during pregnancy and lactation. Acta Paediatr Scand 76:137-142, 1987. [S]

Haxton MJ, Bell J: Fetal anatomical abnormalities and other associated factors in middle-trimester abortion and their relevance to patient counselling. Br J Obstet Gynaecol 90:501-506, 1983. [S]

Hoo JJ, Hadro TA, von Behren P: Possible teratogenicity of sulfasalazine. N Engl J Med 318:1128, 1988. [C]

Jarnerot G, Into-Malmberg MB, Esbjorner E: Placental transfer of sulphasalazine and sulphapyridine and some of its metabolites. Scand J Gastroenterol 16:693-697, 1981. [E]

Mogadam M, Dobbins WO, Korelitz BI, Ahmed SW: Pregnancy in inflammatory bowel disease: Effect of sulfasalazine and corticosteroids on fetal outcome. Gastroenterology 80:72-76, 1981. [E]

Newman NM, Correy JF: Possible teratogenicity of sulphasalazine. Med J Aust 1:528-529, 1983. [C]

Nielsen OH, Andreasson B, Bondesen S, Jarnum S: Pregnancy in ulcerative colitis. Scand J Gastroenterol 18:735-742, 1983. [E]

Willoughby CP, Truelove SC: Ulcerative colitis and pregnancy. Gut 21:469-474, 1980. [E]

SULFATHIAZOLE

Synonyms

Cibazol, Norsulfazolum, Sulfamul, Sulfanilamidothiazole, Thiazamide

Summary

Sulfathiazole is a sulfonamide that is used topically in the treatment of vaginal infections.

Magnitude of Teratogenic Risk

None To Minimal

Quality and Quantity of Data

Poor To Fair

Comment

None

The frequency of congenital anomalies was no greater than expected among the children of 100 women who were treated with sulfathiazole during the first four lunar months of pregnancy or among the children of 124 women treated with this drug anytime in pregnancy in the Collaborative Perinatal Project (Heinonen et al., 1977).

No animal teratology studies of sulfathiazole have been published.

Please see agent summary on sulfamethoxazole for information on a related drug that has been more thoroughly studied.

Key References

Heinonen OP, Slone D, Shapiro S: Birth Defects and Drugs in Pregnancy. Littleton, Mass.: John Wright-PSG, 1977, pp 298, 301, 434-435. [E]

SULFINPYRAZONE

Synonyms

Anturane

Summary

Sulfinpyrazone is a uricosuric agent. It is used to treat chronic gout.

Comment

None

Magnitude of Teratogenic Risk

Undetermined

Quality and Quantity of Data

None

Comment

None

No epidemiological studies of congenital anomalies in infants born to women who used sulfinpyrazone during pregnancy have been reported.

No animal teratology studies of sulfinpyrazone have been published.

Please see agent summary on phenylbutazone for information on a chemically related drug that has been studied.

Key References

None available.

SULFISOXAZOLE

Synonyms

Acetyl Sulphafurazole, Chemovag, Gantrisin, Koro-Sulf, Lipo Gantrisin, Novosoxazole, SK-Soxazole, Sosol, Soxa, Soxomide, Sulfafurazole, Urizole, Velmatrol

Summary

Sulfisoxazole is a sulfonamide used in the treatment of urinary tract and other infections.

Magnitude of Teratogenic Risk

None To Minimal

Quality and Quantity of Data

Fair To Good

Comment

None

The frequencies of congenital anomalies in general, of major malformations, of minor anomalies, and of major classes of congenital anomalies were no greater than expected among the children of 796 women who were treated with sulfisoxazole during the first four lunar months of pregnancy in the Collaborative Perinatal Project (Heinonen et al., 1977). The frequency of congenital anomalies was not increased among the infants of 4287 women who were treated with this drug anytime during pregnancy in this study. Similarly, the frequency of congenital anomalies was no greater than expected among the children of more than 100 and 215 women, respectively, who had been treated with sulfisoxazole during the first trimester of pregnancy in two separate cohorts of the Boston Collaborative Drug Surveillance Program (Jick et al., 1981; Aselton et al., 1985).

Increased frequencies of cleft palate and other facial malformations have been observed among the offspring of mice and rats treated with eight times the usual human dose of sulfisoxazole during pregnancy (Kato & Katagawa, 1973a, b; Lee & Chun, 1975). The relevance of this observation to the therapeutic use of sulfisoxazole in human pregnancy is unknown.

Key References

Aselton P, Jick H, Milunsky A, Hunter JR, et al.: First-trimester drug use and congenital disorders. Obstet Gynecol 65:451-455, 1985. [S]

Heinonen OP, Slone D, Shapiro S: Birth Defects and Drugs in Pregnancy. Littleton, Mass.: John Wright-PSG, 1977, pp 306, 472, 485. [E]

Jick H, Holmes LB, Hunter JR, Madsen S, et al.: First-trimester drug use and congenital disorders. JAMA 246:343-346, 1981. [S]

Kato T, Kitagawa S: Production of congenital anomalies in fetuses of rats and mice with various sulfonamides. Congenital Anomalies (Senten Ijo) 13:7-15, 1973. [A]

Kato T, Kitagawa S: Production of congenital skeletal anomalies in the fetuses of pregnant rats and mice treated with various sulfonamides. Congenital Anomalies (Senten Ijo) 13:17-23, 1973. [A]

Lee KH, Chun KH: [Studies on the effects of sulfisoxazole on developing rat fetuses.] Ch'Oesin Uihak 18:295-300, 1975. [A]

SULFURATED LIME

Synonyms

Calcium Monosulfide, Calcium Sulfide, Vlemasque

Summary

Sulfurated lime is a mixture of calcium sulphate and calcium sulphide. It is used topically as a treatment for acne.

Magnitude of Teratogenic Risk

Undetermined

Quality and Quantity of Data

None

Comment

A small risk cannot be excluded, but a high risk of congenital anomalies in the children of women treated with sulfurated lime during pregnancy is unlikely.

No epidemiological studies of congenital anomalies in infants born to women who used sulfurated lime during pregnancy have been reported.

No animal teratology studies of sulfurated lime have been published.

Key References

None available.

SULINDAC

Synonyms

Clinoril

Summary

Sulindac is a nonsteroidal anti-inflammatory agent with analgesic and antipyretic action. It is commonly used in the treatment of rheumatic and other musculoskeletal disorders.

Magnitude of Teratogenic Risk

Undetermined

Quality and Quantity of Data

None To Poor

Comment

None

No epidemiological studies of congenital anomalies in children born to women treated with sulindac during pregnancy have been reported.

An increased frequency of cleft palate and other malformations was observed among the offspring of mice treated during pregnancy with sulindac in doses similar to those used in humans (Montenegro & Palomino, 1990). A typical dose-response relationship is said to have been observed with doses in and slightly above the human therapeutic range.

In utero constriction or closure of the ductus arteriosus has been observed in rats exposed to 1-100 times the usual human dose of sulindac late in pregnancy (Momma & Takeuchi, 1983a, b). This effect has not been reported for sulindac in humans, but premature closure of the ductus arteriosus has been associated with maternal use of chemically related nonsteroidal anti- inflammatory agents (Grella & Zanor, 1978).

Please consult agent summary on indomethacin for information on a similar agent that has been more thoroughly studied.

Key References

Grella P, Zanor P: Premature labor and indomethacin. Prostaglandins 16:1007-1017, 1978. [S]

Momma K, Takeuchi H: Constriction of fetal ductus arteriosus by nonsteroidal antiinflammatory drugs. Adv Prostaglandin Thromboxane Leukotriene Res 12:499-503, 1983a. [A]

Momma K, Takeuchi H: Constriction of fetal ductus arteriosus by non-steroidal anti-inflammatory drugs. Prostaglandins 26:631-643, 1983b. [A]

Montenegro MA, Palomino H: Induction of cleft palate in mice by inhibitors of prostaglandin synthesis. J Craniofac Genet Dev Biol 10:83-94, 1990. [A]

SUMATRIPTAN

Synonyms

GR 43175

Summary

Sumatriptan is a serotonin receptor agonist used in the treatment of migraine headache. It is administered orally or, in a much smaller dose, subcutaneously.

Magnitude of Teratogenic Risk

Undetermined

Quality and Quantity of Data

None

Comment

None

No epidemiological studies of congenital anomalies among infants born to women treated with sumatriptan during pregnancy have been reported.

No animal teratology studies of sumatriptan have been published, although the manufacturer reports that they have been done in the rat and rabbit and were negative (Humphrey et al., 1991).

Key References

Humphrey PPA, Feniuk W, Marriott AS, et al.: Preclinical studies on the anti-migraine drug, sumatriptan. Eur Neurol 31:282-290, 1991. [R]

SUTILAINS

Synonyms

Travase

Summary

Sutilains is a topical preparation containing proteolytic enzymes derived from Bacillus subtilis. It is used as a debriding agent for burns and other wounds.

Magnitude of Teratogenic Risk

Undetermined

Quality and Quantity of Data

None

Comment

A small risk cannot be excluded, but a high risk of congenital anomalies in the children of women treated with sutilains during pregnancy is unlikely.

No epidemiological studies of congenital anomalies in infants whose mothers were treated with sutilains during pregnancy have been reported.

No animal teratology studies of sutilains have been published.

Key References

None available.

TALBUTAL

Synonyms

Lotusate

Summary

Talbutal is an intermediate-acting barbiturate that is administered orally as a sedative and hypnotic.

Magnitude of Teratogenic Risk

Undetermined

Quality and Quantity of Data

None

Comment

A small risk cannot be excluded, but a high risk of congenital anomalies in the children of women treated with talbutal during pregnancy is unlikely.

No epidemiological studies of congenital anomalies in infants whose mothers were treated with talbutal during pregnancy have been reported.

No animal teratology studies of talbutal have been published.

Key References

None available.

TAMOXIFEN

Synonyms

Nolvadex

Summary

Tamoxifen is a nonsteroidal antiestrogenic agent that also has some estrogenic activity. It is given orally to induce ovulation and to treat breast cancer.

Magnitude of Teratogenic Risk

Undetermined

Quality and Quantity of Data

Poor

Comment

A small risk cannot be excluded, but a high risk of congenital anomalies in the children of women treated with tamoxifen during pregnancy is unlikely.

No epidemiological studies of congenital anomalies among infants born to women treated with tamoxifen during pregnancy have been reported. No congenital anomalies were observed among nine infants born to women whose pregnancies occurred after ovulation induction with tamoxifen; five other pregnancies conceived after ovulation induction with tamoxifen in this series were spontaneously aborted (Ruiz-Velasco et al., 1979).

The frequency of malformations in the offspring was not altered but the frequency of embryonic loss or fetal death was increased after maternal treatment of pregnant rabbits or rats with tamoxifen in doses similar to those used in humans (Esaki & Sakai, 1980; Furr et al., 1976, 1979; Furr & Jordan, 1984). Frequent miscarriage or failure of implantation was also observed in dogs treated early in pregnancy with tamoxifen in doses similar to those used in humans (Bowen et al., 1988). No fetal abnormalities were noted among the offspring of marmosets treated during pregnancy with tamoxifen in doses about 6 times greater than those used in humans (Furr et al., 1979; Furr & Jordan, 1984).

Epithelial abnormalities have been observed in human fetal genital tract tissue grown in nude mice injected with tamoxifen pellets

(Cunha et al., 1987). Studies of vaginal cytology in girls and women born after tamoxifen-induced ovulation have not yet been reported.

Please see agent summary on clomiphene for information on a closely related drug that has been more thoroughly studied.

Key References

Bowen RA, Olson PN, Young S, Withrow SJ: Efficacy and toxicity of tamoxifen citrate for prevention and termination of pregnancy in bitches. Am J Vet Res 49:27-31, 1988. [A]

Cunha GR, Taguchi O, Namikawa R, et al.: Teratogenic effects of clomiphene, tamoxifen, and diethylstilbestrol on the developing human female genital tract. Hum Pathol 18:1132-43, 1987. [A]

Esaki K, Sakai Y: Influence of oral administration of tamoxifen on the rabbit fetus. Jitchuken Zenrinsho Kenkyuho 6:217-232, 1980. [A]

Furr BJA, Jordan VC: The pharmacology and clinical uses of tamoxifen. Pharmacol Ther 25:127-205, 1984. [R]

Furr BJ, Patterson JS, Richardson DN, et al.: Tamoxifen. In: Goldberg ME (ed). Pharmacological and Biochemical Properties of Drug Substances, Vol 2. Washington, D.C.: American Pharmaceutical Association, 1979, pp 355-399. [R]

Furr BJA, Valcaccia B, Challis JRG: The effects of nolvadex (tamoxifen citrate; ICI 46,474) on pregnancy in rabbits. J Reprod Fert 48:367-369, 1976. [A]

Ruiz-Velasco V, Rosas-Arceo J, Matute MM: Chemical inducers of ovulation: Comparative results. Int J Fertil 24:61-64, 1979. [S]

TAZOLOL

Synonyms

RS-6245

Summary

Tazolol is a nonspecific beta andrenoreceptor blocker used as a cardiotonic agent.

Magnitude of Teratogenic Risk

Undetermined

Quality and Quantity of Data

None

Comment

None

No epidemiological studies of congenital anomalies in infants born to women who used tazolol during pregnancy have been reported.

No animal teratology studies of tazolol have been published.

Key References

None available.

TEFLURANE

Synonyms

DA-708

Summary

Teflurane is a general anesthetic administered by inhalation.

Magnitude of Teratogenic Risk

Undetermined

Quality and Quantity of Data

None

Comment

None

No epidemiological studies of congenital anomalies in children born to women exposed to teflurane during pregnancy have been reported.

No studies of teratologic effects of teflurane in experimental mammals have been published.

Please see agent summary on halothane for information on a related agent that has been studied.

Key References

None available.

TEMAZEPAM

Synonyms

Cerepax, Euhypnos, Hydroxydiazepam, Lenal, Levanxol, Maeva, Normison, Remestan, Restoril

Summary

Temazepam is a benzodiazepine derivative that is used as a hypnotic.

Magnitude of Teratogenic Risk

Undetermined

Quality and Quantity of Data

None

Comment

None

No epidemiological studies of congenital anomalies among the children of women treated with temazepam during pregnancy have been reported.

No animal teratology studies of temazepam have been published.

Please see agent summary on diazepam for information on a chemically related drug which has been studied.

Key References

None available.

TERAZOSIN

Synonyms

Hytrin

Summary

Terazosin is an alpha-1-adrenergic receptor blocking agent that is administered orally in the treatment of hypertension.

Magnitude of Teratogenic Risk

Undetermined

Quality and Quantity of Data

None

Comment

None

No epidemiological studies of congenital anomalies among infants born to women treated with terazosin during pregnancy have been reported.

No animal teratology studies of terazosin have been published.

Please see agent summary on prazosin for information on a related agent that has been studied.

Key References

None available.

TERBUTALINE

Synonyms

Brethaire, Brethine, Bricanyl, Feevone, Fil-air, Terbasmin

Summary

Terbutaline is a direct-acting sympathomimetic agent. It is used as a bronchodilator and to inhibit premature labor.

Magnitude of Teratogenic Risk

Undetermined

Quality and Quantity of Data

None To Poor

Comment

None

No epidemiological studies of congenital anomalies in infants born to women who took terbutaline during early pregnancy have been reported. Normal weight and development were observed among 21 18-month old children born of pregnancies complicated by premature labor treated with terbutaline (Karlsson et al., 1980).

No adverse effect on fetal survival was seen after treatment of rats with 7-33 times the human dose of terbutaline late in pregnancy (Kudlacz et al., 1989, 1990; Hou & Slotkin, 1989). Decreased neonatal weight was observed in some of these studies at the higher dose.

Fetal tachycardia and transient neonatal hypoglycemia have been observed following short-term maternal terbutaline therapy late in pregnancy (Ingemarsson, 1976; Wallace et al., 1978; Epstein et al., 1979; Sharif et al., 1990). Maternal terbutaline therapy has been used successfully to treat acute intrapartum fetal distress (Tejani et al., 1983; Ingemarsson et al., 1985; Mendez-Bauer et al., 1987; Shekarloo et al., 1989).

Please see agent summary on metaproterenol for information on a similar drug that has been more thoroughly studied .

Key References

Epstein MG, Nicholls E, Stubblefield PG: Neonatal hypoglycemia after beta-sympathomimetic tocolytic therapy. J Pediatr 94:449-453, 1979. [C]

Hou Q-C, Slotkin TA: Effects of prenatal dexamethasone or terbutaline exposure on development of neural and intrinsic control of heart rate. Pediatr Res 26(6):554-557, 1989. [A]

Ingemarsson I: Effect of terbutaline on premature labor. A double-blind placebo-controlled study. Am J Obstet Gynecol 125:520-524, 1976. [E]

Ingemarsson I, Arulkumaran S, Ratnam SS: Single injection of terbutaline in term labor. I. Effect on fetal pH in cases with prolonged bradycardia. Am J Obstet Gynecol 153(8):859-864, 1985. [S]

Karlsson K, Krantz M, Hamberger L: Comparison of various betamimetics on preterm labor, survival and development of the child. J Perinat Med 8:19-26, 1980. [S]

Kudlacz EM, Navarro HA, Eylers JP, et al.: Effects of prenatal terbutaline exposure on cellular development in lung and liver of neonatal rat: Ornithine decarboxylase activity and macromolecules. Pediatr Res 25(6):617-622, 1989. [A]

Kudlacz EM, Navarro HA, Slotkin TA: Regulation of beta-adrenergic receptor-mediated processes in fetal rat lung: Selective desensitization caused by chronic terbutaline exposure. J Dev Physiol 14:103-108, 1990. [A]

Mendez-Bauer C, Shekarloo A, Cook V, Freese U: Treatment of acute intrapartum fetal distress by beta2-sympathomimetics. Am J Obstet Gynecol 156:638-642, 1987. [S]

Sharif DS, Huhta JC, Moise KJ, et al.: Changes in fetal hemodynamics with terbutaline treatment and premature labor. J Clin Ultrasound 18:85-89, 1990. [E]

Shekarloo A, Mendez-Bauer C, Cook V, Freese U: Terbutaline (intravenous bolus) for the treatment of acute intrapartum fetal distress. Am J Obstet Gynecol 160:615-618, 1989. [S]

Tejani NA, Verma UL, Chatterjee S, Mittelmann S: Terbutaline in the management of acute intrapartum fetal acidosis. J Reprod Med 28:857-861, 1983. [S]

Wallace RL, Caldwell DL, Ansbacher R, Otterson WN: Inhibition of premature labor by terbutaline. Obstet Gynecol 51:387-393, 1978. [S]

TERCONAZOLE

Synonyms

Terazol, Triaconazole

Summary

Terconazole is an antifungal agent.

Magnitude of Teratogenic Risk

Undetermined

Quality and Quantity of Data

None To Poor

Comment

None

No epidemiological studies of congenital anomalies in infants born to women who had been treated with terconazole during pregnancy have been reported.

No animal teratology studies of terconazole have been published.

Key References

None available.

TERFENADINE

Synonyms

Seldane

Summary

Terfenadine is an antihistamine used to relieve seasonal allergic reactions such as sneezing, rhinorrhea, pruritis, and lacrimation.

Magnitude of Teratogenic Risk

Undetermined

Quality and Quantity of Data

Poor

Comment

A small risk cannot be excluded, but a high risk of congenital anomalies in the children of women treated with terfenadine during pregnancy is unlikely.

No epidemiological studies of congenital anomalies in infants whose mothers took terfenadine during pregnancy have been reported.

No increased frequency of malformations was found in rats or rabbits born to mothers orally given 30-300 and 30-500 times the usual therapeutic dose of terfenadine during embryonic development, despite the fact higher doses were toxic to some mothers (Gibson et al., 1982).

Key References

Gibson JP, Huffman KW, Newborne JW: Preclinical safety studies with terfenadine. Arzneimittelforsch 22:1179-1184, 1982. [A]

TERPIN HYDRATE

Synonyms

Terpene Hydrate, Terpinol

Summary

Terpin hydrate is an cyclic alcohol that is taken orally as an oral expectorant.

Magnitude of Teratogenic Risk

None

Quality and Quantity of Data

Fair To Good

Comment

None

The frequency of congenital anomalies was no greater than expected among the infants of more than 244 women who took terpin hydrate during the first trimester of pregnancy in two cohorts of the Boston Collaborative Drug Surveillance Program (Jick et al., 1981; Aselton et al., 1985). Similarly, the frequency of congenital anomalies was not significantly increased among the children of 146 women who took terpin hydrate during the first four lunar months of pregnancy or among the children of 1762 women who took this medication anytime during pregnancy in the Collaborative Perinatal Project (Heinonen et al., 1977). No association with maternal use of terpin hydrate during the first trimester of pregnancy was observed in a case-control study involving 266 infants with congenital anomalies (Mellin, 1964).

No animal teratology studies of terpin hydrate have been published.

Key References

Aselton P, Jick H, Milunsky A, Hunter JR, et al.: First-trimester drug use and congenital disorders. Obstet Gynecol 65:451-455, 1985. [S]

Jick H, Holmes LB, Hunter JR, Madsen S, et al.: First-trimester drug use and congenital disorders. JAMA 246:343-346, 1981. [S]

Heinonen OP, Slone D, Shapiro S: Birth Defects and Drugs in Pregnancy. Littleton, Mass.: John Wright-PSG, 1977, pp 378-380, 383, 438, 442, 478, 496. [E]

Mellin GW: Drugs in the first trimester of pregnancy and the fetal life of Homo sapiens. Am J Obstet Gynecol 90:1169-1180, 1964. [E]

TESTOLACTONE

Synonyms

1-Dehydrotestololactone, Fludestrin, Teslac

Summary

Testolactone is a derivative of testosterone that is given orally in the treatment of breast cancer. Testolactone has virtually no virilizing activity but is an inhibitor of estrogen synthesis.

Magnitude of Teratogenic Risk

Undetermined

Quality and Quantity of Data

None

Comment

None

No epidemiological studies of congenital anomalies among infants born to women treated with testolactone during pregnancy have been reported.

No animal teratology studies of testolactone have been published.

Key References

None available.

TESTOSTERONE

Synonyms

Andro 100, Andronaq, Delatestryl, Depotestosterone, Malogen L.A., Oreton, Primoteston, Restandol, Sustanon, Virormone

Summary

Testosterone, the principle androgen synthesized by the testis, ovary, and adrenal gland, normally functions in male embryos to virilize the external genitalia. Testosterone is used medically to treat postpartum breast engorgement and as a palliative therapy for breast cancer. Testosterone is also employed to promote body building.

Magnitude of Teratogenic Risk

Virilization Of Female Genitalia: Moderate

Nongenital Malformations: Undetermined

Quality and Quantity of Data

Virilization Of Female Genitalia: Fair To Good

Nongenital Malformations: Poor

Comment

A small risk cannot be excluded, but a high risk of nongenital malformations in the children of women who used testosterone during pregnancy is unlikely.

No epidemiological studies of congenital anomalies among infants born to women treated with testosterone during pregnancy have been reported, but there are at least 16 reports of female infants with virilization of the external genitalia who were born to women treated with testosterone or methyltestosterone during pregnancy (Grumbach & Ducharme, 1960; Schardein, 1985). Similar cases have been reported with maternal use of other androgenic hormones during pregnancy. Affected female infants exhibit clitoral hypertrophy with or without labioscrotal fusion. The uterus, tubes, and ovaries are normal, and normal female secondary sexual development occurs at puberty (Reschini et al., 1985).

Virilization of external genital structures has been demonstrated among the female offspring of pregnant monkeys, rodents, rabbits, and other mammals treated with testosterone, usually in doses considerably larger than those used in humans (Raynaud, 1937; Hamilton & Wolfe, 1938; Jost, 1947; Wells & van Wagenen, 1954; Phoenix et al., 1959; Schardein, 1985; Ford & Christenson, 1987; Goy et al., 1988; Eaton et al., 1990). In some species, fetal loss is frequently seen (Jost, 1947; Fritz et al., 1984; Sarkar et al., 1986). Nongenital malformations were generally not reported, but most of these studies were not designed to look for nongenital defects. Alternations of sexually dimorphic behavior have been observed in female guinea pigs, rats, and monkeys exposed to testosterone prenatally (Phoenix et al., 1959; Goy et al., 1964, 1988; Huffman & Hendricks, 1981; Hoepfner & Ward, 1988; Eaton et al., 1990).

Key References

Eaton GG, Worlein JM, Glick BB: Sex differences in Japanese macaques (Macaca fuscata): Effects of prenatal testosterone on juvenile social behavior. Horm Behav 24(2):270-283, 1990. [A]

Ford JJ, Christenson RK: Influences of pre- and postnatal testosterone treatment on defeminization of sexual receptivity in pigs. Biol Reprod 36:581-587, 1987. [A]

Fritz H, Giese K, Suter HP: Prenatal and postnatal development of rats following the maternal treatment with testosterone during the late period of embryogenesis. Arzneimittelforsch 34:780-782, 1984. [A]

Goy RW, Bercovitch FB, McBrair MC: Behavioral masculinization is independent of genital masculinization in prenatally androgenized female rhesus macaques. Horm Behav 22(4):552-571, 1988. [A]

Goy RW, Bridson WE, Young WC: Period of maximal susceptibility of the prenatal female guinea pig to masculinizing actions of testosterone propionate. J Comp Physiol Psychol 57(2):166-174, 1964. [A]

Grumbach MM, Ducharme JR: The effects of androgens on fetal sexual development. Androgen-induced female pseudohermaphrodism. Fertil Steril 11:157-180, 1960. [A]

Hamilton JB, Wolfe JM: The effect of male hormone substances upon birth and prenatal development in the rat. Anat Rec 70(Suppl 3):433-440, 1938. [A]

Hoepfner BA, Ward IL: Prenatal and neonatal androgen exposure interact to affect sexual differentiation in female rats. Behav Neurosci 102(1):61-65, 1988. [A]

Huffman L, Hendricks SE: Prenatally injected testosterone propionate and sexual behavior of female rats. Physiol Behav 26(5):773-778, 1981. [A]

Jost A: Studies about the sexual differentiation of the rabbit embryo. 2. Effect of synthetic androgens on genital histogenesis. Arch Anat Microsc Morphol Exp 36:242-270, 1947. [A]

Phoenix CH, Goy RW, Gerall AA, et al.: Organizing action of prenatally administered testosterone propionate on the tissues mediating mating behavior in the female guinea pig. Endocrinology 65:369-382, 1959. [A]

Raynaud A: Intersexuality produced in the female mouse by injection of male hormone to the pregnant mother. C R Soc Biol 126:866-868, 1937. [A]

Reschini E, Giustina G, D'Alberton A, Candiani GB: Female pseudohermaphroditism due to maternal androgen administration: 25-year follow-up. Lancet 1:1226, 1985. [C]

Sarkar K, Kinson GA, Rowsell HC: Embryo resorption following administration of steroidal compounds to rats in mid pregnancy. Can J Vet Res 50:433-437, 1986. [A]

Schardein JL: Chemically Induced Birth Defects. New York: Marcel Dekker, 1985, pp 260-265. [R]

Wells LJ, van Wagenen G: Androgen-induced female pseudohermaphroditism in the monkey (Macaca mulatta): Anatomy of the reproductive organs. Carnegie Contrib Embryol 35:93-106, 1954. [A]

TETANUS IMMUNE GLOBULIN

Synonyms

Hyper-Tet, TIG

Summary

Tetanus immune globulin is the gamma globulin fraction of plasma derived from humans who have been immunized with tetanus vaccine. It is administered intramuscularly to provide immunization against tetanus and in the treatment of tetanus.

Magnitude of Teratogenic Risk

Undetermined

Quality and Quantity of Data

None

Comment

A small risk cannot be excluded, but a high risk of congenital anomalies in the children of women treated with tetanus immune globulin during pregnancy is unlikely.

No epidemiological studies of congenital anomalies in infants whose mothers were treated with tetanus immune globulin during pregnancy have been reported.

No animal teratology studies of tetanus immune globulin have been published.

Key References

None available.

TETRACAINE

Synonyms

Amethocaine, Anethaine, Contralgine, Pantocain, Pontocaine

Summary

Tetracaine is a local anesthetic of the ester class.

Magnitude of Teratogenic Risk

Undetermined

None To Poor

Comment

A small risk cannot be excluded, but there is no indication that the risk of congenital anomalies in the children of women treated with tetracaine during pregnancy is likely to be great.

The frequency of congenital anomalies was not increased among the offspring of 23 women treated with tetracaine during the first four lunar months of pregnancy in the Collaborative Perinatal Project (Heinonen et al., 1977).

No studies of teratologic effects of tetracaine in experimental mammals have been published.

Please see agent summary on lidocaine for information on a related agent that has been more thoroughly studied.

Key References

Heinonen OP, Slone D, Shapiro S: Birth Defects and Drugs in Pregnancy. Littleton, Mass.: John Wright-PSG, 1977, pp 358, 360. [E]

1,2,2,2-TETRA-CHLOROETHANE

Synonyms

Acetylene Tetrachloride, Symtetrachloroethane

Summary

1,1,2,2-tetrachloroethane is a solvent and insecticide. The eight hour time-weighted average threshold limit value for occupational exposure is 1 ppm (6.9 mg/cu m) (HSDB, 1993). 1,1,2,2-tetrachloroethane is readily absorbed through the skin.

Magnitude of Teratogenic Risk

Undetermined

Quality and Quantity of Data

None

Comment

None

No epidemiological studies of congenital anomalies among infants whose mothers were exposed to 1,1,2,2-tetrachloroethane during pregnancy have been reported.

No animal teratology studies of 1,1,2,2-tetrachloroethane have been published.

Key References

HSDB [database online]. Bethesda, Md.: National Library of Medicine; 1985- [updated 1993 April 30]. Available from: National Library of Medicine; BRS Information Technologies, McLean, Va. [O]

TETRACYCLINE

Synonyms

Achromycin, Cefracycline, Cyclopar, Medicycline, Novotetra, Panmycin, Retet-S, Robitet, Sumycin, Topicycline

Summary

Tetracycline is a broad-spectrum antibiotic. It is frequently used in treatment of respiratory tract infections, acne, and other infections.

Magnitude of Teratogenic Risk

Dental Staining: High

Malformations: None To Minimal

Quality and Quantity of Data

Dental Staining: Excellent

Malformations: Fair

Comment

Tetracycline causes staining of the primary dentition in fetuses exposed during the second or third trimesters of pregnancy (Toaff & Ravid, 1966; Cohlan, 1977).

The frequencies of congenital anomalies in general, of major malformations, and of minor anomalies were no greater than expected among the children of 341 women treated with tetracycline during the first four lunar months of pregnancy in the Collaborative Perinatal Project (Heinonen et al., 1977). Similarly, the frequency of congenital anomalies was not increased among the children of 1336 women treated with this medicine anytime during pregnancy. No increase in malformations was found among more than 274 infants of women who took tetracycline during the first trimester of pregnancy in two cohorts of the Boston Collaborative Drug Surveillance Program (Jick et al., 1981; Aselton et al., 1985). An association with maternal use of tetracycline during pregnancy was observed among 46 infants with transposition of the great arteries in one case-control study (Zierler & Rothman, 1985).

The dental staining caused by in utero exposure to tetracycline appears to be only of cosmetic significance, not affecting development of the enamel or the likelihood of forming caries (Genot et al., 1970; Rebich et al., 1985). Similar staining has been found in the bones and lenses of fetuses whose mothers were treated with tetracycline during gestation (Cohlan et al., 1963; Totterman & Saxen, 1969; Krejci & Brettschneider, 1983). Tetracycline administration has been associated with decreased rates of bone growth in premature infants (Cohlan et al., 1963).

Tetracycline exposure during the first trimester of gestation was reported for four babies with congenital or infantile cataracts (Farrar & Mackie, 1964; Harley et al., 1964). These observations were not made in controlled studies, and no definite conclusion can be drawn regarding a possible association between maternal tetracycline exposure and development of cataracts.

One study has been reported in which cleft palate and limb defects were observed among the offspring of pregnant rats treated with therapeutic doses of tetracycline (Filippi, 1967). This finding has not been confirmed in other investigations in rats despite the use of dosages 12-62 times those employed in humans (Mennie, 1962; Hurley et al., 1963). No teratogenic effect was observed among the offspring of rabbits treated during pregnancy with tetracycline in a dose similar to that used in humans (Brown et al., 1968). Treatment of pregnant rats with tetracycline in doses similar to those used clinically results in intense staining of the fetal skeleton (Bevelander & Cohlan, 1962), but the clinical significance of this observation is uncertain (Cohlan, 1980). Staining of the cornea and lens of the eye has also been observed among the fetuses of pregnant rats treated with therapeutic doses of tetracycline (Krejci et al., 1980).

Key References

Aselton P, Jick H, Milunsky A, et al.: First-trimester drug use and congenital disorders. Obstet Gynecol 65:451-455, 1985. [S]

Bevelander G, Cohlan SQ: The effect on the rat fetus of transplacentally acquired tetracycline. Biol Neonat 4:365-370, 1962. [A]

Brown DM, Harper KH, Palmer AK, Tesh SA: Effect of antibiotics upon pregnancy in the rabbit. Toxicol Appl Pharmacol 12:295, 1968. [A]

Cohlan SQ: Drugs and pregnancy. Prog Clin Biol Res 44:77-96, 1980. [A]

Cohlan SQ: Tetracycline staining of teeth. Teratology 15:127-130, 1977. [R]

Cohlan SQ, Bevelander G, Tiamsic T: Growth inhibition of prematures receiving tetracycline. Am J Dis Child 105:453-461, 1963. [C], [S], & [A]

Farrar JF, Mackie IJ: Survey of possible causes of congenital malformation. Med J Aust 2:702-704, 1964. [C]

Filippi B: Antibiotics and congenital malformations: Evaluation of the teratogenicity of antibiotics. Adv Teratol 2:239-256, 1967. [A]

Genot MT, Golan HP, Porter PJ, Kass EH: Effect of administration of tetracycline in pregnancy on the primary dentition of the offspring. J Oral Med 25:75-79, 1970. [E]

Harley JD, Farrar JF, Gray JB, et al.: Aromatic drugs and congenital cataracts. Lancet 1:472-473, 1964. [S]

Heinonen O, Slone D, Shapiro S: Birth Defects and Drugs in Pregnancy. Littleton, Mass.: John Wright-PSG, 1977, pp 296-313. [E]

Hurley LS, Tuchmann-Duplessis H: Influence of tetracycline on the pre- and postnatal development of the rat. C R Acad Sci [D] (Paris) 257:302-304, 1963. [A]

Jick H, Holmes LB, Hunter JR, et al.: First trimester drug use and congenital disorders. JAMA 246:343-346, 1981. [E]

Krejci L, Brettschneider I: Congenital cataract due to tetracycline. Animal experiments and clinical observation. Ophthalmic Paediatr Genet 3(1):59-60, 1983. [A] & [S]

Krejci L, Brettschneider I, Triska J: Eye changes due to systemic use of tetracycline in pregnancy. Ophthalmic Res 12:73-77, 1980. [A]

Mennie AT: Tetracycline and congenital limb abnormalities. Br Med J 2:480, 1962. [A]

Rebich T, Kumar J, Brustman B: Dental caries and tetracycline-stained dentition in an American Indian population. J Dent Res 64(3):462-464, 1985. [E]

Rogers JM, Chernoff N: Chemically induced cataracts in the fetus and neonate. In: Kacew S & Lock S (eds). Toxicologic and Pharmacologic Principles in Pediatrics. New York: Hemisphere Publishing Corp., 1988, pp 255-276. [R]

Toaff R, Ravid R: Tetracyclines and the teeth. Lancet 2:281-282, 1966. [S]

Totterman LE, Saxen L: Incorporation of tetracycline into human foetal bones after maternal drug administration. Acta Obstet Gynecol Scand 48:542-549, 1969. [S]

Zierler S, Rothman KJ: Congenital heart disease in relation to maternal use of Bendectin and other drugs in early pregnancy. N Engl J Med 313:347-352, 1985. [E]

TETRAHYDROZOLINE

Synonyms

Cleer, Collyrium, Murine Plus, Tetryzoline Hydrochloride, Tyzine, Visine

Summary

Tetrahydrozoline is an alpha-adrenergic sympathomimetic agent. It is used topically as a nasal and conjunctival decongestant.

Magnitude of Teratogenic Risk

Undetermined

Quality and Quantity of Data

None

Comment

A small risk cannot be excluded, but a high risk of congenital anomalies in the children of women treated with tetrahydrozoline during pregnancy is unlikely.

No epidemiological studies of congenital anomalies among infants born to women who used tetrahydrozoline during pregnancy have been reported.

No animal teratology studies of tetrahydrozoline have been published.

Please see agent summary on ephedrine for information on a related agent that has been studied.

Key References

None available.

THEOPHYLLINE

Synonyms

Aerolate, Bronkodyl, Constant-T, Elixophyllin, Quibron-T, Slo-Bid, Slo-Phyllin, Somophyllin, Sustaire, Theo-Dur, Theobid, Theo-clear

Summary

Theophylline is a xanthine derivative with strong diuretic action. It is used as a bronchodilator and as a stimulant of myocardial and respiratory function. Theophylline is found in many teas.

Magnitude of Teratogenic Risk

None To Minimal

Quality and Quantity of Data

Poor To Fair

Comment

None

The frequency of congenital anomalies was no greater than expected among the children of 193 women who took medications containing theophylline during the first four lunar months of pregnancy or among the children of 653 women who took such medicines anytime during pregnancy in the Collaborative Perinatal Project (Heinonen et al., 1977). The frequency of stillbirth was not increased among the pregnancies of 253 asthmatic women treated with theophylline in this study (Neff & Leviton, 1990). Three infants with various severe cardiovascular malformations who were born to asthmatic women treated with theophylline throughout pregnancy have been reported (Park et al., 1990), but no cause and effect relationship can be inferred from these anecdotal observations.

An increased frequency of congenital anomalies was observed among the offspring of pregnant mice and rats treated with theophylline in doses 6-25 times those used therapeutically in humans (Georges & Denef, 1968; Fujii & Nishimura, 1969, Tucci & Skalko, 1978; Lindstrom et al., 1990). Cleft palate and skeletal anomalies were most frequently observed. A typical dose-response relationship was demonstrated. The relevance

of these observations to the clinical use of theophylline in human pregnancy is unknown.

Transient theophylline toxicity characterized by jitteriness and tachycardia has been observed in neonates born shortly after maternal ingestion of theophylline (Turner et al., 1980; Spector, 1984).

Key References

Fujii T, Nishimura H: Teratogenic actions of some methylated xanthines in mice. Okajimas Fol Anat Jap 46:167-175, 1969. [A]

Georges A, Denef J: [Digital anomalies: Teratogenic manifestations from xanthine derivatives administered to rats]. Arch Int Pharmacodyn Ther 172:219-222, 1968. [A]

Heinonen OP, Slone D, Shapiro S: Birth Defects and Drugs in Pregnancy. Littleton, Mass.: John Wright-PSG, 1977, pp 366-370. [E]

Lindstrom P, Morrissey RE, George JD, et al.: The developmental toxicity of orally administered theophylline in rats and mice. Fundam Appl Toxicol 14:167-178, 1990. [A]

Neff RK, Leviton A: Maternal theophylline consumption and the risk of stillbirth. Chest 97:1266-1267, 1990. [E]

Park JM, Schmer V, Myers TL: Cardiovascular anomalies associated with prenatal exposure to theophylline. South Med J 83(12):1487-1488, 1990. [C]

Spector SL: Reciprocal relationship between pregnancy and pulmonary disease. Chest 86(S):1S-5S, 1984. [R]

Tucci SM, Skalko RG: The teratogenic effects of theophylline in mice. Toxicol Lett 1:337-341, 1978. [A]

Turner ES, Greenberger PA, Patterson R: Management of the pregnant asthmatic patient. Ann Intern Med 6:905-918, 1980. [R]

THIABENDAZOLE

Synonyms

Foldan, Lombristop, Mintezol, Minzolum, Nomoxiur, Tiabendazole, Triasox

Summary

Thiabendazole is an antihelmintic used to treat a variety of parasitic infections.

Magnitude of Teratogenic Risk

Undetermined

Quality and Quantity of Data

Poor

Comment

None

No epidemiological studies of congenital anomalies in infants born to women who took thiabendazole during pregnancy have been reported.

An increased frequency of malformations including cleft palate, limb reduction defects, and vertebral fusion defects was observed among the offspring of mice treated with 5-48 times the usual human dose of thiabendazole during pregnancy (Ogata et al., 1984, 1989). This effect exhibited typical time- and dose-dependence. In contrast, no teratogenic effect was observed among the offspring of rats, rabbits, or lambs treated respectively with 1.5-10, 2-16, or 4 times the human dose of thiabendazole during pregnancy (Delatour & Richard, 1976; Robinson et al., 1978; Khera et al., 1979; Szabo et al., 1974). The relevance of these findings to clinical use of thiabendazole in human pregnancy is uncertain.

Key References

Delatour P, Richard Y: Proprietes embryotoxiques et antimitotiques en serie benzimidazole. Therapie 31:505-515, 1976. [A]

Khera KS, Whalen C, Trivett G, Angers G: Assessment of the teratogenic potential of biphenyl, ethoxyquin, piperonyl butoxide, diuron, thiabendazole, phosalone, and lindane in rats. Toxicol Appl Pharmacol 48:A33, 1979. [A]

Ogata A, Ando H, Kubo Y, Hiraga K: Teratogenicity of thiabendazole in ICR mice. Food Chem Toxicol 22:509-520, 1984. [A]

Ogata A, Fujitani T, Yoneyama M, et al.: Glutatione and cysteine enhance and diethylmaleate reduces thiabendazole teratogenicity in mice. Food Chem Toxicol 27(2):117-123, 1989. [A]

Robinson HJ, Phares HF, Graessle OE: The toxicological and antifungal properties of thiabendazole. Ecotoxicol Environ Safety 1:471-476, 1978. [A]

Szabo KT, Miller CR, Scott GC: The effects of methyl-5(6)-butyl-2-benzimidazole carbamate (parbendazole) on reproduction in sheep and other animals. II. Teratological study in ewes in the United States. Cornell Vet 64 (Suppl. 4):41-55, 1974. [A]

THIALBARBITONE

Synonyms

Natrium Cyclohexenylallylthiobarbituricum, Thialbarbital Sodium

Summary

Thialbarbitone is a barbiturate that has been used as an intravenous general anesthetic.

Magnitude of Teratogenic Risk

Undetermined

Quality and Quantity of Data

None

Comment

None

No epidemiological studies of congenital anomalies in children born to women exposed to thialbarbitone during pregnancy have been reported.

No investigations of teratologic effects of thialbarbitone in experimental animals have been published.

Please see agent summary on thiopental for information on a related agent that has been studied.

Key References

None available.

THIAMINE

Synonyms

Aberil, Aneurine Hydrochloride, BayBee-1, Benerva, Betalin S, Betaxin, Vitamin B_1

Summary

Thiamine (vitamin B_1) is an essential dietary component. It is used as a coenzyme in intermediary metabolism. The U.S. Recommended Dietary Allowance of thiamine in pregnancy is 1.4 mg/day. Doses more than 200 times greater than this are used to treat severe deficiency states.

Magnitude of Teratogenic Risk

Undetermined

Quality and Quantity of Data

None To Poor

Comment

A small risk cannot be excluded, but there is no indication that the risk of congenital anomalies in the children of women who take large amounts of thiamine during pregnancy is likely to be great.

No epidemiological studies of congenital anomalies in infants born to mothers who took excessive amounts of thiamine during pregnancy have been reported.

Survival and weight gain of newborn rats were not affected by treatment of the mother with thiamine during pregnancy in doses about 130 times the human recommended daily al-lowance (Schumacher et al., 1965) or about 50 times the rat daily requirement (Morrison & Sarett, 1959).

Maternal thiamine deficiency has been associated with fetal death and decreased fetal weight gain in rats (Nelson & Evans, 1955; Roecklein et al., 1985).

Key References

Morrison AB, Sarett HP: Effects of excess thiamine and pyridoxine on growth and reproduction in rats. J Nutr 69:111-116, 1959. [A]

Nelson MM, Evans HM: Relation of thiamine to reproduction in the rat. J Nutr 55:151-163, 1955. [A]

Roecklein B, Levin SW, Comly M, Mukherjee AB: Intrauterine growth retardation induced by thiamine deficiency and pyrithiamine during pregnancy in the rat. Am J Obstet Gynecol 151:455-460, 1985. [A]

Schumacher MF, Williams MA, Lyman RL: Effect of high intakes of thiamine, riboflavin and pyridoxine on reproduction in rats and vitamin requirements of the offspring. J Nutr 86:343-349, 1965. [A]

THIAMPHENICOL

Synonyms

Dextrosulphenidol, Flogotisol, Glitisol, Neomyson, Racephenicol, Thiamcol, Tiamfenicol, Urfamycine

Summary

Thiamphenicol is a broad spectrum antibiotic.

Magnitude of Teratogenic Risk

Undetermined

Quality and Quantity of Data

Poor

Comment

A small risk cannot be excluded, but there is no indication that the risk of congenital anomalies in the children of women treated with thiamphenicol during pregnancy is likely to be great.

No epidemiological studies of congenital anomalies in children born to women who took thiamphenicol during pregnancy have been reported.

In one series of studies, the frequency of congenital anomalies was no greater than expected among the offspring of mice or rats treated during pregnancy with thiamphenicol in doses, respectively, 1-33 and 1-3 times those used clinically (Suzuki et al., 1973a, b). Fetal loss occurred at the higher doses which were toxic to the mothers. In contrast, an increased frequency of skeletal malformations was reported among the offspring of rats treated with 2 times the usual human dose of thiamphenicol very early in pregnancy in another study (Silva & Andrade, 1970).

Please see agent summary on chloramphenicol for information on a related drug that has been more thoroughly studied.

Key References

Silva NOG, Andrade ATL: The effects of thiophenicol upon the rat conceptus. Fertil Steril 21:431-433, 1970. [A]

Suzuki Y, Kondo S, Okada F, Suzuki I, et al.: [Effects of thiamphenicol administered to the pregnant animals upon the development of their fetuses and neonates.] Oyo Yakuri 7:41-51, 1973a. [A]

Suzuki Y, Okada F, Kondo S, Suzuki I, et al.: [Effects of thiamphenicol glycinate hydrochloride administered to the pregnant animals upon the development of their fetuses and neonates.] Oyo Yakuri 7:859-870, 1973b. [A]

THIAMYLAL

Synonyms

Surital

Summary

Thiamylal is a short-acting barbiturate used intravenously to induce general anesthesia.

Magnitude of Teratogenic Risk

None To Minimal

Quality and Quantity of Data

None To Poor

Comment

None

The frequency of congenital anomalies was not increased among the offspring of 21 women treated with thiamylal during the first four lunar months of pregnancy in the Collaborative Perinatal Project (Heinonen et al., 1977).

An increased frequency of limb and digital anomalies was observed in the offspring of mice treated during pregnancy with thiamylal in doses 3-7 times the usual human dosage, but no teratogenic effect was seen with 1-2 times the human dose (Tanimura, 1965).

Please see agent summary on thiopental for information on a similar agent that has been more thoroughly studied.

Key References

Heinonen OP, Slone D, Shapiro S: Birth Defects and Drugs in Pregnancy. Littleton, Mass.: John Wright-PSG, 1977, pp 336-337. [E]

Tanimura T: The effect of thiamylal sodium administration to pregnant mice upon the development of their offspring. Kaibogaku Zasshi (Acta Anat Nippon) 40:323-328, 1965. [A]

THIETHYLPERAZINE

Synonyms

Norzine, Torecan

Summary

Thiethylperazine is a phenothiazine that is used in the treatment of nausea and vertigo.

Magnitude of Teratogenic Risk

Undetermined

Quality and Quantity of Data

None To Poor

Comment

A small risk cannot be excluded, but a high risk of congenital anomalies in the children of women treated with thiethylperazine during pregnancy is unlikely.

No adequate epidemiological studies of congenital anomalies among infants born to women treated with thiethylperazine during pregnancy have been reported.

The frequency of cleft palate was substantially increased among the offspring of mice and rats treated during pregnancy with thiethylperazine in doses respectively 83-670 and 330 times those used in humans (Szabo & Brent, 1974). The relevance of this observation to clinical use of thiethylperazine in human pregnancy is unknown.

Please see agent summary on chlorpromazine for information on a related agent that has been more thoroughly studied.

Key References

Szabo KT, Brent RL: Species differences in experimental teratogenesis by tranquillising agents. Lancet 1:565, 1974. [A]

THIMEROSAL

Synonyms

Colluspray, Mercurothiolate, Merseptyl, Merthiolate, Nutramersal, Thimerosalate, Thiomersal

Summary

Thimerosal (merthiolate) is a bacteriostatic and fungistatic mercurial compound that is used as a preservative, disinfectant, and topical antiseptic.

Magnitude of Teratogenic Risk

Minimal

Quality and Quantity of Data

Poor

Comment

None

The frequency of congenital anomalies was greater than expected among 56 children born to women who used thimerosal topically during the first four lunar months of pregnancy in the Collaborative Perinatal Project (RR=2.69, p<0.05) (Heinonen et al., 1977). The risk of congenital anomalies of a type that could occur anytime during pregnancy was similar among 60 infants whose mothers were reported to have used topical thimerosal, but this was not statistically significant (RR=3.13, 95% confidence interval 0.87-7.60).

The frequency of malformations was not increased but fetal death was seen more often than expected among the offspring of rats given daily intraperitoneal injections of 1 ml of a thimerosal solution 2-20 times stronger than that used topically in humans (Gasset et al., 1975). Fetal death was seen with increased frequency among the offspring of rabbits in which a thimerosal solution 0.2-20 times as strong as that used topically in humans was instilled into the eyes repeatedly each day (Ito et al., 1972; Gasset et al., 1975). The clinical relevance of these observations is uncertain.

Key References

Gasset AR, Itoi M, Ishii Y, Ramer RM: Teratogenicities of ophthalmic drugs. II. Teratogenicities and tissue accumulation of thimerosal. Arch Ophthalmol 93:52-55, 1975. [A]

Heinonen OP, Slone D, Shapiro S: Birth Defects and Drugs in Pregnancy. Littleton, Mass.: John Wright-PSG, 1977, pp 298, 300, 302, 313, 434-435. [E]

Ito M, Ishii T, Kaneko N: Teratogenicities of antiviral opthalmics on experimental animals. Rinsho Ganka 26:631-640, 1972. [A]

THIOPENTAL

Synonyms

Farmotal, Intraval Sodium, Leopental, Pentothal, Thiobarbital, Tiobarbital

Summary

Thiopental is a fast-acting barbiturate that is used as an intravenous general anesthetic. It is sometimes also administered rectally.

Magnitude of Teratogenic Risk

None To Minimal

Quality and Quantity of Data

Fair

Comment

None

The frequency of congenital anomalies was no greater than expected among the children of 152 women treated with thiopental during the first four lunar months of pregnancy in the Collaborative Perinatal Project (Heinonen et al., 1977).

The frequency of malformations was not increased among the offspring of mice or rats treated during pregnancy with 1.5-3 times the usual human dose of thiopental (Persaud, 1965; Tanimura et al., 1967).

Transient alterations of neonatal behavior have been observed among infants born to women anesthetized with thiopental during delivery (Celleno et al., 1989). Alterations of fetal movement have been noted during maternal anesthesia with thiopental during the first trimester of pregnancy (Jorgensen & Marsal, 1988).

Please see agent summary on phenobarbital for information on a related agent that has been more thoroughly studied.

Key References

Celleno D, Capogna G, Tomassetti M, et al.: Neurobehavioural effects of propofol on the neonate following elective caesarean section. Br J Anaesth 62:649-654, 1989. [E]

Heinonen OP, Slone D, Shapiro S: Birth Defects and Drugs in Pregnancy. Littleton, Mass.: John Wright-PSG, 1977, pp 336-337. [E]

Jorgensen NP, Marsal K: Influence of thiopental anaesthesia on fetal motor behaviour in early pregnancy. Early Hum Dev 17:71-78, 1988. [E]

Persaud TVN: Tiererperimentelle untersuchungen zur frage der teratogenen wirkung von barbituraten. Acta Biol Med Ger 14:89-90, 1965. [A]

Tanimura T, Owaki Y, Nishimura H: Effect of administration of thiopental sodium to pregnant mice upon the development of their offspring. Okajimas Folia Anat Jpn 43:219-226, 1967. [A]

THIORIDAZINE

Synonyms

Mallorol, Mellaril, Melleretten, Novoridazine, Thioril

Summary

Thioridazine is a phenothiazine tranquilizer. It is used in the treatment of psychoses, moderate and severe emotional disorders, and severe behavioral problems.

Magnitude of Teratogenic Risk

Undetermined

Quality and Quantity of Data

Poor To Fair

Comment

None

No adequately controlled epidemiological studies of malformations in children born to women treated with thioridazine during pregnancy have been published. No congenital anomalies were found in a series of 23 infants born to women treated with thioridazine during the first trimester of pregnancy (Scanlan, 1972).

Increased frequencies of cleft palate were observed among the offspring of rats and mice treated respectively with 50 times and more than 12 times the usual human dose of thioridazine during pregnancy (Szabo & Brent, 1974), but the effect appeared to be attributable largely to a drug-induced reduction of maternal feeding (Szabo & Brent, 1975). No alteration of litter size, neonatal mortality, or neonatal weight gain was noted among the offspring of rats treated during pregnancy with thioridazine in doses equivalent to those used in humans (Murphree et al., 1962).

Please see agent summary on chlorpromazine for information on a related agent that has been more thoroughly studied.

Key References

Murphree OD, Monroe BL, Seager LD: Survival of offspring of rats administered phenothiazines during pregnancy. J Neuropsychiatry 3:295-297, 1962. [A]

Scanlan FJ: The use of thioridazine (Melleril) during the first trimester. Med J Aust 1:1271-1272, 1972. [S]

Szabo KT, Brent RL: Reduction of drug-induced cleft palate in mice. Lancet 1:1296-1297,1975. [A]

Szabo KT, Brent RL: Species differences in experimental teratogenesis by tranquillising agents. Lancet 1:565, 1974. [A]

THIOTHIXENE

Synonyms

Navane, Tiotixene

Summary

Thiothixene is a thioxanthine tranquilizer and is used to treat psychosis.

Magnitude of Teratogenic Risk

Undetermined

Quality and Quantity of Data

None To Poor

Comment

None

No epidemiological studies of congenital anomalies in infants born to mothers treated with thiothixene during pregnancy have been reported.

The frequency of malformations was not increased among the offspring of mice or rabbits treated during pregnancy with 20-180 times the usual human dose of thiothixene (Owaki et al., 1969a, b).

Please see agent summary on chlorpromazine for information on a related drug that has been more thoroughly studied.

Key References

Owaki Y, Momiyama H, Yokoi Y: [Teratological studies on thiothixene (NavaneR) in mice]. Oyo Yakuri 3:315-320, 1969a. [A]

Owaki Y, Momiyama H, Yokoi Y: [Teratological studies on thiothixene (NaveneR) in rabbits]. Oyo Yakuri 3:321-324, 1969b. [A]

THIRAM

Synonyms

Arasan, Fernasan, Methyl Thiuramdisulfide, Nomersan, Pomarsol, Puralin, Rezifilm, Thiurad, Thiuramyl, Thylate

Summary

Thiram is used as an agricultural fungicide and in the manufacture of rubber.

Magnitude of Teratogenic Risk

Undetermined

Quality and Quantity of Data

Poor

Comment

None

No epidemiological studies of congenital anomalies among the infants of women exposed to thiram during pregnancy have been reported.

Increased frequencies of fetal death and of skeletal, central nervous system, and other anomalies have been observed among the offspring of mice, rats, and hamsters treated during pregnancy with very large doses (more than 100 mg/kg/day) of thiram, but such doses were generally also toxic to the mothers (Robens, 1969; Roll, 1971; Short et al., 1976). Typical dose and time-of-gestation dependence of the teratogenic effect was evident. Behavioral alterations have been observed among the offspring of rats treated during pregnancy with somewhat smaller (25 mg/kg/d) doses of thiram (Hinkova & Vergieva, 1976). All of these studies deal with treatments that are

hundreds to thousands of times greater than permissible exposure levels, so the relevance of such investigations to thiram exposure occurring in human pregnancy is uncertain.

Key References

Hinkova L, Vergieva T: Functional toxicity and environmental factors. I. Behavioural studies on the progeny of pesticide-treated rats during pregnancy. Adverse Eff Environ Chem Psychotropic Drugs 2:215-218, 1976. [A]

Robens JF: Teratologic studies of carbaryl, diazinon, norea, disulfiram, and thiram in small laboratory animals. Toxicol Appl Pharmacol 15:152-163, 1969. [A]

Roll R: Teratologic studies with thiram (TMTD) on two strains of mice. Arch Toxikol 27:173-186, 1971. [A]

Short Jr RD, Russel JQ, Minor JL and Lee C-C: Developmental toxicity of ferric dimethyldithiocarbamate and bis(dimethylthiocarbamoyl) disulfide in rats and mice. Toxicol Appl Pharmacol 35:83-94, 1976. [A]

TICARCILLIN

Synonyms

Tarcil, Ticar, Ticarpen

Summary

Ticarcillin is a carboxypenicillin that is administered parenterally in the treatment of severe Gram-negative infections.

Magnitude of Teratogenic Risk

Undetermined

Quality and Quantity of Data

None To Poor

Comment

A small risk cannot be excluded, but a high risk of congenital anomalies in the children of women treated with ticarcillin during pregnancy is unlikely.

No epidemiological studies of congenital anomalies among infants born to women treated with ticarcillin during pregnancy have been reported.

No teratogenic effects are said to have occurred among the offspring of mice and rats treated with ticarcillin during pregnancy, but data supporting this statement have not been published (Jackson et al., 1985).

Please see agent summary on penicillin for information on a related agent that has been more thoroughly studied.

Key References

Jackson D, Cockburn A, Cooper DL, et al.: Clinical pharmacology and safety evaluation of timentin. Amer J Med 79(Suppl 5B):44-55, 1985. [S] & [A]

TICLATONE

Synonyms

Landromil

Summary

Ticlatone is an antifungal and antibacterial agent. It is used topically to treat mycotic infections of the skin.

Magnitude of Teratogenic Risk

Undetermined

Quality and Quantity of Data

None

Comment

None

No epidemiological studies of congenital anomalies in infants born to women who used ticlatone during pregnancy have been reported.

No animal teratology studies of ticlatone have been published.

Key References

None available.

TILACTASE

Synonyms

Hydrolact, Lactase, Maxilact

Summary

Tilactase (beta-D-galactosidase) is an enzyme involved in the hydrolysis of lactose. It is administered orally or added to milk in the management of tilactase deficiency.

Magnitude of Teratogenic Risk

Undetermined

Quality and Quantity of Data

None

Comment

A small risk cannot be excluded, but a high risk of congenital anomalies in the children of women treated with tilactase during pregnancy is unlikely.

No epidemiological studies of congenital anomalies in infants whose mothers used tilactase during pregnancy have been reported.

No animal teratology studies of tilactase have been published.

Key References

None available.

TILETAMINE

Synonyms

CI-634

Summary

Tiletamine is an injectable anesthetic that has been used in veterinary medicine.

Magnitude of Teratogenic Risk

Undetermined

Quality and Quantity of Data

None

Comment

None

No epidemiological studies of congenital anomalies in children born to women exposed to tiletamine during pregnancy have been reported.

No studies of teratologic effects of tiletamine in experimental animals have been published.

Key References

None available.

TIMOLOL

Synonyms

Betim, Blocadren, Proflax, Temserin, Timacor, Timoptic, Timoptol

Summary

Timolol is a beta-adrenergic receptor blocking agent. It is used for treating hypertension, myocardial infarction, and glaucoma.

Magnitude of Teratogenic Risk

Undetermined

Quality and Quantity of Data

None To Poor

Comment

None

No epidemiological studies of congenital anomalies among infants born to women treated with timolol during pregnancy have been reported.

No animal teratology studies of timolol have been published.

Fetal bradycardia and blockage of the fetal response to hypoxia were observed in pregnant sheep given timolol during the third trimester of pregnancy in doses less than those used clinically (Cottle et al., 1983). The relevance of this observation to the use of timolol in human pregnancy is unknown.

Please see agent summary on propranolol for information on a related agent that has been more thoroughly studied.

Key References

Cottle MKW, Van Petten GR, van Muyden P: Maternal and fetal cardiovascular indices during fetal hypoxia due to cord compression in chronically cannulated sheep. I. Responses to timolol. Am J Obstet Gynecol 146:678-685, 1983. [A]

TIN

Synonyms

Potassium Stannate, Sodium Stannate, Stannic Chloride, Stannic Oxide, Stannous Chloride, Stannous Sulfate, Tin Tetrachloride

Summary

Tin is a heavy metal that is widely used in industry.

Magnitude of Teratogenic Risk

Undetermined

Quality and Quantity of Data

None

Comment

None

No human epidemiological studies of congenital anomalies in infants born to mothers who were exposed to tin during pregnancy have been reported.

No animal teratology studies of metallic tin or inorganic tin salts have been published.

Key References

None available.

TIOCONAZOLE

Synonyms

Vagistat

Summary

Tioconazole is an imidazole antifungal agent used topically.

Magnitude of Teratogenic Risk

Undetermined

Quality and Quantity of Data

None To Poor

Comment

None

No epidemiological studies of congenital anomalies in infants whose mothers were treated with tioconazole during pregnancy have been reported.

The frequency of malformations was not increased among the offspring of rats treated systemically during pregnancy with high doses of tioconazole (Noguchi et al., 1982).

Key References

Noguchi Y, Tochibana M, Nabatake H, Iijima M, et al.: [Preclinical safety evaluation of tioconazole]. Yakuri to Chiryo (Basic Pharmacol Therap) 10:3849-3861, 1982. [A]

TOBRAMYCIN

Synonyms

Gernebcin, Nebramycin Factor 6, Obramycin, Tobradex, Tobradistin, Tobramicina, Tobramycetin, Tobrex

Summary

Tobramycin is an aminoglycoside antibiotic that is used parenterally to treat bacterial infections.

Magnitude of Teratogenic Risk

Undetermined

Quality and Quantity of Data

Poor

Comment

Because it is an aminoglycoside, maternal tobramycin treatment during pregnancy may produce a risk for fetal auditory nerve damage.

No epidemiological studies of congenital anomalies among infants born to women treated with tobramycin during pregnancy have been reported.

The frequency of malformations was not increased among the offspring of mice, rats, or rabbits treated during pregnancy with tobramycin in doses respectively 3-12, 3-12, and 2.5-5 times the maximum dose used in humans (Welles et al., 1973; Hasegawa et al., 1975). Evidence of ototoxicity was observed among the offspring of guinea pigs treated during the last half of pregnancy with tobramycin in doses 12 times the maximum used in humans; this was not seen with treatment during the first four weeks of pregnancy (Akiyoshi, 1978).

Key References

Akiyoshi M: Evaluation of ototoxicity of tobramycin in guinea pigs. J Antimicrob Chemother 4 (Suppl A):69-72, 1978. [A]

Hasegawa Y, Yoshida T, Kozen T, et al.: Teratological studies on tobramycin in mice and rats. Chemotherapy 23(3):1544-1553, 1975. [A]

Welles JS, Emmerson JL, Gibson WR, et al.: Preclinical toxicology studies with tobramycin. Toxicol Appl Pharm 25:398-409, 1973. [A]

TOCAINIDE

Synonyms

Tonocard

Summary

Tocainide is an antiarrhythmic agent that can be administered orally.

Magnitude of Teratogenic Risk

Undetermined

Quality and Quantity of Data

None

Comment

None

No epidemiological studies of congenital anomalies among infants born to women treated with tocainide during pregnancy have been reported.

No animal teratology studies of tocainide have been published.

Please see agent summary on lidocaine for information on a related agent that has been studied.

Key References

None available.

TOLAZAMIDE

Synonyms

Ronase, Tolinase

Summary

Tolazamide is a sulfonyluria. It is used as an oral hypoglycemic agent.

Magnitude of Teratogenic Risk

Undetermined

Quality and Quantity of Data

None

Comment

None

No epidemiological studies have been reported regarding malformations in the offspring of women treated with tolazamide during pregnancy.

No experimental animal teratology studies of tolazamide have been published.

Please see agent summary on chlorpropamide for information on a chemically related drug which has been more thoroughly studied.

Key References

None available.

TOLAZOLINE

Synonyms

Benzazoline Hydrochloride, Priscoline

Summary

Tolazoline is an imidazoline derivative that acts as a peripheral vasodilator and alpha adrenergic blocking agent. Tolazoline has been used in the treatment of peripheral vascular disease.

Magnitude of Teratogenic Risk

Undetermined

Quality and Quantity of Data

None

Comment

None

No epidemiological studies of congenital anomalies among infants born to women treated with tolazoline during pregnancy have been reported.

No animal teratology studies of tolazoline have been published.

Key References

None available.

TOLBUTAMIDE

Synonyms

Butamidum, Glyconon, Mobenol, Novobutamide, Oramide, Orinase, Rastinon, Tolglybutamide

Summary

Tolbutamide is a sulfonylurea compound that is used as an oral hypoglycemic agent.

Magnitude of Teratogenic Risk

None To Minimal

Quality and Quantity of Data

Poor To Fair

Comment

None

The frequency of congenital anomalies was no greater than expected among the children of 42 women who had been treated with tolbutamide during pregnancy in the Collaborative Perinatal Project; only 13 of these women were treated during the first trimester (Heinonen et al., 1977). Clinical series suggest that malformations among infants born to women treated with tolbutamide during pregnancy are not substantially more frequent than expected among infants of diabetic mothers (Dolger et al., 1969; Notelovitz, 1971; Coetzee & Jackson, 1984).

The frequency of malformations was no greater than expected among the offspring of mice, rats, or rabbits treated with tolbutamide during pregnancy in doses 5-20 times those used in humans, although increased rates of fetal death and delayed skeletal maturation were seen in some studies (Lazarus & Volk, 1963; McColl et al., 1965, 1967; Belisle & Long, 1976). Fetal malformations including exencephaly were induced by maternal treatment with tolbutamide in one study in mice, but the dose used, about 50 times the human therapeutic dose, often killed the mothers (Smithberg & Runner, 1963).

Key References

Belisle RJ, Long SY: Tolbutamide treatment of pregnant mice: Repeated administration reduces fetal lethality. Teratology 13:65-70, 1976. [A]

Coetzee EJ, Jackson WPU: Oral hypoglycaemics in the first trimester and fetal outcome. S Afr Med J 65:635-637, 1984. [E]

Dolger H, Bookman JJ, Nechemias C: Tolbutamide in pregnancy and diabetes. J Mt Sinai Hosp 36:471-474, 1969. [S]

Heinonen OP, Slone D, Shapiro S: Birth Defects and Drugs in Pregnancy. Littleton, Mass.: John Wright-PSG, 1977, p 443. [E]

Lazarus SS, Volk BW: Absence of teratogenic effect of tolbutamide in rabbits. J Clin Endocrinol Metab 23:597-599, 1963. [A]

McColl JD, Globus M, Robinson S: Effect of some therapeutic agents on the developing rat fetus. Toxicol Appl Pharmacol 7:409-417, 1965. [A]

McColl JD, Robinson S, Globus M: Effect of some therapeutic agents on the rabbit fetus. Toxicol Appl Pharmacol 10:244-252, 1967. [A]

Notelovitz M: Sulphonylurea therapy in the treatment of the pregnant diabetic. S Afr Med J 45:226-229, 1971. [E]

Smithberg M, Runner MN: Teratogenic effects of hypoglycemic treatments in inbred strains of mice. Am J Anat 113:479-489, 1963. [A]

TOLCICLATE

Synonyms

Fungifos, Kilmicene, Tolmicen

Summary

Tolciclate is a topical antifungal agent used to treat dermatomycoses.

Magnitude of Teratogenic Risk

Undetermined

Quality and Quantity of Data

None

Comment

None

No epidemiological studies of congenital anomalies in infants born to women who used tolciclate during pregnancy have been reported.

No teratogenic effects were found among the offspring of rats or rabbits treated systemically with very large doses of tolciclate during pregnancy (deCarneri et al., 1976; Harakawa et al., 1981).

Key References

deCarneri I, Monti G, Bianchi A, Castellino S, et al.: Tolciclate against dermatophytes. Arzneimittelforsch 26:769-772, 1976. [A]

Harakawa T, Suzuki T, Hayashizaki A, Nishimura N, et al.: [Reproductive studies of tolciclate.] Kiso to Rinsho 15:2413-2425, 1981. [A]

TOLINDATE

Synonyms

Dalnate

Summary

Tolindate is an antifungal agent.

Magnitude of Teratogenic Risk

Undetermined

Quality and Quantity of Data

None

Comment

None

No epidemiological studies of congenital anomalies in infants born to women who used tolindate during pregnancy have been reported.

No animal teratology studies of tolindate have been published.

Key References

None available.

TOLMETIN

Synonyms

Tolectin, Tolmex

Summary

Tolmetin is a nonsteroidal anti-inflammatory agent with analgesic and antipyretic action. It is used in the treatment of rheumatic and musculoskeletal disorders.

Magnitude of Teratogenic Risk

Undetermined

Quality and Quantity of Data

None To Poor

Comment

Alterations of perinatal cardiopulmonary adaptation have been reported in infants born to mothers who took pharmacologically related nonsteroidal anti-inflammatory agents shortly before delivery (Manchester et al., 1976; Llevin et al., 1978; Itskovitz et al., 1980). Premature closure of the ductus arteriosus has been observed among the offspring of rats treated with tolmetin just prior to delivery in doses 1-4 times those used in humans (Momma et al., 1983; Nishimura et al., 1984.)

No epidemiological studies of congenital anomalies among children of women treated with tolmetin during pregnancy have been published.

No increase in the frequency of malformations was observed among the offspring of pregnant rabbits treated with tolmetin in doses less than 1-4 times the usual human dose (Nishimura et al., 1977). Increased fetal mortality occurred at the high dose levels, but such doses were toxic to the mothers.

Alterations of perinatal cardiopulmonary adaptation have been reported in infants born to mothers who took pharmacologically related nonsteroidal anti-inflammatory agents shortly before delivery (Manchester et al., 1976; Levin et al., 1978; Itskovitz et al., 1980). Premature closure of the ductus arteriosus has been observed among the offspring of rats treated with tolmetin just prior to delivery in doses 1-4 times those used in humans (Momma et al., 1983; Nishimura et al., 1984).

Please see agent summary on indomethacin for information on a related agent that has been studied.

Key References

Itskovitz J, Abramovici H, Brandes JM: Oligohydramnion, meconium and perinatal death concurrent with indomethacin treatment in human pregnancy. J Reprod Med 24:137-140, 1980. [C]

Levin DL, Fixler DE, Morriss FC, Tyson J: Morphologic analysis of the pulmonary vascular bed in infants exposed in utero to prostaglandin synthetase inhibitors. J Pediatr 92:478-483, 1978. [C]

Manchester D, Margolis HS, Sheldon RE: Possible association between maternal indomethacin therapy and primary pulmonary hypertension of the newborn. Am J Obstet Gynecol 126:467-469, 1976. [C]

Momma K, Takeuchi H: Constriction of fetal ductus arteriosus by non-steroidal anti-inflammatory drugs. Prostaglandins 26(4):631-643, 1983. [A]

Nishimura K, Fukagawa S, Shigematsu K, Mukumoto K, et al.: Teratogenicity study of 1-methyl-5-p-toluoylpyrrole-2-acetate sodium dihydrate (tolmetin sodium) in rabbits. Iyakuhin Kenkyu 8:158-164, 1977. [A]

Nishimura K, Sato K, Nanto T, Yoshida K: Constriction of fetal ductus arteriosus by anti-inflammatory agents in rats. Teratology 30:35A, 1984. [A]

TOLNAFTATE

Synonyms

Aftate, Tinactin

Summary

Tolnaftate is a topical antifungal agent.

Magnitude of Teratogenic Risk

Undetermined

Quality and Quantity of Data

None To Poor

Comment

A small risk cannot be excluded, but a substantial risk of congenital anomalies in the children of women who used tolnaftate during pregnancy is unlikely.

No epidemiological studies of congenital anomalies among infants born to women treated with tolnaftate during pregnancy have been reported.

The frequency of malformations was not increased among the offspring of mice or rats treated systemically during pregnancy with tolnaftate in doses of 50-2000 or 25-500 mg/kg/d (Noguchi et al., 1966).

Key References

Noguchi T, Hashimoto Y, Makita T, et al.: Teratogenesis study of tolnaftate, an antitrichophyton agent. Toxicol Appl Pharmacol 8:386-397, 1966. [A]

TOLUENE

Synonyms

Methyl Benzene, Phenylmethane, Toluol

Summary

Toluene is an organic solvent that is widely used, especially in the paint, printing, and adhesive industries. Toluene is also abused by inhalation. Maternal exposure can be monitored by measuring toluene in the blood or its major metabolite, hippuric acid, in the urine (Low et al., 1988). The U.S. permissible exposure level for toluene is 100 ppm (375 mg/cu m) as an 8-hour time-weighted average (Hathaway et al., 1991).

Magnitude of Teratogenic Risk

For Usual Occupational Exposure: None To Minimal

For Abuse: Undetermined

Quality and Quantity of Data

For Usual Occupational Exposure: Poor To Fair

For Abuse: Poor To Fair

Comment

1) Commercial products ordinarily contain a mixture of volatile hydrocarbons, and rarely contain pure toluene.

2) Case reports indicate that there is a phenotype associated with maternal toluene abuse (see below) and therefore a small risk is possible.

No epidemiological studies have been reported of congenital anomalies in children born to women who abused toluene by inhalation during pregnancy. More than a dozen children whose mothers frequently abused toluene during pregnancy have been reported with a similar pattern of congenital anomalies (Hersh et al., 1985; Hersh, 1989; Wilkins-Haug & Gabow, 1991; Lindemann, 1991; Seaver et al., 1991). The children exhibited central nervous system dysfunction, developmental delay, attention deficit disorder, microcephaly, growth deficiency, short palpebral fissures, deep-set eyes, blunt fingers, and small fingernails. It has been suggested that the anomalies in such children constitute a "toluene embryopathy". Another eight infants with similar phenotypic features whose mothers inhaled large amounts of spray paint fumes containing toluene during pregnancy have been reported but not described in detail (Goodwin, 1988). Among 21 pregnancies in women who chronically abused tolune in one series, there were three perinatal deaths. Most of the infants had fetal growth retardation and neonatal hyertonia. Growth retardation was present in eight of 13 of these children followed to at least one year of age, microcephaly occurred in seven of 13, and developmental delay in six of 13 (Wilkins-Haug & Gabow, 1991). Toluene abuse is known to produce neurotoxicity in adults (King, 1982; Low et al., 1988) and had apparently done so in two of the mothers reported by Hersh et al. (1985). It is reasonable to believe that a similar effect may be produced in the fetus.

An increased frequency of occupational exposure to aromatic solvents was found in one case-control study of the mothers of 301 infants with major congenital anomalies; the excess exposure was attributable almost entirely to toluene (McDonald et al., 1987). The malformations in infants of mothers who had aromatic solvent exposure in this study were quite heterogeneous, and the exposures reported by the women were low level.

Toluene exposure during pregnancy was no more frequent than expected in a case-control study of 38 women who had miscarriages while working in pharmaceutical factories (Taskinen et al., 1986). Similarly, the frequency of miscarriage was no greater than expected among 166 pregnancies of women who were exposed to toluene while working in university laboratories (Axelsson et al., 1984). In a cohort study of women with occupational exposure to high levels of tolune (50-150 ppm), an increased rate of spontaneous abortion was observed (Ng et al., 1992). However, the rate among the exposed group is similar to what would normally be expected (12.4%), while the rates in the comparison groups were inexplicably low.

The frequency of malformations was not increased among the offspring of rats, mice, or rabbits treated respectively by toluene inhalation in chronic doses equivalent to 1-20, 1-10, or <1-5 times the U.S. permissible exposure level (Hudak & Ungvary, 1978; Shigeta et al., 1982; Ungvary et al., 1983; Anonymous, 1984, 1985; Ungvary & Tatrai, 1985; Courtney et al., 1986; Klimish et al., 1992). Fetal growth and developmental retardation or fetal death were sometimes seen at the higher doses, often in association with signs of maternal toxicity.

Transient neonatal hyperchloremic acidosis has been observed in infants of women who chronically abused toluene during pregnancy (Goodwin, 1988; Lindmann, 1991). Renal tubular dysfunction with consequent hyperchloremic acidosis is a frequent manifestation of chronic toluene toxicity in pregnant women as well (Wilkins-Haug and Gabow, 1991).

Key References

Anonymous: Two generation inhalation reproduction/fertility study on a petrolem derived hydrocarbon with toluene with submittal letter dated 082085. EPA/OTS; Doc #FYI-AX-0885-0294, 1985. [A]

Anonymous: Two generation inhalation study on a petroleum-derived hydrocarbon with cover letter dated 021384 and EPA acknowledgement dated 031984. EPA/OTS; Doc #FYI-AX-0284-0294 Initial Sequence A, 1984. [A]

Axelsson G, Lutz C, Rylander R: Exposure to solvents and outcome of pregnancy in university laboratory employees. Br J Ind Med 41:305-312, 1984. [E]

Courtney KD, Andrews JE, Springer J, et al.: A perinatal study of toluene in CD-1 mice. Fundam Appl Toxicol 6:145-154, 1986. [A]

Goodwin TM: Toluene abuse and renal tubular acidosis in pregnancy. Obstet Gynecol 71(5):715-718, 1988. [S]

Hathaway GJ, Proctor NH, Hughes JP, Fischman ML (eds): Proctor and Hughes' Chemical Hazards of the Workplace, 3rd ed. New York: Van Nostrand Reinhold, 1991, p 103. [R]

Hersh JH: Toluene embryopathy: Two new cases. J Med Genet 26(5):333-337, 1989. [C]

Hersh JH, Podruch PE, Rogers G, Weisskopf B: Toluene embryopathy. J Pediatr 106:922-927, 1985. [C]

Hudak A, Ungvary G: Embryotoxic effects of benzene and its methyl derivatives: Toluene, xylene. Toxicology 11:55-63, 1978. [A]

King MD: Neurological sequelae of toluene abuse. Human Toxicol 1:281-287, 1982. [S]

Klimisch H-J, Hellwig J, Hofmann A: Studies on the prenatal toxicity of toluene in rabbits following inhalation exposure and proposal of a pregnancy guidance value. Arch Toxicol 66:373-381, 1992. [A]

Lindemann R: Congenital renal tubular dysfunction associated with maternal sniffing of organic solvents. Acta Paediatr Scand 80:882-884, 1991. [C]

Low LK, Meeks JR, Mackerer CR: Health effects of the alkylbenzenes. I. Toluene. Toxicol Ind Health 4:49-76, 1988. [R]

McDonald JC, Lavoie J, Cote R, et al.: Chemical exposures at work in early pregnancy and congenital defect: A case-referent study. Br J Ind Med 44:527-533, 1987. [E]

Ng TP, Foo SC, Yoong T: Risk of spontaneous abortion in workers exposed to toluene. Br J Ind Med 49:804-808, 1992. [E]

Seaver LH, Pearson MA, Rimsza ME, Hoyme HE: Toluene embryopathy: Elucidation of phenotype and mechanism of teratogenesis in 12 patients. Am J Hum Genet 49(Suppl 4):237, 1991. [S]

Shigeta S, Aikawa H, Misawa T: Effects of maternal exposure to toluene during pregnancy on mouse embryos and fetuses. Tokai J Exp Clin Med 7:265-270, 1982. [A]

Taskinen H, Lindbohm M-L, Hemminki K: Spontaneous abortions among women working in the pharmaceutical industry. Br J Ind Med 43:199-205, 1986. [E]

Ungvary G, Tatrai E: On the embryotoxic effects of benzene and its alkyl derivatives in mice, rats and rabbits. Arch Toxicol (Suppl 8):425-430, 1985. [A]

Ungvary GY, Tatrai E, Lorincz M, Barcza GY: Combined embryotoxic action of toluene, a widely used industrial chemical, and acetylsalicylic acid (Aspirin). Teratology 27:261-269, 1983. [A]

Wilkins-Haug L, Gabow PA: Toluene abuse during pregnancy: Obstetric complications and perinatal outcomes. Obstet Gynecol 77:504-509, 1991. [S]

TOLYCAINE

Summary

Tolycaine is a local anesthetic that has been used topically.

Magnitude of Teratogenic Risk

Undetermined

Quality and Quantity of Data

None

Comment

None

No epidemiological studies of congenital anomalies in children born to women exposed to tolycaine during pregnancy have been reported.

No investigations of teratologic effects of tolycaine in experimental animals have been published.

Please see agent summary on procaine for information on a related agent that has been studied.

Key References

None available.

TOXOPLASMOSIS

Synonyms

Toxoplasma gondii

Summary

Toxoplasmosis is caused by the intracellular protozoan parasite, Toxoplasma gondii. Infections in adults are usually asymptomatic or associated with localized lymphadenopathy and are acquired by eating undercooked infected meat or by handling soil or cat feces containing the organism. About one-third of adult Americans have serological evidence of past Toxoplasma infection (Remington, 1974; Dubey & Beattie, 1988).

Magnitude of Teratogenic Risk

Moderate

Quality and Quantity of Data

Good To Excellent

Comment

Risk assessment pertains to primary infection during pregnancy.

The clinical features of congenital toxoplasmosis were first recognized in 1923, and transplacental transmission of the parasite was established by 1940 (Remington & Desmonts, 1990). The spectrum of illness in infants with congenital toxoplasmosis is very broad (Eichenwald, 1960; Couvreur et al., 1984; Dubey & Beattie, 1988). Most infected babies appear completely normal clinically. Severely affected infants may die in the neonatal period or manifest encephalitis, hydrocephalus, intracranial calcifications, chorioretinitis, erythroblastosis, anemia, jaundice, hepatosplenomegaly, glomerulitis, myocarditis, and myositis. Central nervous system involvement is almost always present in such babies (Remington & Desmonts, 1990). Long term sequellae may include seizures, mental retardation, cerebral palsy, deafness, and blindness. In some infants, manifestations of the disease do not appear until after the neonatal period. Later reactivation of neonatal disease may also occur.

Congenital toxoplasmosis usually occurs after a primary maternal infection during pregnancy. The likelihood of fetal infection varies with the time in gestation the maternal infection occurs, with a much higher risk for transmission later than earlier. The risk of transmission ranges from less than 1% for maternal infection prior to conception to more than 90% with infection near term (Remington

& Desmonts, 1990; Desmonts, 1982; Desmonts et al., 1985; Daffos et al., 1988). On the other hand, clinical manifestations of the disease are more likely and more severe with infections earlier in pregnancy. Overall, the highest risk for having a baby with severe manifestations occurs with maternal infection between 10 and 24 weeks of gestation (Desmonts, 1982). In a prospective study of 542 women who acquired toxoplasmosis during pregnancy, severe congenital toxoplasmosis occurred in 6% and perinatal death in 5% of infants whose mothers were infected in the first trimester, in 2% and 2% of infants whose mothers were infected in the second trimester, and in none of 128 infants whose mothers were infected in the third trimester (Remington & Desmonts, 1990). Three percent of the infants whose mothers acquired toxoplasmosis in the first trimester, 25% of infants whose mothers acquired the infection in the second trimester, 59% of infants whose mothers acquired the infection in the third trimester had mild or subclinical infections. Many of these infants are likely to develop chorioretinitis or neurological abnormalities later in childhood if not treated (Wilson et al., 1980; Koppe et al., 1986). Among 210 prospectively identified infants with congenital toxoplasmosis infection, 40% of those with maternal infection during the first trimester, 18% of those with maternal infection in the second trimester, and 3% of those with maternal infection in the the third trimester had severe disease (Couvreur et al., 1984).

Diagnosis of primary maternal infection by Toxoplasma during pregnancy is usually based on serological studies. Several tests are in use, and all have limitations that may make interpretation difficult in some cases (Fuccillo et al., 1987; Remington & Desmonts, 1990). In general, however, recent infection is diagnosed by the presence of specific IgM antibodies and a very high dye test titer (1:1000 or more) or a substantial rise in the dye test titer over two to three weeks, particularly if associated with a typical pattern of lymphadenopathy (Remington & Desmonts, 1990). Prenatal diagnosis of fetal infection in pregnant women found to have primary Toxoplasma infection during pregnancy can be performed by amniocentesis and fetal blood sampling with testing by parasite isolation and specific IgM antibody measurement (Desmonts et al., 1985; Daffos et al., 1988; Foulon et al., 1990). High-resolution ultrasound examination is useful in identifying hydrocephalus, hydrops, and some other severe manifestations of fetal infection, but is not a reliable means of determining whether or not transmission of Toxoplasma to the fetus has occurred. Screening and treatment of primary toxoplasmosis during pregnancy are advocated by some authorities but not by others (Remington & Desmonts, 1990; Hohlfeld et al., 1989; Daffos et al., 1988; McCabe & Remington, 1988; Thorp et al., 1988; McCabe & Oster, 1989; Anonymous, 1990; Foulon et al., 1990; Jeannel et al., 1990).

Transmission of Toxoplasma organisms during gestation occurs both naturally and experimentally in a variety of species (Dubey & Beattie, 1988; Remington & Desmonts, 1990). Congenital toxoplasmosis is seen in domesticated cats, dogs, pigs, goats and sheep. The infection is especially common in sheep where it causes abortion, embryonic or fetal death, stillbirth, and illness in the neonatal period. Experimental transplacental Toxoplasma infections have also been produced in mice, rats, guinea pigs, and rabbits.

Key References

Anonymous: Antenatal screening for toxoplasmosis in the UK. Lancet 336:346-348, 1990. [O]

Couvreur J, Desmonts G, Tournier G, et al.: Etude d'une serie homogene de 210 cas de toxoplasmose congenitale chez des nourrissons ages de 0 a 11 mois et depistes de facon prospective. Ann Pediatr (Paris) 31:815-819, 1984. [E]

Daffos F, Forestier F, Capella-Pavlovsky M, et al.: Prenatal management of 746 pregnancies at risk for congenital toxoplasmosis. N Engl J Med 318(5):271-275, 1988. [E]

Desmonts G: Toxoplasmose acquise de la femme enceinte. Estimation du risque de transmission du parasite et de toxoplasmose congenitale. Lyon Med 248:115-123, 1982. [E]

Desmonts G, Forestier G, Thulliez PH, et al.: Prenatal diagnosis of congenital toxoplasmosis. Lancet 1:500-504, 1985. [E]

Dubey JP, Beattie CP: Toxoplasmosis of Animals and Man. Boca Raton: CRC Press, 1988. [O]

Eichenwald H: A study of congenital toxoplasmosis. In: Siim JC (ed). Human Toxoplasmosis. Copenhagen: Munksgaard, 1960, pp 41-49. [R]

Foulon W, Naessens A, Mahler T, et al.: Prenatal diagnosis of congenital toxoplasmosis. Obstet Gynecol 76(5):769-772, 1990. [S]

Fuccillo DA, Madden DL, Tzan N, et al.: Difficulties associated with serological diagnosis of toxoplasma gondii infections. Diagn Clin Immunol 5:8-13, 1987. [S]

Hohlfeld P, Daffos F, Thulliez P, et al.: Fetal toxoplasmosis: Outcome of pregnancy and infant follow-up after in utero treatment. J Pediatr 115(5):765-769, 1989. [S]

Jeannel D, Costagliola D, Niel G, et al.: What is known about the prevention of congenital toxoplasmosis? Lancet 336:359-361, 1990. [R]

Koppe JG, Loewer-Sieger DH, de Roever-Bonnet H: Results of 20-year follow-up of congenital toxoplasmosis. Lancet 1:254-255, 1986. [S]

McCabe RE, Oster S: Current recommendations and future prospects in the treatment of toxoplasmosis. Drugs 38(6):973-987, 1989. [R]

McCabe R, Remington JS: Toxoplasmosis: The time has come. N Engl J Med 318(5):313-315, 1988. [O]

Remington JS: Toxoplasmosis in the adult. Bull NY Acad Med 50:211-227, 1974. [R]

Remington JS, Desmonts G: Toxoplasmosis. In: Remington JS & Klein JO (eds). Infectious Diseases of the Fetus and Newborn Infant. Philadelphia: W.B. Saunders Co., 1990, pp 89-195. [O]

Thorp JM, Seeds JW, Herbert WNP, et al.: Prenatal management and congenital toxoplasmosis [Letter]. N Engl J Med 319:372, 1988. [O]

Wilson CB, Remington JS, Stagno S, et al.: Development of adverse sequelae in children born with subclinical congenital toxoplasma infection. Pediatrics 66(5):767-774, 1980. [S]

TRAMAZOLINE

Synonyms

Biciron, Ellatun, Rhinaspray, Rhinogutt, Spray-Tish

Summary

Tramazoline is an alpha adrenergic stimulant used topically to treat allergic rhinitis.

Magnitude of Teratogenic Risk

Undetermined

Quality and Quantity of Data

None

Comment

A small risk cannot be excluded, but a high risk of congenital anomalies in the children of women treated with tramazoline during pregnancy is unlikely.

No epidemiological studies of congenital anomalies among infants whose mothers were treated with tramazoline during pregnancy have been reported.

No animal teratology studies of tramazoline have been published.

Please see agent summary on ephedrine for information on a related agent that has been studied.

Key References

None available.

TRANYLCYPROMINE

Synonyms

Parnate, Transamine Sulphate

Summary

Tranylcypromine is a monoamine oxidase inhibitor that is used orally in the treatment of depressive illness.

Magnitude of Teratogenic Risk

Undetermined

Quality and Quantity of Data

None To Poor

Comment

A small risk cannot be excluded, but a high risk of congenital anomalies in the children of women treated with tranylcypromine during pregnancy is unlikely.

No adequate epidemiological studies of congenital anomalies among infants born to women treated with tranylcypromine during pregnancy have been reported.

No reduction in the number of viable fetuses was observed among the offspring of pregnant mice treated with tranylcypromine in doses much smaller than those used in humans (Poulson & Robson, 1963).

Key References

Poulson E, Robson JM: The effect of amine oxidase inhibitors on pregnancy. J Endocrin 27:147-152, 1963. [A]

TRAZODONE

Synonyms

Deprax, Desyrel, Manegan, Molipaxin, Pragmarel, Thombran, Tramensan, Trittico

Summary

Trazodone is an antidepressant with sedative action.

Magnitude of Teratogenic Risk

Undetermined

Quality and Quantity of Data

None To Poor

Comment

None

No epidemiological studies of malformations in the children of women who used trazodone during pregnancy have been reported.

The frequency of malformations was not signficantly increased among the offspring of pregnant rats and rabbits treated with trazodone in doses 8-38 times that used in humans (Barcellona, 1970; Rivett & Barcellona, 1974; Suzuki, 1974). Fetal death and growth retardation were seen in association with maternal toxicity at the higher doses.

Key References

Barcellona PS: Investigations on the possible teratogenic effects of trazodone in rats and rabbits. Boll Chim Farm 109:323-332, 1970. [A]

Rivett KF, Barcellona PS: Toxicology of trazodone. Mod Probl Pharmacopsychiat 9:76-86, 1974. [A]

Suzuki Y: Teratogenicity and placental transfer of trazodone. Mod Probl Pharmacopsychiat 9:87-94, 1974. [A]

TRETINOIN

Synonyms

A-Acido, Acretin, all-trans-Retinoic acid, Retin A, Retinoic Acid, Trans-Retinoic Acid, Vitamin A Acid

Summary

Tretinoin (all-trans-retinoic acid) is a vitamin A congener used topically in the treatment of acne and other dermatologic diseases. Systemic absorption of tretinoin from the skin does occur, but only to a limited degree.

Magnitude of Teratogenic Risk

Undetermined

Quality and Quantity of Data

Poor

Comment

1) A small risk cannot be excluded, but a high risk of congenital anomalies in the children of women treated with tretinoin during pregnancy is unlikely.

2) Risk assessment is for topical use only. There may be a substantial risk with systemic use of this agent.

No epidemiological studies of congenital anomalies among infants born to women treated with tretinoin during pregnancy have been reported. A child with low birth weight and a dysplastic auricle who was born to a mother who used tretinoin cream throughout the first 11 weeks of pregnancy has been described (Camera & Pregliasco, 1992). No causal relationship can be determined on the basis of this anecdotal observation.

Teratogenic effects similar to those demonstrated with other retinoids have been observed among the offspring of pregnant monkeys, rabbits, mice, rats, and hamsters treated systemically with tretinoin in doses of 2-10 mg/kg/d or greater (Zbinden, 1975; Newell-Morris et al., 1980; Kamm, 1982; Willhite & Shealy, 1984; Rosa et al., 1986; Alles & Sulik, 1989, 1990; Granstom & Kullaa-Mikkonen, 1990; Hendrickx & Hummler, 1992). Malformations observed among affected fetuses include those of the ear, face, palate, limb, central nervous system, and heart. Fetal death was frequent. Typical dependence of the teratogenic effect on dose and time of gestation has been demonstrated in mice (Kochhar et al., 1984).

Studies have been also been done of the teratogenicity of topical tretinoin preparations applied to the skin of experimental animals. It is difficult to compare the dosages used in these studies to those used in humans because the experimental investigations involve relatively large areas of application and conditions which promote absorption of the drug. It seems likely that the absorbed dose of tretinoin in all of these studies is substantially greater than that usually encountered therapeutically in humans. Increased rates of fetal death have been observed among pregnant rabbits treated topically with tretinoin (Zbinden, 1975). Skeletal malformations were seen with increased frequency among the offspring of rats treated topically with large amounts of tretinoin in some studies but not others (Zbinden, 1975; Seegmiller et al., 1990; Chahoud et al., 1989, 1991). Cleft palate was seen with increased frequency among the offspring of mice treated topically with tretinoin during pregnancy (Caldwell & Seegmiller, 1991). The relevance of these observations to use of topical tretinoin preparations in human pregnancy is uncertain. No teratogenic effect was observed among the offspring of pregnant hamsters treated with topical tretinoin (Willhite et al., 1990).

Please see agent summary on isotretinoin for information on a closely related agent that has been more thoroughly studied . It should be noted, however, that isotretinoin is given orally so that systemic absorption is much greater than with topical adminstration of tretinoin.

Key References

Alles AJ, Sulik KK: Retinoic-acid-induced limb-reduction defects: Perturbation of zones of programmed cell death as a pathogenetic mechanism. Teratology 40:163-171, 1989. [A]

Alles AJ, Sulik KK: Retinoic acid-induced spina bifida: Evidence for a pathogenetic mechanism. Development 108:73-81, 1990. [A]

Caldwell AP, Seegmiller RE: Evaluation of the teratognic potential of topically applied all-trans

retinoic acid (RA) in mice. Teratology 43(5):443, 1991. [A]

Camera G, Pregliasco P: Ear malformation in baby born to mother using tretinoin cream. Lancet 339:687, 1992. [C]

Chahoud I, Lofberg B, Mittmann B, Nau H: Teratogenicity and pharmacokinetics of vitamin A acid (tretinoin, all-trans retinoic acid) after dermal application in the rat. Naunyn Schmiedebergs Arch Pharmacol 339(Suppl):R30, 1989. [A]

Chahoud I, Nau H, Tzimas G, et al.: Teratogenicity und pharmacokinetics of tretinoin after topical und oral application in the rat. Teratology 44(3):15A, 1991. [A]

Granstrom G, Kullaa-Mikkonen A: Experimental craniofacial malformations induced by retinoids and resembling branchial arch syndromes. Scand J Plast Reconstr Hand Surg 24:3-12, 1990. [A]

Hendrickx AG, Hummler H: Teratogenicity of all-trans retinoic acid during early embryonic development in the cynomolgus monkey (Macaca fascicularis). Teratology 45:65-74, 1992. [A]

Kamm JJ: Toxicology, carcinogenicity, and teratogenicity of some orally administered retinoids. J Am Acad Dermatol 6:652-659, 1982. [A]

Kochhar DM, Penner JD, Tellone CI: Comparative teratogenic activities of two retinoids: Effects on palate and limb development. Teratogenesis Carcinog Mutagen 4:377-387, 1984. [A]

Newell-Morris L, Sirianni JE, Shepard TH, et al.: Teratogenic effects of retinoic acid in pigtail monkeys (Macaca nemestrina). II. Craniofacial features. Teratology 22:87-101, 1980. [A]

Rosa FW, Wilk AL, Kelsey FO: Teratogen update: Vitamin A congeners. Teratology 33:355-364, 1986. [R]

Seegmiller RE, Carter MW, Ford WH, White RD: Induction of maternal toxicity in the rat by dermal application of retinoic acid and its effect on fetal outcome. Reprod Toxicol 4(4):277-281, 1990. [A]

Willhite CC, Sharma RP, Allen PV, Berry DL: Percutaneous retinoid absorption and embryotoxicity. J Invest Dermatol 95:523-529, 1990. [A]

Willhitc CC, Shealy YF: Amelioration of embryotoxicity by structural modification of the termainal group of cancer chemopreventive retinoids. J Natl Cancer Inst 71:689-695, 1984. [A]

Zbinden G: Investigations on the toxicity of tretinoin adminstered systemically to animals. Acta Derm Venereol (Suppl) 74:36-40, 1975. [A]

TRIACETIN

Synonyms

Enzactin, Fungacetin, Glycerol Triacetate, Glyped

Summary

Triacetin is an antifungal agent. It is used topically to treat superficial infections and as a fungistatic additive to foods.

Magnitude of Teratogenic Risk

Undetermined

Quality and Quantity of Data

None

Comment

None

No epidemiological studies of congenital anomalies in infants born to women treated with triacetin during pregnancy have been reported.

No animal teratology studies of triacetin have been published.

Key References

None available.

TRIAFUNGIN

Summary

Triafungin is an antifungal agent.

Magnitude of Teratogenic Risk

Undetermined

Quality and Quantity of Data

None

Comment

None

No epidemiological studies of congenital anomalies in infants born to women who used triafungin during pregnancy have been reported.

No animal teratology studies of triafungin have been published.

Key References

None available.

TRIAMCINOLONE

Synonyms

Adcortyl, Aristocort, Aristospan, Azmacort, Cenocort Forte, Cinonide, Fluoxiprednisolonum, Kenacort, Ledercort, Triam, Triamolone 40

Summary

Triamcinolone is a synthetic glucocorticoid used to treat allergic and inflammatory conditions. It is employed in systemic form as well as in local injectable and topical preparations, from which substantial absorption may occur.

Magnitude of Teratogenic Risk

Undetermined

Quality and Quantity of Data

Poor

Comment

Chronic use of triamcinolone at high doses may be associated with fetal growth retardation.

No epidemiological studies of congenital anomalies in children of women treated with triamcinolone during pregnancy have been reported. Severe fetal growth retardation has been observed in the infant of a woman who was treated chronically with large amounts of topical triamcinolone during pregnancy (Katz et al., 1990). This anecdotal report is of concern because similar findings have been observed in nonhuman primates (see below).

An increased frequency of malformations was found among the offspring of three species of nonhuman primates treated during pregnancy with triamcinolone in doses <1-20 times those used clinically (Hendrickx et al., 1980; Parker & Hendrickx, 1983; Tarara et al., 1988; Bacher & Michejda, 1988; Jerome & Hendrickx, 1988; Hendrickx & Tarara, 1990). Neural tube defects and other central nervous system abnormalities, craniofacial malformations, and skeletal anomalies were seen most often; fetal growth retardation and fetal or neonatal death also occurred commonly. The teratogenic effect was shown to exhibit typical dependence on dose and time of exposure (Tarara et al., 1989).

Cleft palate occurs with increased frequency among the offspring of mice, rats, and hamsters treated during pregnancy with triamcinolone in doses within the human therapeutic range or greater (Walker, 1965; Shah & Kilistoff, 1976; Melnick et al., 1981; Rowland & Hendrickx, 1983; Marazita et al., 1988). Typical dose and time dependence of this effect have been demonstrated. The relevance of these findings to the risk of malformations in children of women treated with triamcinolone during pregnancy is unknown.

Please see agent summary on prednisone for information on a related agent.

Key References

Bacher JD, Michejda M: Allogeneic fetal bone cranioplasty in Macaca mulatta. Fetal Ther 3:108-117, 1988. [A]

Hendrickx AG, Pellegrini M, Tarara R, Parker R, et al.: Craniofacial and central nervous system malformations induced by triamcinolone acetonide in nonhuman primates: I. General teratogenicity. Teratology 22:103-114, 1980. [A]

Hendrickx AG, Tarara RP: Triamcinolone acetonide-induced meningocele and meningoencephalocele in rhesus monkeys. Am J Pathol 136(3):725-727, 1990. [A]

Jerome CP, Hendrickx AG: Comparative teratogenicity of triamcinolone acetonide and dexamethasone in the rhesus monkey (Macaca mulatta). J Med Primatol 17:195-203, 1988. [A]

Katz VL, Thorp JM, Jr, Bowes WA, Jr: Severe symmetric intrauterine growth retardation associated with the topical use of triamcinolone. Am J Obstet Gynecol 162(2):396-397, 1990. [C]

Marazita ML, Jaskoll T, Melnick M: Corticosteroid-induced cleft palate in short-ear mice. J Craniofac Genet Dev Biol 8:47-51, 1988. [A]

Melnick M, Jaskoll T, Slavkin HC: Corticosteroid-induced cleft palate in mice and H-2 Haplotype: Maternal and embryonic effects. Immunogenetics 13:443-450, 1981. [A]

Parker RM, Hendrickx AG: Craniofacial and central nervous system malformations induced by triamcinolone acetonide in nonhuman primates: II. Craniofacial pathogenesis. Teratology 28:35-44, 1983. [A]

Rowland JM, Hendrickx AG: Teratogenicity of triamcinolone acetonide in rats. Teratology 27:13-18, 1983. [A]

Shah RM, Kilistoff A: Cleft palate induction in hamster fetuses by glucocorticoid hormones and their synthetic analogues. J Embryol Exp Morphol 36:101-108, 1976. [A]

Tarara RP, Cordy DR, Hendrickx AG: Central nervous system malformations induced by triamcinolone acetonide in nonhuman primates: Pathology. Teratology 39:75-84, 1989. [A]

Tarara RP, Wheeldon EB, Hendrickx AG: Central nervous system malformations induced by triamcinolone acetonide in nonhuman primates: Pathogenesis. Teratology 38:259-270, 1988. [A]

Walker BE: Cleft palate produced in mice by human-equivalent dosage with triamcinolone. Science 149:862-863, 1965. [A]

TRIAMTERENE

Synonyms

Diesse, Diucelpin, Dyrenium, Dytac, Jatropur, Natrium, Teriam, Triamteril, Urocaudal

Summary

Triamterene is a mild diuretic with potassium-sparing effects.

Magnitude of Teratogenic Risk

Undetermined

Quality and Quantity of Data

None To Poor

Comment

None

The frequency of congenital anomalies was no greater than expected among the children of 271 women treated with triamterine during pregnancy in the Collaborative Perinatal Project (Heinonen et al., 1977). Only five of these women were treated during the first four lunar months of gestation.

The frequency of malformations was not increased among the offspring of rats treated during pregnancy with triamterine in a dose more than 10 times that used in humans (Ellison & Maren, 1972). In another study in rats, maternal treatment with as much as 5 times the human dose of triamterene during pregnancy did not increase the frequency of cleft palate in the offspring (Posner, 1972).

Key References

Ellison AC, Maren TH: The effect of potassium metabolism on acetazolamide-induced teratogenesis. Johns Hopkins Med J 130:105-115, 1972. [A]

Heinonen OP, Slone D, Shapiro S: Birth Defects and Drugs in Pregnancy. Littleton, Mass.: John Wright-PSG, 1977, pp 372, 341. [E]

Posner HS: Significance of cleft palate induced by chemicals in the rat and mouse. Food Cosmet Toxicol 10:839-855, 1972. [A]

TRIAZOLAM

Synonyms

Halcion

Summary

Triazolam is a benzodiazepine derivative used as a hypnotic.

Magnitude of Teratogenic Risk

None To Minimal

Quality and Quantity of Data

None To Poor

Comment

None

No epidemiological studies of congenital anomalies in infants born to mothers who took triazolam during pregnancy have been reported.

The frequency of malformations was not increased among the offspring of rats or rabbits treated, respectively, with 60-60,000 and 60-10,000 times the usual human dose of triazolam during pregnancy (Matsuo et al., 1979).

Please see agent summary on diazepam for information on a related agent that has been more thoroughly studied.

Key References

Matsuo A, Kast A, Tsunenari Y: Reproduction studies of triazolam in rats and rabbits. Iyakuhin Kenkyu 10:52-67, 1979. [A]

TRIBROMOETHANOL

Synonyms

Avertin, Bromethol, Tribromoethyl Alcohol

Summary

Tribromoethanol is a general anesthetic that is administered rectally.

Magnitude of Teratogenic Risk

Undetermined

Quality and Quantity of Data

None

Comment

None

No epidemiological studies of congenital anomalies in children born to women exposed to tribromoethanol during pregnancy have been reported.

No studies of teratologic effects of tribromoethanol in intact experimental animals have been published. An increased frequency of embryonic loss was observed among pregnant mice treated with 4-6 times the human anesthetic dose of tribromoethanol prior to the time of implantation (Kaufman, 1977). The relevance of this observation to the clinical use of tribromoethanol in human pregnancy is unknown.

Use of tribromoethanol in women during labor has been associated with profound and prolonged depression of the newborn infant (Baker, 1960).

Key References

Baker JBE: The effects of drugs on the fetus. Pharmacol Rev 12:37-90, 1960. [R]

Kaufman MH: Effect of anesthesia on the outcome of pregnancy in female mice. J Reprod Fertil 49:167-168, 1977. [A]

1,1,2-TRICHLOROETHANE

Synonyms

Beta-Trichloroethane, Ethanetrichloride, TCE Vinyltrichloride

Summary

1,1,2-trichloroethane is used as a solvent. Occupational exposures occur primarily in steel manufacturing, telecommunication, and scientific instrument manufacturing industries (HSDB, 1993). The eight hour time-weighted average threshold limit value for occupational exposure is 10 ppm (45 mg/cu m) (HSDB, 1993).

Magnitude of Teratogenic Risk

Undetermined

Quality and Quantity of Data

None

Comment

None

No epidemiological studies of congenital anomalies among the infants of women who were exposed to 1,1,2-trichloroethane during pregnancy have been reported.

No animal teratology studies of 1,1,2-trichloroethane have been published.

Key References

HSDB [database online]. Bethesda, Md.: National Library of Medicine; 1985- [updated 1993 April 30]. Available from: National Library of Medicine; BRS Information Technologies, McLean, Va. [O]

No animal teratology studies of trichlormethiazide have been published.

Please see agent summary on hydrochlorothiazide for information on a related agent that has been more thoroughly studied.

Key References

Heinonen OP, Slone D, Shapiro S: Birth Defects and Drugs in Pregnancy. Littleton, Mass.: John Wright-PSG, 1977, pp 372, 441. [E]

TRICHLORMETHIAZIDE

Synonyms

Esmarin, Fluitran, Metahydrin, Naqua, Triazide

Summary

Trichlormethiazide is a thiazide diuretic that is used orally in the treatment of edema and hypertension.

Magnitude of Teratogenic Risk

Undetermined

Quality and Quantity of Data

Poor

Comment

A small risk cannot be excluded, but a high risk of congenital anomalies in the children of women treated with trichlormethiazide during pregnancy is unlikely.

The frequency of congenital anomalies was not increased among the children of 405 women who were treated with trichlormethiazide anytime during pregnancy in the Collaborative Perinatal Project (Heinonen et al., 1977). Only two of these women were treated during the first four lunar months of gestation.

TRICHLOROETHYLENE

Synonyms

Algylen, Chlorylen, Ethinyl Trichloride, Germalgene, Trethylene, Triclene, Trimar

Summary

Trichloroethylene is widely used as an industrial solvent and cleaning agent. Trichloroethylene has also limitedly been used as a general anesthetic administered by inhalation. The threshold limit value for occupational exposure to trichloroethylene is 50 ppm (270 mg/cu m) as a time-weighted average (HSDB, 1993). The short-term exposure level is 200 ppm (1080 mg/cu m). For comparison, the dose used in anesthesia is 0.5 - 2% (5000 to 20,000 ppm). Urine measurement of trichloroethanol can be used for biological monitoring of exposure to trichloroethylene.

Magnitude of Teratogenic Risk

Occupational Exposure: None To Minimal

Anesthesia: Undetermined

Quality and Quantity of Data

Occupational Exposure: Poor

Anesthesia: None To Poor

Comment

None

An association with parental work or residence in an area in which drinking water was contaminated by trichloroethylene was observed in a series of 707 children with congenital heart disease (Goldberg et al., 1990). The study design did not permit conventional statistical analysis, and no cause-and-effect relationship can be inferred from this investigation. In a case control study of 361 women with spontaneous abortions, no association with occupational use of solvents was observed (Windham et al., 1991). The odds ratio was 3.1 (95% confidence interval 0.92-10.4) for occupational use of trichloroethylene in this study.

The frequency of malformations was not increased among the offspring of mice, rats, or rabbits chronically treated with tricholoroethylene vapor during pregnancy in concentrations below those used for anesthesia but at or several times greater than the occupational exposure limits for humans (Schwetz et al., 1975; Dorfmueller et al., 1979; Hardin et al., 1981; Healy et al., 1982). In some studies, fetal weight was reduced in exposed pregnancies.

No major malformations were observed among the offspring of rats fed 10-1000 mg/kg/d of trichloroethylene throughout pregnancy (Manson et al., 1984). Neonatal death was increased among the offspring of pregnant rats treated with the highest dose, but this dose was also toxic to the mothers. In another study, the frequencies of fetal death and microopthalmia or anophthalmia were increased among the offspring of pregnant rats treated with 475-1500 mg/kg/d of trichoroethylene (Narotsky et al., 1990). All of these doses also produced maternal toxicity. Increased frequencies of heart malformations were observed among the offspring of rats, the uteri of which had been continually infused with trichloroethylene during pregnancy (Dawson et al., 1990).

No teratogenic effect was observed among the offspring of mice fed 24-240 mg/kg/d of tricholoroethylene during pregnancy in one study (Cosby & Dukelow, 1992). Fetal death and malformations, especially cleft palate, were observed with increased frequency among the offpring of mice treated with 2-2.5 ml/kg on one day during pregnancy in another investigation (Hayasaka et al., 1991). This treatment induced toxicity in the mothers as well.

Key References

Cosby NC, Dukelow WR: Toxicology of maternally ingested trichloroethylene (TCE) on embryonal and fetal development in mice and of TCE metabolites on in vitro fertilization. Fundam Appl Toxicol 19:268-274, 1992. [A]

Dawson BV, Johnson PD, Goldberg SJ, Ulreich JB: Cardiac teratogenesis of trichloroethylene and dichloroethylene in a mammalian model. J Am Coll Cardiol 16:1304-1309, 1990. [A]

Dorfmueller MA, Henne SP, York RG, Bornschein RL, et al.: Evaluation of teratogenicity and behavioral toxicity with inhalation exposure of maternal rats to trichloroethylene. Toxicology 14:153-166, 1979. [A]

Goldberg SJ, Lebowitz MD, Graver EJ, Hicks S: An association of human congenital cardiac malformations and drinking water contaminants. J Am Coll Cardiol 16(1):155-164, 1990. [E]

Hardin BD, Bond GP, Sikov MR, Andrew FD, et al.: Testing of selected workplace chemicals for teratogenic potential. Scand J Work Environ Health 7(Suppl 4):66-75, 1981. [A]

Hayasaka S, Inouye M, Yamamura H: Teratogenicity of oral administrations of trichloroethylene in mice. Environ Med 35:139-142, 1991. [A]

Healy TEJ, Poole TR, Hopper A: Rat fetal development and maternal exposure to trichloroethylene 100 p.p.m. Br J Anaesth 54:337-341, 1982. [A]

HSDB [database online]. Bethesda (Md): National Library of Medicine; 1985- [updated 1993 April 30]. Available from: National Library of Medicine; BRS Information Technologies, McLean, Va. [O]

Manson JM, Murphy M, Richdale N, et al.: Effects of oral exposure to trichloroethylene on female reproductive function. Toxicology 32:229-242, 1984. [A]

Narotsky MG, Schlicht M, Berman E, Elder JA, et al.: Effects of trichloroethylene in an in vivo developmental toxicity screen. Teratology 41(5):580, 1990. [A]

Schwetz BA, Leong BKJ, Gehring PJ: The effect of maternally inhaled trichloroethylene, perchloroethylene, methyl chloroform, and methylene chloride on embryonal and fetal development in mice and rats. Toxicol Appl Pharmacol 32:84-96, 1975. [A]

Windham GC, Shusterman D, Swan SH, Fenster L, et al.: Exposure to organic solvents and adverse pregnancy outcome. Am J Ind Med 20:241-259, 1991. [E]

TRIDIHEXETHYL

Synonyms

Pathilon

Summary

Tridihexethyl is a quaternary ammonium antimuscarinic agent. It is given orally in the treatment of peptic ulcers and gastrointestinal spasms.

Magnitude of Teratogenic Risk

Undetermined

Quality and Quantity of Data

None

Comment

None

No epidemiological studies of congenital anomalies among infants born to women treated with tridihexethyl during pregnancy have been reported.

No animal teratology studies of tridihexethyl have been published.

Please see agent summary on isopropamide for information on a related agent that has been studied.

Key References

None available.

TRIENTINE

Synonyms

Trien, Triethylenetetramine

Summary

Trientine is a chelating agent that is given orally in the treatment of Wilson's disease. Trientine (triethylenetetramine) is also used in the plastic and petrochemical industries.

Magnitude of Teratogenic Risk

Undetermined

Quality and Quantity of Data

Poor

Comment

A small risk cannot be excluded, but a high risk of congenital anomalies in the children of women treated with trientine during pregnancy is unlikely.

No congenital anomalies were observed among six children born to women who were treated with trientine for Wilson's disease during pregnancy (Walshe, 1982).

Fetal death and congenital anomalies, primarily massive hemorrhage and edema, were increased among the offspring of rats treated during pregnancy with trientine in doses 2-4 times those used in humans (Keen et al., 1983). Such doses also produced maternal toxicity; no teratogenic effect was noted with doses within the human therapeutic range.

Key References

Keen CL, Cohen NL, Lonnerdal B, et al.: Teratogenesis and low copper status resulting from triethylenetetramine in rats (41693). Proc Soc Exp Biol Med 173:598-605, 1983. [A]

Walshe JM: Treatment of Wilson's disease with trientine (triethylene tetramine) dihydrochloride. Lancet 1:643-647, 1982. [S]

TRIFLUOPERAZINE

Synonyms

Stelazine

Summary

Trifluoperazine is a phenothiazine used to treat psychoses and other psychiatric illnesses.

Magnitude of Teratogenic Risk

None To Minimal

Quality and Quantity of Data

Fair

Comment

None

The frequency of congenital anomalies was no higher than expected among the children of 42 women who took trifluoperazine during the first four lunar months of pregnancy in the Collaborative Perinatal Project (Heinonen et al., 1977). Similarly, the frequency of congenital anomalies was not increased among the infants of 59 women treated with trifluoperazine during the first trimester of pregnancy (General Practitioner Research Group, 1963). The incidence of malformations did not appear to be increased in a survey of infants born to 480 pregnant women treated with trifluoperazine (Moriarty & Nance, 1963).

The frequency of malformations was no higher than expected among the offspring of rabbits and mice treated during pregnancy with 20-80 and 290-1150 times those used clinically (Khan & Azam, 1969). A dose-dependent reduction of fetal weight occurred among the rabbits and an increased frequency of fetal loss occurred among the mice in this study. Szabo & Brent (1974) reported an increased frequency of cleft palate in the offspring of mice treated with 70-300 times the usual human dose of trifluoperazine during pregnancy. The relevance of these observations to the clinical use of this drug in human pregnancy in unknown.

Please see agent summary on chlorpromazine for information on a related agent that has been more thoroughly studied.

Key References

General Practitioner Research Group: Drugs in pregnancy survey. Practitioner 191:775-780, 1963. [S]

Heinonen OP, Slone D, Shapiro S: Birth Defects and Drugs in Pregnancy. Littleton, Mass.: John Wright-PSG, 1977, pp 323-325. [E]

Khan I, Azam A: Study of teratogenic activity of trifluoperazine, amitriptyline, ethionamide and thalidomide in pregnant rabbits and mice. Proc Eur Soc Study Drug Toxic 10:235-242, 1969. [A]

Moriarty AJ, Nance MR: Trifluoperazine and pregnancy. Can Med Assoc J 88:375-376, 1963. [O]

Szabo KT, Brent RL: Species differences in experimental teratogenesis by tranquillising agents. Lancet 1:565, 1974. [A]

TRIFLURIDINE

Synonyms

F3T, Trifluorothymidine, Viroptic

Summary

Trifluridine is a nucleotide analog used topically in the treatment of herpes simplex infections of the eye. Systemic absorption of trifluridine following topical application is negligible (Carmine et al., 1982).

Magnitude of Teratogenic Risk

Undetermined

Quality and Quantity of Data

None To Poor

Comment

A small risk cannot be excluded, but a high risk of congenital anomalies in the children of women treated with trifluridine during pregnancy is unlikely.

No epidemiological studies of congenital anomalies among infants born to women treated with trifluridine during pregnancy have been reported.

The frequency of malformations was not increased among the offspring of rats or rabbits treated with trifluridine during pregnancy (Itoi et al., 1972, 1975). The dosages used were large, being similar to that given to humans without correction for the difference in the size of the species.

Key References

Carmine AA, Brogden RN, Heel RC, et al.: Trifluridine: A review of its antiviral activity and therapeutic use in the topical treatment of viral eye infections. Drugs 23:329-353, 1982. [R]

Itoi M, Gefter JW, Kaneko N, et al.: Teratogenicities of ophthalmic drugs. I. Antiviral ophthalmic drugs. Arch Ophthalmol 93:46-51, 1975. [A]

Itoi M, Ishii Y, Kaneko N: Teratogenicities of antiviral ophthalmics on experimental animals. Rinsho Ganka(Jpn J Clin Opthal) 26:631-640, 1972. [A]

TRIMECAINE

Summary

Trimecaine is a local anesthetic.

Magnitude of Teratogenic Risk

Undetermined

Quality and Quantity of Data

None

Comment

A small risk cannot be excluded, but there is no indication that the risk of congenital anomalies in the children of women treated with trimecaine during pregnancy is likely to be great.

No epidemiological studies of congenital anomalies in children born to women exposed to trimecaine during pregnancy have been reported.

No investigations of teratologic effects of trimecaine in experimental animals have been published.

Key References

None available.

TRIMETHADIONE/ PARAMETHADIONE

Synonyms

Paramethadione, Tridione, Trimedone, Trimethadione, Trioxanona, Troxidone

Summary

Trimethadione and paramethadione are closely related oral anticonvulsant agents used to treat petit mal seizures.

Magnitude of Teratogenic Risk

High

Quality and Quantity of Data

Good To Excellent

Comment

This risk assessment is for chronic use in the treatment of seizure disorders.

Studies of malformations in infants born to women who took trimethadione or paramethadione during pregnancy are difficult to interpret because assessment of the effects of anticonvulsant drug exposure is confounded by many other factors (Friis et al., 1989; Dansky & Finnell, 1991; Kaneko, 1991). Among these confounders are the facts that most women with seizures are treated with some anticonvulsant drug, that many women are treated with more than one drug, that women who are not treated or are treated with a single agent probably have milder disease, and that trimethadione or paramethadione use rarely occurs in women without seizures.

A characteristic pattern of malformations called the "fetal trimethadione syndrome" occurs among children of women treated with trimethadione or paramethadione during pregnancy (German et al., 1970; Zackai et al., 1975; Feldman et al., 1977; Smith, 1977; Goldman & Yaffe, 1978; Rosen & Lightner, 1978; Dansky & Finnell, 1991). Frequent features of this syndrome include growth retardation, microcephaly, cleft lip and/or palate, and unusual facies with V-shaped eyebrows, broad nasal bridge, epicanthal folds, and anteverted nostrils. Cardiovascular malformations, especially ventricular septal defect, tetralogy of Fallot, patent ductus arteriosus, and transposition of the great vessels, are common. Genitourinary and gastrointestinal anomalies may also occur. Many affected pregnancies are miscarried, and stillbirth or death in infancy appears unusually frequent. Surviving affected children often are short and mentally retarded; speech difficulty and conductive hearing loss are common. The precise risk of fetal trimethadione syndrome in exposed pregnancies is unknown but appears to be relatively high. Congenital anomalies were observed in 30% of 61 infants born to women treated with trimethadione (usually in combination with another anticonvulsant) during the first trimester of pregnancy in one study (Nakane et al., 1980).

A variety of malformations were observed among the offspring of mice treated during pregnancy with trimethadione in doses 8-22 times those used in humans (Brown et al., 1979; Wells et al., 1989). Typical dose and time dependence of the teratogenic effect were observed. The malformations seen include cardiovascular, vertebral, and palatal defects. Malformations have also been observed among the offspring of rats and rhesus monkeys treated during pregnancy with 2-10 and 1-2 times the human therapeutic dose of trimethadione (Vorhees, 1983; Fradkin et al., 1981). Persistent behavioral alterations occur among the offspring of rats treated with trimethadione in 5 times the human dose (Vorhees, 1983).

Key References

Brown NA, Shull G, Fabro S: Assessment of the teratogenic potential of trimethadione in the CD-1 mouse. Toxicol Appl Pharmacol 51:59-71, 1979. [A]

Dansky LV, Finnell RH: Parental epilepsy, anticonvulsant drugs, and reproductive outcome: Epidemiologic and experimental findings spanning three decades. 2: Human studies. Reprod Toxicol 5(4):301-335, 1991. [R]

Feldman GL, Weaver DD, Lovrien EW: The fetal trimethadione syndrome. Am J Dis Child 131:1389-1392, 1977. [C]

Fradkin R, Scott WJ, Wislon JG: Trimethadione teratogenesis in the rat and rhesus monkey. Teratology 24:39-40A, 1981. [A]

Friis ML: Facial clefts and congenital heart defects in children of parents with epilepsy: Genetic and environmental etiologic factors. Acta Neurol Scand 79:433-459, 1989. [R]

German J, Kowal A, Ehlers KH: Trimethadione and human teratogenesis. Teratology 3:349-362, 1970. [C]

Goldman AS, Yaffe SJ: Fetal trimethadione syndrome. Teratology 17:103-106, 1978. [R]

Kaneko S: Antiepileptic drug therapy and reproductive consequences: Functional and morpholologic effects. Reprod Toxicol 5:179-198, 1991. [R]

Nakane Y, Okuma T, Takahashi R, Sato Y, et al.: Multi-institutional study on the teratogenicity and fetal toxicity of antiepileptic drugs: A report of a collaborative study group in Japan. Epilepsia 21:663-680, 1980. [E]

Rosen RC, Lightner ES: Phenotypic malformations in association with maternal trimethadione therapy. J Pediatr 92:240-244, 1978. [C]

Smith DW: Teratogenicity of anticonvulsive medications. Am J Dis Child 131:1337-1339, 1977. [R]

Vorhees CV: Fetal anticonvulsant syndrome in rats: Dose- and period-response relationships of prenatal diphenylhydantoin, trimethadione and phenobarbital exposure on the structural and functional development of the offspring. J Pharmacol Exp Ther 227:274-287, 1983. [A]

Wells PG, Nagal MK, Greco GS: Inhibition of trimethadione and dimethadione teratogenicity by the cyclooxygenase inhibitor acetylsalicylic acid: A unifying hypothesis for the teratologic effects of hydantoin anticonvulsants and structurally related compounds. Toxicol Appl Pharmacol 97:406-414, 1989. [A]

Zackai EH, Mellman WJ, Neiderer B, Hanson JW: The fetal trimethadione syndrome. J Pediatr 87:280-284, 1975. [C]

TRIMETHOBENZAMIDE

Synonyms

Bio-Gan, Stemetic, Tebamide, T-Gen, Ticon, Tigan, Tiject

Summary

Trimethobenzamide is an ethanolamine derivative with weak antihistamine properties. It is used as an antinauseant and antiemetic.

Magnitude of Teratogenic Risk

None To Minimal

Quality and Quantity of Data

Fair To Good

Comment

None

The frequencies of congenital anomalies in general, of major malformations, and of minor anomalies were no greater than expected among the infants of 340 women treated with trimethobenzamide during the first four lunar months of pregnancy in the Collaborative Perinatal Project (Heinonen et al., 1977). Similarly, the frequency of congenital anomalies was not increased among the children of 700 women treated with this drug anytime in pregnancy. No malformations were observed among the infants of more than 120 women treated with trimethobenzamide during the first trimester of pregnancy in the Boston Collaborative Drug Surveillance Program (Jick et al., 1981; Aselton et al., 1985). Milkovich & van den Berg (1976) observed a weak association between maternal use of trimethobenzamide during the first 84 days of pregnancy and the occurrence of congenital anomalies (broadly defined) in a cohort of 194 children evaluated at five years of age. This relationship is unlikely to be causal because no such association was observed among these children at one month or one year of age, there was no specificity or pattern in the anomalies that occurred, and no such association was observed in the other cohort studies cited above. In a case-control study of 325 infants with pyloric stenosis, no association was found with maternal use of trimethobenzamide during pregnancy (Mitchell et al., 1983).

No animal teratology studies of trimethobenzamide have been published.

Key References

Aselton P, Jick H, Milunsky A, Hunter JR, et al.: First-trimester drug use and congenital disorders. Obstet Gynecol 65:451-455, 1985. [S]

Heinonen OP, Slone D, Shapiro S: Birth Defects and Drugs in Pregnancy. Littleton, Mass.:

John Wright-PSG, 1977, pp 323-324, 327, 330, 437, 489. [E]

Jick H, Holmes LB, Hunter JR, Madsen S, et al.: First-trimester drug use and congenital disorders. JAMA 246:343-346, 1981. [S]

Milkovich L, van den Berg BJ: An evaluation of the teratogenicity of certain antinauseant drugs. Am J Obstet Gynecol 125:244-248, 1976. [S]

Mitchell AA, Schwingl PJ, Rosenberg L, et al.: Birth defects in relation to Bendectin use in pregnancy. II. Pyloric stenosis. Am J Obstet Gynecol 147(7):737-742, 1983. [E]

TRIMETHOPRIM

Synonyms

Abaprim, Ipral, Monotrim, Proloprim, Syraprim, Tiempe, Trimethoxyprim, Trimogal, Trimpex

Summary

Trimethoprim is a competitive inhibitor of dihydrofolate reductase with specificity for microbial rather than mammalian systems (Mandell & Sande, 1990). It is used as an oral antimicrobial agent, often in combination with a sulfonamide.

Magnitude of Teratogenic Risk

None To Minimal

Quality and Quantity of Data

Poor To Fair

Comment

None

The frequency of congenital anomalies was no greater than expected among the infants of 89 women treated with trimethoprim in combination with sulfamethoxazole during the first trimester of pregnancy or of 211 treated with this agent anytime during pregnancy in one cohort study (Colley et al., 1982). No congenital anomalies were observed among the infants of 42 women treated with trimethoprim in combination with sulfamethoxazole in a clinical trial of treatment for bacteriuria in the first trimester of pregnancy (Bailey, 1984). In another trial, the frequency of congenital anomalies was no higher than expected among the infants of 120 women treated with trimethoprim and sulfamethoxazole, but only 10 of these women were treated during the first trimester (Williams et al., 1969). An association with maternal use of a trimethoprim-sulfamethoxazole during pregnancy was observed in a case-control study of 6228 infants with congenital anomalies (Czeizel, 1990). The association was seen with treatment at all gestational ages including the first trimester (OR=2.3, 95% confidence interval 1.22-4.00) and involved a variety of congenital anomalies. No characteristic pattern was observed among exposed cases that had multiple congenital anomalies. The author concluded that the association between maternal exposure to trimethoprim-sulfamethoxazole and congenital anomalies was probably due to the underlying maternal disorder and not to the drugs per se.

No teratogenic effect was observed among the offpring of rats treated during pregnancy with trimethoprim in doses 3 times those used in humans, but treatment with doses 6-60 times those used clinically produced increased frequencies of embryonic malformations and death (Udall, 1969; Kreutz, 1981). Maternal toxicity was also observed at the higher doses. The anomalies seen primarily affected the skeleton and were similar to those that occur with folate antagonists such as aminopterin and methotrexate. The relevance of these observations to the use of trimethoprim in therapeutic doses in human pregnancy is uncertain.

Key References

Bailey RR: Single-dose antibacterial treatment for bacteriuria in pregnancy. Drugs 27:183-186, 1984. [S]

Colley DP, Kay J, Gibson GT: Study of the use in pregnancy of co-trimoxazole sulfamethizole. Aust J Pharm 63:570-575, 1982. [S]

Czeizel A: A case-control analysis of the teratogenic effects of co-trimoxazole. Reprod Toxicol 4(4):305-313, 1990. [E]

Kreutz VR: Investigation on the influence of trimethoprim at the intrauterine development in the rat. Anat Anz 149:151-159, 1981. [A]

Mandell GL, Sande MA: Antimicrobial agents (continued). Sulfonamides, trimethoprim-sulfamethoxazole, quinolones, and agents for urinary tract infections. In: Gilman AG, Rall TW, Nies AS, Taylor P (eds). Goodman and Gilman's The Pharmacological Basis of Therapeutics, 8th ed. New York: Pergamon Press, 1990, pp 1047-1064. [O]

Udall V: Toxicology of sulphonamide-trimethoprim combinations. Postgrad Med J 45:42-45, 1969. [A]

Williams JD, Brumfitt W, Condie AP, Reeves DS: The treatment of bacteriuria in pregnant women with sulphamethoxazole and trimethoprim: A microbiological, clinical and toxicological study. Postgrad Med J 45(Suppl):71-76, 1969. [S]

TRIMIPRAMINE

Synonyms

Stangyl, Surmontil, Trimeprimine

Summary

Trimipramine is a tricyclic antidepressant.

Magnitude of Teratogenic Risk

Undetermined

Quality and Quantity of Data

None To Poor

Comment

A small risk cannot be excluded, but a high risk of congenital anomalies in the children of women treated with trimipramine during pregnancy is unlikely.

No epidemiological studies of congenital anomalies in infants whose mothers were treated with trimipramine during pregnancy have been reported.

An increased frequency of central nervous system malformations was observed among the offspring of pregnant mice treated with trimipramine in a dose about 25 times that used in humans (Jurand, 1980).

Please see agent summary on amitriptyline for information on a related agent that has been more thoroughly studied.

Key References

Jurand A: Malformations of the central nervous system induced by neurotropic drugs in mouse embryos. Develop Growth Differ 22:61-78, 1980. [A]

TRIPROLIDINE

Synonyms

Actidil, Actifed Capsules, Actiphyll, Pro-Actidil, Tripyrolidine

Summary

Triprolidine is an antihistamine used to treat allergic conditions.

Magnitude of Teratogenic Risk

None To Minimal

Quality and Quantity of Data

Poor To Fair

Comment

None

The frequency of congenital anomalies was no greater than expected among the infants of 628 women treated with triprolidine during the first trimester of pregnancy in two cohorts of the Boston Collaborative Drug Surveillance Program (Jick et al., 1981; Aselton et al., 1985).

No animal teratology studies of triprolidine have been published.

Key References

Aselton P, Jick H, Milunsky A, Hunter JR, Stergachis A: First-trimester drug use and congenital disorders. Obstet Gynecol 65:451-455, 1985. [E]

Jick H, Holmes LB, Hunter JR, Madsen S, Stergachis A: First-trimester drug use and congenital disorders. JAMA 246:343-346, 1981. [E]

TROLAMINE

Synonyms

Mobisyl, Triethanolamine, Trihydroxytriethy-lamine

Summary

Trolamine (triethanolamine) is used as an emulsifying agent in the textile, chemical, wood, paper, and dye industries, among others. It is employed in ear drops to remove impacted wax and, combined with salicylate, in topical anesthetics.

Magnitude of Teratogenic Risk

Undetermined

Quality and Quantity of Data

None

Comment

A small risk cannot be excluded, but a high risk of congenital anomalies in the children of women treated with trolamine during pregnancy is unlikely.

No epidemiological studies of congenital anomalies among infants born to women ex-posed to trolamine during pregnancy have been reported.

No animal teratology studies of trolamine have been published.

Key References

None available.

TRYPTOPHAN

Synonyms

Tryptoplex

Summary

Tryptophan, an amino acid, is an essential dietary component. Large doses of tryptophan have been used as a hypnotic and appetite suppressant.

Magnitude of Teratogenic Risk

Undetermined

Quality and Quantity of Data

Poor

Comment

Although the risk associated with this agent is unknown, animal studies raise concern about the possibility of a substantial risk at high doses. (see below).

No epidemiological studies of congenital anomalies in infants born to women who took large amounts of tryptophan during pregnancy have been reported. Unexplained eosinophilia, thrombocytosis and leukocytosis in association with recurrent low-grade fevers were observed for the first several months of life in an infant whose mother took 1 gram of supplemental tryptophan daily throughout the second and third trimester of pregnancy (Hatch et al.,

1991). No causal relationship can be inferred on the basis of this anecdotal observation.

Increased rates of fetal loss and fetal growth retardation have been observed among the offspring of pregnant hamsters given diets containing tryptophan in amounts equivalent to those used to treat insomnia in humans (Meier & Wilson, 1983). Decreased fetal body and brain weight have been observed among the offspring of rats fed diets containing 5-7% but not 1.4-2.8% tryptophan during pregnancy (Matsueda & Niyama, 1982; Funk et al., 1991). The effective treatment would be expected to provide a dose of tryptophan 20-30 times greater than that used to treat insomnia in humans. The rate of congenital anomalies was not affected by this treatment although there was an increased frequency of fetal resorptions among rats fed diets containing 2.8% but not 7.5% tryptophan (Funk et al., 1991). The relevance of these observations to the clinical use of tryptophan in human pregnancy is unknown.

Key References

Funk DN, Worthington-Roberts B, Fantel A: Impact of supplemental lysine or tryptophan on pregnancy course and outcome in rats. Nutr Res 11:501-512, 1991. [A]

Hatch DL: Persistent eosinophilia in an infant with probable intrauterine exposure to L-tryptophan-containing supplements. Pediatrics 88:810-813, 1991. [C]

Matsueda S, Niiyama Y: The effects of excess amino acids on maintenance of pregnancy and fetal growth in rats. J Nutr Sci Vitaminol 28:557-573, 1982. [A]

Meier AH, Wilson JM: Tryptophan feeding adversely influences pregnancy. Life Sci 32:1193-1196, 1983. [A]

TUBOCURARINE

Synonyms

Curarin, Jexin, Tubarine, Tubocuran

Summary

Tubocurarine is a non-depolarizing muscle relaxant that produces paralysis of voluntary muscle. Tubocurarine is used as an adjunct to anesthesia and assisted ventilation.

Magnitude of Teratogenic Risk

Undetermined

Quality and Quantity of Data

Poor

Comment

1) A small risk cannot be excluded, but a high risk of congenital anomalies in the infants of women who received acute treatment with tubocurarine during pregnancy is unlikely.

2) Chronic maternal treatment with tubocurarine as part of ventilatory therapy may be associated with the development of fetal contractures.

No epidemiological studies of congenital anomalies among infants born to women treated with tubocurarine during pregnancy have been reported. No adverse effects were noted among about 25 infants born after receiving in utero intramuscular injections of 1.5-3 mg/kg of tubocurarine for diagnostic or therapeutic procedures in the second or third trimester of gestation (Moise et al., 1987). An infant with multiple congenital contractures was born to a woman who was treated with tubocurarine repeatedly over 10 days in the late first or early second trimester of pregnancy (Jago, 1970). No cause and effect relationship can be inferred from this case report because the mother had also attempted instrumental abortion, had tetanus, and suffered repeated episodes of severe hypoxia during the pregnancy.

Multiple joint contractures, pulmonary hypoplasia, growth retardation, and other features of fetal akinesia were seen among newborn rats that had been injected in utero with 2-4 mg/kg/d of tubocurarine late in gestation (Shoro, 1977; Moessinger, 1983). The relevance of these observations to maternal treatment with tubocurarine in human pregnancy is unknown.

Key References

Jago RH: Arthrogryposis following treatment of maternal tetanus with muscle relaxants. Arch Dis Child 45:277-279, 1970. [C]

Moessinger AC: Fetal akinesia deformation sequence: An animal model. Pediatr 72:857-863, 1983. [A]

Moise KJ, Carpenter RJ, Deter RL, et al.: The use of fetal neuromuscular blockade during intrauterine procedures. Am J Obstet Gynecol 157(4):874-879, 1987. [S]

Shoro AA: Intra-uterine growth retardation and limb deformities produced by neuromuscular blocking agents in the rat fetus. J Anat 123(2):341-350, 1977. [A]

UBIQUINONE

Synonyms

Caomet, Coenzyme Q10, Decarene, Decorenone, Mitocor, Neuquinone, Ubidecarenone, Ubione

Summary

Ubiquinones are a series of naturally occurring benzoquinones involved in mitochondrial electron transport. Individual ubiquinones are specified by an appended number that indicates the length of the side chain. Ubiquinones have been used as dietary supplements and in the treatment of congestive heart failure.

Magnitude of Teratogenic Risk

Undetermined

Quality and Quantity of Data

None To Poor

Comment

A small risk cannot be excluded, but a high risk of congenital anomalies in the children of women treated with ubiquinone during pregnancy is unlikely.

No epidemiological studies of congenital anomalies among infants born to women treated with large doses of ubiquinone during pregnancy have been reported.

No teratogenic effect was observed among the offspring of pregnant mice or rats treated with "ubiquinone-9" in doses of 20-4000 or 20-2000 mg/kg/d (Nakazawa et al., 1969).

Key References

Nakazawa M, Ohzeki M, Takahashi N, Tsuchida T: Toxicity tests of ubiquinone-9. II. Teratogenicity. Oyo Yakuri 3:155-159, 1969. [A]

UNDECYLENIC ACID

Synonyms

Calcium Undecylenate, Caldesene, Cruex, Desenex, Kool Foot, Merlenate, Pedi-Dry, Quinsana Plus, Undoguent

Summary

Undecylenic acid is used as a topical antifungal agent.

Magnitude of Teratogenic Risk

Undetermined

Quality and Quantity of Data

None

Comment

None

No epidemiological studies of congenital anomalies in infants born to women treated with undecylenic acid during pregnancy have been reported.

No animal teratology studies of undecylenic acid have been published.

Key References

None available.

URETHANE

Synonyms

Ethyl Carbamate, Ethyl Urethane

Summary

Urethane is an antineoplastic agent that is rarely used now. It also has a hypnotic action and is employed as an anesthetic for animals. Urethane is used in the chemical, textile, pesticide and cosmetic industries.

Magnitude of Teratogenic Risk

Undetermined

Quality and Quantity of Data

Poor

Comment

None

No epidemiological studies of congenital anomalies in children born to mothers who took urethane during pregnancy have been reported. A few anecdotal descriptions of normal infants born to mothers who were treated with urethane at various times in pregnancy have been reported (Gililland & Weinstein, 1983).

Lung, skeletal, and craniofacial malformations have been found with increased frequency in the offspring of mice treated with urethane in doses 8 or more times greater than those

used in humans (Nomura & Okamoto, 1972; Nomura, 1974, 1977; Collins & Sotomayor, 1989). Typical dose- and time-dependence of this teratogenic effect was demonstrated. Only skeletal variations were observed with significantly increased frequency among the offspring of pregnant rats treated with urethane in doses 8 times those used in humans in one study (Takaori et al., 1966). In another, the frequency of malformations was not increased but fetal weight was reduced and skeletal variations were more frequent among the offspring of pregnant rats treated with 25 times the human dose of urethane, a dose that was maternally toxic (Daston et al., 1991). Central nervous system and cardiac malformations were reported among the offspring of hamsters treated during pregnancy with 2-8 times the human dose of urethane (Ferm, 1966).

Treatment of mice with urethane during pregnancy in doses 4-8 times those used in humans produced an increased frequency of hepatomas, pulmonary adenomas, ovarian tumors, and other neoplasms in the offspring (Vesselinovitch et al., 1967; Nomura & Okamoto, 1972; Field & Lang, 1988; Collins & Sotomayor, 1989). The relevance of these findings to the risks associated with the use of urethane in human pregnancy is unknown.

Key References

Collins TFX, Sotomayor RE: Developmental toxicity of urethan. Toxicol Ind Health 5(6):1045-1060, 1989. [R]

Daston GP, Overmann GJ, Taubeneck MW, Lehman-McKeeman LD, et al.: The role of metallothionein induction and altered zinc status in maternally mediated developmental toxicity: Comparison of the effects of urethane and styrene in rats. Toxicol Appl Pharmacol 110:450-463, 1991. [A]

Ferm VH: Severe developmental malformations. Arch Pathol 81:174-177, 1966. [A]

Field KJ, Lang CM: Hazards of urethane (ethyl carbamate): A review of the literature. Lab Anim 22:255-262, 1988. [R]

Gililland G, Weinstein L: The effects of cancer chemotherapeutic agents on the developing fetus. Obstet Gynecol Surv 38:6-13, 1983. [R]

Nomura T: An analysis of the changing urethan response of the developing mouse embryo in relation to mortality, malformation, and neoplasm. Cancer Res 34:2217-2231, 1974. [A]

Nomura T: Similarity of the mechanism of chemical carcinogen-initiated teratogenesis and carcinogenesis in mice. Cancer Res 37:969-973, 1977. [A]

Nomura T, Okamoto E: Transplacental carcinogenesis by urethan in mice: Teratogenesis and carcinogenesis in relation to organogenesis. Gann 63:731-742, 1972. [A]

Takaori S, Tanabe K, Shimamoto K: Developmental abnormalities of skeletal system induced by ethylurethan in the rat. Jpn J Pharmacol 16:63-73, 1966. [A]

Vesselinovitch SD, Mihailovich N, Pietra G: The prenatal exposure of mice to urethan and the consequent development of tumors in various tissues. Cancer Res 27:2333-2337, 1967. [A]

UROFOLLITROPIN

Synonyms

Metrodin

Summary

Urofollitropin is a follicle-stimulating hormone extracted from the urine of postmenopausal women. It is administered parenterally in the treatment of infertility.

Magnitude of Teratogenic Risk

Undetermined

Quality and Quantity of Data

None

Comment

A small risk cannot be excluded, but a high risk of congenital anomalies in the children of women treated with urofollitropin during pregnancy is unlikely.

No epidemiological studies of congenital anomalies in infants whose mothers were treated with urofollitropin during pregnancy have been reported.

No animal teratology studies of urofollitropin have been published.

Key References

None available.

VALPROIC ACID

Synonyms

Convulex, Depakene, Depakote, Epilim, Sodium Dipropylacetate, Sodium 2-Propylvalerate, Sodium Valproate, Valproate

Summary

Valproic acid is a commonly used oral anticonvulsant.

Magnitude of Teratogenic Risk

Neural Tube Defects: Small To Moderate

Other Congenital Anomalies: Small To Moderate

Quality and Quantity of Data

Neural Tube Defects: Good

Other Congenital Anomalies: Poor To Fair

Comment

These risks are additive

Epidemiological studies of malformations in infants born to women who took valproic acid during pregnancy are difficult to interpret because assessment of the effects of anticonvulsant treatment is confounded by many other factors (Kelly, 1984; Kallen, 1986; Lammer et al., 1987; Dansky & Finnell, 1991; Kaneko, 1991). Among these confounders are the facts that most women with seizures are treated with some anticonvulsant drug, that many women are treated with more than one anticonvulsant at a time, that women who are not treated or are treated with a single agent probably have milder disease, and that valproic acid treatment is uncommon in women without seizures.

An association between the occurrence of spina bifida in infants and maternal use of valproic acid in the first trimester of pregnancy has been observed in a case-control study involving 337 affected children (Anonymous, 1983; Robert et al., 1983; Robert, 1988). Many other epidemiological studies and clinical series support the existence of this association (Jeavons, 1982; Koch et al., 1983; Mastroiacovo et al., 1983; Lindhout & Meinhardi, 1984; Bertollini et al., 1985; Jager-Roman et al., 1986; Lindhout & Schmidt, 1986; Lammer et al., 1987; Kallen et al., 1989; Martinez-Frias, 1990, 1991; Rosa, 1991; Battino et al., 1992; Dravet et al., 1992; Kaneko et al., 1992; Omtzigt et al., 1992a; Lindhout et al., 1992a, 1992b). The defect observed is usually lumbar or sacral spina bifida; it is often associated with hydrocephalus (Linhout et al., 1992b). Anencephaly is rarely seen. In one study, the valproic acid doses and serum levels were significantly higher in five women with epilepsy who had children with spina bifida than in 84 epileptic women who took valproic acid during pregnancy but had unaffected children (Omtzigt et al., 1992a, 1992b). The best available estimate of the risk of spina bifida among the children of women treated with valproic acid during the first trimester of pregnancy is 1-2% in populations in which the background rate of spina bifida is about 1/1000. The risk may be greater in populations with a higher background rate. Spina bifida can be detected prenatally by high-resolution ultrasonography and measurement of amniotic fluid or maternal serum alpha-feto-protein concentration (Weinbaum et al., 1986; Serville et al., 1989).

A distinctive pattern of minor anomalies of the face and digits, i.e., a "fetal valproate syndrome," has been described in infants born to women treated with valproic acid during pregnancy (DiLiberti et al., 1984; Winter et al., 1987; Ardinger et al., 1988; Martinez-Frias, 1990). This syndrome involves postnatal growth retardation, microcephaly, developmental delay, midface hypoplasia, epicanthal folds, short nose, broad nasal bridge, thin upper lip, thick lower lip, and micrognathia.

An association (OR=4.48, 95% confidence interval 1.5-18.2) with maternal use of valproic acid during pregnancy was observed in a case-control study involving 12,506 children with congenital anomalies other than spina bifida (Martinez-Frias et al., 1989). An increased frequency of congenital anomalies in general (OR=1.95, 95% confidence interval 1.11-3.46) was observed in a cohort study of 79 infants born to women who were treated with valproic acid for seizure disorders during pregnancy (Dravet et al., 1992). The validity of this association is difficult to determine because different methods were used to identify congenital anomalies in the study and control groups. Cleft palate, congenital heart disease, hypospadias, club feet and defects of the radius and related digital rays have been observed in children born to women who were treated with valproic acid for seizure disorders during pregnancy, but it is unclear whether or not these defects are attributable directly to maternal treatment with valproic acid (Thomas & Buchanan, 1981; Jeavons, 1982; Koch et al., 1983; Mastroiacovo et al., 1983; Bertollini et al., 1987; Lammer et al., 1987; Kallen et al., 1989; Martinez-Frias, 1990; Vanfleteren et al., 1990; Verloes et al., 1990; Lindhout et al., 1992a, 1992b). In one study, serum levels of valproic acid in the first trimester of pregnancy were significantly higher in women with epilepsy who had children with congenital anomalies than in epileptic women who took valproic acid during pregnancy but had unaffected children (Battino et al., 1992). A similar trend was observed in another study, but statistical analysis of the effect was not provided (Lindhout et al., 1992a).

Increased frequencies of craniofacial and skeletal anomalies as well as of fetal death have been observed among the offspring of rhesus monkeys treated during pregnancy with <1-10 times the maximum human therapeutic dose of valproic acid (Mast et al., 1986; Hendrickx et al., 1988). The effect exhibited typical dose-dependence. Exposure of pregnant mice or rats to valproic acid in doses that are associated with blood levels above the human therapeutic range causes embryonic death and malformations in the offspring (Nau & Loscher, 1986; Nau & Scott, 1986; Vorhees, 1987a; Ritter et al., 1987; Binkerd et al., 1988; Finnell et al., 1988; Sonodo et al., 1990; Turner et al., 1990; Collins et al., 1990, 1991; Cotariu & Zaidman, 1991; Finnell & Dansky, 1991; Nau et al., 1991; Khera, 1992). Exencephaly and skeletal anomalies are among the most common malformations observed in mice; cardiac, skeletal, and urinary tract anomalies are seen most often in rats. The teratogenic effect exhibits a typical dose-response relationship in both species. In rats, no increase in malformations was observed when dams were treated during pregnancy with doses of valproic acid which produced blood levels within the human therapuetic range (Vorhees, 1987a). Spina bifida can be produced among the offspring of pregnant mice by treatment with valproic acid in doses 15-25 times those used in humans (Ehlers et al., 1992a, b). Increased frequencies of neural tube defects have also been observed among the offspring of hamsters treated with five times the maximum human dose of valproic acid during pregnancy (Moffa et al., 1984). The rate of valproic acid-induced exencephaly in the mouse can be reduced by concurrent treatment of the mother with folic acid analogues (Wegner & Nau, 1991).

Behavioral alterations have been reported among the offspring of rats treated with valproic acid during pregnancy in doses equivalent to those used in humans (Sobrian & Nandedkar, 1986; Vorhees, 1987b).

Perinatal distress and unusual neonatal behavior have been noted in infants born to women treated with valproic acid or a variety of other anticonvulsants during pregnancy (Koch et al., 1985; Jager-Roman et al., 1986, 1987). There are also anecdotal reports of afibrinogenemia and hepatic failure in infants born to women who were treated with valproic acid during pregnancy (Majer & Green, 1987; Legius et al., 1987). Similar compications have been reported in children and adults on such therapy.

Key References

Anonymous: Valproate: A new cause of birth defects: Report from Italy and follow-up from France. MMWR 32:438-439, 1983. [R]

Ardinger HH, Atkin JF, Blackston RD, Elsas LJ, et al.: Verification of the fetal valproate syndrome phenotype. Am J Med Gen 29:171-185, 1988. [S]

Battino D, Binelli S, Caccamo ML, Canevini MP, et al.: Malformations in offspring of 305 epileptic women: a prospective study. Acta Neurol Scand 85:204-207, 1992. [E]

Bertollini R, Kallen B, Mastroiacovo P, Robert E: Anticonvulsant drugs in monotherapy. Effect on the fetus. Eur J Epidemiol 3(2):164-171, 1987. [E]

Bertollini R, Mastroiacovo P, Segni G: Maternal epilepsy and birth defects: A case-control study in the Italian Multicentric Registry of Birth Defects (IPIMC). Eur J Epidemiol 1:67-72, 1985. [E]

Binkerd PE, Rowland JM, Nau H, Hendricks AG: Evaluation of valproic acid (VPA) developmental toxicity and pharmacokinetics in Sprague-Dawley rats. Fundam Appl Toxicol 11:485-493, 1988. [A]

Collins MD, Fradkin R, Scott WJ Jr.: Induction of postaxial forelimb ectrodactyly with anticonvulsant agents in A/J mice. Teratology 41:61-70, 1990. [A]

Collins MD, Walling KM, Resnick E, Scott WJ Jr.: The effect of administration time on malformations induced by three anticonvulsant agents in C57BL/6J mice with emphasis on forelimb ectrodactyly. Teratology 44:617-627, 1991. [A]

Cotariu D, Zaidman JL: Minireview. Developmental toxicity of valproic acid. Life Sciences 48(14):1341-1350, 1991. [R]

Dansky LV, Finnell RH: Parental epilepsy, anticonvulsant drugs, and reproductive outcome: Epidemiologic and experimental findings spanning three decades. 2: Human studies. Reprod Toxicol 5(4):301-335, 1991. [R]

DiLiberti JH, Farndon PA, Dennis NR, Curry CJR: The fetal valproate syndrome. Am J Med Genet 19:473-481, 1984. [S]

Dravet C, Julian C, Legras C, Magaudda A, ct al.: Epilepsy, antiepileptic drugs, and malformations in children of women with epilepsy: A French prospective cohort study. Neurology 42(Suppl 5):75-82, 1992. [E]

Ehlers K, Sturje H, Merker H-J, Nau H: Spina bifida aperta induced by valproic acid and by all-trans-retinoic acid in the mouse: Distinct differences in morphology and periods of sensitivity. Teratology 46:117-130, 1992b. [A]

Ehlers K, Sturje H, Merker H-J, Nau H: Valproic-acid induced spina bifida: A mouse model. Teratology 45:145-154, 1992a. [A]

Finnell RH, Bennett GD, Karras SB, Mohl VK: Common hierarchies of susceptibility to the induction of neural tube defects in mouse embryos by valproic acid and its 4-propyl-4-pentenoic acid metabolite. Teratology 38:313-320, 1988. [A]

Finnell RH, Dansky LV: Parental epilepsy, anticonvulsant drugs, and reproductive outcome: Epidemiologic and experimental findings spanning three decades; 1: Animal studies. Reprod Toxicol 5(4):281-299, 1991. [R]

Hendrickx AG, Binkerd P, Rowland JM, Rowland JR, et al.: Valproic acid developmental toxicity and pharmacokinetics in the rhesus monkey: An interspecies comparison. Teratology 38:329-345, 1988. [A]

Jager-Roman E, Deichl A, Jakob S, Hartmann A-M, et al: Fetal growth, major malformations, and minor anomalies in infants born to women receiving valproic acid. J Pediatr 108:997-1004, 1986. [S]

Jager-Roman E, Koch S, Helge H: Gentamicin pharmacokinetics in cystic fibrosis. [Reply to the Editor] J Pediatr 111:309-310, 1987. [S]

Jeavons PM: Sodium valproate and neural tube defects. Lancet 2:1282-1283, 1982. [S]

Kallen B: Maternal epilepsy, antiepileptic drugs and birth defects. Pathologica 78:757-768, 1986. [R]

Kallen B, Robert E, Mastroiacovo P, Martinez-Frias ML, et al.: Anticonvulsant drugs and malformations: Is there a drug specificity? Eur J Epidemiol 5(1):31-36, 1989. [E]

Kaneko S: Antiepileptic drug therapy and reproductive consequences: Functional and morphologic effects. Reprod Toxicol 5(3):179-198, 1991. [R]

Kaneko S, Otani K, Kondo T, Fukushima Y, et al.: Malformation in infants of mothers with epilepsy receiving antiepileptic drugs. Neurology 42(Suppl 5):68-74, 1992. [E]

Kelly TE: Teratogenicity of anticonvulsant drugs. I: Review of the literature. Am J Med Genet 19:413-434, 1984. [R]

Khera KS: Valproic acid-induced placental and teratogenic effects in rats. Teratology 45:603-610, 1992. [A]

Koch S, Gopfert-Geyer I, Hauser I, Hartmann A, et al.: Neonatal behavior disturbances in infants of epileptic women treated during pregnancy. In: Prevention of Physiology and Mental Congenital Defects. B. Epidemiology, Early Detection and Therapy, and Environmental Factors. Prog Clin Biol Res 163B:453-461, 1985. [E]

Koch S, Jager-Roman E, Rating D, Helge H: Possible teratogenic effect of valproate during pregnancy. J Pediatr 103:1007-1008, 1983. [S]

Lammer EJ, Sever LE, Oakley GP: Teratogen update: Valproic acid. Teratology 35:465-473, 1987. [R]

Legius E, Jaeken J, Eggermont E: Sodium valproate, pregnancy, and infantile fatal liver failure. Lancet 2:1518-1519, 1987. [C]

Lindhout D, Meinardi H: Spina bifida and in-utero exposure to valproate. Lancet 2:396, 1984. [S]

Lindhout D, Meinardi H, Meijer JWA, Nau H: Antiepileptic drugs and teratogenesis in two consecutive cohorts: Changes in prescription policy paralleled by changes in pattern of malformations. Neurology 42(Suppl 5):94-110, 1992a. [E]

Lindhout D, Omtzigt JGC, Cornel MC: Spectrum of neural-tube defects in 34 infants prenatally exposed to antiepileptic drugs. Neurology 42(Suppl 5):111-118, 1992b. [E]

Lindhout D, Schmidt D: In-utero exposure to valproate and neural tube defects. Lancet 1:1392-1393, 1986. [S]

Majer RV, Green PJ: Neonatal afibrinogenaemia due to sodium valproate. Lancet 2:740-741, 1987. [C]

Martinez-Frias ML: Clinical manifestation of prenatal exposure to valproic acid using case reports and epidemiologic information. Am J Med Genet 37:277-282, 1990. [E]

Martinez-Frias ML: Valproate and spina bifida. Lancet 1:611-612, 1989. [E]

Martinez-Frias ML: Valproic acid and spina bifida. Lancet 338:196-197, 1991. [O]

Mast TJ, Cukierski MA, Nau H, Hendrickx AG: Predicting the human teratogenic potential of the anticonvulsant, valproic acid, from a non-human primate model. Toxicol 39:111-119, 1986. [A]

Mastroiacovo P, Bertollini R, Morandini S, Segni G: Maternal epilepsy, valproate exposure, and birth defects. Lancet 2:1499, 1983. [E]

Moffa AM, White JA, MacKay EG, Frias JL: Valproic acid, zinc and open neural tubes in 9 day-old hamster embryos. Teratology 29:47A, 1984. [A]

Nau H, Hauck R-S, Ehlers K: Valproic acid-induced neural tube defects in mouse and human: Aspects of chirality, alternative drug development pharmacokinetics and possible mechanisms. Mini review. Pharmacol Toxicol 69:310-321, 1991. [R]

Nau H, Loscher W: Pharmacologic evaluation of various metabolites and analogs of valproic acid: Teratogenic potencies in mice. Fundam Appl Toxicol 6:669-676, 1986. [A]

Nau H, Scott WJ: Weak acids may act as teratogens by accumulating in the basic milieu of the early mammalian embryo. Nature 323:276-278, 1986. [A]

Omtzigt JGC, Los FJ, Grobbee DE, Pijpers L, et al.: The risk of spina bifida aperta after first-trimester exposure to valproate in a prenatal cohort. Neurology 42(Suppl 5):119-125, 1992a. [E]

Omtzigt JGC, Nau H, Los FJ, Pijpers L, et al.: The disposition of valproate and its metabolites in the late first trimester and early second trimester of pregnancy in maternal serum, urine, and amniotic fluid: Effect of dose, co-medication, and the presence of spina bifida. Eur J Clin Pharmacol 43:381-388, 1992b. [E]

Ritter EJ, Scott WJ, Randall JL, Ritter JM: Teratogenicity of Di(2-ethylhexyl) phthalate, 2-ethylhexanol, 2-ethylhexanoic acid, and valproic acid, and potentiation by caffeine. Teratology 35:41-46, 1987. [A]

Robert E: Valproic acid as a human teratogen. Congen Anom 28(Suppl):S71-S80, 1988. [E]

Robert E, Robert JM, Lapras C: Is valproic acid teratogenic? Rev Neurol 139:445-447, 1983. [E]

Rosa FW: Spina Bifida in infants of women treated with carbamazepine during pregnancy. N Engl J Med 324(10):674-677, 1991. [E]

Serville F, Carles D, Guibaud S, Dallay D: Fetal valproate phenotype is recognisable by mid pregnancy. J Med Genet 26:348-349, 1989. [C]

Sobrian SK, Nandedkar AKN: Prenatal antiepileptic drug exposure alters seizure susceptibility in rats. Pharmacol Biochem Behav 24:1383-1391, 1986. [A]

Sonoda T, Ohdo S, Ohba K, Okishima T, et al.: Teratogenic effects of sodium valproate in the Jcl:ICR mouse fetus. Acta Paediatr Jpn 32:502-507, 1990. [A]

Thomas D, Buchanan N: Teratogenic effects of anticonvulsants. J Pediatr 99:163, 1981. [C]

Turner S, Sucheston ME, De Philip RM, Paulson RB: Teratogenic effects on the neuroepithelium of the CD-1 mouse embryo exposed in utero to sodium valproate. Teratology 41:421-442, 1990. [A]

Vanfleteren M, Crolla D, Vermeulen J, Devos E: Depakine-induced embryopathy. J Belge Radiol 73(6):532-533, 1990. [C]

Verloes A, Frikiche A, Gremillet C, Paquay T, et al.: Proximal phocomelia and radial ray aplasia in fetal valproic syndrome. Eur J Pediatr 149:266-267, 1990. [C]

Vorhees CV: Behavioral teratogenicity of valproic acid: Selective effects on behavior after prenatal exposure to rats. Psychopharmacology 92:173-179, 1987b. [A]

Vorhees CV: Teratogenicity and developmental toxicity of valproic acid in rats. Teratology 35:195-202, 1987a. [A]

Wegner C, Nau H: Diurnal variation of folate concentrations in mouse embryo and plasma: The protective effect of folinic acid on valproic-acid-induced teratogenicity is time dependent. Reprod Toxicol 5(6):465-471, 1991. [A]

Weinbaum PJ, Cassidy SB, Vintzileos AM, Campbell WA, et al.: Prenatal detection of a neural tube defect after fetal exposure to valproic acid. Obstet Gynecol 67:31S-33S, 1986. [C]

Winter RM, Donnai D, Burn J, Tucker SM: Fetal valproate syndrome: Is there a recognisable phenotype? J Med Genet 24:692-695, 1987. [C]

VANCOMYCIN

Synonyms

Vancocin, Vancoled, Vancor

Summary

Vancomycin is an antibiotic used to treat staphylococcal or streptococcal infections. It is administered intravenously for systemic therapy and orally for intralumenal therapy of the gastrointestinal tract, from which it is not absorbed.

Magnitude of Teratogenic Risk

Undetermined

Quality and Quantity of Data

None

Comment

None

No epidemiological studies of congenital anomalies in infants born to women who took vancomycin during pregnancy have been reported. No evidence of auditory or renal damage was found among 10 infants whose mothers had been treated with vancomycin during the second or third trimester of pregnancy (Reyes et al., 1989).

No animal teratology studies of vancomycin have been published.

Key References

Reyes MP, Ostrea EM, Cabinian AE, et al.: Vancomycin during pregnancy: Does it cause hearing loss or nephrotoxicity in the infants? Am J Obstet Gynecol 161(4):977-981, 1989. [S]

VARICELLA-ZOSTER VIRUS

Synonyms

Chicken Pox

Summary

Varicella-zoster virus (VZV) is a member of the herpes virus group. It is the causative agent of chickenpox and of herpes zoster. Varicella occurs as a primary infection; latent persistence of VZV infections may develop, and zoster represents a reactivation of such latent infection (Gershon, 1990).

Magnitude of Teratogenic Risk

Small

Quality and Quantity of Data

Fair To Good

Comment

1) Fetal viraemia is more common than embryopathy.

2) Varicella-zoster immunoglobulins should be provided to infants born to women who develop chicken pox 4-6 days prior to delivery and to susceptible women who are exposed but have not yet developed rash (Anonymous, 1984).

More than three dozen children have been reported with a characteristic and highly unusual pattern of anomalies who were born to women who had symptoms of VZV infection during pregnancy (Laforet & Lynch, 1947; Enders, 1984; Brunell, 1984; Broomhead, 1985; Higa et al., 1987; Alkalay et al., 1987; Grose & Itani, 1989; Gershon, 1990). Typical features include congenital cicatricial skin lesions that correspond to a dermatome distribution, fetal growth retardation, limb anomalies, and brain and eye defects. Cerebral, cortical, and cerebellar atrophy, seizures, developmental delay, and nerve palsies are common. Chorioretinitis, cataracts, optic atrophy, and microphthalmia are the most frequent ocular abnormalities; gastrointestinal and genitourinary anomalies are often observed. Many affected individuals die in infancy.

The most severely involved infants appear to be those born of mothers who have varicella during the first trimester of gestation (Brunell, 1984; Enders, 1984; Gershon, 1990), although similar manifestations have been reported among the offspring of women who had varicella during the second trimester (Brice, 1976; Grose & Itani, 1989; Gershon, 1990).

Infants with similar congenital anomalies have also been reported after maternal zoster in pregnancy, but this is much less common than with maternal varicella (Brazin et al., 1979; Eyal et al., 1983; Gershon, 1990).

The risk of major congenital anomalies among infants born to women who had chickenpox in the first trimester of pregnancy has been estimated to be 2.3% over the background rate (Preblud et al., 1986). This estimate is based on a total of 131 cases pooled from four prospectively ascertained series (Siegel, 1973; Enders, 1984; Paryani & Arvin, 1986; Preblud et al., 1986). The risk for fetal anomalies was estimated to be 0.6% over the background rate for second or third trimester exposure, based on a total of 461 cases. No cases of VZV embryopathy were observed among the liveborn children of 91 women who developed varicella during pregnancy in a more recent prospective series; most of these women had chickenpox in the first trimester (Jones et al., 1990).

There appears to be an increased frequency of cancer, especially leukemia, among the children of women who had varicella during pregnancy (Adelstein & Donovan, 1972; Vianna & Polan, 1976; Fine et al., 1985). Nine cases of malignancy were observed among some 400 young people whose mothers had varicella during pregnancy. Data from a case-control study of children with malignancies and comparisons of secular trends of varicella infection and leukemia occurrence support the validity of this association (Bithell et al., 1973; Vianna & Polan, 1976, Till et al., 1979). If varicella exposure during gestation does predispose to the development of childhood leukemia, the risk of this occurring is probably no more than a few percent.

Zoster may occur in infants who have not had chickenpox but whose mothers had varicella during pregnancy, even if the children have no manifestations of VZV embryopathy (Brunell & Kotchmar, 1981; Gershon, 1990).

It has been recommended that passive immunization with varicella-zoster immune globulin (VZIG) be provided to pregnant women who have been closely exposed to someone with varicella or zoster and who are seronegative and have no history of having had chickenpox themselves (Anonymous, 1984; Broomhead, 1985; Greenspoon & Masaki, 1989; Gershon, 1990; Prober et al., 1990). Passive immunization seems unlikely to prevent transplacental passage of VZV in a pregnant woman who has already developed clinical manifestations of chickenpox (Prober et al., 1990; Gershon, 1990).

Some severe manifestations of fetal VZV infection may be apparent on ultrasound examination in the second or third trimester of pregnancy (Alexander, 1979; Essex-Carter & Heggarty, 1983; Cuthbertson et al., 1987; Byrne et al., 1990), but such prenatal testing appears unlikely to detect most affected fetuses. Although chorionic villus sampling and fetal blood sampling to identify VZV or specific antibody response to it have been reported (Cuthbertson et al., 1987; Grose et al., 1989; Isada et al., 1991), such studies have not been shown to be reliable means of diagnosing VZV embryopathy (Gershon, 1990).

Maternal varicella infections within three weeks of delivery may be associated with manifestations of varicella in the newborn infant (Pearson, 1964; Brunell, 1984; Miller et al., 1989; Gershon, 1990; Sterner et al., 1990). The prognosis for these infants is generally good, but pneumonitis or even death may occur, especially in infants whose mothers developed chickenpox less than six days before delivery.

No animal teratology studies of maternal VZV infection have been published.

Key References

Adelstein AM, Donovan JW: Malignant disease in children whose mothers had chickenpox, mumps, or rubella in pregnancy. Br Med J 1:629-631, 1972. [E]

Alexander I: Congenital varicella. Br Med J 2:1074, 1979. [C]

Alkalay AL, Pomerance JJ, Rimoin DL: Fetal varicella syndrome. J Pediatr 111:320-323, 1987. [S]

Anonymous: Varicella-zoster immune globulin for the prevention of chickenpox. MMWR 33:84-100, 1984. [R]

Bithell JF, Draper GJ, Gorbach PD: Association between malignant disease in children and maternal virus infections. Br Med J 1:706-708, 1973. [E]

Brazin SA, Simkovich JW, Johnson WT: Herpes zoster during pregnancy. Obstet Gynecol 53:175-181, 1979. [C]

Brice JEH: Congenital varicella resulting from infection during second trimester of pregnancy. Arch Dis Child 51:474-476, 1976. [C]

Broomhead I: Varicella-zoster infections. Major Probl Clin Pediatr 17:161-173, 1985. [R]

Brunell PA: Fetal and neonatal varicella-zoster infections. Semin Perinatol 7(1):47-56, 1983. [R]

Brunell PA, Kotchmar GS: Zoster in infancy: Failure to maintain virus latency following intrauterine infection. J Pediatr 98;71-73, 1981. [C]

Byrne JLB, Ward K, Kochenour NK, Dolcourt JL: Prenatal sonographic diagnosis of fetal varicella syndrome. Am J Hum Genet 47:A270, 1990. [C]

Cuthbertson G, Weiner CP, Giller RH, et al.: Prenatal diagnosis of second trimester congenital varicella syndrome by virus-specific IgM. J Pediatr 111:592-595, 1987. [C]

Enders G: Varicella-zoster virus infection in pregnancy. Prog Med Virol 29:166-196, 1984. [R]

Essex-Cater A, Heggarty H: Fatal congenital varicella syndrome. J Infect 7:77-78, 1983. [C]

Eyal A, Friedman M, Peretz BA, Paldi E: Pregnancy complicated by herpes zoster. J Reprod Med 28:600-603, 1983. [C] & [R]

Fine PEM, Adelstein AM, Snowman J, Clarkson JA, et al.: Long term effects of exposure to viral infections in utero. Br Med J 290:509-511, 1985. [E]

Gershon AA: Chickenpox, measles and mumps. In: Remington JS & Klein JO (eds). Infectious Diseases of the Fetus and Newborn Infant. Philadelphia: W.B. Saunders Co., 1990, pp 395-420. [R]

Greenspoon JS, Masaki DI: Screening for varicella-zoster immunity and the use of varicella zoster immune globulin in pregnancy. Am J Obstet Gynecol 160:1020-1022, 1989. [R]

Grose C, Itani O: Pathogenesis of congenital infection with three diverse viruses: Varicella-zoster virus, human parvovirus, and human immunodeficiency virus. Semin Perinatol 13(4):278-293 1989. [R]

Grose C, Itani O, Weiner CP: Prenatal diagnosis of fetal infection: Advances from amniocentesis to cordocentesis--congenital toxoplasmosis, rubella, cytomegalovirus, varicella virus, parvovirus and human immunodeficiency virus. Pediatr Infect Dis J 8:459-468, 1989. [R]

Higa K, Dan K, Manabe H: Varicella-zoster virus infections during pregnancy: Hypothesis concerning the mechanisms of congenital malformations. Obstet Gynecol 69:214-222, 1987. [S]

Isada NB, Paar DP, Johnson MP, et al.: In utero diagnosis of congenital varicella zoster virus infection by chorionic villus sampling and polymerase chain reaction. Am J Obstet Gynecol 165:1727-1730, 1991. [C]

Jones KL, Johnson KA, Chambers TA: Prospective follow-up of offspring born to women infected with varicella during pregnancy. Teratology 41:569, 1990. [S]

Laforet EG, Lynch CL: Multiple congenital defects following maternal varicella. N Engl J Med 236:534-537, 1947. [C]

Miller E, Cradock-Watson JE, Ridehalgh MKS: Outcome in newborn babies given anti-varicella-zoster iummunoglobulin after perinatal maternal infection with varicella-zoster virus. Lancet 2:371-373, 1989. [S]

Paryani SG, Arvin AM: Intrauterine infection with varicella-zoster virus after maternal varicella. N Eng J Med 314:1542-1546, 1986. [S]

Pearson HE: Parturition varicella-zoster. Obstet Gynecol 23:21-27, 1964. [S]

Preblud SR, Cochi SL, Orenstein WA: Varicella-zoster infection in pregnancy. [Letter to the editor] N Engl J Med 315:1415-1418, 1986. [O]

Prober CG, Gershon AA, Grose C, et al.: Consensus: Varicella-zoster infections in pregnancy and the perinatal period. Pediatr Infect Dis J 9(12):865-869, 1990. [C]

Siegel M: Congenital malformations following chickenpox, measles, mumps, and hepatitis. JAMA 226:1521-1524, 1973. [E]

Sterner G, Forsgren M, Enocksson E, et al.: Varicella-zoster infections in late pregnancy. Scand J Infect Dis (Suppl 71):30-35, 1990. [S]

Till M, Rapson N, Smith PG: Family studies in acute leukaemia in childhood: A possible association with autoimmune disease. Br J Cancer 40:62-71, 1979. [E]

Vianna NJ, Polan AK: Childhood lymphatic leukemia: Prenatal seasonality and possible association with congenital varicella. Am J Epidemiol 103:321-332, 1976. [S]

VECURONIUM

Synonyms

Norcuron, ORG NC 45

Summary

Vecuronium is a non-depolarizing neuromuscular blocking agent that is administered intravenously to induce muscle relaxation during surgery.

Magnitude of Teratogenic Risk

Undetermined

Quality and Quantity of Data

None

Comment

None

No epidemiological studies of congenital anomalies among infants born to women treated with vecuronium during pregnancy have been reported.

No animal teratology studies of vecuronium have been published.

Vecuronium has been administered directly to the fetus in the second or third trimester to facilitate intrauterine transfusion (Leveque et al., 1992). No adverse fetal effect of such treatment was observed.

Please see agent summary on tubocurarine for information on a related agent that has been studied.

Key References

Leveque C, Murat I, Toubas F, et al.: Fetal neuromuscular blockade with vecuronium bromide: Studies during intravascular intrauterine transfusion in isoimmunized pregnancies. Ancsthesiology 76(4):642-644, 1992. [C]

VERAPAMIL

Synonyms

Berkatens, Calan, Cordilox, Iproveratril, Isoptin, Securon

Summary

Verapamil is a calcium channel blocker that is used to treat cardiac arrhythmias and angina pectoris.

Magnitude of Teratogenic Risk

Undetermined

Quality and Quantity of Data

None

Comment

None

No epidemiological studies of malformations in infants born to women treated with verapamil during pregnancy have been reported. No adverse drug-related effects were observed among the infants of 90 or 47 hyptertensive women treated with verapamil in late pregnancy in two therapeutic trials (Orlandi et al., 1986; Marlettini et al., 1990).

Decreased litter size and reduced fetal weight were observed among rats treated parenterally with verapamil during pregnancy in doses similar to those used in humans (Spatz et al., 1986). This treatment produced maternal toxicity in the rats.

Verapamil has been employed in combination with other tocolytic agents in the therapy of premature labor in women (Gummerus, 1977; Carstensen et al., 1983). Verapamil has also been used to treat fetal cardiac arrhythmias during the second and third trimesters of pregnancy (Wladimiroff & Stewart, 1985; Gembruch et al., 1988). Unexplained fetal death has occurred after successful therapy of fetal supraventricular tachycardia with verapamil (Owen et al., 1988).

Key References

Carstensen MH, Bahnsen J, Sterzing E: Tocolysis with beta-sympathicomimetics alone or combined with the calcium antagonist verapamil. Geburtshilfe Frauenheilkd; 43:431-437, 1983. [S]

Gembruch U, Hansmann M, Bald R: Direct intrauterine fetal treatment of fetal tachyarrhythmia with severe hydrops fetalis by antiarrhythmic drugs. Fetal Ther 3:210-215, 1988. [C]

Gummerus M: Treatment of premature labour and antagonization of the side effects of tocolytic therapy with verapamil. Z Geburtshife Perinatol 181:334-340, 1977. [S]

Marlettini MG, Crippa S, Morselli-Labate AM, et al.: Randomized comparison of calcium antagonists and beta-blockers in the treatment of pregnancy-induced hypertension. Curr Ther Res 48(40):684-692, 1990. [S]

Orlandi C, Marlettini MG, Cassani A, et al.: Treatment of hypertension during pregnancy with the calcium antagonist verapamil. Curr Ther Res 39(6):884-893, 1986. [S]

Owen J, Colvin EV, Davis RO: Fetal death after successful conversion of fetal supraventricular tachycardia with digoxin and verapamil. Am J Obstet Gynecol 158:1169-1170, 1988. [C]

Spatz RJ, Pillalamari ED, Diab GM, Abadir AR, et al.: Verapamil effect on fetus in rat. Proc West Pharmacol Soc 29:319-320, 1986. [A]

Wladimiroff JW, Stewart PA: Treatment of fetal cardiac arrhythmias. Br J Hosp Med 34:134-140, 1985. [R]

VIDARABINE

Synonyms

Adenine Arabinoside, Ara-A, Vira-A

Summary

Vidarabine is a DNA synthesis inhibitor that is employed as an antiviral agent. It is used systemically to treat disseminated infections and locally to treat ophthalmic infections.

Magnitude of Teratogenic Risk

Undetermined

Quality and Quantity of Data

Poor

Comment

None

No epidemiological studies of congenital anomalies in infants born to women treated with vidarabine during pregnancy have been reported.

Increased frequencies of central nervous system, skeletal, and other anomalies occurred in the offspring of rats treated during pregnancy with vidarabine in parenteral doses 2-40 times those used in humans, but such doses also produced maternal toxicity (Schardein et al., 1977; Klug et al., 1991). Similar teratogenic effects and maternal toxicity occurred among pregnant rabbits given vidarabine parenterally in doses within the human therapeutic range (Schardein et al., 1977). An increased frequency of malformations was also observed in rabbits when very large doses of the drug were applied to the mother's skin during pregnancy. Among the offspring of five rhesus monkeys treated parenterally with vidarabine in a dose equivalent to that used therapeutically in humans, three viable offspring without gross malformations, one macerated stillbirth, and one spontaneous abortion were found (Schardein et al., 1977). The relevance of these observations to the clinical use of vidarabine in human pregnancy is uncertain.

Key References

Klug S, Lewandowski C, Merker H-J, Stahlmann R, et al.: In vitro and in vivo studies on the prenatal toxicity of five virustatic nucleoside analogues in comparison to aciclovir. Arch Toxicol 65:283-291, 1991. [A]

Schardein JL, Hentz DL, Petrere JA, Fitzgerald JE, et al.: The effect of vidarabine on the development of the offspring of rats, rabbits, and monkeys. Teratology 15:231-242, 1977. [A]

VIDEO DISPLAY UNITS

Synonyms

VDT, VDU, Video Display Screens

Summary

Video display units (VDUs) are commonly used to provide output on computer terminals and microcomputers. Although VDUs produce electromagnetic radiation of various frequencies, the levels of radiation emitted are much less than current environmental and occupational standards and are often no greater than background amounts (Bergqvist, 1984; Lee, 1985; Marriott & Stuchly, 1986; Kavet & Tell, 1991).

Magnitude of Teratogenic Risk

None

Quality and Quantity of Data

Good

Comment

None

Several large epidemiological studies of congenital anomalies and spontaneous abortion among women who used VDUs during pregnancy have been reported. These data have recently been reviewed, and the important methodological limitations of the studies discussed (Marcus, 1990; Kavet & Tell, 1991; Juutilainen, 1991). The frequency of congenital anomalies was no greater than expected among cohorts of 4517, 4731, 2748, and 1757 infants born to women who used VDUs extensively during pregnancy (Ericson & Kallen, 1986a; Westerholm & Ericson, 1987; McDonald et al., 1988). Similarly, no association was found with maternal VDU use during early pregnancy in a case-control study of 235 children with congenital anomalies (Kurppa et al., 1985). In another case-control study that included 102 children with various malformations, an association with maternal use of VDUs during pregnancy was observed (OR=1.7, 95% confidence interval 1.1-2.6), but much of this effect may have been due to confounding factors (Ericson & Kallen, 1986b).

Cohort studies of 2748, 2249, 2291, 1056, and 366 pregnancies among women exposed frequently to VDUs found no consistent association with spontaneous abortion (Westerholm & Ericson, 1987; Ericson & Kallen, 1986a; McDonald et al., 1988; Schnorr et al., 1991). In one case-control study involving 355 women who had had a spontaneous abortion, a weak association with maternal VDU use during pregnancy was noted (Goldhaber et al., 1988), but four other case-control studies of similar or larger size found no such association (Bryant & Love, 1989; Ericson & Kallen, 1986b; Nielsen & Brandt, 1990; Windham et al., 1990).

At least two dozen instances have been noted in which an apparent cluster of adverse pregnancy outcomes (spontaneous abortions or congenital anomalies) occurred among women who used VDUs while pregnant (Bergqvist, 1984; Abenhaim et al., 1988; Abenhaim & Lert, 1991). Each of these apparent clusters involved small groups of women (usually fewer than 30), and, given the frequency of occupational VDU use, many such observations would be expected to occur due to chance alone.

Several teratology studies have been performed in rodents using prolonged exposures to time-varying magnetic fields similar to those produced by VDUs but several times more intense (Juutilainen, 1991; Kavet & Tell, 1991). Most of these investigations found no effect of the exposure on the frequency of either malformations or fetal death. One study in mice found a slightly increased rate of congenital anomalies among the offspring of exposed animals (Tribukait et al., 1987); another study did not find this but found an increased rate of fetal death which was not seen in the first study (Frolen et al., 1993). In a third study in mice, neither effect was seen (Wiley et al., 1990).

Key References

Abenhaim L, Lert F: Methodological issues for the assessment of clusters of adverse pregnancy outcomes in the workplace: The case of video display terminal users. J Occup Med 33:1091-1096, 1991. [R]

Abenhaim L, Lert F, Kaminski M, Mammelle N, et al.: Travail sur terminal a ecran et grossesse. Evaluation des risques par consensus. Rapport d'un group de travail de l'INSERM. Rev Epidemiol Sante Publique 36:235-245, 1988. [S]

Bergqvist U: Video display terminals and health. Scand J Work Environ Health 10(Suppl 2):56-87, 1984. [S]

Bryant HE, Love EJ: Video display terminal use and spontaneous abortion risk. Int J Epidemiol 18:132-138, 1989. [E]

Ericson A, Kallen B: An epidemiological study of work with video screens and pregnancy outcome: I. A registry study. Am J Ind Med 9:447-457, 1986a. [E]

Ericson A, Kallen B: An epidemiological study of work with video screens and pregnancy outcome: II. A case-control study. Am J Ind Med 9:459-475, 1986b. [E]

Frolen H, Svedenstal BM, Paulsson LE: Effects of pulsed magnetic fields on the developing mouse embryo. Bioelectromagnetics 14(3):197-204, 1993. [A]

Goldhaber MK, Polen MR, Hiatt RA: The risk of miscarriage and birth defects among women who use visual display terminals during pregnancy. Am J Ind Med 13:697-706, 1988. [E]

Juutilainen J: Effects of low-frequency magnetic fields on embryonic development and pregnancy. Scand J Work Environ Health 17:149-158, 1991. [R]

Kavet R, Tell RA: VDTs: Field levels, epidemiology, and laboratory studies. Health Physics 61(1):47-57, 1991. [R]

Kurppa K, Holmberg PC, Rantala K, Nurminen T, et al.: Birth defects and exposure to video display terminals during pregnancy. Scand J Work Environ Health 11:353-356, 1985. [E]

Lee WR: Working with visual display units. Br Med J 291:989-991, 1985. [R]

Marcus M: Epidemiologic studies of VDT use and pregnancy outcome. Reprod Toxicol 4(1):51-56, 1990. [R]

Marriott IA, Stuchly MA: Health aspects of work with visual display terminals. J Occup Med 28:833-848, 1986. [R]

McDonald AD, McDonald JC, Armstrong B, Cherry N, et al.: Work with visual display units in pregnancy. Br J Ind Med 45:509-515, 1988. [E]

Nielsen CV, Brandt LPA: Spontaneous abortion among women using video display terminals. Scand J Work Environ Health 16:323-328, 1990. [E]

Schnorr TM, Grajewski BA, Hornung RW, et al.: Video display terminals and the risk of spontaneous abortion. N Engl J Med 324:727-733, 1991. [A]

Tribukait B, Cekan E, Paulsson LE: Effects of pulsed magnetic fields on embryonic development in mice. In: Knave B & Wideback P-G (eds). Work with Display Units 86. Amsterdam: Elsevier Science Publishers, 1987, pp 129-134. [A]

Westerholm P, Ericson A: Pregnancy outcome and VDU-work in a cohort of insurance clerks. In: Knave B & Wideback P-G (eds). Work with Display Units 86. Amsterdam: Elsevier Science Publishers, 1987, pp 104-110. [E]

Wiley M, Agnew D, Harvey S, et al.: The effects of maternal exposure to VDT-like magnetic fields throughout pregnancy on the prenatal development of CD-1 mice. Teratology 41(5):599-600, 1990. [A]

Windham GC, Fenster L, Swan SH, Neutra RR: Use of video display terminals during pregnancy and the risk of spontaneous abortion, low birthweight, or intrauterine growth retardation. Am J Ind Med 18:675-688, 1990. [E]

VINBLASTINE

Synonyms

Velban, Velbe, Velsar, Vincaleucoblastine

Summary

Vinblastine is a periwinkle alkaloid that is administered intravenously as an antineoplastic agent. It acts to arrest dividing cells in metaphase.

Magnitude of Teratogenic Risk

Undetermined

Quality and Quantity of Data

Poor To Fair

Comment

Although the teratogenic risk of vinblastine is unknown, it may be substantial because it is cytotoxic.

No epidemiological studies of congenital anomalies among infants born to women treated with vinblastine during pregnancy have been published. At least 26 apparently normal infants have been reported whose mothers were treated with vinblastine, often in combination with other antineoplastics, during pregnancy (Lacher & Geller, 1966; Goguel, 1970; Johnson & Filshie, 1977; Doll et al., 1988; Christman et al., 1990; Aviles et al., 1991). In 17 of these cases, exposure occurred during the first trimester. Two infants with congenital anomalies have been reported whose mothers received cancer chemotherapy including vinblastine during the first trimester of pregnancy (Garrett 1974; Mulvihill et al., 1987). Lack of comparison groups in these cases makes it difficult to ascertain the role of vinblastine in the etiology of these malformations.

There is no evidence that cancer chemotherapy with vinblastine in either parent prior to conception measurably alters the risk of congenital anomalies in subsequent children (Green et al., 1991; Zuazu et al., 1991).

Fetal death and craniofacial, eye, neural tube, and abdominal wall malformations occur with increased frequency among the offspring of rats treated during pregnancy with vinblastine in doses 1-5 times those used in humans (DeMyer, 1964; Cohlan & Kitay, 1965). An increased frequency of fetal death was observed among pregnant mice treated with 100-1000 times the maximum human therapeutic dose of vinblastine (Joneja & LeLiever, 1974). Increased frequencies of eye, skeletal, and visceral anomalies were observed at 700 times the human dose, but higher doses caused death of all fetuses. Increased frequencies of fetal death and of eye, neural tube, and skeletal malformations were seen among the offspring of hamsters treated during pregnancy with vinblastine in doses 2-5 or more times greater than those used in humans (Ferm, 1963). Fetal death also is seen in pregnant rabbits given doses of vinblastine similar to those used in humans (Morris et al., 1967).

Key References

Aviles A, Diaz-Maqueo JC, Talavera A, et al.: Growth and development of children of mothers treated with chemotherapy during pregnancy: Current status of 43 children. Am J Hematol 36;243-248, 1991.

Christman JE, Teng NNH, Lebovic GS, Sikic BI: Delivery of a normal infant following cisplatin, vinblastine, and bleomycin (PVB) chemotherapy for malignant teratoma of the ovary during pregnancy. Gynecol Oncol 37:292-295, 1990. [C]

Cohlan SQ, Kitay D: The teratogenic effect of vincaleukoblastine in the pregnant rat. J Pediatr 66(3):541-544, 1965. [A]

DeMyer W: Vinblastine-induced malformations of face and nervous system in two rat strains. Neurology 14:806-808, 1964. [A]

Doll DC, Ringenberg QS, Yarbro JW: Management of cancer during pregnancy. Arch Intern Med 148:2058-2064, 1988. [R]

Ferm VH: Congenital malformations in hamster embryos after treatment with vinblastine and vincristine. Science 141:426, 1963. [A]

Garrett MJ: Teratogenic effects of combination chemotherapy. Ann Intern Med 80:667, 1974. [C]

Goguel A: Hodgkin's disease and pregnancy. La Presse Med 78:1507-1510, 1970.

Green DM, Zevon MA, Lowrie G, et al.: Congenital anomalies in children of patients who received chemotherapy for cancer in childhood and adolescence. N Engl J Med 325(3):141-146, 1991. [E]

Johnson IR, Filshie GM: Hodgkin's disease diagnosed in pregnancy. Br J Obstet Gynaecol 84:791-792, 1977. [C]

Joneja MG, LeLiever WC: Effects of vinblastine and podophyllin on DBA mouse fetuses. Toxicol Appl Pharmacol 27:408-414, 1974. [A]

Lacher MJ, Geller W: Cyclophosphamide and vinblastine sulfate in Hodgkin's disease during pregnancy. JAMA 195(6):192-194, 1966. [C]

Morris JM, vanWagenen G, Hurteau GD, et al.: Compounds interfering with ovum implantation and development. I. Alkaloids and antimetabolites. Fertil Steril 18(1):7-17, 1967. [A]

Mulvihill JJ, McKeen EA, Rosner F, Zarrabi MH: Pregnancy outcome in cancer patients. Cancer 60:1143-1154, 1987. [C]

Zuazu J, Julia A, Sierra J, et al.: Pregnancy outcome in hematologic malignancies. Cancer 67(3):703-709, 1991. [E]

VINCRISTINE

Synonyms

LCR, Leurocristine Sulfate, Oncovin, VCR, Vincasar, Vincrisul

Summary

Vincristine is an alkaloid of the periwinkle plant that is administered intravenously as an antineoplastic agent. Vincristine blocks mitosis by inhibiting assembly of microtubules.

Magnitude of Teratogenic Risk

Undetermined

Quality and Quantity of Data

Poor To Fair

Comment

Although the teratogenic risk of vincristine is unknown, it may be substantial because it is cytotoxic.

No epidemiological studies of congenital anomalies among infants born to women treated with vincristine during pregnancy have been reported. The frequency of congenital anomalies does not appear to be excessive among infants whose mothers were treated during pregnancy with vincristine in combination with other antineoplastic agents in reported clinical series (Gililland & Weinstein, 1983; Catanzarite & Ferguson, 1984; Sutcliffe & Chapman, 1986; Zuazu et al., 1991; Aviles et al., 1991). Such anecdotal reports include more than 20 cases with first trimester treatment and more than 30 with treatment in pregnancy after the first trimester. However, because comparison cases are not included in the studies, it is difficult to determine the clinical significance of these findings. An association with maternal occupational exposure to vincristine and other antineoplastic drugs observed in a case-control study of 124 miscarriages in nurses (Selevan et al., 1985) cannot be interpreted without independent confirmation because of methodological limitations and concern about biological plausibility.

Increased frequencies of central nervous system, skeletal, facial, body wall, and other malformations were observed among the offspring of pregnant mice treated with 6.7-13 times the usual human dose of vincristine (Joneja & Ungthavorn, 1969; Sieber et al., 1978; Svoboda & O'Shea, 1984). Increased rates of fetal growth retardation and fetal death were also noted. Similar teratogenic effects have been observed among the offspring of rhesus monkeys, hamsters, and rats treated during pregnancy with vincristine in doses respectively 5-17, 3 or more, and 5 times those used in humans (Ferm, 1963; Courtney & Valerio, 1968; Wilson, 1971).

Key References

Aviles A, Diaz-Maqueo JC, Talavera A, et al.: Growth and development of children of mothers treated with chemotherapy during pregnancy: Current status of 43 children. Am J Hematol 36:243-248, 1991. [S]

Catanzarite VA, Ferguson II JE: Acute leukemia and pregnancy: A review of management and outcome, 1972-1982. Obstet Gynecol Surv 39(11):663-678. [C] & [R]

Courtney KD, Valerio DA: Teratology in the Macaca mulatta. Teratology 1:163-172, 1968. [A]

Ferm VH: Congenital malformations in hamster embryos after treatment with vinblastine and vincristine. Science 141:426, 1963. [A]

Gililland J, Weinstein L: The effects of cancer chemotherapeutic agents on the developing fetus. Obstet Gynecol Surv 38(1):6-13, 1983. [C] & [R]

Joneja M, Ungthavorn S: Teratogenic effects of vincristine in three lines of mice. Teratology 2:235-240, 1969. [A]

Selevan SG, Lindbohn M-L, Hornung RW, Hemminki K: A study of occupational exposure to antineoplastic drugs and fetal loss in nurses. N Engl J Med 313(19):1173-1178, 1985. [E]

Sieber SM, Whang-Peng J, Botkin C, Knutsen T: Teratogenic and cytogenetic effects of some plant-derived antitumor agents (vincristine, colchicine, maytansine, VP-16-213 and VM-26) in mice. Teratology 18:31-48, 1978. [A]

Sutcliffe SB, Chapman RM: Lymphomas and leukemias. In: Cancer in Pregnancy. Therapeutic Guidelines. Allen HH, Nisker JA (eds). Mt. Kisco, NY: Futura Publishing Co., 1986. [R]

Svoboda KK, O'Shea KS: Optic vesicle defects induced by vincristine sulfate: An in vivo and in vitro study in the mouse embryo. Teratology 29:223-239, 1984. [A]

Wilson JG: Use of rhesus monkeys in teratological studies. Fed Proc 30(1):104-109, 1971. [A]

Zuazu J, Julia A, Sierra J, et al.: Pregnancy outcome in hematologic malignancies. Cancer 67(3):703-709, 1991. [S]

VINYL ETHER

Synonyms

Aether Vinylicus, Divinyl Ether, Vinydan, Vinesthene

Summary

Vinyl ether is a general anesthetic administered by inhalation.

Magnitude of Teratogenic Risk

Undetermined

Quality and Quantity of Data

None

Comment

None

No epidemiological studies of congenital anomalies in children born to women exposed to vinyl ether during pregnancy have been reported.

No investigations of teratologic effects of vinyl ether in experimental animals have been published.

Key References

None available.

VIRIDOFULVIN

Summary

Viridofulvin is an antifungal agent.

Magnitude of Teratogenic Risk

Undetermined

Quality and Quantity of Data

None

Comment

None

No epidemiological studies of congenital anomalies in infants born to women who used viridofulvin during pregnancy have been reported.

No animal teratology studies of virido-fulvin have been published.

Key References

None available.

VITAMIN A

Synonyms

Alphalin, Antixerophthalmic Vitamin, Aquasol A, Arovit, Axeropholum, Oleovitamin A, Pedi-Vit A, Retinol, Ro-A-Vit, Vi-Dom A

Summary

Vitamin A, a fat-soluble nutrient, is essential for normal vision. Large doses of vitamin A are used to treat deficiency states and certain skin diseases. Vitamin A has been taken in amounts 20-40 or more times the U.S. Recommended Dietary Allowance (RDA) by some individuals for various purported health benefits, but this use is not generally accepted. Retinoids, including retinol, retinaldehyde, and retinoic acid, possess vitamin A activity directly; carotenoids such as beta-carotene can be metabolized to form vitamin A. One international unit (IU) of vitamin A is equivalent to 0.3 mcg of all-trans retinol or 0.6 mcg of beta-carotene. The current U.S. RDA for vitamin A in pregnant women is the equivalent of 800 mcg (2667 IU) of retinol or 4800 mcg (8000 IU) of beta-carotene per day. Vitamin A has a long biological half-life and bioaccumulates (Hathcock et al., 1990).

Magnitude of Teratogenic Risk

Low Dose (<10,000 IU): None

High Dose (>25,000 IU): Undetermined

Quality and Quantity of Data

Low Dose (<10,000 IU): Good

High Dose (>25,000 IU): Poor

Comment

1) Although the teratogenic risk of high doses (>25,000 IU) of vitamin A is unknown, experimental studies in animals and an analogy with the effects of chemically related compounds raise concern that it may be substantial.

2) Intake of vitamin A as beta-carotene appears to be associated with a much smaller (or nonexistent) teratogenic risk in comparison with intake of an equivalent dose of vitamin A as retinol (Anonymous, 1987).

3) Large amounts of vitamin A may be found in some food sources (e.g., liver) (Sanders, 1990).

No significant association was observed with maternal use of high-dose (10,000 IU per day or more) vitamin A in a case-control study that included 11,293 children with minor and major congenital anomalies, but the statistical power of this study was poor because of a very low rate of exposure (Martinez-Frias and Salvador, 1988, 1990). A trend toward association with doses of 40,000 IU or greater was seen but did not reach statistical significance. No recurrent pattern of congenital anomalies was observed among the 16 exposed cases.

Several instances of congenital anomalies in infants born to mothers who took large amounts of vitamin A during pregnancy have been reported (Pilotti & Scorta, 1965; Bernhardt & Dorsey, 1974; Mounoud et al., 1975; Rosa et al., 1986), but no recurrent pattern of anomalies has been observed. Although such cases are of concern, the number reported is far less than would be expected to occur by chance even if vitamin A is not teratogenic in humans with "megadose" exposures (Rosa, 1987). No congenital anomalies were observed in 14 pregnancies with first-trimester exposures to high doses (25,000 IU or greater) of vitamin A (Zuber et al, 1987). In the same clinical series, three other similarly exposed pregnancies resulted in spontaneous abortion.

Increased frequencies of fetal death and congenital anomalies have consistently been observed among the offspring of rats, mice,

654

and hamsters treated during pregnancy with 750 to many thousands of times the human RDA of vitamin A (Cohlan, 1954; Kalter & Warkany, 1961; Marin-Padilla & Ferm, 1965; Kochhar, 1967; Willhite, 1984; Eckhoff et al, 1989). Typical dependence of the teratogenic effect on time of treatment during pregnancy has been demonstrated in all three species, and typical dose dependence has been shown in hamsters. Many different malformations are seen in affected offspring, but craniofacial, central nervous system, and skeletal anomalies are most frequent. Cardiac and eye anomalies have been reported in the offspring of pigs and cleft palate in the offspring of dogs treated during pregnancy with very large doses of vitamin A (Palludan, 1966; Wiersig & Swenson, 1967). Malformations have been produced in the offspring of pregnant rabbits treated with vitamin A in a doses about 300 times greater than the human RDA (Kamm, 1982). Behavioral abnormalities have been observed among physically normal offspring of rats treated with 1500 or more times the human RDA of vitamin A during pregnancy (Mooney et al., 1981).

Although the teratogenicity of vitamin A (retinol) has not been established in humans, there is reason to suspect that the risk of congenital anomalies may be increased among the children of women who take very large amounts of this substance early in pregnancy. Very high doses of vitamin A are teratogenic in many species of experimental animals, and isotretinoin, a closely related compound, has been shown to be a human teratogen. Teratogenic dosages of vitamin A in experimental animals are hundreds to thousands of times greater than the human RDA (Kamm, 1982; Anonymous, 1987); such doses are rarely if ever encountered among pregnant women, even those who take "megadose" vitamins.

Please see agent summary on isotretinoin for more information on this closely related compound.

Key References

Anonymous: Teratology Society position paper: Recommendations for vitamin A use during pregnancy. Teratology 35:269-275, 1987. [R]

Bernhardt IB, Dorsey DJ: Hypervitaminosis A and congenital renal anomalies in a human infant. Obstet Gynecol 43:750-755, 1974. [C]

Cohlan SQ: Congenital anomalies in the rat produced by excessive intake of vitamin A during pregnancy. Pediatrics 13:556-569, 1951. [A]

Eckhoff Ch, Lofberg B, Chahoud I, et al.: Transplacental pharmacokinetics and teratogenicity of a single dose of retinol (vitamin A) during organogenesis in the mouse. Toxicol Lett 48:171-184, 1989. [A]

Hathcock JN, Hattan DG, Jenkins MY, et al.: Evaluation of vitamin A toxicity. Am J Clin Nutr 52:183-202, 1990. [R]

Kalter H, Warkany J: Experimental production of congenital malformations in strains of inbred mice by maternal treatment with hypervitaminosis A. Am J Pathol 38:1-21, 1961. [A]

Kamm JJ: Toxicology, carcinogenicity, and teratogenicity of some orally administered retinoids. J Am Acad Dermatol 6(4):652-659, 1982. [A] & [R]

Kochhar DM: Teratogenic activity of retinoic acid. Acta Pathol Microbiol Scand 70:398-404, 1967. [A]

Marin-Padilla M, Ferm VH: Somite necrosis and developmental malformations induced by vitamin A in the golden hamster. J Embryol Exp Morphol 13:1-8, 1965. [A]

Martinez-Frias ML, Salvador J: Megadose vitamin A and teratogenicity. Lancet 1:236, 1988. [E]

Martinez-Frias ML, Salvador J: Epidemiological aspects of prenatal exposure to high doses of vitamin A in Spain. Eur J Epidemiol 6(2):118-123, 1990. [E]

Mooney MP, Hoyenga KT, Hoyenga KB, et al.: Prenatal hypervitaminosis A and postnatal behavioral development in the rat. Neurobehav Toxicol Teratol 3:1-4, 1981. [A]

Mounoud RL, Klein D, Weber F: [A case of Goldenhar syndrome: Acute vitamin A intoxication in the mother during pregnancy.] J Genet Hum 23:135-154, 1975. [C]

Palludan B: Swine in teratological studies. In: Bustad LK , McClellan RO (eds). Swine in Biomedical Research. Columbus, Ohio: Battelle Memorial Institute, 1966, pp 51-78. [A]

Pilotti G, Scorta A: [Hypervitaminosis A during pregnancy and neonatal malformation of the urinary apparatus.] Minerva Gynecol 17:1103-1108, 1965. [C]

Rosa FW: Difficulties with vitamin A human teratology. Teratology 35(3):28A, 1987. [O]

Rosa FW, Wilk AL, Kelsey FO: Teratogen update: Vitamin A congeners. Teratology 33:355-364, 1986. [R]

Sanders TAB: Vitamin A and pregnancy. [Letter] Lancet 336:1375, 1990. [O]

Wiersig DO, Swenson MJ: Teratogenicity of vitamin A in the canine. Fed Proc 26:486, 1967. [A]

Willhite CC: Dose-response relationships of retinol in production of the Arnold-Chiari malformation. Toxicol Lett 20:257-262, 1984. [A]

Zuber C, Librizzi RJ, Vogt BL: Outcomes of pregnancies exposed to high doses Vitamin A. Teratology 35(2):42A, 1987. [S]

VITAMIN D

Synonyms

Alfacalcidol, Calcifediol, Calciferol, Calcitriol, Cholecalciferol, Dichysterol, Dihydrotachysterol, Dihydroxyvitamin D_3, Ergocalciferol, Oleovitamin D, Rocaltrol, Tachyrol

Summary

Vitamin D includes a series of compounds that are able to prevent and cure ricketts. Vitamin D synthesis occurs in the skin in the presence of sunlight. Many foods also contain this fat-soluble vitamin. The current U.S. Recommended Dietary Allowance (RDA) of vitamin D in pregnancy is 10 mcg (400 Units) per day (NRC, 1989).

Magnitude of Teratogenic Risk

None To Minimal

Quality and Quantity of Data

Poor

Comment

This assessment refers to risks associated with very high doses of vitamin D. Vitamin D in small doses is a necessary dietary component.

No epidemiological studies of malformations in infants born to women who took large amounts of vitamin D during pregnancy have been reported. In one clinical series, no malformations were observed among 15 children born to hypoparathyroid women who ingested an average of more than 200 times the recommended daily allowance of vitamin D throughout pregnancy (Goodenday & Gordon, 1971).

Administration of vitamin D to pregnant rabbits and rats in doses hundreds to thousands of times greater than the human recommended daily allowance produces cardiovascular and craniofacial anomalies in the offspring similar to those seen in the human Williams syndrome (supravalvular aortic stenosis, unusual facies, and infantile hypercalcemia) (Friedman & Roberts, 1966; Friedman & Mills, 1969; Chan et al., 1979). Although it has been suggested that the Williams syndrome in humans may be related to maternal ingestion of large amounts of vitamin D or otherwise altered maternal calcium metabolism (Friedman, 1968), the available evidence provides little support for this hypothesis (Forbes, 1979).

Maternal vitamin D deficiency during pregnancy can produce rachitic skeletal anomalies in newborn humans (Ford et al., 1973; Moncrieff & Fadahunsi, 1974) and rats (Warkany, 1943).

Key References

Chan GM, Buchino JJ, Mehlhorn D, Bove KE, et al.: Effect of vitamin D on pregnant rabbits and their offspring. Pediatr Res 13:121-126, 1979. [A]

Forbes GB: Vitamin D in pregnancy and the infantile hypercalcemic syndrome. [Letter] Pediatr Res 13:1382, 1979. [R]

Ford JA, Davidson DC, McIntosh WB, et al.: Neonatal rickets in Asian immigrant population. Br Med J 3:211-212, 1973. [C]

Friedman WF: Vitamin D and the supravalvular aortic stenosis syndrome. Adv Teratol 3:85-96, 1968. [R]

Friedman WF, Mills LF: The relationship between vitamin D and the craniofacial and dental anomalies of the supravalvular aortic stenosis syndrome. Pediatrics 43:12-18, 1969. [A]

Friedman WF, Roberts WC: Vitamin D and the supravalvar aortic stenosis syndrome. The transplacental effects of vitamin D on the aorta of the rabbit. Circulation 34:77-86, 1966. [A]

Goodenday LS, Gordon GS: No risk from vitamin D in pregnancy. Ann Intern Med 75:807-808, 1971. [S]

Moncrieff M, Fadahunsi TO: Congenital rickets due to maternal vitamin D deficiency. Arch Dis Child 49:810-811, 1974. [C]

NRC (National Research Council): Recommended Dietary Allowances, 10th ed. Report of the Subcommittee on the Tenth Edition of the RDAs, Food and Nutrition Board, Commission on Life Sciences. Washington, D.C.: National Academy Press, 1989. [O]

Warkany J: Effect of maternal rachitogenic diet on skeletal development of young rat. Am J Dis Child 66:511-516, 1943. [A]

VITAMIN E

Synonyms

Alpha Tocopherols, Aquasol E, Eferol, Ephynal, Eprolin, Pheryl E, Tokols, Vita-E, ZE Caps

Summary

Vitamin E is an essential nutrient. This fat-soluble vitamin has been used in large doses as an antioxidant. The U.S. Recommended Dietary Allowance (RDA) of vitamin E in pregnancy is 10 mg per day.

Magnitude of Teratogenic Risk

Undetermined

Quality and Quantity of Data

Poor

Comment

None

No epidemiological studies of congenital anomalies in infants born to women who took large doses of vitamin E during pregnancy have been reported.

In most studies, the frequency of malformations was no greater than expected among the offspring of rats or mice treated with vitamin E during pregnancy in doses hundreds to thousands of times the human recommended daily allowance (Sato et al., 1973; Hook et al., 1974; Krasavage & Terhaar, 1977; Hurley et al., 1983). An increased frequency of cleft palate was observed in the offspring of mice given 750 to 1500 times the human recommended dietary allowance of vitamin E in one investigation (Momose et al., 1972).

Fetal death occurs with very high frequency among the offspring of vitamin E deficient rats (Cheng et al., 1957; King, 1964). Dietary deficiency of vitamin E is rare in humans who eat a calorically adequate diet.

Key References

Cheng DW, Chang LF, Bairnson TA: Gross observations on developing abnormal embryos induced by maternal vitamin E deficiency. Anat Rec 129:167-185, 1957. [A]

Hook EB, Healy KM, Niles AM, Skalko RG: Vitamin E: Teratogen or anti-teratogen? Lancet 1:809, 1974. [O]

Hurley LS, Dungan DD, Keen CL, Lonnerdal B: The effects of vitamin E on zinc deficiency teratogenesis in rats. J Nutr 113:1875-1877, 1983. [A]

King DW: Effect of d-gamma-tocopherol on the incidence of teratogeny in vitamin E-deficient rats. Nature 204:785-786, 1964. [A]

Krasavage WJ, Terhaar CJ: D-alpha-tocopheryl poly(ethylene glycol) 1000 succinate. Acute toxicity, subchronic feeding, reproduction, and teratologic studies in the rat. J Agric Food Chem 25:273-278, 1977. [A]

Momose Y, Akiyoshi S, Mori K, Nishimura N, et al.: On teratogenicity of vitamin E. Mie Kenritsu Daigakubu Igakubu Kaibogaku Kyoshitsu Gyosekishu 20:27-35, 1972. [A]

Sato Y: [Study of developmental pharmacology on vitamin E.] Folia Pharmacol Japon 69:293-298, 1973. [A]

WARFARIN

Synonyms

Coumadin, Marevan, Panwarfin, Sodium Warfarin, Sofarin, Warfilone, Warnerin

Summary

Warfarin is an anticoagulant that depresses synthesis of vitamin K-dependent clotting factors. It is used in treatment of a variety of thromboembolic disorders. Warfarin is also employed as a rodenticide.

Magnitude of Teratogenic Risk

Small To Moderate

Quality and Quantity of Data

Good

Comment

Available data deal with chronic use of warfarin in therapeutic doses.

A very uncommon but strikingly similar pattern of congenital anomalies has been observed in more than 40 children born to women treated with warfarin during pregnancy (Warkany, 1976; Hall et al., 1980; Stevenson et al., 1980; Stein et al., 1984; Zakzouk, 1986; Khera, 1987). Frequent features of this pattern of anomalies, which is called the warfarin embryopathy or fetal warfarin syndrome, include nasal hypoplasia, stippled epiphyses on radiographs, and growth retardation. Although the direct pathogenic role of warfarin in this syndrome has been questioned (Stein et al., 1984; Khera, 1987), the occurrence of similar congenital anomalies in an infant with an inherited deficiency of multiple vitamin K-dependent coagulation factors whose mother did not have heart disease and did not take warfarin during pregnancy favors a causal interpretation (Pauli et al., 1987).

The greatest period of susceptibility to the skeletal features of fetal warfarin syndrome is in the latter half of the first trimester of pregnancy. No adequate epidemiological study is available on which to base risk estimates for this syndrome, but, on the basis of published experience with warfarin use in pregnancy (an obviously biased sample), it has been estimated that about 10% of infants born alive to mothers who take warfarin during pregnancy have warfarin embryopathy (Hall et al., 1980). In one series of 38 children who had been born to women treated with warfarin throughout pregnancy and in whom physical examinations were performed to look for features of warfarin embryopathy, one child had typical features of warfarin embryopathy and two others had mild manifestations of this condition (Salazar et al., 1984). In contrast, none of 20 children born to women treated with a strictly controlled low (5 mg/d or less) dose of warfarin throughout pregnancy had warfarin embryopathy on thorough evaluation (Cotrufo et al., 1991).

Central nervous system (CNS) and eye anomalies have been observed unusually often among the children of mothers who were treated with warfarin during pregnancy (Hall et al., 1980; Stevenson et al., 1980; Kaplan, 1985). These abnormalities may occur in association with other features of warfarin embryopathy or in otherwise unaffected infants whose mothers took warfarin during gestation. These CNS and eye anomalies may occur with maternal use of warfarin after the first trimester. On the basis of published experience, the frequency of CNS structural anomalies among liveborn infants whose mothers took warfarin during pregnancy has been estimated to be about 3% (Hall et al., 1980).

Two infants with fatal diaphragmatic hernia who were born to women treated with warfarin throughout pregnancy have been

658

described (O'Donnell et al., 1985; Normann & Stray-Pedersen, 1989). Neither child was noted to have features of warfarin embryopathy, but the clinical description is quite limited in both reports.

The frequency of stillbirth appears to be substantially increased in warfarin-exposed pregnancies, and spontaneous abortion is also more common than expected (Hall et al., 1980; Sheikhzadeh et al., 1983; Vitali et al., 1986; Sareli et al., 1989). In a series of 128 pregnancies in women who were treated throughout gestation with warfarin because of cardiac valve replacement, the rate of stillbirth was 7% and the rate of miscarriage was 28% (Salazar et al., 1984).

Maternal warfarin use late in pregnancy has been associated with fetal, placental, and neonatal hemorrhage (Stevenson et al., 1980; Salazar et al., 1984; Vitali et al., 1986; Sareli et al., 1989). Such hemorrhage may result from the pharmacologic action of warfarin.

A dose-dependent increased frequency of fetal death has been reported among the offspring of mice treated during pregnancy with warfarin in doses 1-4 times those used in humans (Kronick et al., 1974). An increased frequency of minor skeletal anomalies was also observed in this study, but the effect was not clearly related to dose. No increase in the frequency of major malformations was observed among the offspring of pregnant rabbits treated with 10-100 times the usual human dose of warfarin (Grote & Weinmann, 1973). Increased frequencies of fetal death and of hemorrhages of the brain, face, eyes, ears and occasionally limbs were seen among the offspring of rats treated during pregnancy with warfarin in doses 15-500 times those used in humans (Howe & Webster, 1990). Skeletal anomalies were not seen in the affected fetuses in this study, but similar treatment of the pups postnatally produced marked maxillonasal hypoplasia (Howe & Webster, 1992). Much of the skeletal maturation that occurs prenatally in humans does not occur until after birth in rats.

Key References

Cotrufo M, de Luca TSL, Calabro R, et al.: Coumarin anticoagulation during pregnancy in patients with mechanical valve prostheses. Eur J Cardiothorac Surg 5:300-305, 1991. [S]

Grote VW, Weinmann I: Examination of the active substances coumarin and rutin in a teratogenic trial with rabbits. Arzneimittelforsch 23:1319-1320, 1973. [A]

Hall JG, Pauli RM, Wilson KM: Maternal and fetal sequelae of anticoagulation during pregnancy. Am J Med 68:122-140, 1980. [R]

Howe AM, Webster WS: Exposure of the pregnant rat to warfarin and vitamin K1: An animal model of intraventriuclar hemorrhage in the fetus. Teratology 42:413-420, 1990. [A]

Howe AM, Webster WS: The warfarin embryopathy: A rat model showing maxillonasal hypoplasia and other skeletal disturbances. Teratology 46:379-390, 1992. [A]

Kaplan LC: Congenital Dandy Walker malformation associated with first trimester warfarin: A case report and literature review. Teratology 32:333-337, 1985. [C] & [R]

Khera KS: Maternal toxicity of drugs and metabolic disorders--A possible etiologic factor in the intrauterine death and congenital malformation: A critique on human data. CRC Crit Rev Toxicol 17:345-375, 1987. [R]

Kronick J, Phelps NE, McCallion DJ, Hirsh J: Effects of sodium warfarin administered during pregnancy in mice. Am J Obstet Gynecol 118:819-823, 1974. [A]

Normann EK, Stray-Pedersen B: Warfarin-induced fetal diaphragmatic hernia. Case report. Br J Obstet Gynaecol 96:729-730, 1989. [C]

O'Donnell D, Meyers AM, Sevitz H, et al.: Pregnancy after renal transplantation. Aust NZ J Med 15:320-325, 1985. [E]

Pauli RM, Lian JB, Mosher DF, et al.: Association of congenital deficiency of multiple vitamin K-dependent coagulation factors and the phenotype of the warfarin embryopathy: Clues to the mechanism of teratogenicity of coumarin derivatives. Am J Hum Genet 41:566-583, 1987. [C]

Salazar E, Zajarias A, Gutierrez N, Iturbe I: The problem of cardiac valve prostheses, anticoagulants, and pregnancy. Circulation 70 (Suppl I):I169-I177, 1984. [E]

Sareli P, England JM, Berk MR, et al.: Maternal and fetal sequelae of anticoagulation during pregnancy in patients with mechanical heart valve prostheses. Am J Cardiol 63:1462-1465, 1989. [S]

Sheikhzadeh A, Ghabusi P, Hakim SH, et al.: Congestive heart failure in valvular heart disease in pregnancies with and without valvular prostheses and anticoagulant therapy. Clin Cardiol 6:465-470, 1983. [S]

Stein Z, Kline J, Kharrazi M: What is a teratogen? Epidemiological criteria. Issues Rev Teratol 2:23-66, 1984. [R]

Stevenson RE, Burton M, Furlauto GJ, Taylor HA: Hazards of oral anticoagulants during pregnancy. JAMA 243:1549-1551, 1980. [C]

Vitali E, Donatelli F, Quaini E, et al.: Pregnancy in patients with mechanical prosthetic heart valves. J Cardiovasc Surg 27:221-227, 1986. [S]

Warkany J: Warfarin embryopathy. Teratology 14:205-210, 1976. [C]

Zakzouk MS: The congenital warfarin syndrome. J Laryngol Otol 100:215-219, 1986. [C]

XYLOMETAZOLINE

Synonyms

Neo-Synephrine II, Otrivin, Sinex Long-Acting, Sinutab Sinus Spray

Summary

Xylometazoline is a sympathomimetic agent used topically as a nasal decongestant.

Magnitude of Teratogenic Risk

None To Minimal

Quality and Quantity of Data

Poor To Fair

Comment

None

The frequency of congenital anomalies was not increased among 432 infants born to women who used xylometazoline during the first trimester of pregnancy in two sequential cohorts of a single study (Jick et al., 1981; Aselton et al., 1985).

No animal teratology studies of xylometazoline have been published.

Key References

Aselton P, Jick H, Milunsky A, Hunter JR, et al.: First-trimester drug use and congenital disorders. Obstet Gynecol 65:451-455, 1985. [S]

Jick H, Holmes LB, Hunter JR and Madsen S, et al.: First-trimester drug use and congenital disorders. JAMA 246:343-346, 1981. [S]

YEAST CELL DERIVATIVE

Summary

Yeast cell derivative is the alcohol extract of yeast. It is used topically to promote healing.

Magnitude of Teratogenic Risk

Undetermined

Quality and Quantity of Data

None

Comment

A small risk cannot be excluded, but a high risk of congenital anomalies in the children of women who used yeast cell derivative during pregnancy is unlikely.

No epidemiological studies of congenital anomalies among infants born to women who used yeast cell derivative during pregnancy have been reported.

No animal teratology studies of yeast cell derivative have been published.

Key References

None available.

YELLOW FEVER VACCINE

Synonyms

Arilvax, YF-VAX

Summary

Yellow fever vaccine is a live attenuated virus preparation used to produce immunization to yellow fever (Anonymous, 1990).

Magnitude of Teratogenic Risk

Undetermined

Quality and Quantity of Data

None

Comment

None

No epidemiological studies of congenital anomalies among infants born to women immunized with yellow fever vaccine during pregnancy have been reported.

No animal teratology studies of yellow fever vaccine have been published.

Key References

Anonymous: Yellow fever vaccine: Recommendations of the Immunization Practices Advisory Committee (ACIP). MMWR (Morb Mortal Wkly Rep) 39(RR-6):1-6, 1990. [R]

YOHIMBINE

Synonyms

Aphrodine Hydrochloride, Corynine Hydrochloride, Yocon, Yohimex

Summary

Yohimbine is an indolalkylamine alkaloid that acts as a blocker of alpha-2 adrenergic receptors. It is used in the treatment of erectile impotence and as an aphrodisiac.

Magnitude of Teratogenic Risk

Undetermined

Quality and Quantity of Data

None To Poor

Comment

None

No epidemiological studies of congenital anomalies among infants born to women who took yohimbine during pregnancy have been reported.

No adverse effect was noted among the offspring of rats treated prior to implantation with yohimbine in a dose 62 times that used in humans (Bovet-Nitti & Bovet, 1959). No animal teratology studies of yohimbine have been published.

Please see agent summary on reserpine for information on a related agent that has been more thoroughly studied.

Key References

Bovet-Nitti F, Bovet D: Action of some sympatholytic agents on pregnancy in the rat. Proc Soc Exp Biol Med 100:555-557, 1959. [A]

ZIDOVUDINE

Synonyms

Azidodeoxythymidine, Azidothymidine, AZT, Retrovir

Summary

Zidovudine (AZT) is a thymidine analog that is given orally to treat AIDS or AIDS-related complex.

Magnitude of Teratogenic Risk

Minimal

Quality and Quantity of Data

Poor To Fair

Comment

Please see HIV summary for information on teratogenic risks related to the aids virus.

No congenital anomalies attributable to zidovudine were noted among 45 infants born to pregnant women treated with this medication for HIV infection in one series (Sperling et al., 1992). Twelve of these pregnancies were treated in the first trimester.

Increased rates of embryonic death were observed among pregnant mice given drinking water containing zidovudine in a dose that produced blood levels below those encountered with therapeutic doses in humans (Toltzis et al., 1991). No increase in malformations was observed among the offspring of pregnant rats or rabbits treated with 5-25 or 5-21 times the maximum human dose of zidovudine (Ayers, 1988; Stahlmann et al., 1989). A high rate of postnatal death was observed among the pups born to rats treated with high doses in one study.

Key References

Ayers K: Preclinical toxicology of zidovudine. Am J Med 85:186, 1988. [O]

Sperling RS, Stratton P, O'Sullivan MJ, et al.: A survey of zidovudine use in pregnant women with human immunodeficiency virus infection. N Engl J Med 326(13):857-861, 1992. [S]

Stahlmann R, Rahn U, Baumann-Wilschke I, Thiel R: Pharmacokinetics, prenatal toxicity and hematotoxicity of zidovudine in rats. Nauyn-Sch-miedeberg's Arch Pharmacol 339 (Suppl):R30, 1989. [A]

Toltzis P, Marx CM, Kleinman N, et al.: Zidovudine-associated embryonic toxicity in mice. J Infect Dis 163:1212-1218, 1991. [A]

Zidovudine In Pregnancy Registry

A registry on the inadvertent use of zidovudine during pregnancy has been established by Burroughs Wellcome with collaboration of the Centers for Disease Control and the American Social Health Association. The registry attempts to prospectively follow such pregnancy to ascertain exposure information and the pregnancy outcome.

A report summarizing the progress and findings of the registry is prepared periodically, and is available to health professionals from the address below.

Health professionals are encouraged to report all cases of zidovudine use during pregnancy to Dr. Elizabeth B. Andrews at the address below, or by telephone: (800) 722-9292, ext. 8465.

Elizabeth B. Andrews, Ph.D.
Head, Epidemiology Section
Epidemiology, Surveillance &
    Pharmacoeconomics Division
Burroughs Wellcome Co.
3030 Cornwallis Rd.
Research Triangle Park, NC 27709

ZINC OXIDE

Synonyms

Herisan, Primer, Zincofax

Summary

Zinc oxide is used in dermatological preparations as an astringent, soothing, and protective agent. It is also employed in dental cements. Zinc oxide is practically insoluble in water and common organic solvents.

Magnitude of Teratogenic Risk

None

Quality and Quantity of Data

None

Comment

This risk assessment is based on the poor dermal absorption of zinc oxide

---

No epidemiological studies of congenital anomalies in the children of women who used zinc oxide during pregnancy have been reported.

No animal teratology studies of zinc oxide have been published.

Please see agent summary on zinc salts for information on soluble salts and metallic zinc.

Key References

None available.

ZINC SALTS

Synonyms

Zinc Acetate, Zinc Chloride, Zinc Gluconate, Zinc Sulfate

Summary

Zinc is an essential trace element. The U.S. Recommended Dietary Allowance (RDA) of zinc during pregnancy is 15 mg/d. Zinc salts are used topically as caustic and astringent agents.

Magnitude of Teratogenic Risk

Undetermined

Quality and Quantity of Data

Poor

Comment

None

No epidemiological studies of congenital anomalies in infants born to women who took large amounts of zinc salts during pregnancy have been reported.

Skeletal anomalies were observed with increased frequency among the offspring of mice injected with 6-12 mg/kg/d of zinc during pregnancy (Chang et al., 1977). Abnormal fur and immunosuppression occurred among the offspring of pregnant mink fed a diet containing 50 times the usual amount of zinc (Bleavins et al., 1983). The frequency of congenital anomalies was no greater than expected among the offspring of pregnant rats fed diets containing 10-31 times the usual amount of zinc (Khera & Shah, 1979; Hackman & Hurley, 1984; Reinstein et al., 1984). Similarly, the frequency of congenital anomalies was not increased among the offspring of pregnant mice fed 2.5-25 times the standard amount of zinc during pregnancy (Hackman & Hurley, 1983). The relevance of these observations to the risk associated with maternal ingestion of large amounts of zinc in human pregnancy is unknown.

Key References

Bleavins MR, Aulerich RJ, Hochstein JR, Hornshaw TC, et al.: Effects of excessive dietary zinc on the intrauterine and postnatal development of mink. J Nutr 113:2360-2367, 1983. [A]

Chang CH, Mann DE, Gautieri RF: Teratogenicity of zinc chloride, 1,10-phenanthroline, and a zinc-1,10-phenanthroline complex in mice. J Pharmaceut Sci 66:1755-1758, 1977. [A]

Hackman RM, Hurley LS: Interaction of dietary zinc, genetic strain, and acetazolamide in teratogenesis in mice. Teratology 28:355-368, 1983. [A]

Hackman RM, Hurley LS: Interactions of salicylate, dietary zinc, and genetic strain in teratogenesis in rats. Teratol 30:225-236, 1984. [A]

Khera KS, Shah BG: Failure of zinc acetate to reduce ethylenethiourea-induced fetal anomalies in rats. Toxicol Appl Pharmacol 48:229-235, 1979. [A]

Reinstein NH, Lonnderdal B, Keen CL, Hurley LS: Zinc-copper interactions in the pregnant rat: Fetal outcome and maternal and fetal zinc, copper and iron. J Nutr 114:1266-1279, 1984. [A]

ZINC UNDECYLENATE

Synonyms

Caldesene Powder, Cruex, Tineafax Powder, Zinc Undecenoate

Summary

Zinc undecylenate is an antifungal agent. It is used to treat mycotic infections of the skin.

Magnitude of Teratogenic Risk

Undetermined

Quality and Quantity of Data

None

Comment

A small risk cannot be excluded, but there is no indication that the risk of congenital anomalies in the children of women treated with zinc undecylenate during pregnancy is likely to be great.

No epidemiological studies of congenital anomalies in infants born to women who used zinc undecylenate during pregnancy have been reported.

No animal teratology studies of zinc undecylenate have been published.

Key References

None available.

ZINOCONAZOLE

Synonyms

SC-38390

Summary

Zinoconazole is an antifungal agent.

Magnitude of Teratogenic Risk

Undetermined

Quality and Quantity of Data

None

Comment

None

No epidemiological studies of congenital anomalies in infants born to women who used zinoconazole during pregnancy have been reported.

No animal teratology studies of zinoconazole have been published.

Key References

None available.

ZOLAMINE

Synonyms

Otodyne

Summary

Zolamine is ethylenediamine derivative with antihistaminic and local anesthetic properties.

Magnitude of Teratogenic Risk

Undetermined

No epidemiological studies of congenital anomalies in children born to women exposed to zolamine during pregnancy have been reported.

No investigations of teratologic effects of zolamine in experimental animals have been published.

Key References

None available.

Index

Note: Generic names are capitalized.

Adomal, 195
Adrenaline, 227
Adriamycin, 214
Adriblastin, 214
Adriblastina, 214
Adriblastine, 214
Adrucil, 256
Adsorbocarpine, 502
Adsorbonac, 568
Adumbran, 457
Aduvex 24, 459
Advastab 45, 459
Advastab 47, 203
Advil, 305
AeroBid, 254
Aerolate, 598
Aerolin, 11
Aerolone, 323
Aeroseb-Dex, 176
Aerosporin Powder, 512
Aerrane, 319
Aethambutolum, 233
Aethanolum, 12
Aether Vinylicus, 653
Aethoheptazin, 237
Aethylium Chloratum, 239
Afilan, 355
Afko-Lube, 212
Aflatoxin B1, 9
AFLATOXINS, 9
Afrin, 461
Afrinol, 533
Aftate, 614
Agaricacceae, 534
Agarol, 411
Agent AT 539, 450
Agerite, 417
AHF, 38
AIDS, 291
Airbron, 7
Ak-Dex, 176
AK-Homatropine, 291
Ak-Sulf, 581
AK-Taine, 525
Ak-Tate, 516
Akarpine, 502
Aktivex, 105
ALANINE, 11
Albalon, 428
Albaxin, 56
ALBUMIN, 11

ALBUTEROL, 11
Alcaine, 525
Alcanfor, 88
Alcatrao Mineral, 142
Alchloquin, 133
ALCLOMETASONE
    DIPROPIONATE, 12
Alcobon, 253
ALCOHOL, 12
Alcolec PG, 332
Alcon Opulets Benoxinate, 62
Alcon Opulets Pilocarpine,
    502
Alcool, 12
Aldactone, 576
Aldecin, 58
ALDICARB, 15
Aldifen, 201
Aldomet, 396
Alepam, 457
Alexan, 162
Alfacalcidol, 656
Alfatesin, 20
Alfathesin, 20
Alfatil, 101
Alfenta, 16
ALFENTANIL, 16
Alferon, 18
Alfimid, 268
Algobid, 195
Algopent, 479
Algylen, 626
ALIFLURANE, 17
Aliflurano, 17
Alifluranum, 17
Alisobumalum, 81
Alkeran, 364
all-trans-Retinoic acid, 620
ALLANTOIN, 17
Allantol, 17
Allegron, 447
Aller-eze, 132
Allergefon, 97
Allergon, 538
Allerzine, 206
Allocaine, 521
ALLOPURINOL, 17
Allylbarbital, 81
Allylbarbituric Acid, 81
Allylisopropylmalonylurea, 40
Allypropymal, 40

Almevax, 555
ALOE, 18
Alol, 1
Alophen Pill, 495
Alopresin, 90
Aloquin, 417
Aloral, 17
Alotano, 278
ALPHA INTERFERON, 18
Alpha Tocopherols, 657
ALPHA-1-PROTEINASE
    INHIBITOR, 19
Alpha-Alanine, 11
Alpha-Aminopropionic Acid,
    11
ALPHA-KETOGLUTARIC
    ACID, 19
alpha-Methopterin, 390
Alphalin, 654
Alphapress, 294
AlphaRedisol, 299
Alphatrex, 69
ALPHAXALONE/
    ALPHADOLONE, 20
ALPRAZOLAM, 20
ALPRENOLOL, 21
ALPROSTADIL, 21
Alsadorm, 216
ALTEPLASE, 22
Aluline, 17
Alupent, 379
Alurate, 40
Alvinine Shampoo, 72
Alvinol, 233
Alyrane, 224
Alzapam, 344
Amantadin, 23
AMANTADINE, 23
Amantan, 23
Ambacamp, 56
Ambaxin, 56
Ambaxino, 56
Amben, 26
Ambodryl, 75
AMBRUTICIN, 23
Ambush, 482
Amciderm, 24
Amcill, 34
AMCINONIDE, 24
Amcinonido, 24
Amcinonidum, 24

Amdinocillin Pivoxil, 24
AMDINOCILLIN/
    PIVAMDINOCILLIN, 24
Amekrin, 35
Amen, 361
Amercide, 89
Americaine, 66
Amerlate P, 332
Amersol, 305
Amethocaine, 595
Amethopterin, 390
Ametycine, 413
Amfebutamone, 79
Amfepramone Hydrochloride,
    189
Amforol, 473
Amfotericina B, 33
Amicacin, 25
Amicar, 27
Amicla, 24
Amid-Sal, 560
Amidate, 245
Amidrine, 450
AMIKACIN, 25
Amikacina, 25
Amikacine, 25
Amikacinum, 25
Amikin, 25
Amilnitrit, 36
AMILORIDE, 25
Amimetilina, 533
AMINACRINE, 26
Aminoacridine, 26
AMINOBENZOATE (PARA-
    AMINOBENZOIC
    ACID), 26
Aminobenzoic Acid, 26
AMINOCAPROIC ACID, 27
Aminocyclohexylpenicillin,
    158
AMINOGLUTETHIMIDE, 27
AMINOHIPPURATE, 28
Aminohippuric Acid, 28
Aminophenurobutane, 98
Aminopt, 26
AMINOPTERIN, 29
Aminosidine Sulfate, 470
AMIODARONE, 30
Amipramizide, 25
Amitril, 31
AMITRIPTYLINE, 31

Amizepin, 93
Amjodaronum, 30
Ammoidin, 393
AMMONIUM LACTATE, 32
Amoenol, 133
AMOXAPINE, 32
AMOXICILLIN, 33
Amoxidin, 33
Amoxil, 33
Amphetamine, 179
Ampho-Moronal, 33
AMPHOTERICIN B, 33
Amphozone, 33
AMPICILLIN, 34
Ampicin, 34
Ampilean, 34
Amplibac, 56
AMPT, 407
AMRINONE, 35
Amsa, 35
AMSACRINE, 35
Amsidine, 35
Amsidyl, 35
Amycor, 72
AMYL NITRITE, 36
AMYLASE, 36
Amyleinii Chloridum, 37
AMYLOCAINE, 37
Amylolytic Enzyme, 36
Amylopol P, 36
Amzyme TX 8, 36
Anabactyl, 96
Anacin-3, 2
Anadrol, 461
Anaesthesin, 66
Anaesthesinum, 66
Anafranil, 137
Analgesine, 39
Analgizer, 393
Anamid, 328
Ananda, 402
Anaphranil, 137
Anapolon, 461
Anaprel, 547
Anaprox, 429
Anaspaz, 304
Anasteron, 461
Anasyth, 576
Anavar, 456
Ancobon, 253
Ancosal, 571

Ancotil, 253
Andapsin, 579
Andro 100, 593
Androfluorene, 258
Android, 401
Androlone, 428
Andronaq, 593
Androstanazole, 576
Anecotan, 393
Anestacon, 337
Anethaine, 595
Aneurine Hydrochloride, 601
Angel Dust, 486
Angilol, 528
ANISOTROPINE, 37
Anisotropine Methylbromide,
    37
Anodynon, 239
Anorex, 487
Ansmin, 205
Antabuse, 210
Antadine, 23
Antamon, 388
Antegan, 162
Antepan, 532
Antepar, 505
Antepsin, 579
Anthel, 535
Anthisan, 538
Anthra-Derm, 38
ANTHRALIN, 38
Anti-Hist, 206
ANTI-INHIBITOR
    COAGULANT
    COMPLEX, 39
Anti-Sept, 116
Antibiopto, 107
Antibiotic A 9145, 566
Antibiotic Acid S, 23
Antietanol, 210
Antigen Alpha, 57
Antigen MbaA, 57
ANTIHEMOPHILIC
    FACTOR, 38
Antimalarinae Chlorhydras,
    542
Antiminth, 535
Antipres, 274
Antipress, 307
Antipyrin Salicylate, 39
ANTIPYRINE, 39

671

CHLORDANE, 108
CHLORDANTOIN, 109
CHLORDIAZEPOXIDE, 110
Chlorethazine, 357
Chlorethyl, 239
Chlorhydrate d'Amyleine, 37
Chlorhydroxyquinoline, 116
Chloridin, 538
Chlorimipramine, 137
Chlormethazanone, 111
Chlormethine, 357
CHLORMEZANONE, 111
Chlormezanonum, 111
Chlorobenzoxazolinone, 121
Chlorocain, 370
Chlorodeoxylincomycin, 132
Chloroethane, 239
CHLOROFORM, 112
Chloroiodoquine, 133
Chlorolincomycin, 132
Chloromide, 119
Chloromycetin, 107
Chloronase, 119
Chlorophen, 476
CHLOROPROCAINE, 113
Chloroptic, 107
CHLOROQUINE, 113
CHLOROTHIAZIDE, 115
Chloroxazone, 121
CHLOROXINE, 116
CHLOROXYLENOL, 116
Chloroxyquinoline, 116
Chlorpactin WCS-90, 460
CHLORPHENIRAMINE, 116
CHLORPROMAZINE, 117
CHLORPROPAMIDE, 119
CHLORPYRIFOS, 120
Chlorquinol, 116
Chlorspan, 116
Chlortab, 116
CHLORTHALIDONE, 121
Chlortrimeton, 116
Chlortritylimidazol, 141
Chlorylen, 626
Chlorzide, 295
CHLORZOXAZONE, 121
Chlotride, 115
Cholac, 331
Cholan-DH, 172
Cholecalciferol, 656
CHOLERA VACCINE, 122

Chologon, 172
Choloxin, 335
Chorigon, 122
CHORIONIC
    GONADOTROPIN, 122
Choron 10, 122
Chrome Alum, 124
Chromelin, 198
Chrometrace, 124
Chromic Potassium Sulfate,
    124
Chromium Chloride, 124
CHROMIUM SALTS, 124
Chromium Trichloride, 124
Chromium Trioxide, 124
Chronogyn, 167
Chronulac, 331
Chrysazin, 168
Chrysodermol, 38
CI-634, 608
Cibalith-S, 340
Cibazol, 584
Ciclacillin, 158
Ciclometicaina, 159
CICLOPIROX, 125
Cicloplegyl, 50
Cicloserina, 160
Ciclosporine, 160
Ciclovalidin, 160
Cidomycin, 265
Ciflox, 130
CIGARETTE SMOKING
    (Tobacco), 125
Cignolin, 38
Cigthranol, 38
CILASTATIN, 128
Cimal, 129
CIMETIDINE, 129
Cin-Quin, 543
Cincaine Chloride, 187
Cinchocaine, 187
Cincocaina, 187
Cinecolex R-X, 574
Cinkain, 187
Cinobac, 130
Cinobactin, 130
Cinonide, 622
CINOXACIN, 130
Cipractin, 162
Cipro, 130
Cipro IV, 130

Ciprobay, 130
CIPROFLOXACIN, 130
Ciproxin, 130
Cirantin, 288
Circanol, 229
Circubid, 233
Citanest, 517
Citocillin, 158
CITRATE, 131
Citravescent, 569
Citric Acid, 131
Citroflex A, 7
Citrosodina, 569
CL-719, 265
CLA, 131
Claforan, 102
Claradin, 45
CLARITHROMYCIN, 131
Claversal, 376
Clearasil Acne Treatment, 67
Cleer, 598
Clemanil, 132
CLEMASTINE, 132
Clemastine Fumarate, 132
Cleocin, 132
CLIDINIUM BROMIDE, 132
Clindamicina, 132
CLINDAMYCIN, 132
Clinoril, 586
CLIOQUINOL, 133
Clistin, 97
Cloazepam, 138
Clodantoin, 109
CLOFAZIMINE, 133
Clofuzid, 116
Clomid, 134
CLOMIPHENE, 134
Clomiphene Citrate, 134
Clomipramina, 137
CLOMIPRAMINE, 137
Clomipraminum, 137
CLONAZEPAM, 138
Clonazepamum, 138
CLONIDINE, 139
Clonopin, 138
Cloramin, 357
CLORAZEPATE, 140
Cloridrato de Hidralazina, 294
Clormetina, 357
Closina, 160
Clotride, 115

Dinitrogen Oxide, 438
DINITROPHENOL, 201
Dinofan, 201
DINOSEB, 202
Diocto, 212
Diodoquin, 315
Dioeze, 212
Diosuccin, 212
Diothane Ointment, 204
Dioxyanthrachinonum, 168
DIOXYBENZONE, 203
Diperocaine, 204
DIPERODON, 204
DIPHENHYDRAMINE, 204
DIPHENIDOL, 205
Diphenin, 499
Diphenoxin, 194
DIPHENOXYLATE, 206
Diphenoxylic Acid, 194
Diphenylan, 499
Diphenylhydantoin, 499
DIPHENYLPYRALINE, 206
DIPHTHERIA ANTITOXIN, 207
Dipotassium Chlorazepate, 140
Dipotassium Monophosphate, 207
DIPOTASSIUM PHOSPHATE, 207
Dipramol, 207
Diprivan, 526
Diprolene, 69
Diprosone, 69
DIPYRIDAMOLE, 207
DIPYRITHIONE, 208
Dirythmin, 209
Disalcid, 560
Disalicyclic Acid, 560
Disipal, 453
Disodium Azodisalicylate, 451
Disodium Ethydronate, 245
Disodium Hydrophosphate, 209
Disodium Molybdate, 415
Disodium Orthophosphate, 209
DISODIUM PHOSPHATE, 209
Disodium Phosphoric Acid, 209
DISOPYRAMIDE, 209
Dispamil, 468

Dissenten, 343
Dista, 101
Distaclor, 101
Distamine, 474
DISULFIRAM, 210
Disulone, 169
Disyncran, 387
Dithranol, 38
Ditranol, 38
Ditropan, 459
Diucardin, 297
Diucelpin, 624
Diucene, 67
Diuchlor H, 295
Diulo, 403
Diuramid, 4
Diuret, 115
Diuril, 115
Diurilix, 115
Diurone, 115
DIVALPROEX, 211
Divinyl Ether, 653
Dixarit, 139
Dixina, 196
DM Syrup, 180
DMPA, 361
DMSO, 200
DNBP, 202
DOBUTAMINE, 212
Dobutrex, 212
DOCONAZOLE, 212
DOCUSATE, 212
Dolene, 527
Dolicur, 200
Dolobid, 195
Dolophine, 382
Doloxene, 527
Domical, 31
Domol, 563
Dopa, 334
Dopamet, 396
Dopar, 334
DOPOM, 274
Doral, 541
Dorbane, 168
Dorcol Decongestant, 533
Doriden, 268
Dorimide, 268
Dormel, 107
Dorsacaine, 62
Doryx, 215

Dosalupent, 379
Double Check, 441
DOXEPIN, 213
Doxised, 216
DOXORUBICIN, 214
Doxy-100, 215
Doxy-Caps, 215
Doxy-Lemmon, 215
Doxy-Tabs, 215
DOXYCYCLINE, 215
DOXYLAMINE, 216
Dozic, 276
DPH, 499
Dragnet, 482
Dragocal, 87
Drauxin, 76
Drenison, 259
Drenusil, 512
Dridase, 459
Dridol, 217
DROCODE, 217
Droleptan, 217
Dromisol, 200
Dromoran, 335
Droncit, 515
DROPERIDOL, 217
Droxaryl, 77
Dry and Clear, 67
Drylon, 139
DSP, 209
DTIC, 166
DTIC-Dome, 166
Dubronax, 169
Dufalone, 188
Dulcolax, 73
Duogastril, 129
Duolax, 168
Duotrate, 477
Duphalac, 331
Durabolin, 428
Duracef, 101
Duracralfat, 579
Duranest, 244
Durapental, 481
Duraquin, 543
Duration, 461
Durbis, 209
Duretic, 395
Duromine, 496
Duromorph, 417
Durrax, 303

Fenicol, 107
Fenilefrina Cloridrato, 496
Fenitoina, 499
Fenmetrazina, 489
Fenobarbital, 490
Fenol, 494
Fenolftaleina, 495
FENOPROFEN, 250
Fenopron, 250
Fenoximone, 225
FENTICONAZOLE, 251
Fepron, 250
Feprona, 250
Fernasan, 606
Ferndex, 179
Ferrous Aspartate, 317
Ferrous Carbonate, 317
Ferrous Fumarate, 317
Ferrous Gluconate, 317
Ferrous Lactate, 317
Ferrous Oxalate, 317
Ferrous Succinate, 317
Ferrous Sulfate, 317
Ferrous Tartrate, 317
Ferrum, 317
Fertyl, 134
Fiberall, 535
Fifth Disease, 470
Filair, 591
FILGRASTIM, 251
FILIPIN, 251
Fisalamine, 376
Fladd, 552
Flagyl, 405
Flavitan, 552
Flavossato, 252
FLAVOXATE, 252
Flavoxato, 252
FLECAINIDE, 252
Fleet Relief, 514
Flexartal, 99
Flexazone, 121
Flexeril, 159
Flogotisol, 601
Floraquin, 315
Florasan, 225
Florone, 195
Floxiridina, 253
FLOXURIDINE, 253
Flubason, 175
Flucitosina, 253

FLUCYTOSINE, 253
Fludestrin, 593
Fluidasa, 538
Fluitran, 626
Fluniget, 195
FLUNISOLIDE, 254
FLUOCINONIDE, 254
Fluogen, 312
Fluopan, 278
FLUORIDE, 255
Fluorigard, 255
Fluorineed, 255
Fluoritab, 255
Fluorodeoxyuridine, 253
Fluoroplex, 256
FLUOROURACIL, 256
Fluotestin, 258
Fluothane, 278
FLUOXETINE, 257
Fluoxiprednisolonum, 622
FLUOXYMESTERONE, 258
Flura Drops, 255
Fluracil, 256
FLURANDRENOLIDE, 259
FLURAZEPAM, 259
Fluril, 256
FLUROXENE, 259
Flutone, 195
Fluzone, 312
Foldan, 599
Folex, 390
Follutein, 122
FOMOCAINE, 260
Fonoline White, 483
Fonoline Yellow, 483
Forane, 319
FORMALDEHYDE, 260
Formalin, 260
Formol, 260
Formulex, 189
Formyl Trichloride, 112
Fortasec, 343
Forthion, 350
Fortral, 479
Fortunan, 276
Fortuss, 217
Fospirate, 120
Fostex BPO, 67
Fovane, 67
Fradiomycin Sulphate, 430
FRAMYCETIN, 261

Framygen, 261
Freebase, 143
Freeuril, 67
Frumtosnil, 172
Frusemide, 263
FUDR, 253
Fugacillin, 96
Fulixan, 195
Fulvicin, 272
Fumagon, 186
Fumazone, 186
Fungacetin, 622
Fungaflor, 225
Fungarest, 330
Fungazil, 225
Fungifos, 612
Fungilin, 33
FUNGIMYCIN, 262
Fungizone, 33
Fungo-Hubber, 330
Fungoral, 330
Furacilinum, 437
Furacin, 437
Furacine, 437
Furadantin, 436
Furadoninum, 436
Furamide, 198
Furan, 436
Furaxone, 262
FURAZOLIDONE, 262
Furazosin Hydrochloride, 515
Furesol, 437
FUROSEMIDE, 263

G-CSF, 251
g-Strofantin, 454
Gabbromycin, 470
Gabroral, 470
Gamadiabet, 6
Gamanil, 343
Gamasol 90, 200
Gamma Hexachlor, 339
Gamma OH, 569
Gammistin, 76
Gamulin Rh, 550
Ganphen, 523
Gantanol, 582
Gantrisin, 585
Garamycin, 265
Gardenal, 490
Garranil, 90

681

683

Ivacin, 504
Ivalon, 260
Izoacridina, 26

Jalovis, 293
Janimine, 307
Jatropur, 624
Jelonet, 483
Jexin, 636
Jeypine, 116
Joints, 353
Joulie's Solution, 209
Junk, 283
Juvastigmin, 431

K-Lor, 513
K-Lyte/Cl, 513
K-Tab, 513
Kabikinase, 577
Kainair, 525
KALAFUNGIN, 327
Kalgan, 488
Kalpren, 87
Kampfer, 88
Kamycine, 328
KANAMYCIN, 328
Kantaridin, 88
Kantharidin, 88
Kantrex, 328
Kaochlor, 513
KAOLIN, 328
Kaon Cl, 513
Kaopectate, 328
Kappadione, 365
Kardonyl, 435
Karidium, 255
Karsan, 260
Katapresan, 139
Kato, 513
Kay-Cee-L, 513
Kayexalate, 570
Keal, 579
Keflex, 104
Kefolor, 101
Keforal, 104
Kefroxil, 101
Kefzol, 102
Kelecin, 332
Kemadrin, 523
Kempi, 575
Kenacort, 622

Kerasalicyl, 571
Kerecid, 306
Kerlone, 71
Ketalar, 329
KETAMINE, 329
Ketanrift, 17
Kethamed, 473
Ketocholanic Acid, 172
KETOCONAZOLE, 330
Ketoderm, 330
Ketoisdin, 330
Kidrolase, 43
Kilacar, 522
Killmaster, 120
Kilmicene, 612
Kinaden, 293
Kissing Disease, 228
Klebcil, 328
Klinomycin, 412
Klonopin, 138
Klor-Con, 513
Klotrix, 513
Klucel, 302
Koate-HP, 38
Kolton, 206
Konakion, 365
Kondremul, 411
Konsyl, 535
Konyne-HT, 249
Kool Foot, 637
Koro-Sulf, 585
Koromex, 441
Korostatin, 448
Kortison, 154
Kumarin, 155
Kwell, 339

L-Dopa, 334
l-Nordefrin, 334
L-PAM, 364
L-Sarcolysin, 364
L-Thyroxine Sodium, 335
Lac-Hydrin, 32
Lacrisert, 302
Lactase, 607
Lactated Pepsin, 481
LACTIC ACID (LACTATE),
    330
LACTULOSE, 331
Ladakamycin, 52
Ladogar, 167

Lady, 143
Lagaquin, 113
Lamoxactam, 419
Lampocef, 102
Lampren, 133
Lamprene, 133
Lanatigen C, 331
Lanatosid C, 331
LANATOSIDE C, 331
Lanceotic, 39
Landromil, 607
Laniazid, 321
Lanogels, 332
LANOLIN, 332
Lanoxicaps, 196
Lanoxin, 196
Laractone, 576
Larapam, 506
Largactil, 117
Lariam, 363
Larodopa, 334
Larotid, 33
Lasan, 38
Lasix, 263
Laspar, 43
Latamoxef, 419
Latamoxefum, 419
Latiazem Hydrochloride, 198
Latoral, 104
Laudicon, 298
Laughing Gas, 438
Laurex 16, 105
LCR, 652
LECITHINS, 332
Ledercort, 622
Ledermicina, 173
Ledermycin, 173
Ledertrexate, 390
Legatrin, 544
Lemoran, 335
Lenal, 590
Lentard, 313
Leopental, 604
Lergefin, 97
Lergine, 523
Lergoban, 206
Lesterol, 520
LEUCINOCAINE, 333
Leucinocaine Mesylate, 333
Leucodinine, 417
Leucogen, 43

Leukaemomycin C, 169
Leunase, 43
LEUPROLIDE, 333
Leuprorelin, 333
Leupurin, 373
Leurocristine Sulfate, 652
Levanxol, 590
Levate, 31
Levicor, 380
Levo-Dromoran, 335
LEVODOPA, 334
Levofalan, 364
LEVONORDEFRIN, 334
Levorfanol, 335
Levorphan Tartrate, 335
Levorphanal, 335
LEVORPHANOL, 335
Levothroid, 335
LEVOTHYROXINE, 335
LEVOXADROL, 337
Levsin, 304
Levsinex, 304
Lexinor, 446
Li-Ban Lice Control Spray,
    160
Libritabs Tablets, 110
Librium, 110
Lidanar, 377
Lidanil, 377
Lidase, 293
Lidemol, 254
Lidex, 254
LIDOCAINE, 337
LidoPen, 337
Lignocaine, 337
Limbatril, 31
LINDANE, 339
Linestrenol, 346
Linitul, 483
Linituss, 316
Linodil, 313
Linoral, 235
Lip-Sed Jel, 465
Lip-Sed Stick, 465
Lipo Gantrisin, 585
Liquaemin, 280
Liquid Paraffin, 411
Liquisulf, 572
Lisacef, 104
Lisolipin, 181
Litaler, 302

Litarex, 340
Lithane, 340
LITHIUM, 340
Lithobid, 340
Lithonate, 340
Lithostat, 6
Lithotabs, 340
Livera, 515
Lobamine, 388
Lobatox, 342
LOBELINE, 342
Lobidan, 342
Lobnico, 342
Locapred, 175
Locus Purgat, 59
Lodosyn, 97
Lombristop, 599
Lomidine, 478
LOMOFUNGIN, 342
Lomupren, 156
Lomusol, 156
LOMUSTINE, 343
Longacef, 101
Longifene, 77
Loniten, 412
LOPERAMIDE, 343
Lopid, 265
Lopirin, 90
Lopremone, 532
Lopressor, 404
Lopril, 90
Loprox, 125
Lopurin, 17
LORAZEPAM, 344
Lorelco, 520
Lorexane, 339
Lotrimin, 141
Lotusate, 588
LOVASTATIN, 344
LSD, 347
Lucidol, 67
Lucostine, 343
Lucrin, 333
Ludiomil, 352
Luforan, 271
Luminal, 490
Lupron, 333
Lurselle, 520
Lutal, 271
Lutamin, 271
Lutrol, 511

Lyderm, 254
LYDIMYCIN, 345
Lyme borrelia, 345
LYME DISEASE, 345
LYNESTRENOL, 346
Lysanxia, 514
Lysergic Acid Diethylamide,
    347
LYSERGIDE, 347
Lysodren, 414
Lyteers, 301

M & B 693, 582
M & B-800, 478
M-Dihydroxybenzene, 549
Maclicine, 187
Macmiror, 435
Macrodantin, 436
Macrogols, 511
Madurox, 53
Maeva, 590
MAFENIDE, 348
MAGALDRATE, 349
Magic Mushrooms, 534
Magis-Ciclina, 173
Magmilor, 435
MAGNESIUM SULFATE,
    349
Magrilan, 355
Malarivon, 113
MALATHION, 350
Malfamin, 348
Malipur, 89
Mallorol, 604
Malogen L.A., 593
Maloprim Tablets, 538
Man-Gro, 351
Mandelamine, 387
Manegan, 619
Mangan, 351
MANGANESE, 351
Manna Sugar, 352
MANNITOL, 352
Mantadan, 23
Mantadine, 23
Mantadix, 23
Maphenide, 348
Maprofix LK, 569
MAPROTILINE, 352
Marcain, 78
Marevan, 658

Marfanil, 348
MARIJUANA, 353
Mariquita, 353
Maroxol-50, 201
Masdil, 198
Maternal Stress, 220
Maxeran, 402
Maxidex, 176
Maxiflor, 195
Maxilact, 607
Maximed, 533
Maxiton, 179
Maxolon, 402
Maxtrex, 390
Maynar, 8
Mazanor, 355
Mazepine, 93
Mazildene, 355
MAZINDOL, 355
MDL 19205, 507
Measles Vaccine, German, 555
MEASLES VACCINE, LIVE, 356
Measurin Tablets, 45
Meaverin, 370
Mebaral, 370
MEBENDAZOLE, 356
Mebubarbital Sodium, 480
Mebumal Sodium, 480
Mecamilamina, 357
Mecamine, 357
MECAMYLAMINE, 357
MECHLORETHAMINE, 357
Mechothane, 72
Mecillinam, 24
Meclan, 360
MECLIZINE, 359
Meclociclina, 360
MECLOCYCLINE, 360
Mecloderm, 360
MECLOFENAMATE, 360
Meclomen, 360
Meclutin Semplice, 360
Medaron, 262
Medazole, 356
Medianox, 107
Medichol, 172
Medicoal, 106
Medicort, 296
Medicycline, 596
Medihaler Iso, 323

Medihaler-Epi, 227
Medipren, 305
Medomet, 396
Medrol, 400
MEDROXYPROGES-
    TERONE, 361
MEFENAMIC ACID, 363
Mefenesina, 368
MEFLOQUINE, 363
Mefolin, 489
Megace, 364
Megacef, 104
MEGESTROL, 364
Megral, 229
Mekamine, 357
Meladinin, 393
Meladoxen, 393
Melitoxin, 188
Mellaril, 604
Melleretten, 604
MELPHALAN, 364
MENADIOL, 365
MENINGOCOCCAL
    POLYSACCHARIDE
    VACCINE, 365
Menomune-A/C/Y/W-135,
    365
Menospasm, 189
Menrium Tablets, 110
MENTHOL, 366
Mepacrine, 542
Mepacrini Hydrochloridum,
    542
MEPARTRICIN, 366
MEPENZOLATE, 367
MEPERIDINE, 367
Mephenamine Hydrochloride,
    453
MEPHENESIN, 368
MEPHENYTOIN, 369
MEPHOBARBITAL, 370
Mephyton, 365
MEPIVACAINE, 370
Mepivastesin, 370
Mepred, 400
MEPROBAMATE, 371
Meprospan, 371
MEPRYLCAINE, 373
Meprylcaini Chloridum, 373
Mepyramine, 538
Meravil, 31

Merbentyl, 189
Mercaleukin, 373
MERCAPTOPURINE, 373
Mercaptothion, 350
Mercapurin, 373
Mercurothiolate, 603
MERCURY (ELEMENTAL),
    375
Mereprime, 216
Merlenate, 637
Merpan, 89
Merseptyl, 603
Merthiolate, 603
Meruvax II, 555
MESALAMINE, 376
Mesalazine, 376
Mesantoin, 369
Mesatonum, 496
Mescal Buttons, 377
MESCALINE, 377
Mesontoin, 369
MESORIDAZINE, 377
Mestinon, 537
MESTRANOL, 378
Mesuximide, 394
Met-HGH, 573
METABUTETHAMINE, 379
METABUTOXYCAINE, 379
Metaciclina, 381
Metacortandralone, 516
Metacycline, 381
Metaderm, 69
Metaglucina, 6
Metahydrin, 626
Metallic Mercury, 375
Metamucil, 535
Metandren, 401
Metaoxedrini Chloridum, 496
Metaprel, 379
METAPROTERENOL, 379
Metaradrine, 380
METARAMINOL, 380
Metarbital, 386
Metasep, 116
Metassalone, 380
METAXALONE, 380
Meteros, 404
Methabol, 461
METHACRYLATES, 381
METHACYCLINE, 381
METHADONE, 382

687

Midamor, 25
MIDAZOLAM, 409
Midone, 518
Mifegyne, 409
MIFEPRISTONE (RU-486),
   409
Migrenin, 39
Milchsaure, 330
Milk Acid, 330
Milontin, 495
MILRINONE, 410
Miltown, 371
MINAXOLONE, 411
Mindiab, 267
Mineral Jelly, 483
MINERAL OIL, 411
Mini-Gamulin, 550
Mini-Pill, 443
Minidiab, 267
Minihep, 280
Minims Pilocarpine, 502
Minims Sodium Chloride, 568
Minipres, 515
Minirin, 174
Minirin/DDAVP, 174
Minizide Capsules, 515
Minociclina, 412
Minocine, 412
Minocrin, 26
MINOCYCLINE, 412
Minodiab, 267
Minodyl, 412
Minomycin, 412
Minoral, 6
Minoran, 390
MINOXIDIL, 412
Mintezol, 599
Minurin, 174
Minzolum, 599
Mioblock, 466
Mioxom, 99
Mirciclina, 173
Miroseryn, 160
Mist, 486
Mithracin, 509
Mithramycin, 509
Mitocin-C, 413
Mitocor, 637
MITOMYCIN, 413
MITOTANE, 414
MJ-9067, 224

MK 0787, 307
MK-130, 159
Moban, 414
Mobenol, 611
Mobilan, 309
Mobisyl, 635
Moccasin Antitoxic Serum, 39
Modamide, 25
Modane Bulk, 535
Moderil, 547
Modulan, 332
Moebiquin, 315
Molatoc, 212
MOLINDONE, 414
Molipaxin, 619
Molson, 1
Molybdate, 415
MOLYBDENUM, 415
Molybdic Acid, 415
MOMETASONE FUROATE,
   416
Monacolin K, 344
Monacrin, 26
Monelan, 416
Monensic Acid, 416
MONENSIN, 416
Monistat, 408
Mono-Gesic, 560
MONOBENZONE, 417
Monocaine, 82
Monochloroethane, 239
Monoclate, 38
Monocor, 74
Mononucleosis, 228
Monoparin, 280
Monosodium Azlocillin, 55
Monosodium Carbonate, 567
Monotard, 313
Monotrim, 633
More Attenuated Enders
   Strain, 356
Morfina, 417
MORPHINE, 417
MORRHUATE, 419
Motiax, 249
Motrin, 305
Motussin, 273
MOXALACTAM, 419
Moxam, 419
MPA, 361
MS Contin, 417

MSIR, 417
MSTA, 420
Mucinase, 293
Mucomyst, 7
Mucosal, 7
Mucoxin, 458
Mucret, 7
Multiparin, 280
Multipax, 303
Multitest CMI, 567
MUMPS SKIN TEST
   ANTIGEN, 420
MUMPS VIRUS, 420
MUMPS VIRUS VACCINE,
   422
Mumpsvax, 422
MUPIROCIN, 422
Murine Monoclonal Antibody,
   423
Murine Plus, 598
Muro-128, 568
Murode, 195
MUROMONAB-CD3, 423
Muscaran, 72
Muskel Trancopal, 111
Mustargen, 357
Mustine, 357
Mutabase, 185
Mutamycin, 413
Mutesa, 458
Mutrulen, 243
Myambutol, 233
Myanesin, 368
Mycanden, 278
Mycardol, 477
Mycelex, 141
Mychel, 107
Mycifradin Sterile Powder,
   430
Myciguent Ointment, 430
Mycilan, 278
Mycospor, 72
Mycostatin, 448
Mydfrin, 496
Mydriasine, 50
Mydriatin, 498
Mykrox, 403
Mylase 100, 36
Mylicon, 566
Mylosar, 52
Mynocine, 412

Myo Hermes, 72
Myocholine, 72
Myochrysine, 270
Myoflexine, 121
Myoinositol, 313
Myolespen, 111
Myotonachol, 72
Myotonine, 72
Myotrope, 473
Mysoline, 518
Mysteclin-F, 33
Mytrex F Cream, Ointment, 272

N-Ethyl-O-Crotonotoluide, 157
N-Formimidoylthienamycin, 307
N-Sulphanilylacetamide, 581
NABILONE, 423
Nadisan, 98
NADOLOL, 424
Nadrothyron D, 181
Nafcil, 424
NAFCILLIN, 424
Nafrine, 461
NAFTIFINE, 425
Naftin, 425
Naftopen, 424
NALBUPHINE, 425
Nalcrom, 156
Nalfon, 250
Nalgesic, 250
NALIDIXIC ACID, 426
Nalidixinic acid, 426
Nalidixol, 426
Nallpen, 424
Nalonee, 426
Nalossone, 426
NALOXONE, 426
NALTREXONE, 427
Nalurin, 426
Nandrobolic, 428
NANDROLONE, 428
Nansius, 140
NAPHAZOLINE, 428
Naphcon, 428
Naphtha Coal Tar, 142
Naphtha Solvents, 142
Naphthicillin, 424
Naphthidone, 365

Naprilene, 222
Naprosyn, 429
Naprosyne, 429
NAPROXEN, 429
Naptall, 1
Naqua, 626
Narcan, 426
NARCOBARBITAL, 430
Narcotile, 239
Nardelzine, 488
Nardil, 488
NaSal, 568
Nasalcrom, 156
Nasalide, 254
Nastenon, 461
Natrimax, 295
Natrium, 624
Natrium
    Cyclohexenylallylthio-
    barbituricum, 600
Natrium Phosphoricum, 209
Natriummolybdat, 415
Natriuran, 121
Natrosol, 301
Naturacil, 535
Nature's Remedy, 18
Naturetin, 61
Naturon, 395
Navane, 605
Nebramycin Factor 6, 609
Neg-Gram, 426
NegGram, 426
Nehydrin, 229
Nemabrom, 186
Nemafume, 186
Nemagon, 186
Nemanax, 186
Nemapaz, 186
Nemasole, 356
Nematox, 186
Nembutal, 480
Nemocid, 535
Neo-Betalin, 299
Neo-Calme, 182
Neo-Cobefrin, 334
Neo-Codema, 295
Neo-Cultol, 411
Neo-Cytamen, 299
Neo-Medrol, 400
Neo-NaClex, 61
Neo-Renal, 263

Neo-Synephrine II, 660
Neo-Tears, 301
Neocalglucon, 87
Neocholan, 172
Neocin, 430
Neofazol, 102
Neolexina, 104
NEOMYCIN, 430
Neomyson, 601
Neophryn, 496
Neosone, 154
NEOSTIGMINE, 431
Neosyn, 497
Neothesin, 505
Nepenthe, 417
Nephril, 512
Neptal, 1
Neptazane, 386
Neracid, 89
Nesacaine, 113
Netillin, 431
NETILMICIN, 431
Netilyn, 431
Netrocin, 431
Netromicine, 431
Netromycin, 431
Nettacin, 431
Neupogen, 251
Neuquinone, 637
Neuramate, 371
Neurosyn, 518
Neurotol, 93
Neut, 567
NF-71, 435
NIACIN, 432
NIACINAMIDE, 432
Niagestin, 364
Niamine, 435
Nibromin-A, 522
Nicamide, 435
Niclocide, 433
NICLOSAMIDE, 433
Nico-400, 432
Nicobid, 432
Nicolar, 432
Nicorine, 435
Nicotinamide, 432
Nicotinex, 432
Nicotinic Acid, 432
Nicotinic Acid Amide, 432

Nicotinoyldiaethylamidum, 435
Nicotylamide, 432
Nidazol, 405
NIFEDIPINE, 433
Nifedipinum, 433
Nifelat, 433
NIFURATEL, 435
Nifuratel, 435
Nifurazolidone, 262
NIFURMERONE, 435
NIKETHAMIDE, 435
Nikoban, 342
Nilidrine, 448
Niloric Tablets, 229
Nilstat, 448
Nipasol, 530
Nipazol, 530
Niran, 108
Nirulid, 25
NITRALAMINE, 436
Nitramyl, 36
Nitro Kleenup, 201
Nitro-Bid, 437
Nitro-Dur, 437
Nitroendipine, 433
Nitrofural, 437
NITROFURANTOIN, 436
NITROFURAZONE, 437
Nitrogen Monoxide, 438
Nitrogen Mustard Oxide, 357
Nitrogenol, 105
NITROGLYCERIN, 437
Nitroglycerol, 437
Nitroglyn, 437
Nitrol, 437
Nitrolingual, 437
Nitrophene, 201
Nitrostat, 437
NITROUS OXIDE, 438
Nivaquine, 113
Nix, 482
NIZATIDINE, 441
Nizoral, 330
Nizovules, 330
No Doz, 84
Nobensine-75, 189
Noctec, 107
Nolahist, 488
Noludar, 402
Nolvadex, 588

Nomersan, 606
Nomoxiur, 599
NONOXYNOLS, 441
Nor-QD, 443
Norcuron, 647
Nordefrin, 334
Nordotol, 93
NORETHINDRONE, 443
Norethinodrel, 445
Norethisterone, 443
NORETHYNODREL, 445
Norflex, 453
NORFLOXACIN, 446
NORFLURANE, 446
Norgestin, 443
NORGESTREL, 447
Norisodrine, 323
Norit, 106
Norlestrin, 235
Norlutate, 443
Norlutin, 443
Normison, 590
Normosan, 233
Normoten, 274
Norodin, 385
Noroxin, 446
Noroxycodone, 460
Norpace, 209
Norplant, 447
Norsulfazolum, 584
Nortestosterone Decanoate, 428
North American Coral Snake Antivenin, 40
NORTRIPTYLINE, 447
Norzine, 603
Nossacin, 130
Nostril, 497
Nova-Rectal, 480
Novafed, 533
Novasen, 45
Novasmasol, 379
Novestrol, 235
Novobetamet, 69
Novobutamide, 611
Novocain, 521
Novochlorhydrate, 107
Novochlorocap, 107
Novochlorpromazine, 117
Novocimetine, 129
Novocloxin, 141

Novodigal, 196
Novodipam, 182
Novohydrazide, 295
Novolin, 313
Novolorazem, 344
Novomedopa, 396
Novopheniram, 116
Novopirocam, 506
Novopramine, 307
Novopranol, 528
Novopropamide, 119
Novopropoxyn, 527
Novopurol, 17
Novoridazine, 604
Novosemide, 263
Novoserin, 160
Novosoxazole, 585
Novotetra, 596
Novothalidone, 121
Novotriptyn, 31
Novoxapin, 213
Noxiron, 268
Noxyron, 268
NSC-102816, 52
NSC-107041, 561
Nubain, 425
Numal, 40
Numotac, 319
Nupercainal, 187
Nuprin, 305
Nuran, 162
Nutramersal, 603
Nutrasweet, 44
Nycodenz, 316
Nydrazid, 321
NYLIDRIN, 448
Nyodid, 295
NYSTATIN, 448
Nystex, 448
Nytilax, 564
Nytol, 204

O-V Statin, 448
Obramycin, 609
Ocean Mist, 568
Ocean-A/S, 50
Octachlor, 108
Octamide, 402
Octanil, 320
OCTANOIC ACID, 449
Octine, 320

Peroxyl, 297
Perperine, 233
PERPHENAZINE, 482
Persantin, 207
PERUVIAN BALSAM, 483
Petavlon, 478
Pethadol, 367
Pethidine Hydrochloride, 367
Petinimid, 238
Petinutin, 394
Petnidan, 238
Petogasrin, 478
Petro-Phylic, 483
Petrol, 264
PETROLATUM, 483
Petrolatum, Liquid, 411
Petroleum Benzin, 264
Petroleum Ether, 264
Petroleum Jelly, 483
Petroleum Solvents, 142
Petroleum Spirit, 264
Peyote, 377
Peyote Buttons, 377
Peyote Cactus, 377
Peyotl, 377
Pfizerpen for Injection, 476
PGE1, 21
Phasal, 340
Phaseomannitol, 313
PHENACAINE, 484
PHENACETIN, 484
Phenantoin, 369
Phenazo, 485
Phenazone, 39
PHENAZOPYRIDINE, 485
Phencen, 523
PHENCYCLIDINE, 486
PHENDIMETRAZINE, 487
PHENELZINE, 488
Phenergan, 523
Phenethylhydrazine, 488
PHENINDAMINE, 488
PHENIRAMINE, 488
PHENMETRAZINE, 489
PHENOBARBITAL, 490
Phenobarbitone, 490
PHENOL, 494
Phenolaine, 37
Phenolax, 495
PHENOLPHTHALEIN, 495
PHENSUXIMIDE, 495

PHENTERMINE, 496
Phentermyl, 496
Phenyl Hydrate, 494
Phenyl Hydride, 64
Phenylalanine Mustard, 364
PHENYLBUTAZONE, 496
PHENYLEPHRINE, 496
Phenylethylmalonylurea, 490
Phenylisohydantoin, 473
Phenylmercuric Acetate, 375
Phenylmethane, 614
PHENYLPROPANOL-
    AMINE, 498
Phenylpseudohydantoin, 473
PHENYLTOLOXAMINE, 498
PHENYTOIN, 499
Pheramin, 204
Pheryl E, 657
Phiaquin, 299
Phiasol, 465
pHisoHex, 289
Phos-Flur, 255
Phosphate, 552
Phospholine, 218
Phospholinjodid, 218
Phospholutein, 332
Phygiene, 330
Physiomycine, 381
Phytonadione Tablets, 365
Pilocar, 502
PILOCARPINE, 502
Pilopine, 502
PIMOZIDE, 503
PINDOLOL, 503
PIPERACILLIN, 504
Piperasol, 505
PIPERAZINE, 505
PIPEROCAINE, 505
PIPERONYL BUTOXIDE,
    505
Pipracil, 504
Pipril, 504
Pirantel, 535
Piridane, 120
Piridossina Cloridrato, 537
Pirimetamina, 538
PIROXICAM, 506
PIROXIMONE, 507
Pirrolnitrina, 540
PITCHER PLANT
    DISTILLATE, 507

Pitocin, 464
Piton-S, 464
Pivamdinocillin, 24
Pivmecillinam, 24
Placidyl, 233
Placinoral, 344
PLAGUE VACCINE, 508
Plantago Seed, 535
Plaquenil, 300
Plasdone, 513
PLASMA PROTEIN
    FRACTION, 508
Plasma-Plex, 508
Plasmanate, 508
Plasmatein, 508
Plestrovis, 542
PLICAMYCIN, 509
Plurigram, 381
PNEUMOCOCCAL
    VACCINE, 509
Pneumovax 23, 509
Polik, 278
Poliomyelitis Vaccine (Salk),
    509
POLIOVIRUS VACCINE,
    INACTIVATED, 509
POLIOVIRUS VACCINE,
    LIVE, 510
Polistine, 97
Politiazida, 512
Polmiror, 435
Poly-Histine D Capsules, 498
Polycillin, 34
POLYESTRADIOL
    PHOSPHATE, 511
POLYETHYLENE GLYCOL,
    511
Polyhydroxyethylene, 511
Polymixin E, 152
Polymox, 33
POLYMYXIN B, 512
Polyoxyethylene Glycols, 511
POLYTHIAZIDE, 512
Polyvalent Antivenin, 39
Polyvidone, 513
Polyvinylpyrrolidone, 513
Pomarsol, 606
Ponstel, 363
Pontel, 515
Pontocaine, 595
Pot, 353

693

Potassium Stannate, 608
Potassium Biphosphate, 207
POTASSIUM CHLORIDE, 513
Potassium Monophosphate, 207
Poudre Velours, 306
Pounce, 482
POVIDONE, 513
Pragmarel, 619
Prame Gel, 514
Praminil, 307
Pramocaine Hydrochloride, 514
PRAMOXINE, 514
Prax, 514
Prazene, 514
PRAZEPAM, 514
Prazi, 515
PRAZIQUANTEL, 515
Prazite, 515
PRAZOSIN, 515
Predalone T.B.A., 516
Predate, 516
Prednacinolone, 175
Prednicen-M, 516
PREDNISONE/PREDNISOLONE, 516
Prefrin, 497
Preglandin, 264
Pregnyl, 122
Prelis, 404
Prelone, 516
Prelu-2, 487
Preludin, 489
Premerge, 202
Premesyn, 465
Prent, 1
Pres, 222
Presinol, 396
Pressonex, 380
Presun 4, 465
Priadel, 340
PRILOCAINE, 517
Primaclone, 518
Primafen, 102
Primamycin, 280
Primatene, 227
Primer, 662
PRIMIDOLOL, 518
PRIMIDONE, 518

Primobolan, 364
Primogyn, 235
Primoteston, 593
Primoxin, 446
Primperan, 402
Principen, 34
Prioderm, 350
Priscoline, 611
Pristacin, 105
Privine, 428
Pro-Actidil, 634
Pro-Sof, 212
Proaqua, 67
PROBENECID, 520
Probese-P, 489
PROBUCOL, 520
PROCAINAMIDE, 521
PROCAINE, 521
Procamide, 521
Procan SR, 521
Procapan, 521
Procardia, 433
Prochlorpemazine, 522
PROCHLORPERAZINE, 522
Prociclidina, 523
PROCLONOL, 522
Procrin, 333
Proctofoam, 514
PROCYCLIDINE, 523
Prodigox, 196
Profasi, 122
Profilate, 38
Profilnine Heat-Treated, 249
Proflax, 608
Progeril, 229
Progesic, 250
Proglicem, 185
Proglycem, 185
Progynon C, 235
Proheptatriene Hydrochloride, 159
Proladone, 460
Prolamine, 498
Prolastin, 19
Proloprim, 633
Promapar, 117
Promazin, 117
Promet, 523
PROMETHAZINE, 523
Promide, 119
Pronestyl, 521

Propaderm, 58
Propaesin, 554
Propagest, 498
PROPANIDID, 524
PROPANOCAINE, 525
PROPARACAINE, 525
Propazyl, 554
Properidol, 217
Propesin, 554
Prophenpyridamine Maleate, 488
PROPIONATE, 526
Propionic Acid, 526
Proplex SX-T, 249
Proplex T, 249
PROPOFOL, 526
PROPOXYCAINE, 527
PROPOXYPHENE, 527
PROPRANOLOL, 528
Propycil, 530
Propyl-p-Hydroxybenzoate, 530
Propyl-Thyracil, 530
PROPYLPARABEN, 530
Propylparasept, 530
PROPYLTHIOURACIL, 530
Proscillan, 532
PROSCILLARIDIN, 532
Proserinum, 431
Prostaglandin E1, 21
Prostaphlin, 455
Prostigmin, 431
Prostin VR Pediatric, 21
Protaphane, 313
Protein VP 1, 470
Protein VP 2, 470
Protemate, 508
Protexin, 23
Prothazine, 523
PROTIRELIN, 532
Protivar, 456
Protostat, 405
PROTRIPTYLINE, 533
Protropin, 574
Proventil, 11
Provera, 361
Provitar, 456
Proxagesic, 527
Proxine, 429
Proxymetacaine, 525
Prozac, 257

Prulet, 495
Pruralgan, 200
Pruralgin, 200
PSEUDOEPHEDRINE, 533
Pseudomonic Acid A, 422
PSILOCYBINE, 534
Psoradrate, 38
Psoralen, 393
Psorcon, 195
Psoriderm, 142
Psorox, 142
PSYLLIUM, 535
PTU, 530
Pump-Hep, 280
Punktyl, 344
Puralin, 606
Purinethol, 373
PVP, 513
Pyknolepsinum, 238
Pymal, 538
Pynol, 116
Pynosect, 482
Pyocianil, 96
Pyopen, 96
Pyquiton, 515
PYRANTEL, 535
PYRAZINAMIDE, 536
Pyrazine Carboxylamide, 536
Pyrazinoic Acid Amide, 536
PYRETHRINS, 536
Pyrethrum, 536
Pyridacil, 485
Pyridium, 485
PYRIDOSTIGMINE, 537
PYRIDOXINE, 537
Pyridoxinium Chloride, 537
PYRILAMINE, 538
Pyrilene, 474
PYRIMETHAMINE, 538
Pyrinex, 120
Pyrisept, 105
PYRITHIONE, 539
Pyroace, 540
PYRROCAINE, 540
PYRROLNITRIN, 540

Quarzan, 132
Quarzan Bromide, 132
QUAZEPAM, 541
QUAZINONE, 541
QUAZODINE, 541

Quellada, 339
Quench Cream, 26
Quesyl, 116
Quibron-T, 598
Quick Silver, 375
Quiess, 303
Quin-Amino, 544
QUINACRINE, 542
Quinaglute, 543
Quinalbarbitone Sodium, 563
Quinaminoph, 544
Quinate, 543
Quindan, 544
Quine, 544
QUINESTROL, 542
Quinetazona, 543
QUINETHAZONE, 543
Quinidex, 543
QUINIDINE, 543
QUININE, 544
Quinisocaine Hydrochloride, 200
Quinolor, 116
Quinora, 543
Quinsana Plus, 637
Quiphile, 544
Quitaxon, 213
Quixaline, 116
Quotane, 200

R 134a, 446
R 34000, 212
R 38486, 409
R 39,500, 469
R 818, 252
R-Gen, 315
RABIES ANTISERUM, 545
RABIES IMMUNE GLOBULIN, 546
Racephenicol, 601
RADON, 546
Ramses, 441
RANITIDINE, 547
Rastinon, 611
Rattex, 155
Raythesin, 554
Reapam, 514
REC 15/1476, 251
Recef, 102
Recombivax HB, 282
Rectules, 107

Redoxon, 42
Refined Naphtha, 142
Refrane, 342
Refusal, 210
Regenon Retard, 189
Regibon, 189
Reglan, 402
Regletin, 21
Regonol, 537
Regulane, 343
Regulon, 67
Regutol, 212
Rela, 99
Relatin, 98
Relax Llano, 389
Relaxant, 252
Relaxar, 368
Reldan, 120
Releaxo-Powel, 99
Relefact LH-RH, 271
Relefact TRH, 532
Relisorm L, 271
Relizon, 111
Remedacen, 217
Remestan, 590
Remsed, 523
Renese, 512
Renflos, 195
Renidone, 121
Renitec, 222
Reniten, 222
Rentylin, 481
Reomax, 232
RESCINNAMINE, 547
Resectisol, 352
RESERPINE, 547
Resochin, 113
Resorcin, 549
RESORCINOL, 549
Respihaler Decadron, 176
Respramin, 27
Restandol, 593
Restoril, 590
Retet-S, 596
Retin A, 620
Retinoic Acid, 620
Retinol, 654
Retrovir, 661
Reudene, 506
Revertina, 357
Rexan, 111

Tiject, 632
TILACTASE, 607
Tildiem, 198
TILETAMINE, 608
Timacor, 608
TIMOLOL, 608
Timonil, 93
Timoptic, 608
Timoptol, 608
TIN, 608
Tin Tetrachloride, 608
Tinactin, 614
Tindurin, 538
Tineafax Powder, 664
Tiobarbital, 604
TIOCONAZOLE, 609
Tiotil, 530
Tiotixene, 605
Tixair, 7
Tobacco, 125
Tobradex, 609
Tobradistin, 609
Tobramicina, 609
Tobramycetin, 609
TOBRAMYCIN, 609
Tobrex, 609
TOCAINIDE, 610
Tofranil, 307
Togamycin, 575
Tokols, 657
TOLAZAMIDE, 610
TOLAZOLINE, 611
TOLBUTAMIDE, 611
TOLCICLATE, 612
Tolectin, 613
Tolglybutamide, 611
Tolinase, 610
TOLINDATE, 612
TOLMETIN, 613
Tolmex, 613
Tolmicen, 612
TOLNAFTATE, 614
TOLUENE, 614
Toluol, 614
TOLYCAINE, 616
Tonilen, 172
Tonka Bean Camphor, 155
Tonocard, 610
Tonsillosan, 330
Topex, 67
Topicaine, 66

Topicort, 175
Topicycline, 596
Topiderm, 175
Topifug, 175
Topisolon, 175
Topocaine, 159
TOPV, 510
Torecan, 603
Torelle, 120
Torental, 481
Tosmicil, 172
Tosmilen, 172
Tosmilene, 172
Totacillin, 34
Totocillin, 187
Toxichlor, 108
Toxoplasma gondii, 616
TOXOPLASMOSIS, 616
Tracrium, 49
Tral, 289
Tralanta, 367
Traline, 289
TRAMAZOLINE, 619
Tramensan, 619
Trans-Retinoic Acid, 620
Transamine Sulphate, 619
Transderm Scop, 561
Transderm-Nitro, 437
Transene, 140
Tranxene, 140
Tranxilium, 140
TRANYLCYPROMINE, 619
Traumatociclina, 360
Travase, 587
Travenon, 181
TRAZODONE, 619
Trecator, 237
Tredemine, 433
Tremaril, 389
Tremarit, 389
Tremoforat, 59
Tremonil, 389
Tremoquil, 389
Trendar, 305
Trental, 481
Trescatyl, 237
Trest, 389
Trethylene, 626
TRETINOIN, 620
Trexan, 427
TRH-Roche, 532

Triacetaldehyde, 468
TRIACETIN, 622
Triaconazole, 592
TRIAFUNGIN, 622
Triam, 622
TRIAMCINOLONE, 622
Triaminic Chewables, 498
Triamolone 40, 622
TRIAMTERENE, 624
Triamteril, 624
Triasox, 599
Triazide, 626
TRIAZOLAM, 624
Tribavirin, 551
TRIBROMOETHANOL, 625
Tribromoethyl Alcohol, 625
Tributyl Acetylcitrate, 7
Tributyl Citrate Acetate, 7
Tricandil, 366
Trichlormethan, 112
TRICHLORMETHIAZIDE, 626
Trichlorochromium, 124
TRICHLOROETHYLENE, 626
Trichloroform, 112
Trichloromethane, 112
Triclene, 626
Triclorometano, 112
Tricodein, 149
Tricoloid, 523
Tricyclamol, 523
Tridesilon, 175
TRIDIHEXETHYL, 628
Tridil, 437
Tridione, 630
Trien, 628
TRIENTINE, 628
Triethanolamine, 635
Triethylenetetramine, 628
TRIFLUOPERAZINE, 629
Trifluorothymidine, 629
TRIFLURIDINE, 629
Trifonazole, 72
Trihydroxytriethylamine, 635
Triketocholanic Acid, 172
Trilafon, 482
Trimar, 626
TRIMECAINE, 630
Trimedone, 630
Trimegol, 89

Trimeprimine, 634
Trimethadione, 630
TRIMETHADIONE/
    PARAMETHADIONE,
    630
TRIMETHOBENZAMIDE,
    632
TRIMETHOPRIM, 633
Trimethoxyprim, 633
Trimethylene, 160
Trimeton, 116
TRIMIPRAMINE, 634
Trimogal, 633
Trimox, 33
Trimpex, 633
Trimtabs, 487
Trimysten, 141
Trioxanona, 630
TRIPROLIDINE, 634
Triptil, 533
Tripyrolidine, 634
Trisodium Orthophosphate,
    570
Trittico, 619
Triulose, 198
Trobicin, 575
Trochin, 113
TROLAMINE, 635
Trombovar, 572
Tronolane Cream, 514
Tronothane, 514
Tropax, 459
Tropium, 110
Troxidone, 630
TRYPTOPHAN, 635
Tryptoplex, 635
Tubarine, 636
Tubocuran, 636
TUBOCURARINE, 636
Tuss-Ornade Liquid, 498
Tuttomycin, 261
Tydantil, 435
Tylenol, 2
Tyzine, 598

Ubidecarenone, 637
Ubione, 637
UBIQUINONE, 637
UK 11-443, 518
Ulcedine, 129
Ulcerone, 73

Ultandren, 258
Ultandrene, 258
Ultracain, 42
Ultracef, 101
Ultracil, 158
Ultralente, 313
Ultralexin, 104
Ultramycin, 412
UNDECYLENIC ACID, 637
Undoguent, 637
Uniderm A, 17
Unilex, 332
Unimycin, 463
Uniparin, 280
Unipen, 424
Unisal, 195
Unitop, 157
Uppers, 179
Uracid, 388
Urade, 569
Uranap, 388
Urantoin, 436
Urecholine, 72
URETHANE, 638
Urfamycine, 601
Uri-Tet, 463
Uriben, 426
Uricemil, 17
Uridon, 121
Urimor, 395
Urispas, 252
Uritol, 263
Uritone, 387
Urizole, 585
Urocaudal, 624
UROFOLLITROPIN, 639
Urolene Blue, 397
Uronefrex, 6
Uronorm, 130
Uropyrine, 485
Uroxacin, 130
Urozide, 295
Utimox, 33
UV Absorber-3, 450
UV Sun Block, 450
UV Sun Filter, 450
Uvasorb DMO, 465
Uvilon, 505
Uvinul N 539, 450

V-Gan, 523

Vaderm, 12
Vagilia, 580
Vaginyl, 405
Vagistat, 609
Vagosin, 523
Valadol, 2
Valamin, 235
Valaminetten, 235
Valdorm, 259
Valisone, 69
Valium, 182
Valmid, 235
Valmidate, 235
Valpin 50, 37
Valproate, 639
Valproate Semisodico, 211
Valproate Semisodique, 211
Valproate Semisodium, 211
VALPROIC ACID, 639
Valrelease, 182
Vanclay, 328
Vancocin, 643
Vancoled, 643
VANCOMYCIN, 643
Vancor, 643
Vansil, 456
Vapo-Iso, 323
Vaponefrin, 227
Vaporole, 36
Vaporpac, 450
VARICELLA-ZOSTER
    VIRUS, 644
Vaseline, 483
Vaseline Oil, 411
Vasoclear, 428
Vasocon, 428
Vasodilan, 326
Vasorome, 456
Vasoton, 21
Vasoxine Hydrochloride, 392
Vasoxyl, 392
Vastcillin, 158
Vatracin, 158
VCR, 652
VDT, 649
VDU, 649
Vectrin, 412
VECURONIUM, 647
Velardon, 467
Velbacil, 56
Velban, 650

701